Business
Aspects of
Optometry

Second Edition

Business Aspects of Optometry

John G. Classé, OD, JD

Lawrence S. Thal, OD, MBA

Roger D. Kamen, OD, MS

Ronald S. Rounds, OD

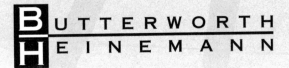

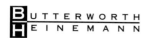

An Imprint of Elsevier Inc.

625 Walnut Street
Philadelphia, PA 19106

NOTICE

Optometry is an ever-changing field. Standard safety precautions must be followed, but as new research and clinical experience broaden our knowledge, changes in treatment and drug therapy may become necessary or appropriate. Readers are advised to check the most current product information provided by the manufacturer of each drug to be administered to verify the recommended dose, the method and duration of administration, and contraindications. It is the responsibility of the licensed prescriber, relying on experience and knowledge of the patient, to determine dosages and the best treatment for each individual patient. Neither the publisher nor the author assumes any liability for any injury and/or damage to persons or property arising from this publication.

Previous edition copyrighted 1997

Library of Congress Cataloging-in-Publication Data

Business aspects of optometry / John G. Classé ... [et al.].–2nd ed.
    p. ; cm
  Includes bibliographical references and index.
  ISBN 0-7506-7385-0
   1. Optometry–Practice. I. Classé, John G.
   [DNLM: 1. Optometry–organization & administration. 2. Professional
  Practice–organization & administration. WW 704 B979 2003]
  RE959.3.B87 2003
  617.7′5′068–dc21

                                                    2003051880

Acquisitions Editor: Christie Hart
Developmental Editor: Christie Hart
Publishing Services Manager: John Rogers
Project Manager: Doug Turner
Designer: Amy Buxton

Printed in the United States of America.

Last digit is the print number: 9 8 7 6 5 4 3 2 1

Contributing Authors

Craig Bowen, OD
Adjunct Clinical Professor of Optometry
Pacific University College of Optometry
Forest Grove, Oregon

Jack Bridwell, OD
Visiting Associate Professor of Optometry
University of Houston College of Optometry

John G. Classé, OD, JD
Professor of Optometry
University of Alabama at Birmingham School
  of Optometry

John Crane, OD
Clinical Assistant Professor of Optometry
University of Missouri-St. Louis College of Optometry

C. Thomas Crooks III, OD
Associate Clinical Professor of Optometry
University of Alabama at Birmingham School
  of Optometry

Richard D. Hazlett, OD, PhD
Professor of Optometry
Southern College of Optometry
Memphis, Tennessee

Craig Hisaka, OD, MPH
Clinical Professor of Optometry
University of California School of Optometry, Berkeley

C. Denise Howard, OD
Clinical Assistant Professor
Indiana University School of Optometry, Bloomington

Janice M. Jurkus, OD, MBA
Professor
Illinois College of Optometry, Chicago

Roger D. Kamen, OD, MS
Associate Professor of Optometry
Michigan College of Optometry, Ferris State University
Big Rapids, Michigan

Harry Kaplan, OD
Assistant Professor of Optometry
Pennsylvania College of Optometry, Philadelphia

David Kirschen, OD, PhD
Professor of Optometry
Southern California College of Optometry, Fullerton

Greg Luce, OD
Adjunct Assistant Professor of Optometry
Pacific University College of Optometry
Forest Grove, Oregon

W. Howard McAlister, OD, MA, MPH
Associate Professor of Optometry
University of Missouri-St. Louis College of Optometry

Gary L. Moss, OD, MBA
Associate Professor of Optometry
New England College of Optometry
Boston, Massachusetts

Sam Quintero, OD
Associate Professor of Optometry
University of Houston College of Optometry
Houston, Texas

Daisy Rampolla, OD
Assistant Professor
Inter American University School of Optometry
San Juan, Puerto Rico

Diane Robbins-Luce, OD
Adjunct Assistant Professor of Optometry
Pacific University College of Optometry
Forest Grove, Oregon

Maria Robles, OD
Adjunct Professor
Inter American University School of Optometry
San Juan, Puerto Rico

Ronald S. Rounds, OD
Associate Professor of Optometry
Northeastern State University College of Optometry
Tahlequah, Oklahoma

Stuart M. Rothman, OD
Associate Clinical Professor of Optometry
State University of New York, State College of
  Optometry, New York City

Peter G. Shaw-McMinn, OD
Assistant Professor of Optometry
Southern California College of Optometry, Fullerton

Morton W. Silverman, OD
Professor of Optometry
Nova Southeastern University College of Optometry
Fort Lauderdale, Florida

Lawrence S. Thal, OD, MBA
Associate Clinical Professor of Optometry
University of California School of Optometry, Berkeley

Mark R. Wight, OD
Assistant Clinical Professor of Optometry
Ohio State University School of Optometry, Columbus

In memory of our colleagues
Michael Usdan, OD
and
Jack W. Bennett, OD
in recognition of their many contributions to
practice management education and to
the creation of this text
and
George W. Mertz, OD
in appreciation for his efforts to advance optometry
and improve the education of optometrists

Preface to the First Edition

This textbook represents a unique achievement in optometric education. Never before have all the educators in a subject area worked together to provide a common textbook. *Business Aspects of Optometry* represents such an effort—an effort that was motivated by the need to provide a core body of knowledge for students and to provide a common curriculum among the schools. This textbook achieves both goals, because it will be used by the practice management educators—and students—at all schools and colleges of optometry.

The cooperation to produce this book exhibited by faculty members who teach practice management has been extraordinary. It is the product of a decade of collaboration intended to improve the quality of practice management education in the schools and to elevate the standing of practice management as a discipline. The seminal event in this effort was the decision by the Association of Schools and Colleges of Optometry (ASCO) and the American Optometric Association to sponsor a meeting of practice management educators in the mid-1980s. This meeting produced recommendations for a model practice management curriculum, a curriculum that was subsequently adopted by ASCO. Financial support—initially from Allergan and then from Vistakon—allowed subsequent meetings to be held, which in turn led to the formation of an organization to promote practice management education, the Association of Practice Management Educators (APME). This organization set as one of its first goals the creation of a practice management textbook to be used at all schools. This book represents the achievement of that goal.

Business Aspects of Optometry describes the career choices available to optometry school graduates, the many steps that must be taken to initiate a private practice, and the administrative and business issues that must be understood to successfully operate such a practice. It is intended to serve as the companion volume to *Legal Aspects of Optometry*, which describes complementary legal issues. Using both books, optometry students will find the encouragement and information needed to make the large step into a professional career after graduation.

The effort to write this book was largely due to the inspiration of two individuals. The first is Dr. Richard Hopping, President of the Southen California College of Optometry. Long a champion of practice management education, Dr. Hopping was the individual who was not only most responsible for the decision to bring practice management educators together but was also able to obtain the necessary financial support for annual meetings. His contributions to the advancement of practice management education have been invaluable. We must also acknowledge Dr. Harris Nussenblatt, who tragically passed away before the textbook was completed. Dr. Nussenblatt sought to create a cohesive and collegial organization of practice management educators, and his leadership led to the initiation of this project. Therefore, this book is dedicated to his memory.

It is our sincere hope that students and practitioners will find this text both informative and useful. Practice management is not a subject that can be readily taught in the classroom; to be meaningfully learned, practical experience is needed. Yet there are technical aspects of law and business administration that must be mastered before practical application is feasible. It is to those subjects, and to the broader principles of business management, that this book has been directed.

John G. Classé, O.D., J.D.
Craig Hisaka, O.D., M.P.H.
Donald H. Lakin, O.D.
Ronald S. Rounds, O.D.
Lawrence S. Thal, O.D., M.B.A.

Preface to the Second Edition

This updated edition of *Business Aspects of Optometry* is a reaffirmation of the commitment made—now well over a decade ago—by practice management educators to produce a definitive textbook that could be used at all schools and colleges of optometry. The intent of the book is to incorporate all the necessary elements of the practice management curriculum into one resource, and with the second edition that goal has been realized. New chapters describing business organizations, insurance, contracts, taxes, financial planning, record keeping, and other topics have been added, and the chapters from the first edition have been updated, resulting in a text that addresses all facets of practice management.

Like the first edition, this book represents a collaborative effort by practice management educators, and among the twenty-five contributors are representatives of all U.S. schools and colleges of optometry as well as colleagues from Inter American University in Puerto Rico. The textbook represents a unique achievement in optometric education and is a key part of the commitment made by the Association of Practice Management Educators (APME) to elevate the teaching of practice management and standardize the curriculum taught in optometry schools.

Since the 1980s the efforts of APME to improve practice management education have received outstanding support from industry, initially from Allergan and for the past decade from Vistakon. These companies have made it possible for APME members to meet annually and share ideas for teaching, constructing a model curriculum, conducting research, and writing this book. To these corporate supporters we express our gratitude and extend our sincere thanks. Their encouragement and assistance have been invaluable in helping us realize our organization's goals over these many years.

The efforts of individual APME members have also been essential to the creation of this textbook, but since the publication of the first edition we have suffered the loss of Drs. Michael Usdan of Southern College of Optometry and Jack Bennett of the University of Missouri, St. Louis. In addition we have lost our greatest supporter at Vistakon, Dr. George W. Mertz. Because of their many contributions to APME and dedication to practice management education, it is fitting that we dedicate the second edition of *Business Aspects of Optometry* to their memory.

It is our hope that this textbook will enable optometry school graduates to set out upon rewarding careers as primary eyecare providers and to devote themselves to serving the public competently, professionally, and efficiently, with full knowledge of the business and legal issues so vital to individual success. It is to this larger enterprise, and in support of those beginning our profession, that this book is also dedicated.

John G. Classé, OD, JD
Lawrence S. Thal, OD, MPH
Roger D. Kamen, OD, MS
Ronald S. Rounds, OD

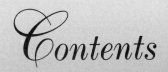

Contents

Introduction

Lawrence S. Thal

Although "optometry" is a uniquely American invention, the profession's antecedents reach back to antiquity and to the science of optics.

The early Greeks possessed some knowledge of optics; Plato, Aristotle, and Euclid all wrote about it.

Plato's comments on optics date back to 400 B.C. Aristotle seemed familiar with what we know today as myopia. Archimedes discovered the relationship between a sphere and a cylinder. He was aware of the importance of this discovery, attested to by the fact that he directed that a sphere and a cylinder be engraved on his tombstone. Archimedes was the ingenious Greek who destroyed the Roman fleet by the use of burning mirrors.

Ptolemy of Egypt knew and wrote about refraction in the 2nd century. He wrote 13 volumes on the refraction of light and the function of vision. In the 11th century, Alhazen, an Arabian philosopher, wrote about the anatomy of the eye and about optics.

The Chinese claim that the use of spectacles began in China in very ancient times. However, the Englishman Roger Bacon (Figure 1) was the first to write about convex lenses for presbyopia ("old sight"), describing their use in 1276. He may have invented the use of lenses for near vision. Allasandre de la Spina, an Italian monk, is credited with "perfecting spectacles"; however, an inscription on the tomb of Salvino D'Armato (in 1317, the date of his death) credits him with the invention. Actual credit, therefore, is uncertain, but spectacles appeared in Europe sometime between 1275 and 1285.

The clinical application of the science of optics began in Europe. Christopher Scheiner, a Jesuit priest, is often called the "Father of Optometry." He described the vision of myopic individuals in 1625.

The ancestors of U.S. optometrists are the European opticians who, like other skilled craftsmen of the time, organized themselves into guilds. The origin of the guilds is lost in the history of the Dark Ages. It is certain that originally guilds were organizations of congenial people, tied together by some common activity or background, for the purpose of ensuring that fellow members received a Christian burial when they died and that their widows and orphans received adequate care. In the 11th and 12th centuries, the possibility that a loved one might spend eternity in purgatory unless that person received proper death rites was a tremendous force in predominantly Christian Europe.

In time, the common activity that bound members of guilds together became more and more important and led to the establishment of craft guilds in the 14th and 15th centuries. These guilds set up standards and price controls for their products, to which each guild member had to adhere. They also set up an educational system so that the skill of the craft could be continued from year to year and to maintain a limit on the number of skilled men in that craft. One learned a craft by first becoming an apprentice to a master. The number of apprentices each master could have was limited. The length of time and the condition of servitude as an apprentice were carefully established. When the apprenticeship was successfully concluded, the worker became a journeyman. His skill was attested to by the guild. As a journeyman he had some freedom of employment, and under certain conditions could change from one master to another. After serving as a journeyman for a definite period, a skilled craftsman

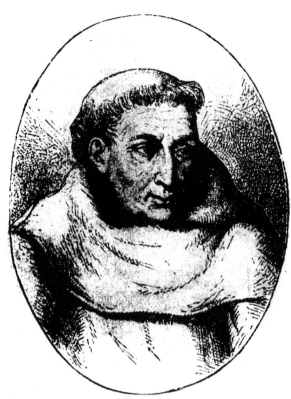

Figure 1 Etching of Friar Roger Bacon, by William H.W. Bicknell, after a painting by Howard Pyle. (Reprinted with permission from the New York Public Library, New York, New York.)

could present his masterpiece to the guild. If it was accepted and approved, he became a master and could establish his own shop.

Apparently the first separate spectacle makers' guild was established in France in 1465; the second was begun in Germany in 1577. This does not mean that there were no spectacle makers before this time, but merely that spectacle makers were members of other guilds. An example of such a guild was the Worshipful Company of Spectacle Makers, an English guild chartered by King Charles I in 1629 (Figure 2).

In April 1628, Robert Alt, citizen and brewer, in concert with 15 other London Spectacle Makers—12 of whom were members of the Brewers' Company—petitioned the King in Council for a charter of incorporation. This petition reads, in part:

> *"To the Kings Most Excellent Majesty:*
> *"The humble petition of Robert Alt on behalf of himself and other poor spectacle makers in and about the City of London.*

> *"Most humbly shewing: That whereas the mystery of making spectacles hath been and still is of good esteem and repute as well in foreign parts beyond the seas as within this Your Majesty's Realm of England: and daily doth increase; and many who have served as Apprentices thereunto; and others who have remained some small time apprentices and afterwards departed from their Masters service; having by indirect and private means attained unto some small insight of the same profession, Do now use many deceipts in the said mystery in making and uttering bad and hurtful wares whereby Your Majesty's subjects are not only merely cosened, but sometimes much prejudiced; and Your Petitioners who have served seven years apprenticeship to the same profession and are good true workmen*

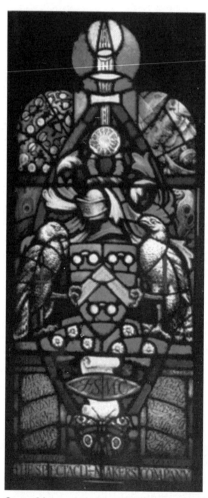

Figure 2 Coat of Arms of the Worshipful Company of Spectacle Makers, found in the Crypt, Guildhall, London. (Reprinted with permission from CJ Eldridge. The Worshipful Company of Spectacle Makers. *J Am Optom Assoc* 50[4]:481–7, 1979.)

(of whom some are charged with wives and children) much wronged in their credit, their profession vilified, and they thereby almost utterly undone, unless Your Majesty's gracious favor be extended towards them for their relief herein. "In tender consideration whereof and forasmuch as all such trade mysteries and manufactures are incorporated into a body politic do still subsist in a comely and commendable manner and those subject to no certain ordinances, rules or government are found by experience to be in short time utterly subverted. And for that your Petitioners conceive a Corporation amongst them to be a means for redress of these their grievances."

It is apparent that little of this petition would need changing to make it suitable for placement on the agenda of an American Optometric Association (AOA) meeting.

The charter granted to "The Master Wardens and Fellowship of Spectacle Makers of London" gave the company very broad powers. It established a means of government for the company, allowed the company to establish standards, and set up search and seizure provisions for substandard spectacles and for the punishment of those violating any of the rules set down by the company.

Generally, persons became members of the guild by servitude through apprenticeship. However, sons of members could become members directly by patrimony. Later on, certain individuals were allowed to purchase membership, called *redemption*. During the 15th century, both on the continent of Europe and in Great Britain, it was almost essential that a craftsman of any kind be a freeman of the city in which he practiced his craft. The only way a person could be a freeman of the city was to obtain this status through membership in a guild. Therefore, before the Worshipful Company of Spectacle Makers was formed, spectacle makers had to be members of some other guild. A nucleus was found in the Brewers' Company, probably through the action of the law of patrimony. It is known that the father of Robert Alt, for example, was a member of the Brewers' Company.

As the number of journeymen increased and as knowledge regarding the mysteries of the various crafts spread, the guilds began to lose power; eventually, their ability to control their craft was lost. The guilds in Great Britain gradually became largely social institutions, until near the close of the 19th century, when the old companies began again to take an interest in regulatory activities. The spectacle makers established an examination that ophthalmic opticians could take vol-

untarily. Those who passed the examination became members of the company, but—more importantly—their competency was attested to by the Worshipful Company of Spectacle Makers.

Much of the craft background in spectacle making was lost by the craft's mere transfer from Europe to America. In the United States, spectacles were sold primarily by peddlers, with customers selecting their own glasses by trial and error methods. Refractive testing of the eye did not make its appearance as a scientific application of optics until the 19th century. The primary advances occurred in Europe.

In the early 1800s the English scientist Thomas Young (Figure 3) discovered astigmatism; in 1827 Sir George Beddell Airy, an English astronomer, measured the astigmatism in his own eyes and had a cylindrical lens ground.

In 1843, Christoph Fronmüller of Germany invented the trial case, making possible the use of subjective examination and the creation of custom-made spectacles. Edward Jaeger, in 1854, published his reading card. In the middle of the 19th century the principles of skiascopy (retinoscopy) were discovered and explained, and in the latter part of the century Hermann Snellen (Figure 4) invented his squared test type. Another key event was the invention of the direct ophthalmoscope by Hermann von Helmholtz in 1850.

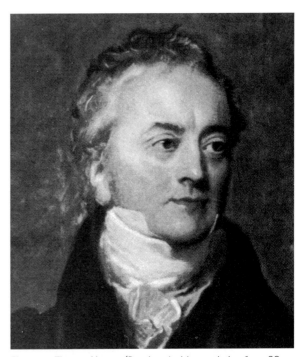

Figure 3 Thomas Young. (Reprinted with permission from CG Mueller, M Rudolph. *Light and vision.* New York, 1966, Time.)

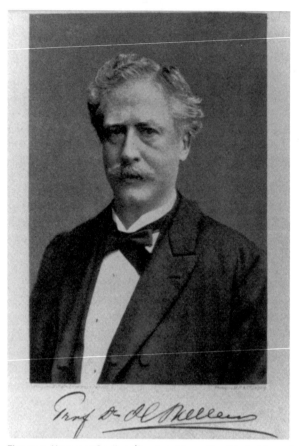

Figure 4 Hermann Snellen. (Reprinted from *Graefe's Archives of Ophthalmology* 667[3];379, 1980.)

Medicine entered the field around 1860, with the Dutch physician Frans Donders publishing his seminal book—*On the Anomalies of Accommodation and Refraction of the Eye*—in 1864. Until this time, eye physicians—called *oculists*—opposed the fitting of spectacles except for "old sight." Oculists began to take an interest in refraction during the late 1800s, and it was urged by some that the important matter of fitting glasses should not be left to opticians. The jealousies that were started then have yet to be outlived.

During the middle of the 19th century, American companies began to produce lenses and frames on a large-scale basis; leading companies included American Optical, Bausch and Lomb, and Shuron. Some of these early manufacturers set up training courses for medical and nonmedical refractionists as a means of boosting the sales of their frames and lenses. Courses ran from 1 to 2 weeks, with the awarding of a gold-embossed certificate at graduation.

Early courses in refraction were a far cry from those found in today's professional curricula. One of the

most advanced courses was given by the Northern Illinois College of Ophthalmology and Otology in 1895; it required 3 months. The Johnston Optical Institute offered four courses, each complete in itself, and maintained that all four together constituted "a university course of instruction in optics" that taught "everything up to the use of the ophthalmoscope." The Klein Optical School (the present New England College of Optometry) had a tuition fee of $25 for the full term. In June 1896, Dr. Theodore F. Klein announced a course of lectures to be given in a tent in a pine grove at the edge of a lake near his summer home. A camping outfit could be purchased for $10, and fish and berries were plentiful, so the students could bring their families while incurring very little expense in their quest to become refracting opticians.

As in medicine, numerous correspondence courses were available, and diplomas were awarded upon successful completion of the course of study.

Despite these shortcomings, by the close of the 1800s refracting opticians had become firmly established as technical experts who were providing a needed and previously neglected service required by modern civilization. The medical profession had almost completely ignored, and even opposed, this necessary service.

Charles F. Prentice (Figure 5) has been called the "Father of Optometry" in the United States. He was a mechanical engineer, optician, and refractionist. He led the fight for the legal recognition of optometry in New York. His efforts were based on the conviction that the refractive services of the time were entirely inadequate; that the refractionists—both medical and nonmedical—were, in general, incompetent; and that it was necessary to establish a professional group separate from medicine to take care of the needs of the public in the field of vision care.

That modern optometry's career has always been attended by controversy is not at all surprising, for the profession was born in controversy. In 1892 Prentice referred a patient to Henry D. Noyes, MD, a leading ophthalmologist and otologist in New York City, for care of an inflammation of one eye. Noyes sent Prentice a letter, ostensibly thanking him for the referral, but in fact reprimanding him for having charged the patient a fee for refractive services in addition to the charge for glasses. Noyes held this to be a serious matter, one that would antagonize the oculists, since they would consider Prentice's actions to have put him in competition with them. Noyes further objected that, by charging for services, Prentice would cause the public to assume that he had the qualifications that entitled him to a fee for advice.

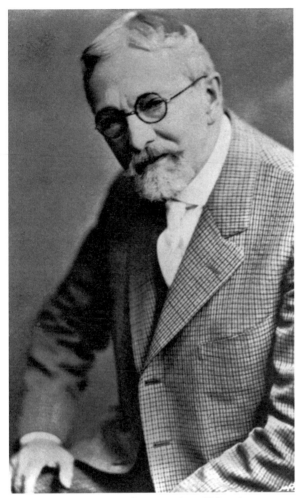

Figure 5 Charles Prentice. (Reprinted from CF Prentice. *Legalized optometry and memoirs.* Seattle, 1926, Casperin Fletcher Press.)

these legislative struggles are well worth reading and are as valid today as they were a century ago.

Before 1903, the AOA was known as the American Association of Opticians, an organization that included in its membership both refracting opticians (the precursors of optometrists) and dispensing opticians (known today as "opticians"). By 1903, however, the dispensing opticians had separated from the organization, and it became necessary to find a name for the refracting opticians. In 1904 the terms "optometry" and "optometrist" were adopted and a campaign was started to popularize them. In 1919 the organization changed its name to the AOA.

With the advent of the optometry laws, schools and colleges of optometry were chartered to provide students with the education and training necessary to meet the requirements set forth in these laws for the practice of optometry. Standards continued to improve as optometry elevated itself through education, organized legislative efforts, and the adoption of codes of practice and codes of ethics.

Today, optometry in the United States has reached a position of recognition and acceptance that is closely equaled only in Britain, Australia, and Canada. Optometry is recognized as a health care profession in all of the states and by the agencies of the federal government. Use of ophthalmic drugs by optometrists is approved in all states. Optometrists and ophthalmologists work together in schools, multidisciplinary clinics, the military, referral centers, and private practice. Interprofessional referrals between members of the two disciplines have become common. Despite the political differences between the two professions, they have in fact come to more closely resemble one another, with optometry emerging as the provider of primary care and ophthalmology continuing to emphasize training for secondary and tertiary care.

Optometrists render a vital service that was borne of medicine's refusal to recognize the widespread public need for refractive care. The profession has always acknowledged an obligation to examine for pathologic factors when rendering this care, an obligation that now includes the treatment of pathologic conditions. Optometrists have every right to be proud of the unique heritage that has led to this combination of knowledge and skills. Optometry cannot be considered a restricted form of ophthalmology; it is a primary health care profession with its own body of knowledge and with unmatched expertise in the area of vision care.

Today's optometry school graduates receive an enlightened and unexcelled education in vision

The controversy gained momentum, and the New York Medical Society agreed to adopt a resolution to expel any member who would send patients to opticians for a refraction. When Prentice and his colleagues submitted to the New York Legislature a bill to regulate the practice of optometry in the state, the medical society vigorously opposed it, ensuring that it would not pass.

Despite the bill's defeat, the idea of legislative recognition caught on among optometrists, and in 1901 Minnesota became the first state to enact an optometry law. After 12 years of continuous effort, led by Andrew J. Cross and Prentice, in 1908 the New York Legislature passed an optometry law. The last jurisdiction, the District of Columbia, completed the "legalization" of optometry by enacting a law in 1924. The many arguments put forth by Prentice and his colleagues during science and in the art and science of health care. Optometry's position that the dispensing of ophthalmic materials is an integral part of this care and is best performed by the practitioner who has examined the patient has withstood the test of time. Even so, emphasis on health care services continues to grow, challenging practitioners to maintain an adequate balance between the traditional refractive services of the past and the health care services of the future. Graduates who seek to enter the practice of optometry will find career choices significantly affected by this dichotomy in services. Some career opportunities will emphasize the sale of ophthalmic materials, with vision and health care services minimal and incidental to the sale; others will emphasize eye and vision care services, with little or no attention paid to the dispensing of ophthalmic materials; and still others will offer a balance between the two skills. Graduates must choose between these options, which are the hallmark of a free-enterprise system.

It is the intent of this book to explore some of the vital issues necessary to the making of these choices and to consider the alternative ways by which graduates may engage in the practice of optometry. In so doing, it is hoped that graduates will be better able to meet their responsibilities to the public and to more adequately serve the health care needs of our country.

Bibliography

Arrington E: *History of optometry*. Chicago, 1929, White Printing House.

Champness R: *A short history of the Worshipful Company of Spectacle Makers*. London, 1965, Apothecaries' Hall.

Classé JG: *Legal aspects of optometry*. Boston, 1989, Butterworth.

Cox M: *Optometry: the profession*. Philadelphia, 1947, Chilton.

Eldridge CJ: The Worshipful Company of Spectacle Makers. *J Am Optom Assoc* 50(4):481–7, 1979.

Gregg J: The Story of Optometry. New York, 1965, Ronald Press.

Gregg J: *A history of the American Optometric Association*. St. Louis, 1972, American Optometric Association.

Hirsch M, Wick R: *The optometric profession*. Philadelphia, 1968, Chilton.

Hofstetter H: *Optometry*. St. Louis, 1948, Mosby.

Prentice CF: *Legalized optometry and memoirs*. Seattle, 1926, Casperin Fletcher Press.

Section One

Practice Options

Chapter *1*

Practice Demographics

Morton W. Silverman and John G. Classé

He who has begun his task has half done it.

Horace *Epistles*

To begin the study of practice management in optometry, it is appropriate to review the status of the profession. *Optometry* is a clinical discipline, primarily composed of private practitioners, and so it is not surprising that the overwhelming majority of optometry school graduates seek to enter the practice of optometry immediately after graduation. To understand the opportunities available in optometry today, it is necessary to examine current demographic information, particularly the number and distribution of optometrists, modes of practice, ophthalmic market, number of eye examinations performed annually by optometrists, types of services optometrists offer, income optometrists receive, and practice patterns of optometry school graduates. The data presented in this chapter are primarily based on surveys conducted by the American Optometric Association (AOA), the Association of Schools and Colleges of Optometry (ASCO), and the Association of Practice Management Educators (APME).

Number and Distribution of Optometrists

The number of practicing optometrists has grown steadily during the past few decades. In 1978 there were fewer than 20,000 practitioners, but–according to the *Optometric Workforce Study*–in 2000 there were 32,485 optometrists in practice, which by 2002 had increased to 33,825.

The major demographic change during these decades has been an increase in the proportion of female optometrists. In 1973 only 3% of practicing optometrists were women. In 1995–for the first time–the majority of Doctor of Optometry recipients were women. By 2000 it was estimated that slightly more than one in five practicing optometrists were women. For optometrists younger than 40, about 43% are women, compared with about 10% of optometrists 40 and older (Table 1-1). This increase in female optometrists has affected patterns of practice for the profession. The other significant change has been in the percent of Asian-American students enrolled in Doctor of Optometry programs, which rose from 5.4% in 1981 to 24.2% in 1999.

Approximately 1125 optometry school graduates annually enter the practice of optometry from the 17 schools and colleges of optometry in the United States (this figure is adjusted for the number of foreign students who graduate but do not practice in the United States). As of 2000, about 550 optometrists were estimated to retire annually, and the number of projected retirees should continue to increase each year, reaching more than 800 by 2015 and steadily increasing through 2030. Based on these projections, the number of practicing optometrists should continue to grow moderately during the next few decades.

The distribution of optometrists varies across the country, with the heaviest ratio of optometrists-to-population in the Midwest (13.8 per 100,000 population) and West (13.6 per 100,000) and the lowest ratio in the Northeast (12.9 per 100,000) and South (10.1 per 100,000). The growing popularity of the West and Northeast during the past two decades has affected practice patterns in those areas, reflected in the growing number of employed optometrists and a trend toward partnership and group practices. The overall optometrist-to-population ratio in the United States is 12.3 per 100,000 population.

As of 1999, the majority of optometrists–approximately 44%–practiced in areas of 25,000 to 100,000

Table 1-1 Distribution of Optometrists and Practice Characteristics by Age and Gender, 1996
N=30,510

	AGE			
	<40	40-54	55-64	65+
Male Optometrists				
Number	6682	12146	2329	2316
Avg Weekly Patient Care hours	42.2	40.4	38.3	30.7
Percentage in Solo Practice	33.7	53.3	57.3	60.1
Percentage TPA Certified	86.7	79.6	62.6	33.1
Female Optometrists				
Number	5082	1832	89	34
Avg Weekly Patient Care hours	37.4	34.2	35.7	30.9
Percentage in Solo Practice	21.6	35.0	60.0	53.1
Percentage TPA Certified	80.4	71.3	51.7	28.6

Data from American Optometric Association: Workforce study of optometrists, *St. Louis, 1997, Author.*
TPA, therapeutic pharmaceutical agents.

population, with approximately 20% in areas of less than 25,000 population and an equal percentage in areas of 100,000 to 250,000 population; the smallest percentage of optometrists—approximately 16%—practiced in areas of greater than 250,000 population.

Modes of Practice

The backbone of the private practice of optometry has traditionally been the individual practitioner, an entrepreneur who invests the capital to begin a practice and serves as its sole owner and clinician. During the 1960s, more than 7 out of 10 optometrists were in solo practice. During the subsequent decades, however, the preeminence of individual proprietorships waned, declining to less than half of practices by 2000 (Table1-2). The major shift in private practice patterns has been toward partnerships, which have gradually increased in popularity from less than 10% of practices in the 1960s to more than one out of three practices by 2000. According to the 2001 AOA Economic Survey, approximately 22% of practicing optometrists were in partnerships of two practitioners and 16% were in partnerships consisting of three to six persons.

Private practice is the choice of about two thirds of practitioners. Based on AOA survey results, it is estimated that 65.4% of practicing optometrists are in private practice; 18.5% in commercial settings; 7.1% in multidisciplinary clinics or hospitals; 6.7% employed

by ophthalmologists or other physicians; and 2.3% in government agencies, including the armed forces. Surveys also have indicated that about 76.8% of optometrists are self-employed, with the remaining 23.2% primarily in employed positions.

The Ophthalmic Market

There are approximately 147 million wearers of corrective lenses (either eyeglasses or contact lenses) in the United States, representing about 55% of the population. More than 158 million Americans wear some type of eyewear. It is estimated that the size of the ophthalmic market in 2000 was approximately $23.4 billion (Figure 1-1). This is a significant increase from a

Table 1-2 Primary Practice Type, 1964-2000

TYPE OF PRACTICE	PERCENTAGE OF OPTOMETRISTS BY YEAR				
(SELF-EMPLOYED)	1964	1979	1987	1995	2000
Sole proprietor	71%	62%	54%	48%	48%
Partnership	8%	13%	17%	7%	22%
Group	—	3%	5%	14%	16%

Data from AOA: 2001 economic Survey. *St. Louis, 2001, Author;* and Classé JG: *Legal Aspects of Optometry. Boston, 1989, Butterworth.*

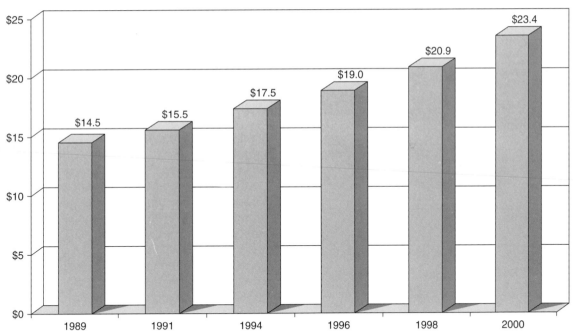

Figure 1-1 Estimated size of the ophthalmic market (in billion $), 1989-2000. (From American Optometric Association: *Caring for the eyes of America—a profile of the optometric profession.* St. Louis, 2002, Author. Reproduced with permission.)

decade earlier, when it was $14.5 billion. The AOA estimates that $5.4 billion of this market represents expenditures for comprehensive eye examinations, follow-up eye care visits, and the treatment of anterior segment conditions by eye doctors. The major share of the ophthalmic market has been held by optometrists in private practice, who in 2000 earned 35.6% of market income (Figure 1-2).

It is estimated that 88 million primary eye care examinations were performed in the United States in 1997, with optometrists conducting approximately 70% of them. Because of the effects of presbyopia on the "baby boom" generation, it is anticipated that most growth in eye care will involve persons in the 45-year-old and older bracket. Corrective lens wear will inevitably be affected by the aging of this generation: currently, about 44% of lenses sold by U.S. optometrists are single vision; 26% are bifocals or trifocals; and 30% are progressives, with progressive lenses being the fastest-growing part of the market.

As of 2000 there were about 34 million contact lens wearers in the United States, an increase of 8% in soft lens wear from the previous year. The contact lens market is not expected to expand significantly in the next few years, primarily because of the impact of refractive surgery. Laser vision correction procedures (one eye) in the United States for 2000 were estimated to be 1.55

million—up 48% from 1999 projected figures of 980,000—and in 2000 approximately $2.5 billion was paid for these procedures.

Number of Annual Eye Examinations

The number of complete eye examinations performed annually by optometrists has grown steadily since the mid-1980s, when parity legislation passed by the U.S. Congress gave optometrists the same standing as physicians under Medicare. This amendment of the Medicare law allowed optometrists to receive reimbursement for medical eye services performed for Medicare-eligible patients. Before the amendment, only ophthalmologists were eligible to provide these services under Medicare.

According to AOA surveys, as of 1998 the mean number of eye examinations per year per optometrist was 2235 (Figure 1-3). This total was 50% greater than the total for 1982, which was 1413. In the year 2000, however, optometrists worked slightly fewer hours, and the average (mean) number of complete eye examinations (including refractions) was slightly less at 2168, which still represents a rise of 16% during the 1990s. In addition, the mean number of all "other" visits performed by optometrists rose from 947 in 1990 to 1073 in 2000, an increase of almost 16% (Table 1-3). As

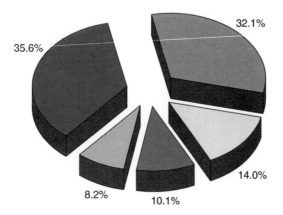

- ■ Private Optometrists
- ■ Chains, Super-Opticals, Mass Merchandisers
- ☐ Private Ophthalmologists
- ■ Managed Care Plans, Clinics
- ☐ Private Opticians

Figure 1-2 Ophthalmic market shares, 2000. (From American Optometric Association: *Caring for the eyes of America—a profile of the optometric profession.* St. Louis, 2002, Author. Reproduced with permission.)

the number of services that may be performed by optometrists expands—because of further changes in state scope of practice laws—it is expected that "other" types of visits also will continue to grow.

Services Offered by Optometrists

With respect to services, AOA surveys indicate that contact lens services are the most common, provided by 96.9% of practicing optometrists in 1999. These surveys also have found that approximately 91.2% of optometrists provide dispensing services (e.g., spectacles); 44.9%, low-vision services; and 34.6%, vision therapy. In addition it is estimated that as of 1997, 8 of 10 optometrists prescribed pharmaceutical agents for therapeutic purposes.

AOA surveys also have reported that as of 2000 the majority of optometrists offered lens tinting (58.3%), and almost half provided lens edging (47.2%) and lens coating for ultraviolet attenuation (46.3%). Fewer than one-quarter (22.2%) did coating for scratch resistance, and relatively few optometrists (8.7%) performed lens surfacing. These figures indicate that the use of in-office finishing has become popular within the profession and represents a response to consumer demands for speedier delivery of eyewear.

Income

The 2001 AOA Economic Survey (which reported income figures for the year 2000) indicated that the mean individual net income for all optometrists that year was $138,846. That figure is up more than 56% from the 1994 survey, when net income was $88,690 (Box 1-1). In fact, during the course of the 1990s—particularly during

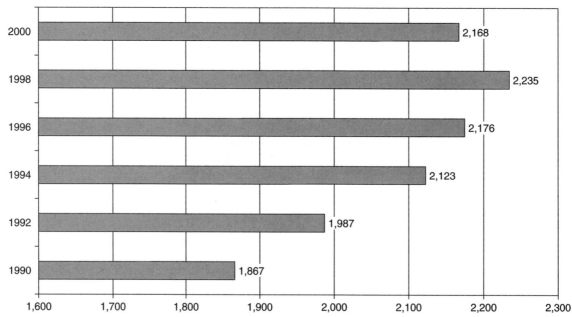

Figure 1-3 Complete eye examinations per year: annual number per optometrist, 1990-2000. (From American Optometric Association: *Caring for the eyes of America—a profile of the optometric profession.* St. Louis, 2002, Author. Reproduced with permission.)

Table 1-3 Hours Worked and Mean Volume of Examinations, 1990-2000

	1990	1992	1994	1996	1998	2000
Weeks worked per year	49.4	49.4	49.5	49.5	49.4	49.0
Complete exams per year	1867	1987	2123	2176	2,235	2168
Other exams per year	947	940	919	896	994	1073

Data from AOA: 2001 AOA economic survey. St. Louis, 2001, Author; and Classé JG, Hisaka C, Lakin DH, Rounds RS, Thal LS: Business aspects of optometry, ed 1. Boston, 1997, Butterworth-Heinemann.

the latter part of the decade—mean net income increased by more than 85%. For individual practitioners the mean gross income in 2000 was $415,623 per optometrist, compared with the 1994 figure of $310,000. That represents a 34% increase during 6 years, but during the past two decades there has been a 341% increase in the gross income of optometrists (in 1978 the mean gross income was $94,195) (Table 1-4). Optometric income also has kept ahead of inflation: during the period 1988 to 2000, the average individual net income of optometrists rose by more than 44%, appreciably faster than inflation (as measured in 1988 dollars).

The 2001 survey also found that the mean net income of female optometrists was about 25% less than that of male optometrists ($140,230 for men and $119,209 for women). This difference has consistently lessened throughout the years: in 1992, women earned 31% less than their male colleagues; in 1994, 29% less; and in 1996, 27% less. The reasons for this disparity appear to be the lengthier mean period in practice for men responding to the AOA survey and the greater number of women who work as employees compared with men.

AOA economic surveys have consistently shown that optometrists in partnerships or groups earn more gross and net income than individual practitioners, and the 2001 survey confirms that this trend is continuing. The mean net income in the year 2000 ranged from $135,340 for solo practitioners to $182,397 for a practice composed of three to five partners (Box 1-2).

For employed optometrists, income for the year 2000 ranged from a high of $123,567 for employment by an ophthalmologist to a low of $88,429 for optometrists employed by a health maintenance organization (HMO). The AOA survey also indicated that there was little difference in the income earned by optometrists employed by an optical chain compared with that of practitioners who worked for an optometrist ($98,667 compared with $95,412, respectively).

For optometrists beginning solo practice, 8 to 10 years are generally required before net income begins to reach the national mean. This length of time is usually needed to build a patient base and pay off educational debts and the costs of initiating a practice. Peak years for income are approximately from 11 to 30 years in practice, after which time the average individual practitioner begins to reduce the time spent at work (Box 1-3). From 30 to 40 years, earnings decrease somewhat, but it is apparent that optometrists may expect to enjoy a lengthy professional career, if they choose to do so.

Expenses of Practice

The expenses of self-employed optometrists in private practice may be divided into the following categories: laboratory costs; wages, benefits, and commissions for employees; rent or mortgage expense; and other costs of doing business.

A practice's net income is the amount remaining after these expenses have been paid. The percentage of

Box 1-1 Individual Mean Net Income, 1988-2000

1988	1990	1992	1994	1996	1998	2000
$66,110	$74,846	$81,571	$88,690	$92,637	$108,262	$138,846

Data from AOA: 2001 AOA economic survey. St. Louis, 2001, Author; and Classé JG, Hisaka C, Lakin DH, Rounds RS, Thal LS: Business aspects of optometry, ed 1. Boston, 1997, Butterworth-Heinemann.

Table 1-4 Self-Employed Mean Gross Income, 1996-2000

	1996	1998	2000
Per Practice	$494,117	$523,645	$648,923
Per Optometrist	$348,134	$364,942	$415,623

Data from AOA: 2001 AOA economic surveys. St. Louis, 2001.

Box 1-3 Individual Mean Net Income by Years in Practice, 2000

YEARS IN PRACTICE	INCOME
5 or less	
6 to 10	$129,200
11 to 15	$158,730
16 to 20	$137,404
21 to 25	$138,908
26 to 30	$157,402
31 to 35	$121,759
36 to 40	$125,576
41 or more	$75,647

Data from AOA: 2001 AOA economic survey. St. Louis, 2001, Author.
Insufficient responses to provide reliable data.

gross income devoted to laboratory expenses has changed relatively little during the past few years; in 1992 these expenses constituted 29% of gross income, whereas subsequent surveys reported that laboratory costs ranged from 26.8% to more than 28% of gross income (Table 1-5). The wages, benefits, and commissions paid to employees have ranged from a low of 14.1% to a high of 16.4%. The cost of rent or mortgage payments, including utilities and telephone, has ranged from 6.3% to 7.1% of gross income. The most important statistic—the ratio of net-to-gross income—has ranged between approximately 31% and 33%.

In 1994, the AOA survey's gross earnings figures for optometrists indicated that income was derived from the following three principal sources: examination fees, the sale of spectacles, and the fitting and sale of contact lenses. The approximate breakdown of those sources of income indicated that examination, diagnosis, and treatment of patients produced 45% of income; the sale of ophthalmic lenses and frames generated 35% of income; and the fitting and sale of contact lenses provided 20% of income. In 1998 statistics from a survey entitled "Jobson's Eye Care Independent 1998 Survey" reported significant differences in the breakdown of services and materials. This survey divided income into the following four sources of revenue: examination fees, including fees for therapeutic care, 29%; spectacles, 36%; contact lenses, 23%; and prescription and plano sunwear and accessories, 12%. These figures indicated that 71% of income in private practice was derived from the dispensing of ophthalmic materials. Both of these surveys illustrate the significance of ophthalmic dispensing and contact lens services, which continue to provide the majority of income in private practices.

An important factor affecting examination income is the influence of government third-party reimbursement plans (e.g., Medicare, Medicaid) and nongovernmental vision medical eye care plans (e.g., vision or medical insurance plans, Vision Service Plan). Although the influence of these plans varies from community to community, the 2001 AOA survey indicated that nearly half (48%) of a typical optometrist's patients are covered by private plans, one fourth (26%) are covered by public programs (such as Medicare or Medicaid), and the balance (26%) have no third-party coverage for optometric services (Table 1-6). According to the 2001 survey, revenue from private plans represented 42% of total practice income, whereas 23% was

Box 1-2 Individual Mean Net Income by Practice Type, 2000

SELF-EMPLOYED	INCOME
Solo	$135,340
Partnership (2 persons)	$151,809
Partnership or group (3-5 persons)	$182,397
Partnership or group (6 or more persons)	$154,500
Optical chain franchisee or lessee	$116,071
Independent contractor	$119,375
Other self-employed	$84,429

EMPLOYED BY	INCOME
Optometrists	$95,412
Ophthalmologists	$123,567
HMOs	$88,429
Hospitals, multidisciplinary clinics	$102,941
Optical chains	$98,667
Armed forces, VA, Public Health Service	$83,500
Other	$112,750

Data from AOA: 2001 AOA economic survey. St. Louis, 2001, Author.

Table 1-5 Median Percentage of Gross Practice Income, Selected Expense Categories, 1990-2000

EXPENSE	1990	1992	1994	1996	1998	2000
Net income	32.7%	32.1%	32.2%	31.0%	31.0%	31.0%
Laboratory expenses	28.9%	29.0%	28.9%	28.0%	26.8%	28.0%
Non-optometrist wages	14.1%	14.5%	14.7%	15.3%	15.3%	16.4%
Rent	7.1%	6.7%	6.6%	6.7%	6.8%	6.3%
Other expenses	17.2%	17.7%	17.6%	19.0%	20.1%	18.3%

Data from AOA: 2001 AOA economic survey. St. Louis, 2001, Author; and Classé JG, Hisaka C, Lakin DH, Rounds RS, Thal LS: Business aspects of optometry, ed 1. Boston, 1997, Butterworth-Heinemann.

from public plans and 35% was from out-of-pocket payments (including cost-sharing amounts from patients covered by third parties). The percent of total practice income paid to optometrists under managed care plans (e.g., HMOs, preferred provider organizations, Vision Service Plan) was 38%.

Practice Patterns of Beginning Practitioners

Optometry school graduates may choose any of several paths when they enter the profession: they may go directly into private practice as self-employed practitioners; they may seek an employment position with other practitioners, in institutions, or with government or industry; or they may decide to continue their education by selecting a residency position. The reason for making a particular career choice obviously varies from person to person, but according to surveys conducted by APME, most optometry school graduates seek to become private practitioners in a partnership setting in medium-sized communities and most of them believe it will require 5 or more years to realize this opportunity. This finding indicates that many optometry

Table 1-6 Third-Party Participation by Optometrists, 1986-2000

SOURCE OF INCOME	1986	1994	2000
Governmental third-party plans	21.0%	21.0%	23.1%
Non-governmental third-party plans	NA	30.8%	42.0%

Data from AOA: 2001 AOA economic survey. St. Louis, 2001, Author; and Classé JG, Hisaka C, Lakin DH, Rounds RS, Thal LS: Business aspects of optometry, ed 1. Boston, 1997, Butterworth-Heinemann.
NA, data not available. Data from AOA Economic Surveys, 1987-2001.

school graduates do not enter the practice opportunity that they would prefer immediately after graduation.

Self-Employment

Although most graduates aspire to become self-employed, only about 30% do so immediately after graduation. Among the most significant factors influencing the decision to become self-employed are age, previous business experience, amount of educational debt incurred, and family obligations. Male graduates are more likely to enter directly into self-employment than are female graduates. The individual who intends to enter into self-employment immediately must devote time to planning and preparation while in school and must have the financial resources necessary to begin practice or be able to secure the credit necessary for such an undertaking.

Employment

Approximately 60% of optometry school graduates enter the practice of optometry through employment positions. Because of the greater availability of positions in commercial settings and the relative ease (as compared with professional positions) with which they may be found, this type of employment is commonly chosen by optometry school graduates. Ophthalmology positions offer the best economic benefits, but there are relatively few of them available to new graduates. Employment with an optometrist may be preferred because such employment is often the means whereby a graduate eventually joins the practice as a co-owner. Finding such an opportunity, however, can require a significant investment of time. It also may be time-consuming to locate available positions in multidisciplinary clinics, HMOs, or industry. Optometry students who do not begin efforts early to locate and make themselves familiar to a prospective employer are in general not as successful in obtaining these positions as students who take these steps.

Residencies

According to a study by the ASCO, about one third of optometry students express an interest in residency training. As of 2000, there were more than 150 residency programs representing 200 residency positions, and approximately 10% to 15% of optometry school graduates choose to participate in them. Female graduates are more likely than male graduates to select residency training. Residency training better prepares optometrists for private practice–particularly in specialty areas–and is usually a requirement for a career in education or the Veterans Administration or other government service. Competition for residencies can be highly rigorous.

Selection of Practice Opportunity

According to APME surveys, about one third of optometry school graduates do not select a practice opportunity until after graduation from optometry school. These surveys indicate that more female graduates wait until after graduation to choose a practice opportunity than do male graduates. Women are more likely to enter into employment positions and also are more willing to work in two or more modes of practice than are men.

Location of Practice Opportunity

APME surveys have indicated that the majority of optometry school graduates seek to work in areas of less than 100,000 population. Approximately two thirds of optometrists currently practice in areas of this size.

First-Year Income

APME annual surveys in 1994 found that the mean gross income for optometrists in the first-year of practice was approximately $47,300. By 2001 first year income had risen to about $71,000. The lowest income was earned by residents and the highest by employees of commercial entities and ophthalmologists. There were differences between male and female graduates, with men earning somewhat more than women.

The 1999 AOA Economic Survey reported that the individual mean net income for optometrists in the first 5 years of practice was $75,923 (this was an average for all 5 years). The 2001 AOA Economic Survey did not report these data.

Indebtedness at Graduation

Statistics compiled by ASCO for the 2000-2001 academic year indicate that 8 of 10 students enrolled in schools and colleges of optometry received financial aid. In general, the amount of financial aid obtained by students in private schools was greater than that of students in state-supported schools. The average indebtedness for year 2001 optometry school graduates varied from school to school, ranging from $14,203 to $130,407; the median debt was about $78,000. Graduates of private schools tended to have higher levels of indebtedness than did graduates of state-supported schools. The effect of debt on practice choices has become a concern of the AOA and ASCO, which have undertaken educational programs to make optometry school students aware of how to limit debt.

Identifying Practice Opportunities

The process of identifying a practice opportunity should begin in optometry school, with a planned, systematic effort to determine the personal and professional needs of the individual student. This process should come to fruition at graduation, permitting a smooth transition from student to practitioner. To realize such an ambitious goal, however, a new licensee must make the following key decisions:
- Where to practice
- Whether to begin as an employer or employee
- How to satisfy the debts of education or of beginning a practice

Individual decisions should be based on personal preferences and an understanding of the relevant facts. Research is usually necessary to obtain information about a location or community. The status of the state law defining the practice of optometry also is an important consideration. Investigation of the community and its economic standing is important in considering the capacity of a community to absorb another practitioner or to support an optometrist. Visits to the community and to individual practitioners are often crucial.

The decision to begin practice as an employee is usually based on economic necessity or recognition of the need for experience before initiating an individual practice. Graduates should consider carefully the advantages and disadvantages of employee arrangements; if employment is determined to be the best option, a systematic effort to locate a practice opportunity should be started while the student is in optometry school. For graduates who desire immediate self-employment, meticulous planning, the use of competent advisors, and careful financial decision making are obligatory.

Indebtedness should not be permitted to adversely influence goals and career plans. Maintaining educational debt at a minimum is a prerequisite for all graduates. Indebtedness influences earning capacity and the ability to secure loans needed to purchase equipment for the start of a practice, to buy a house and car, or to respond to unexpected financial emergencies.

Planning should be initiated in school so that personal and professional goals can be attained more easily after graduation. A wealth of reference materials is available to students or recent graduates, and they should be obtained and consulted. The AOA has a practice placement service and provides technical information to optometry students and association members. Optometry school alumni associations also may be used as a resource. The most important resource, however, is the initiative of individual students. Visiting practices, assessing communities, and compiling information about practice options are essential tasks that should be performed during optometry school. The prepared graduate is more likely to find an opportunity and to take advantage of it. That alone is reason to devote the necessary effort to the task.

Conclusion

In the chapters that follow, the process of beginning a practice, organizing it, and operating it efficiently are described. It should always be kept in mind, however, that the individual initiative of the clinician is the primary consideration for any practice and that success is more often dependent on initiative than any other factor.

Acknowledgement

The authors of this chapter in the first edition of *Business Aspects of Optometry* were John G. Classé and Jack Bennett.

Bibliography

American Optometric Association: *Workforce study of optometrists.* St. Louis, 1997, Author.

American Optometric Association: *1999 AOA economic survey.* St. Louis, 1999, Author.

American Optometric Association: *Caring for the eyes of America 2000, a profile of the optometric profession.* St. Louis, 2000, Author.

American Optometric Association: *Optometry: the primary eye care profession.* St. Louis, 2000, Author.

American Optometric Association: *The state of the profession 2000.* St. Louis, 2000, Author.

American Optometric Association: *Workforce study of optometrists.* St. Louis, 2000, Author.

American Optometric Association: *2001 AOA economic survey.* St. Louis, 2001, Author.

American Optometric Association: *Caring for the eyes of America 2002, a profile of the optometric profession,* St. Louis, 2002, Author.

American Optometric Association: *The state of the profession 2002.* St. Louis, 2002, Author.

Association of Practice Management Educators: *Annual APME surveys, 1990-2001.* Birmingham, Ala, 2002, Author.

Association of Schools and Colleges of Optometry: *Annual student data report, academic year 2001-2002.* Rockville, Md, 2002, Author.

www.aoa.org. Web site for the American Optometric Association.

www.opted.org. Web site for the Association of Schools and Colleges of Optometry.

Chapter 2

Self-Employment Options

Craig Hisaka and W. Howard McAlister

Liberty means responsibility. That is why most men dread it.
George Bernard Shaw *Maxims for Revolutionists*

The majority of optometrists are in private practice and self-employed (see Chapter 1). Not surprisingly, the decision to enter private practice immediately is one that is made by most optometry school graduates. Surveys conducted in the 1990s by the Association of Practice Management Educators have revealed that approximately 60% of graduates enter private practice as employees and that approximately 30% are self-employed; the remaining 10% enter residencies. These same surveys have shown that most graduates who enter employee positions immediately after graduation intend to become self-employed eventually.

The basic decision that must be made by the new graduate is whether to be an employer or an employee. If self-employment is chosen, another important decision involves the type of business organization to use. This choice affects income, liability exposure, tax considerations, and many other matters. This chapter discusses the advantages and disadvantages of entering the various types of self-employment—as a sole proprietor, as a partner, or as a member of a professional association or corporation. It also describes expense sharing. Employment opportunities are described in Chapter 4.

Sole Proprietorship

Sole proprietorship is the choice of about 10% of optometry school graduates. A sole proprietor owns 100% of the practice (see Chapter 6), even if other optometrists work for the practice as employees or independent practitioners. To enter into sole proprietorship, a graduate may start a new practice or purchase an existing practice.

Starting a Practice

The decision to start a practice is a major one and requires extensive planning. Usually, the greatest drawback to starting a practice is financial. Most optometrists have significant loans and debt when they graduate, and the added debt of opening a new office may prevent such an undertaking from being financially feasible. The optometrist must carefully evaluate income and expense projections for the practice, with emphasis on keeping fixed overhead expenses to a minimum. Projections for income should be conservative. When starting a practice "cold," it is essential to have outside sources of income from other employment opportunities.

In addition, the new practitioner needs to learn and develop excellent business and management skills. It will be helpful to obtain additional education in these areas. Courses in business law, financial management, and marketing are particularly useful. Developing a team of advisors—including a skilled certified public accountant familiar with optometry, an attorney, real estate and insurance agents, and a banker—is essential.

Another key factor in starting a practice is finding the right location. An excellent location can mean more than an increase in earnings; it can be the difference between success and failure. The topic of location is discussed in Chapter 14.

If a graduate is willing to accept the responsibility of managing a business and can overcome the financial risks involved, the pride, rewards, and satisfaction of watching a practice grow and mature can be extremely gratifying. A graduate must be willing to forego immediate financial returns for the long-term benefits that self-employment provides. In financial terms, however, the rewards are much better for self-employed optometrists than for employed practitioners. The American Optometric Association Economic Surveys (see Chapter 1) show that higher levels of income are reported by self-employed optometrists. When starting a new practice, however, about an 8- to 10-year period is needed to achieve mean income levels. Once the practice has been established, it can sustain the practitioner 30 to 40 years. Often a sole practitioner will take on employees or decide to form a partnership, which further increases the size of the practice. Because of the liberty the sole proprietor has in making key decisions, there is considerable flexibility in this form of practice arrangement.

Purchasing a Practice

The purchase of an existing practice can be a better choice than starting a new practice. An established office will have equipment, patient flow, staff, and procedures already in place. Financial planning is much easier because the practice has an established gross income, overhead expenses, and cash flow. Determining the fair value of the practice is usually the most difficult aspect of the purchase agreement and is discussed in Chapter 3.

To pay for the practice, a loan can be taken from a bank or the seller can self-finance the purchase. In either event, the purchaser must pay for the practice, with interest, for a period of years. Such an arrangement can be financially advantageous, however, to starting a new practice. The sole proprietor can often do better financially during the 5 to 10 years of repayment than if a new practice is started. Again, financial and legal advice will be needed to determine whether the arrangement is a fair one, to allocate the practice assets for tax purposes, and to draft the contract of sale. Box 2-1 summarizes the major advantages and disadvantages of a sole proprietorship.

The largest group of practicing optometrists—approximately half of those in private practice—are in sole proprietorships. However, the trend is away from solo.

Partnership

The trend in optometry is toward partnership or group practices, as reflected in the preferences of optometry school graduates, who cite partnership as the preferred mode of practice. Reasons for this trend are partially financial and partially personal. In a partnership, overhead is shared among partners, which increases earnings compared with the solo practice, and—as

---

Box 2-1 Advantages and Disadvantages of Sole Proprietorship

Advantages
- One person rule, with control over decisions and destiny
- Higher long-term income potential and greater equity potential
- Independence, control of the office schedule, time off, vacations, and similar matters
- Choice of optometric specialties to be practiced

Disadvantages
- The pressure of all decisions and management and marketing responsibilities rests on the shoulders of the practitioner
- Multiple financial risks and competitive challenges
- Lower starting income, higher start-up costs
- Lack of office coverage in the event of illness, vacation, and time off
- Fewer specialties to offer

American Optometric Association Economic Surveys illustrate—there is a clear difference in earnings based on the size of the practice. Group practices (three or more partners) earn more per practitioner than partnerships do (two partners), which in turn earn more than sole practitioners (see Chapter 1). There also are the personal benefits of partnership to be considered: specialization, consultation, expanded office hours, and increased coverage. These benefits allow partners to enjoy more time outside the practice, pursuing professional or personal activities without loss of partnership income.

The key to a successful partnership is choosing well and having a mutual appreciation and respect for each other. A well-conceived partnership agreement is another essential requirement. Also, because of the complexities of partnership, establishing a competent team of advisors is important to continued viability and success. Box 2-2 summarizes the major advantages and disadvantages of partnerships.

The partnership terms are described in a written agreement. The type of agreement, and the many legal considerations attendant to the management of the practice, depend on the type of business entity chosen for the partnership: general partnership, limited liability company (LLC), professional association or corpo-

Box 2-2 Advantages and Disadvantages of Partnerships

Advantages

- Generally higher earnings than solo optometrists
- Shared overhead, less capital outlay per partner compared to solo optometrists
- Office coverage during vacations, illness, and personal holidays
- Consultation with partner for business and patient management decisions
- Expanded hours, convenience for patients
- Investment in career protected and equity established for retirement, disability, or death

Disadvantages

- Loss of independence
- Personality conflicts with partners or the spouses of partners
- Differences in professional ideas and philosophies
- Unequal distribution of patient load
- Unequal distribution of income based on productivity of the partners

ration (PA or PC), or S corporation. Because of the complexity of these business entities and because state laws govern many aspects of their operation (these laws differ for general partnerships, LLCs, and corporations), an attorney will be needed to form the partnership (see Chapters 7 and 8).

Partnerships are often formed by the assimilation of an associate into a solo practice or by the merger of two solo practices.

Associateship

Many two-person partnerships are created by an established practitioner taking in a new graduate. There is an initial trial period, usually involving 1 to 2 years. The purpose of the trial period is to see whether the two practitioners are compatible and can work well together.

There are significant advantages for the new graduate who chooses to try associateship in the hopes of entering into partnership. First, there is immediate earning capacity, with the associate usually being paid a salary, a percentage of the income produced, or a combination of the two. The associate also gains valu-

able experience, learning the business side of optometry and the art of practice management. To receive this income, there is little initial investment required of the associate, an especially important consideration when there are educational debts to be paid. Most important, if the associate chooses well, a partnership will be formed, providing practice and financial security for as long as the partners wish to continue the arrangement (see Chapter 5).

Mergers

A merger occurs when two or more established practices join together and the practitioners combine resources to share in profits and losses. In some mergers, the practitioners maintain separate locations, whereas in others they combine practices at one location. Beginning optometrists may find merging with another practitioner to be attractive, but the more disparate the two practices are in terms of size and income, the more complicated the details of the merger become.

Considerable negotiation is often required to achieve a merger because of the number of assets, personnel, and operating procedures. Complicated financial arrangements are usually needed to equalize the contributions to the partnership by the partners. Accountants and attorneys are required participants of the formation process (see Chapter 7).

Limited Liability Companies

A relatively new development in partnership arrangements is the LLC. An LLC is a hybrid organization, composed of elements taken from both partnerships and corporations. Because LLCs may be used to render professional services, two or more optometrists can form an LLC partnership. Special provisions apply to the personal liability of members and to the transferability of members' ownership to successors (these rules are similar to the rules for PAs or PCs).

For tax purposes, the LLC is treated like a partnership. The profit (or loss) is allocated to the members of the LLC just as in a partnership. Members of the LLC are not liable as individuals for the debts or negligence of the LLC or for the debts or negligence of other members. In this respect, the LLC is like a PA or PC. These features are the reason that LLCs are preferred over general partnerships. The formation of LLCs is controlled by state law (the state's Limited Liability Company Act). Legal counsel will be needed to determine whether this form of partnership is appropriate and to ensure that the LLC is properly established (see Chapter 7).

Professional Associations and Corporations

PAs and PCs are rarely the choice of optometry school graduates starting a practice. Corporations are artificial entities endowed by law with the capacity of perpetual succession. The PA or PC may consist of a single individual or several individuals, but in either case there is unity of ownership and management. Because of the unique powers that may be exercised by PAs and PCs, they are accorded a legal status that is akin to that of a separate being. The decision to form a PA or PC is typically a financial one, based on a determination that the tax and retirement benefits offset the additional cost and management time involved. Tax and legal counsel are needed before making this choice (Box 2-3).

The PA or PC must be owned by a professional licensee; laypersons may not hold an ownership interest. The licensee also serves as the chief officer of the PA or PC, responsible for management. Because the PA or PC is a separate entity, it may sign contracts in its own name, borrow money, own property, and exercise other rights normally accorded only to persons. In addition, the PA or PC may contract with individuals to provide services. The No. 1 employee of the PA or PC is the licensee, who is paid a salary and awarded benefits under an employment agreement with the PA or PC. Therefore, an optometrist who forms a PA or PC will be its owner, chief officer, and most important employee. In a PA or PC partnership, there will be some proportionate sharing of ownership, duties, and benefits.

PAs and PCs differ from partnerships in terms of their continuity. In partnerships, if a partner dies the partnership is usually dissolved. In a PA or PC, if a shareholder dies the PA or PC continues because it is a separate legal entity that may be owned by a successor shareholder. To transfer ownership, the successor purchases the shares of stock held by the previous shareholder.

Tax and liability issues are different for corporations than for partnerships (see Chapter 8). Unlike other types of business organizations, PAs and PCs must pay income taxes, which is another matter that adds to their complexity and cost. The employees of the PA or PC also pay income tax on the salary and benefits received from the PA or PC. Accounting and tax advice are essential.

Box 2-3 Advantages and Disadvantages of Corporations

Advantages

- Because corporations are legally recognized as a separate entity, tax deductions that are not available to individual proprietorships and partnerships may be claimed by corporations.
- Corporations can establish tax-deductible medical expenses reimbursement plans for employees.
- Tax-deductible employee insurance programs can be established by corporations.
- The administrative requirements of corporations centralize management and clearly define decision making.
- Corporations have continuity of existence, and the withdrawal of a shareholder will not affect the continuation of the corporation.
- Transferability of ownership is easily accomplished by the sale of corporate stock.
- Employees can participate in a tax-deferred retirement plan established for their benefit.

Disadvantages

- The organizational and operational costs of corporations are more expensive than those of any other type of business organization.
- Corporations, because they are a separate entity under law, must pay taxes (unlike sole proprietorships, partnerships, limited liability companies, and S corporations).
- Corporations are subject to the accumulated earnings tax if a corporation keeps (rather than pays out) profits in excess of an amount deemed reasonable for present or future business plans.
- The greater business complexity of corporations makes them more costly and time-consuming to run than other types of business organizations.
- In corporations that consist of more than one person, there is a loss of autonomy in decision making and management is shared.
- Corporations are subject to more disclosure requirements (governmental and private) than are other types of business organizations.
- Tax-deferred employee retirement plans may not be optimal for all employees.

S Corporations

In some circumstances it may be appropriate to form a special type of corporation, called a subchapter S corporation or S corporation. The typical example is a dispen-

Box 2-4 Basic Requirements for Expense Sharing

- Each practitioner is an individual proprietor.
- Overhead expenses, such as the office lease, utilities, salaries of employees, insurance, and other necessary expenditures are shared on a pro-rata basis.
- Ownership of equipment and furnishings is usually separate, although certain items may be purchased and owned jointly.
- A joint bank account is established for the payment of joint expenses, and each practitioner is required periodically to contribute a certain sum to the account; individual contributions are usually a stated percentage of each practitioner's gross income.
- Records are separate and remain the property of the individual practitioners.
- Payment on accounts, collections, and accounts receivable are independently maintained.
- Personnel are usually jointly supervised, but a sole personnel manager can be designated by the practitioners if they so desire.
- A maximum sum is commonly stipulated for joint obligations unless both practitioners agree to the expenditure in advance.
- Adequate liability insurance is required of all practitioners.
- Arrangements may be made for coverage during absences, including compensation to be awarded for such coverage.
- Certain ethical standards or membership in certain professional organizations may be required of all practitioners.
- Some provision for termination of the arrangement with adequate notice will be included in the agreement.

Box 2-5 Advantages and Disadvantages of Expense Sharing

Advantages

- Decreased overhead per optometrist compared to solo optometrists. With reduced overhead per optometrist, more financial resources are available for equipment and instrument purchases and other assets.
- Possibly some coverage can be obtained for patients in cases of emergency or vacation, although joint coverage is not required and must be agreed on by the practitioners.
- Consultation and referral to the other optometrist may be available if the optometrist has a different area of interest or specialty.
- Each optometrist maintains a separate practice and controls individual policies, decisions, and management.

Disadvantages

- Coverage of patients by the other practitioner is not required in the event of illness, disability, and vacations, and must be agreed on beforehand.
- No value is established for the practice, and there is no built-in buyer as in a partnership or corporation.
- Unlike in a partnership or professional association or corporation, profits are not shared.
- Conflicts over scheduling may occur when using a common receptionist.
- Shared expenses must be divided in a fair and reasonable manner, or conflict will occur.
- Decisions about furnishings, improvements, salaries, and other matters may be sources of disagreement.
- Personnel must be shared on an equal or fair basis, or problems can result.

sary that is separate from the professional practice. The use of an S corporation allows ownership to be shared by laypersons (such as opticians, business people, or spouses), and—unlike PAs and PCs—the S corporation pays no income tax, being treated for tax purposes like a partnership. The income (or loss) is divided by the shareholders, who pay taxes on their distributive shares of earnings. Even though the S corporation pays no taxes, it may still claim certain tax benefits, such as contributions to retirement plans, premiums paid for insurance coverage, and other tax deductions that may otherwise be claimed only by PAs and PCs (see Chapter 8).

Because of state legal requirements, the advice and assistance of a certified public accountant and an attorney will be required whether a partnership, LLC, PA or PC, or S corporation is being formed.

Expense Sharing (Shared-Expense Agreement)

In an expense sharing or share-expense agreement, two or more optometrists share a common location and the expenses of the practice in a manner proportionate to their usage. Each optometrist has a separate patient base, financial and patient records, and some equipment and instruments. In an expense sharing arrangement, the practitioners do not share in profits the way they would in a partnership, and they have separate bookkeeping systems to chart income. Certain expenses are shared, however, in some proportion agreed to by the optometrists. These expenses typically include rent, utilities, repair and maintenance costs, supplies, lease payments on shared equipment, insurance, and the salaries of common employees.

This arrangement falls short of partnership because neither practitioner has any ownership interest in the practice of the other. Instead, it consists of two independent businesses that have found it advantageous to share certain common expenses. The basic requirements of expense sharing are listed in Box 2-4.

Beginning practitioners may be presented with an opportunity to enter into an expense-sharing arrangement with another optometrist or, occasionally, another type of health care provider (e.g., dentist, podiatrist, chiropractor). Most often, however, expense sharing is entered into by two individual practitioners who

believe that the economic benefits make such an arrangement worthwhile. Box 2-5 lists the advantages and disadvantages of expense sharing. As in all business arrangements, an attorney will be needed to draft a contract that reflects the agreement reached by the parties.

Conclusion

Self-employed forms of doing business offer the most long-term opportunity, flexibility, security, and financial return for optometrists (Table 2-1). They also require the most effort, investment, commitment, and risk. For graduates who do not feel prepared to enter directly into self-employment after graduation, various employment options may be considered. In a profession in which a 40-year career as a self-employed practitioner is not unusual, a year or two of employment that is used to learn the art of practice administration and patient management merely diminishes the term of

Table 2-1 Differences Between Practice Arrangements

	PARTNERSHIP, LIMITED LIABILITY COMPANY (LLC), OR S CORPORATION	EXPENSE SHARING	PROFESSIONAL ASSOCIATION OR CORPORATION (PA OR PC)	INDIVIDUAL PROPRIETOR
Assets	Shared equally or shared by partnerships, LLC, or S Corporation	Some shared equally, some not shared	Owned by corporation	Owned by doctor
Expenses	Shared equally or in on agreed upon proportion	Some shared equally, some shared on the basis of use, some not shared	Paid by corporation	Paid by doctor
Net income	Divided equally or according to percentage of ownership	Each doctor gets what he or she earns	Each doctor gets a salary and net income shared on the basis of each doctor's ownership	Doctor gets what he or she earns
Fees	Same for all doctors	Each doctor sets his or her own	Same for all doctors	Set by the doctor
Billing	Combined bill	Separate bill from each doctor	Combined bill	One bill
Disability coverage	Yes	No	Yes	No
Death benefit	Yes	No	Yes	No
Retirement benefits	Yes	No	Yes	Yes
Provision for continuity of practice	Yes	No	Yes	No
Obligations to cover for each other	Mandatory	None	Mandatory	None
Records	Merged	Separate	Merged	Owned by doctor

self-employment to 39 or 38 years. In the long term, this short period of employment may prove to be an excellent investment. Employment opportunities for graduates are discussed in Chapter 4.

Acknowledgement

The authors of this chapter in the first edition of *Business Aspects of Optometry* were James Albright, Craig Hisaka, W. Howard McAlister, and Timothy A. Wingert.

Bibliography

Allergan, Inc: *Pathways in optometry.* Irvine, Calif, 1995, Author.

American Optometric Association: *Career advocate for the new practitioner.* St. Louis, 2001, Author.

American Optometric Association: *Caring for the eyes of America—a profile of the optometric profession.* St. Louis, 2002, Author.

Bennett I: *Management for the eyecare practitioner.* Stoneham, Mass, 1993, Butterworth.

Classé JG: *Legal aspects of optometry.* Boston, 1989, Butterworth.

Chapter 3

Purchasing an Eye Care Practice

Gary L. Moss, John G. Classé, and Stuart M. Rothman

Never buy what you do not want, because it is cheap; its cost will be dear to you.

Thomas Jefferson *Canons for Observation in Practical Life*

Optometry school graduates who want to "be their own boss" should consider the purchase of all or part of a practice. This method of entering optometry can often be preferable to starting a practice "from scratch." Surveys show that within 5 years after graduation a significant percentage of optometrists purchase an ownership interest in a solo or group practice. Unquestionably, purchasing a practice is a complicated process (Box 3-1). If done properly, however, the purchase of an existing practice offers more advantages than disadvantages.

Advantages of Purchasing a Practice

A practitioner who buys an existing practice is purchasing a business with a proven track record. Although there usually will be a minor amount of patient attrition, often less than 5%, patient loss can be minimized by properly implementing the necessary transition procedures. An existing practice allows a prospective owner to project anticipated income and operating expenses with more certainty than a practice opened "cold." The new practitioner can expect to have patients scheduled for examinations from the first day of operation, producing an immediate financial and emotional benefit. The new practitioner will initially incur significant out-of-pocket expenses, such as the down payment for the practice, closing costs, attorney's and accountant's fees, security deposits for the premises and utilities, and initial operating costs (such as payments for stationery, additional equipment, and inventory). Income from the practice helps ease this financial burden. Emotionally, the new practitioner receives the benefits of being busy, helping and satisfying the existing patients of the practice, and using a wide range of skills.

The purchaser of an existing practice also is purchasing an existing location. Usually, the purchaser will assume the existing office lease but should be prepared to negotiate for an extension or change in terms with the landlord. Leasehold improvements probably will not be needed, but if a new practitioner wants to modify an office, it may not be necessary to do so immediately and the cost should be reflected as an adjustment in the purchase price. Because the office has already been used to deliver patient care, any problems related to patient flow have probably been eliminated. The telephone system and other utilities are already connected and operational, and there also is a current telephone listing for the office in the telephone book. Laboratory accounts, as well as accounts for contact lenses, frames, and other materials, already will have been established, making it easier for the new practitioner to obtain credit when opening new accounts.

Purchasing an existing practice in a given area does not change the optometrist-to-population ratio in that area because the new practitioner merely replaces the departing one. In an area that has experienced no growth, new patients will either transfer from another practice or come to the practice as new arrivals to the area. When a practice is purchased, the new practitioner is not totally dependent on drawing these patients to the practice and can use the revenue from existing patients to supplement efforts to attract new patients. The practitioner also can devote more effort toward internal office marketing, which has been shown to be five times less costly than external marketing.

The purchase of an existing practice usually allows the new practitioner to assume command of a trained staff. The staff is familiar with the operation of the practice, the patient population, and the problems encountered by the practice. A familiar staff person answering the phone can ease a patient's fear of being seen by a new, unfamiliar practitioner. Having the selling practitioner remain in the practice for a transition period of several weeks to months facilitates the transfer of patients, enabling the purchasing practitioner to become familiar with office operations. The selling practitioner also can introduce the new practitioner to key people in the area, such as bankers, accountants, lawyers, and other health care professionals.

Disadvantages of Purchasing a Practice

A purchasing optometrist always assumes the initial risk of potential loss of some patients. Because it is difficult to predict whether the previous practice's patients will return to the practice under new ownership, there is considerable financial pressure on the new practitioner. The new practitioner usually will not want to disrupt operations or initially make drastic changes for fear of alienating the existing patients of the practice. Thus, the new practitioner will probably have to incorporate changes gradually until the practice reflects the style of the new practitioner.

If the selling practitioner is retiring after many years of practice, older equipment and the physical layout may need to be updated. Equipment may have to be purchased or improvements made, requiring an outlay of capital. Management information systems incorporating new technologies, such as electronic data transmission, will quite often need to be purchased. The new practitioner will want to keep the existing staff, but this may necessitate paying slightly higher wages. Staff members may require retraining or altering their duties. It may be difficult to change habits or duties if staff members have been with the selling practitioner for some length of time. In addition, provider panels of which the seller is a member may not be easily transferred to a new practitioner.

Purchasing an existing practice affords the new practitioner the luxury of not having to perform the many tasks that are a part of opening "cold." The burden of finding a location; leasing an office; hiring employees; purchasing equipment, supplies, and inventory; setting up accounts; arranging for utilities; and building a patient base are greatly lessened since these tasks already have been performed. Indeed, it is this immediate operational viability that is the appeal of purchasing an existing practice. Unlike the practitioner who opens "cold," however, the purchaser of an existing practice must fully evaluate its potential worth and determine an acceptable fair market value.

Factors Affecting Purchase Feasibility

Many variables, both internal and external to a practice, affect the feasibility, desirability, and ultimate value of a practice. First, the more prominent the local market position and the better the practice reputation, the more willing a buyer should be to pay a higher price. Second, government and managed care regulations affecting provider reimbursement have an impact on value. Third, more efficient and updated office operations and computer systems should make the practice more valuable. Finally, newer equipment and leasehold improvements that offer more of a turnkey operation will add value and facilitate the transfer to a new owner.

Trends that are specific to a practice under consideration will have an influence on a prospective purchaser's decision. Patient volume, ratio of new to former patients, ability to retain former patients, active ongoing recall, patient communications, and various sources that refer patients to the office will all affect the desirability of a practice.

The efficiency of practice operations, including the staff's ability and willingness to offer high-quality service and the way cost savings mechanisms are passed onto the patient as part of the value chain, will impact the desirability of a purchase.

Evaluation of the area in which a practice is located will provide information about the current and future viability of the practice. This area may be defined as the probable drawing area of the practice and it can vary from 8 blocks to 15 miles, depending on whether the practice is located in a city or a suburban or rural area. The potential buyer can evaluate existing patient demographic data to determine the extent of the practice's present drawing area. Since a major portion of the payment for a practice is used to secure goodwill or active patient records, moving from one drawing area to another is not a wise idea. The drawing area should be evaluated as though the purchaser were opening up a new practice rather than maintaining an established one. The goal in buying an existing practice is to expand its patient base and to have it increase in value rather than attempting merely to maintain the status quo. In evaluating the area, the potential buyer must determine whether factors that will support new growth are present.

Evaluating the Current Economic Climate

Economic factors to consider include the employment rate, the viability of other practices, population demographics, key economic indicators, and social factors. Employed people are more likely to have disposable income and health insurance; therefore, employed individuals are more likely to seek and be able to afford health care, including optometric care. Also, areas with large employer groups will have more managed care plans that offer vision services to employees. The employment rate of an area may fluctuate from year to year, but the trends of the area can be compared with

state, regional, and national trends. This information can be obtained from local, state, or federal government statistics.

A survey of other health care providers should be performed to determine the number of practitioners who have full- and part-time practices in the area. Full-time practitioners derive all of their income from the area; part-time practitioners must supplement practice income with income from outside the area. Retail businesses should be evaluated for reinvestment. A reinvestment in new equipment, machinery, and inventory generally is undertaken when business owners are experiencing growth or when there is potential for new growth. Speaking to these health care professionals or small business owners would be time well spent on the part of the prospective new practitioner.

Evaluating the Local Demographic Conditions

The following five demographic factors must be considered: optometrist-to-population ratio, growth rate, population age, income level of the population, and key economic indicators.

Optometrist-to-Population Ratio. It is estimated by American Optometric Association manpower studies that one full-time optometrist is needed for every 7800 people. This statistic may be misleading because it does not take into account the presence of ophthalmologists or opticians who may be duplicating some of the optometrist's services. A more realistic appraisal must consider the setting of the practice: rural, suburban, or urban. The following are the minimum population requirements needed for these settings:
- Rural: 4000 to 6000 people per optometrist
- Suburban: 12,000 to 18,000 people per optometrist
- Urban: 25,000 to 45,000 people per optometrist

Using these ratios as a rough estimate of practice viability, a prospective buyer can evaluate the saturation level of practitioners in the drawing area of the practice. Although these ratios will not be changed by the purchase of an existing practice, the potential for new growth may be affected by an unfavorable ratio.

Growth Rate. The infusion of new people into an area means the arrival of prospective patients with no eye care practitioner. These people will be the most fertile source of growth for the practice. In an area with relatively flat growth, new patients will have to be obtained from the patient population of other practitioners or from new arrivals who have moved into the practice area.

Population Age. The population age of an area should be favorable to the type of services that may be added to the practice by the new practitioner. For example, a new practitioner who wants to add low-vision services to an existing practice needs to have a population that is skewed toward senior citizens.

Income Level of Population. The per capita income of the drawing area needs to be evaluated for the type of services provided and the fee structure of the practice.

Key Economic Indicators. The following economic factors should be reviewed to ascertain the viability of the area:

New business starts. New business in an area generally means that there is a favorable economic climate. The success (or failure) rates of these businesses and the turnover rate of small businesses in the area should be analyzed.
New housing starts. This statistic indicates the movement of new people into an area. It also may signal the movement of new jobs and new businesses into an area.
Home prices. The largest investment that most Americans make is in their homes. When real estate values are favorable, people feel more confident about the economy and are more likely to spend disposable income. Downward trends in real estate generally mean a downward economic trend, which will exert an effect on all businesses in an area.
Industry. Practicing in an area that is tied to a specific industry or a specific company may be favorable when economic times are prosperous. However, it can be disastrous in tighter economic times when the industry or company is not doing well. The ideal situation would be to practice in an area that has a diversified economy and offers jobs in various industries.
Social factors. Even though there is no rule that says a practitioner must live in the same area as the practice, there are geographic limits to the separation of primary residence and practice. Just as with any business, running an optometric practice requires time well beyond that needed to examine patients. The stress and strain of long hours spent commuting to and from the practice will undoubtedly take a toll on the practitioner and may affect the practitioner's willingness to tend to the practice beyond patient care hours. Factors to consider include the quality of the school system, cultural and recreational opportunities, health care facilities, climate, affordability and desirability of housing, religious institutions, and the ability of the spouse to earn an income in his or her field of expertise.

Finding the answer to the following questions will lead a young practitioner on a journey of discovery about any practice that is being considered for purchase.
• Does the practice deliver cost-effective quality care?
• Is it able to document outcomes?
• Can it easily integrate with other practices if needed?
• Has the seller taken steps to eliminate inappropriate care?
Specifically, the practitioner should review patient flow and satisfaction, the level of medical information system, the type and number of communications and recall messages, the ability to schedule an appointment, and the ease with which records can be interpreted by others.

Offering a Proposal

Fully investigating the economic and social factors previously identified requires a significant time commitment when a potential buyer visits the practice area. Information can be obtained from local chambers of commerce, real estate offices, banking institutions, other health care practitioners, other business owners, public service companies, local newspapers, direct mail companies, and friends and relatives who live in the area.

Several documents and forms pertaining to the financial and legal aspect of the eye care business to be transferred should be fully investigated and analyzed by both the purchaser and consultants. Box 3-2 lists the major items that should be described in an offering proposal that a prospective practice purchaser is given. The process of uncovering this information requires "due diligence" and includes a review of the ownership structure of the practice. Is creditor or lender consent required to enter into agreements or transfer assets? If so, the prospective purchaser should consider obtaining a letter of Assurance or Good Standing with a full disclosure from attorneys, accountants, and malpractice insurers.

Financial statements that should be reviewed include the following: 3 to 5 years of federal tax returns for the practice, the most recent profit-and-loss statement, short- or long-term debt (with maturity dates), the amount of accounts receivable and accounts payable, depreciation schedules, and assumed liabilities. Are there any local property taxes for which the purchaser would assume responsibility? Has the seller

---

Box 3-2 Information Required for an Offering Proposal

- Compile a brief history of the practice: age, location, and finances.
- Obtain at least 3 years of tax returns: for a sole proprietorship, schedule C; for a partnership or limited liability company, forms 1065 and K-1; and for a professional service corporation, schedule 1120 (1120S if organized as a subchapter S corporation).
- Get the profit and loss statement or the income and expense statement and balance sheets, if available, for at least 3 years, but as a minimum obtain the current year's quarterly statements.
- Complete a list of the assets that are to be transferred by model, age, and fair market value (if available).
- Complete a list of the wholesale or acquisition cost of the current useable frame, spectacle, and contact lens inventory.
- Plot the competition on a map using a radius of 1 to 2 miles in an urban area, 3 to 5 miles in a suburban area, and 7 to 10 miles in a rural area; differentiate between optometrists, ophthalmologists, opticians, and corporate chains.
- Calculate the current patient volume, using a breakdown of new and former patients by number of visits per year, zip codes, and age (if available).
- List the fee schedules for all services and the percentage of patients seen in specialty areas.
- List the practice promotional materials used.

---

received any unusual legal or financial correspondence recently?

What are the details of the present staff members' terms of employment and fringe benefit plans that are offered? Is a restrictive covenant, noncompete, or liquidated damages clause reasonable? What material contracts, commitments, leases, and consignments is the practice obligated to fulfill? Obtain copies and evaluate any management, third-party, and managed care contracts. Ascertain what licenses or permits are required to operate the business. Are any types of agency filings necessary? Obtain copies of any tangible property liens, liabilities, chattel mortgages, security interests, and Uniform Commercial Code filings that will be assumed by a purchaser.

Factors That Influence Practice Value

To evaluate the worth of a practice, the potential buyer should consider the gross and net income of the practice, scope of practice offered by the selling practitioner, practice location, existing office lease, patient records, transition period, physical resources of the practice, and accounts receivable.

Gross Income

Gross income is the total amount of money taken in by the practice for goods and services. The gross income for the 3 years before the sale should be reviewed in detail. This information can be obtained from form 1120 and the profit and loss statement of the practice if the practice is a professional association or corporation, from form 1065 if it is a partnership or limited lia-

bility company, or from schedule C of the seller's tax return if the practice is a sole proprietorship. The gross income should be evaluated for growth from year to year. A practice with an increase in gross income that is less than the increase in the cost of living index for that same period has actually lost income. A decrease in the gross income from year to year indicates that there may be major changes in the area, the economy, or the perception of the practice or practitioner. If there are increases in fees, they must be considered because an increase in gross income may be related to the change in fees, rather than to real growth of the practice.

Gross income also should be compared with the regional average gross income. This comparison may provide some indication of the economic viability of the practice and the area. The number of hours that the practice is in operation must be considered. A practice that is only open part time may have increased earning potential if hours are expanded; reduced hours may indicate a practice that has peaked in its earning potential. As the gross income of a solo practitioner increases, there will come a point at which further growth in income can only be achieved by the addition of another optometrist, extra technical support, or an increase in space. Practices with lower gross incomes may not be able to support a new practitioner who is required not only to finance the purchase of the practice but also to repay student loans.

Net Income

The prospective buyer should determine both the actual net income that is realized by a practice and the ratio of net income to gross income. Most dispensing optometric practices will have an adjusted net-to-gross income ratio of 25% to 35%. Nondispensing practices that are strictly service based may have a higher net-to-gross income ratio, since the overhead expenses are usually lower. Practices that have a lower-than-average net-to-gross-income ratio may incur higher-than-normal overhead expenses. This may be a result of the area or the location of the practice, or it may indicate that there is inefficient office management. Practices with low net-to-gross-income ratios also may be charging lower-than-normal fees for services and materials or may have incurred considerable debt service.

In looking at a practice's net income, the itemization of office expenditures should be investigated. These expenditures can be found on the profit and loss statement of an incorporated practice or on schedule C of an individual proprietor's tax return. Office expenses should be evaluated relative to national or regional averages. Deviations from average can indicate to the prospective buyer how efficiently the practice has been run and how practice income has been spent. The prospective buyer can use these figures to calculate how expenses might increase or decrease after the purchase of the practice.

When a practice is purchased, there is an inevitable loss of some existing patients. These are patients who, for whatever reason, decide not to see the new practitioner. They will need to be replaced by new ones whom the purchaser will attract to the practice. The potential effect of a loss of patients on practice income should be determined; the economic effect of a 5%, 10%, 15%, and greater loss can be calculated using scenario analysis. Although patient attrition will exert a direct effect on the gross income of the practice, fixed expenses, such as salaries, rent, and utilities, will not be affected. Variable expenses, such as laboratory costs for ophthalmic materials, will change with a decrease in gross income. By calculating the changes in these expenses, a hypothetical net income can be determined as a worst-case scenario should the gross income of the practice initially decrease.

There are certain fixed personal expenses, such as rent or mortgage payments, home utilities, and student loans that must be paid regardless of how successful the practice becomes. These expenses should be deducted from the net income of the practice. The amount that remains is the amount that the new practitioner can use to finance the purchase of the practice.

From these calculations, it should become apparent that the practice with the highest gross income may not necessarily be worth the most. It also should be apparent that a practice with a low gross income must produce sufficient net income to cover the practitioner's expenses, including the financing of the practice. If the practice cannot do so, the new practitioner will have to supplement this income by working outside the practice.

Scope of Practice

The number and type of services provided in the practice and the primary emphasis of the practice (services or materials) constitute the scope of the practice. Full-scope practices, providing the highest level of optometric services and materials, generally possess more up-to-date equipment and thus have a higher value. Many retiring practitioners may not have practiced primary care optometry. For the recent graduate, these practices offer an opportunity for a quick increase in the gross income of an existing practice. This can be achieved through attracting new patients to the practice or—with the addition of services or the expansion of hours to include evenings and weekends—through an increase in income derived from the existing patient population.

Practice Location and Lease

When an established practice is purchased, location usually is not a factor affecting the retention of existing patients. However, location is a primary factor in the ability of the practice to attract new patients. The practice location should be in an accessible, viable, professional or commercial area. In most suburban or rural areas, parking must be readily available. Handicapped and elderly patients require a location that is either on ground level or in a building with elevators. Visibility to street traffic also is desirable. Moving the practice during this initial 2- to 3-year period would create a greater erosion in the existing patient base and would saddle the new practitioner with additional moving and renovation expenses at a time when these expenses could probably be least afforded.

A favorable lease agreement is essential and should include options to renew for specified periods after the expiration of the initial lease term. These options give the prospective buyer the security of a longer lease term while retaining the flexibility to leave if the existing space becomes insufficient.

For the buyer to assume an existing lease, the lease must allow the selling practitioner to assign it to a successor. When evaluating the existing lease, the buyer should be sure that the terms are at least as favorable as could be obtained if a new lease were negotiated. The more favorable the lease terms are, the greater its value to the purchaser.

Patient Records

Having an established patient base is the greatest advantage of purchasing a practice. In evaluating the practice, however, the most difficult factor to assess is the likelihood that patients will remain with the practice after it is sold. A patient record in and of itself has no value for such evaluation. Transfer of records to a successor practitioner allows existing patients to feel that continuity of care will be preserved, while allowing the new practitioner to internally market to the existing patient base. The likelihood that a patient will return to the practice for care is greatest for active patients. Since most patients will return for eye care approximately every 2 years, the greatest value is given to those patients who have received care within that period. Patient records with no activity for more than 2 years but less than 5 years have significantly reduced value. Patient records with no activity for more than 5 years have little or no value to the new practitioner; most of these patients are likely to have moved, passed away, or selected another practitioner.

An active practice will have a 25% to 35% rate of new patient visits each year. This rate can be calculated by determining the number of new patients seen during the preceding 2 years. Appointment books or patient records may be used to make this analysis. A certain number of patients examined in prior years should have returned to the practice for subsequent care. This return rate also should be evaluated to determine how well the practice has performed in retaining patients. Patient records also should be sorted by the percentage paid by third-party payers and the percentage paid directly by patients. Third-party payments will not generate the same gross revenue for the practice as fees for service. Practices that have a large percentage of third-party payments need a larger patient base and can only be transferred successfully if the new practitioner will be able to serve as a provider under the third-party plan. These patients generally have less loyalty to the selling practitioner than fee-for-service patients. Their primary loyalty is to the practitioner who continues to provide them with the same benefits.

The average primary care practice (as of 2000) provides about 2300 examinations per practitioner per year. This statistic can be used as a benchmark to measure patient flow of a prospective practice. Practices with fewer than this number of examinations will require higher fees to generate the average gross income. Practices with higher-than-average examination fees but with average gross incomes result from fewer patients being seen or more third-party patients being treated.

The age range of the patient population should be closely representative of the area in general. If the average age of patients is greater than the average age of the population in the area, it could indicate that the practitioner has done little to attract new patients to the practice. There are regulations created by the Health Insurance Portability and Accountability Act that must be adhered to when dealing with patient records (see Chapter 28). Figure 3-1 provides a sample letter that can be used to notify patients about the transfer of care to another practitioner attendant to the sale of a practice.

Transition Period

The transition period allows the selling practitioner to acquaint the new practitioner with the management of the practice. This process includes review of office procedures, ordering of ophthalmic materials, meeting with suppliers, and working to transfer the loyalty of staff members. It also means introducing the new practitioner to key people in the area, including the main referral sources of the practice.

The transition period also applies to staff. In some instances, having existing staff members remain in the office can be more valuable than having the selling practitioner remain. This is especially true for staff members who have been working in the office for many years and who know all of the patients. Since staff members will be the first source of contact for patients both on the telephone and in the office, they can be a vital part of the effort to ease patient apprehension about a new practitioner and can reassure patients who are hesitant about returning.

The selling practitioner should be provided with financial remuneration for assisting during the transition period. Payment is usually provided on a per diem or weekly basis. The new practitioner also should expect to increase the salaries of staff members who are to be retained. This gesture demonstrates good faith on the part of the new practitioner and will pay for itself many times over in goodwill from the staff members.

Physical Resources

The physical resources of a practice include tangible assets, which usually are the equipment, furnishings,

This letter is to advise you that I am (retiring from, or selling) my practice as of ____(MM/DD/YY)____. The reason for my departure is (describe the reason). At this time I would like to take the opportunity to announce that Dr. _____ will be taking over my practice as of ____(MM/DD/YY)_____ and continue to provide the same quality eye care you have received at this office for so many years. I believe Dr. _____'s ability and knowledge will satisfy your eyecare needs and have personally instructed him/her in the important aspects that have made this practice unique and well appreciated by all of my patients.

Dr. _____ graduated from _____ optometry school and performed a post doctorate residency at _____. I am very confident that you will quickly agree that I am leaving the practice in quite competent hands.

In addition, the same loyal support staff that you are very familiar will be available to take care of your needs, as well as answer any of your questions. Should you wish to make an appointment, simply call the same telephone number _____. Our office hours will be ____.

A copy of your record will stay at this office; however, you are under no obligation to accept Dr._____ as your primary eye care practitioner. Should you desire to have your records transferred to another office, we will need your written authorization and a completed record release, which you can obtain by calling this office. If you wish to continue to use the services of this office, you may authorize the release of your records to Dr. _____ at your next visit.

In closing let me express my appreciation for your many years of loyalty, support and friendship. It has been a pleasure to be your optometrist and I want to take this opportunity to wish you much happiness and good health for future years.

Figure 3-1 Sample letter to patients announcing the transfer of records to another practitioner.

office supplies, inventory, and leasehold improvements. The value of tangible assets is often easier and more accurate to determine than that of the intangible assets, such as restrictive covenants.

Older, fully depreciated equipment will have some fair market value but must be evaluated as to its usefulness. Equipment that is in good working order and not obsolete can be used by the new practitioner and replaced when practice revenues allow. Obsolete or nonfunctional equipment that needs to be replaced should not be included when determining the value of the practice. This same consideration applies to furnishings, office supplies, inventory, and leasehold improvements.

The buyer should make sure that the seller owns all the frame and contact lens inventories that are to be purchased. Many contact lenses are supplied on consignment, and the new practitioner assumes responsibility for the consigned material. Frames usually are not consigned, but frames transferred to the new practitioner may not always be returnable if they had been purchased by the seller.

Accounts Receivable

Any fees for services or materials owed to the practice must be accounted for. The longer a debt is outstanding, the less the chance of its ultimate collection. For this reason, accounts receivable are often sold on a discounted basis, calculated on the age of each account. For example, accounts that are less than 30 days old may be purchased for 70% to 80% of their value; accounts 30 to 60 days old, for 50% to 60% of their value; accounts 60 to 90 days old, for 20% to 40% of their value; and accounts 90 to 120 days old, for 5% to 15% of their value. Accounts in excess of 120 days would not have any value. An alternative method is to pay a flat percentage rate, such as 40% to 60%, for all the accounts receivable.

If possible, it is preferable for the new practitioner not to purchase the existing accounts receivable but, instead, allow them to be collected by the selling practitioner during the transition period. If the transition period is very short, the new practitioner may agree to transfer the amounts collected over a specified period to the seller.

Factors That Decrease Practice Value

There are several factors that can significantly reduce the value of a practice to a potential buyer. Some of the most common are:

- Recent cutbacks on time spent in the office, resulting in reduced practice income.
- Failure to have an active recall system to ensure the buyer of uninterrupted patient flow.
- Inadequate and outdated computer and office management systems.
- Office equipment that has not been updated.
- Lack of participation in third-party vision and eye health reimbursement plans.
- Inadequate use of Medicare.

Despite all of the factors that have been described, the "bottom line" in any transfer of property is the law of supply and demand. The greater the demand for an existing practice, the more valuable it becomes. As a corollary rule, the greater the need and urgency to sell, the lower the price that will be attained. In any event, and no matter what the circumstances, there is always a way to determine whether a proposed price is reasonable.

Practice Appraisal

The basis for analyzing the value of a business can be found in Revenue Ruling 59-60, issued by the Internal Revenue Service. A review of the ruling shows that the following items should be included as part of any appraisal:

- A determination of the legal status of the business (information about the practitioner and the practice).
- How similar practices that have been recently sold compare in price to the practice under consideration; how the local and national economy affect the practice.
- A "book value" adjustment of the balance sheet and the profit and loss statement should be performed to reflect the current fair market value of the depreciated tangible assets.
- An analysis that takes into account both income and excess profits (if any) should be performed using capitalization rate methodology.
- Goodwill, franchises, restrictive covenants, and any other intangible assets of a practice should be examined carefully and assigned reasonable values as a result of thorough analysis.

The *fair market value* of a practice as described by the Internal Revenue Service's Ruling 59-60 and defined by the American Society of Appraisers is "the amount at which a practice would change hands between a willing buyer and a willing seller, each having reasonable knowledge of all the pertinent facts and market conditions, neither being compelled nor obligated to buy or sell, and with an exchange of equal consideration to both parties."

No set formula or easy method exists that can be applied to simplify the fair market valuation process. For this reason, a weighted average of several methods is suggested to estimate fair market value. Revenue Ruling 59-60 states that "a sound valuation will be based on all relevant facts, but the elements of common sense, informed judgment and reasonableness must enter into the process of weighing those facts and determining their aggregate significance." There are several acceptable approaches an appraiser may choose when determining the fair market value of a practice. These methods can be divided into the following three basic categories: asset approach, income approach, and market approach.

The Asset-Based Approach

This method values the two primary components that contribute to practice value: tangible and intangible assets. Tangible assets include equipment, machinery, instruments, furnishings, leasehold improvements, supplies, and inventory. The value of tangible assets is determined by fair market value itemization (using comparable sales data and price listings of used equipment) or "book value" (the value remaining from the original basis after depreciation, obtained from the seller's tax returns). Current and unused inventory also may be valued this way, or the wholesale replacement cost may be used. Intangible assets include goodwill, office lease, telephone number, practice name, income-producing ability, and quality of patient records—all factors that should help minimize patient attrition during and after the transition.

The Income Approach

This method develops a value for the practice using a viewpoint similar to that of a disinterested investor who is considering the purchase of a business with comparable investment characteristics. The current value of the practice is based on what the practice can generate in the future for the new owner. This is determined by calculating the future annual net cash flow of the business for a designated number of years. This total is then "discounted" back to the date of sale using a "present value" formulation (explained later in this chapter). The "discount rate" is equivalent to the estimated rate of return on the purchase of the practice viewed as an investment and its value is reflected in the inherent risk of the purchase.

The Market Approach

This method takes into account the significant benchmark variables of the practice, such as net-to-gross income ratio, percent of income for staff salaries, cost of goods sold, and practice overhead expenses, and then compares these numbers to previous sales of similar practices. Once this analysis is completed, a guideline ratio is calculated as a percentage of the past year's gross revenue to determine practice value. Unfortunately, data about sales of optometric practices are difficult to obtain, since information of this nature is used primarily on a proprietary basis by commercial brokers and research houses.

Using Break-Even Analysis to Determine Whether a Price Is Reasonable

Break-even point analysis will not determine the value of a practice or the price for which a practice should sell. It is a useful tool, however, that all prospective practice purchasers should use. It offers a method of calculating the affordability of monthly payments for the practice, based on current practice revenues and expenses, projected financial performance, desired personal salary, and contracted selling price. An example of how to make such a calculation is found in Box 3-3 (see also Chapter 41).

In the example, the break-even point of $35,649 is less than the average total monthly revenue of $37,500 by $1851, indicating that there is enough income to provide the desired salary, to pay off the debt, and operate the practice at present revenues and expenses. There is a cushion or safety factor of $1851 per month, or $22,212 annually, in this example. If the break-even point had been more than the monthly revenue of $37,500, then the available options would have been to take less income, to reduce the monthly debt service payments by obtaining a longer loan repayment schedule, to reduce the monthly total fixed expenses (which is difficult to do), or to decline the purchase.

The most obvious assets of a practice are its tangible items: equipment, instruments, records, furnishings, supplies, inventories, real estate, and so forth. These items can be assigned a fair market value with a reasonable degree of accuracy. The intangible assets of the practice, such as goodwill, lease value, and restrictive covenants, have a higher degree of variability as to the calculation of their value. This intangible value is sometimes defined as the likelihood that the buyer will be able to enjoy the same economic benefits as the seller.

The price paid for an optometric practice is often in the range of 35% to 65% of the practice's gross income for the year preceding the sale. This price may be more if the net-to-gross income ratio is high or if the practice has exceptional assets, such as a considerable amount of up-to-date equipment. The price may be less if the net-to-gross income ratio is low or if there is little usable equipment.

In the usual case, the proposed buyer and the selling practitioner must negotiate the terms of sale themselves. Because most optometrists are not knowledgeable about the legal, tax, and accounting issues that are part of such a sale, it is necessary to use a team of consultants so that needed technical advice can be obtained.

Restrictive Covenants

When one enters into an agreement for the purchase of a practice, the purchase agreement should include what is known as a restrictive covenant or covenant not to compete. Simply put, this is a clause that prevents the selling optometrist from practicing optometry for a specific period within a specified geographic area. The intent is to prevent economic harm to the buyer. Without this provision the selling optometrist would be free to open an office literally "across the street," thereby significantly lowering the practice goodwill by drawing away patients. An attorney will be required to draft the language of such a covenant so that it will be in compliance with state law and thereby enforceable in court if legal action were to become necessary.

Consultants

The purchase of a practice may be the single largest investment that an optometrist makes. An investment of this magnitude should not be attempted without consulting various experts, including an optometric advisor, an attorney, and an accountant.

Optometric Advisor

This practitioner will have personal knowledge of the demographics of vision and eye care in the area; the value of equipment, inventory, and supplies; and

---

Box 3-3 Sample Break-Even Analysis

For purposes of this example, it is assumed that the practice grosses $450,000 per year and that the agreed-upon sales price is $290,000, of which $250,000 will be financed for 10 years at 9% interest.

Step 1

Average gross monthly income for this practice is $450,000 ÷ 12 = $37,500.

Step 2

Total fixed expenses (TFE) must be determined; TFE includes salary, rent, insurance, utilities, and similar expenses. In this example 40% of gross income will be used as the TFE (which amounts to $180,000 annually, or $15,000 per month).

Step 3

Monthly payments of $3167 for the loan obtained from an amortization schedule.

Step 4

Practitioner income must be calculated; for this example, it will be $90,000 annually, or $7,500 per month.

Step 5

The total fixed cost (TFC) must be determined, which is equal to the sum of TFE, debt service payments, and practitioner income:

$$TFC = TFE + debt\ service + doctor's\ income$$

In this example the total of the three figures is $25,667, expressed as a monthly average.

Step 6

The formula for break-even point (BEP) is: $\dfrac{TFC}{1-VC^*(\%)} = \dfrac{25,667}{1.0-0.28} = \dfrac{25,667}{0.72} = \$35,649$

Answer

The break-even point is $35,649.

*VC, Variable costs (the laboratory bills or the cost of goods sold, which in this example are 28% of the gross income, or 0.28).

---

the reputation of the seller and the practice. This advisor will be able to provide unique support in the transition after the sale. Advisors may be found through local or state optometric societies, through schools and colleges of optometry, or independently through advertisements in professional journals. A qualified practice appraiser will be able to evaluate all of these factors and arrive at a fair price for the value of the practice.

Attorney

The prospective purchaser should hire an attorney who has experience in the sale of optometric practices. The attorney will prepare the contract for the purchase of the practice and will provide any needed documentation. The attorney usually will not negotiate the contract but may provide legal or tax advice concerning the sale.

Accountant

The accountant will review the financial records of the practice and, along with the optometric advisor, determine its fair market value. The accountant also will evaluate the potential payment terms of the purchase, including the allocation of assets for tax purposes. It would be ideal for the accountant to have some experience with optometric or professional practice sales.

Tax Consequences of Purchasing a Practice

Changes in federal tax law have made the apportionment of dollar value to the assets of a practice transfer easier and less contentious to determine. One precaution is to make sure that the allocation is completed as an "arm's length agreement" (one with no hint of

Box 3-4 Tax Implications for the Buyer When Purchasing Practice Assets

ASSET	TAX DEDUCTION
Supplies and inventory	Deducted in the year of purchase
Computers, electronic equipment*	Depreciated over 5 years
Equipment and furnishings	Depreciated over 7 years
Goodwill and patient records	Amortized over 15 years
Covenant not to compete	Amortized over 15 years
Leasehold improvements, building	Depreciated over 39 years

Data from Taxpayer Relief Acts of 1997 and 2000.
*Purchased computer software may be depreciated over 3 years.

Box 3-5 First-Year Adjusted Cash Flow Analysis

Dr. Seller agrees to sell the practice, which has gross revenues of $465,000, for a total of $250,000 to Dr. Buyer. Dr. Buyer will make a 20% down payment, and Dr. Seller will finance the balance due (80% of the sales price) for 6 years at a 9% simple interest rate, which will result in monthly payments of $3600.

Dr. Buyer has inspected Dr. Seller's schedule C forms and tax returns for the business for the past 3 years and is satisfied that the financial data and ratios are favorable. Based on this information, Dr. Buyer is projecting the first year's gross revenues to be $500,000. The relevant practice expenses in this analysis are as follows:

The fixed costs for this practice include a rental lease of $3500 per month, an optician salary of $45,000 per year, a secretary-receptionist who is paid $25,000 per year, and an ophthalmic technician who is paid $30,000 per year. The telephone bill is $1000 per month, which includes an advertisement in the Yellow Pages. The cost of utilities (i.e., water, electricity, and gas) and janitorial services is $15,000 per year. Miscellaneous fixed operating costs are another $1500 per month. Variable expenses for the practice include the wholesale cost of materials sold and average about 30% of gross revenues ($150,000).

Dr. Buyer plans to draw a first-year income of $85,000, with $5000 annual increases thereafter. Dr. Buyer believes that the previous year's annual growth rate of 8% in gross revenue and 4% in total office expenses can be sustained for the next 3 to 5 years, creating a stable practice income. Dr. Buyer's accountant advises that his effective overall income tax payment would be 25%.

Tangible assets to be purchased have a fair market value of $100,000 and will be depreciated $20,000 annually using a 5-year straight line schedule to zero salvage value. Based on this strategy, the first-year adjusted cash flow will be $1960. This "positive" result indicates that there will be a financial cushion for the first year; a "negative" result would necessitate revision of financial projections because there would be a shortfall of cash for either loan obligations or personal income.

Anticipated gross revenue	$500,000
Less fixed costs of operation	−$187,000
Less variable costs of operation	−$150,000
Less depreciation	−$20,000
Less personal income	−$85,000
Pretax income	$58,000
Multiply by effective tax rate of 0.25%	−$14,500
After-tax income	$43,500
Add back depreciation	+$20,000
Net practice cash flow	$63,500
Less annual note payment to seller	−$43,200
Adjusted cash flow for the practice	$20,300

If all practice revenue and expenses are realized as projected, Dr. Buyer can anticipate earning $85,000 plus $20,300 ($105,300 total) the first year. However, if the actual net cash flow for the practice is negative, then that amount would have to be subtracted from the projected personal income of $85,000.

collusion between buyer and seller to minimize the tax implications). Both the buyer and seller are required to report the same values on Internal Revenue Service form 8594 in the year of the sale.

Many practice sales are seller financed. The purchaser pays a certain amount down, and the balance is paid during the course of years to the selling practitioner, who holds a note from the purchaser. Because of this long-term relationship between buyer and seller, the sales agreement needs to be fair. Otherwise, the arrangement will fail, and the selling optometrist (who is usually retired) will not receive the bargained-for value from the buyer.

The note held by the selling practitioner should specify a reasonable amount of simple interest to be applied to the unpaid balance. Over the course of years, the interest adds significantly to the total amount received by the seller. It is a tax-deductible expense for the buyer.

One important aspect of the sale of a practice is the tax ramifications of the sale. Technical rules must be followed, particularly when allocating value to the practice assets for tax purposes. Tax advice is necessary to ensure that all requirements have been complied with. Current depreciation periods that affect the purchaser are listed in Box 3-4 for various assets.

To calculate the after-tax net cash flow for the first year, a sample practice sale cash flow analysis is provided in Box 3-5.

Bibliography

Barresi B, Scott C: Internet research: improving traditional community analysis before launching a practice. *J Am Optom Assoc* 71(1):55-8, 2000.

Dietrich MO: *Medical practice valuation guidebook 2001/2002*, ed 2, San Diego, 2001, Windsor Professional Information.

Fox YM, Levine BA: *How to join, buy, or merge a physician's practice*. St. Louis, 1997, Mosby.

Internal Revenue Service publication 537, *Installment sales*.

Internal Revenue Service Ruling 59-60, as applied to the purchase of a medical practice. Available at: *www.physiciansnews.com/business/202.html*.

Keene RD: *How to value a medical practice*. Alpharetta, Ga, 1999, Robert D. Keene.

Moss G: Financial decisions in a managed care era. *Optom Economics* 2(1):25-30,1996.

Moss G, Shaw-McMinn P: *Eyecare business marketing and strategy*. Boston, 2001, Butterworth-Heinemann.

Pratt S, Reilly R, Schweihs R: *Valuing small businesses and professional practices*, ed 3, New York, 1998, McGraw-Hill.

Schryver DL: How to determine fair market value. *Med Group Manage J* 45(6):6, 1998.

Tinsley R, Sides R, Anderson G: *Valuation of medical practice*. New York, 1999, Wiley.

www.aoa.org. Web site for the American Optometric Association.

www.irs.ustreas.gov. Web site for the Internal Revenue Service, which contains forms and publications that can be downloaded.

Chapter *4*

Employment Options

Craig Hisaka and W. Howard McAlister

Work expands so as to fill the time available for its completion.
Cyril Parkinson *Parkinson's Law*

Approximately 60% of the graduates from optometry school enter the practice of optometry as employees, even though the majority of these graduates ultimately intend to become self-employed. Surveys begun in the 1990s by the Association of Practice Management Educators indicate that 50% of optometry school graduates enter a practice setting that is not intended to be their ultimate choice and that they expect to spend up to 5 years in that setting before switching to the desired form of practice. These graduates invariably choose employee positions rather than starting or purchasing a practice. The usual reasons that graduates cite for choosing employment are inadequate business experience, significant debt at graduation, and overriding family obligations or other commitments.

Lack of meaningful business experience is a common concern among optometry school graduates. By working for others, graduates can participate in optometric practices but are not financially accountable for them. Many students overcome this lack of experience by working with private practitioners during summers or vacation periods and by planning externships in practice settings that are similar to the setting desired at graduation. During these periods, patient care and practice administration can be learned so that the student is able to feel confident about both types of management skills at graduation.

Another common concern of graduates is lack of the financial resources needed to start a practice, usually because of educational debts. Although the cost of schooling can be high and loans may be required to pay for the years of professional education, students can and should limit debt as much as possible. Surveys conducted at schools and colleges of optometry have shown that some groups of students are good at minimizing debt, whereas other groups are not. These surveys indicate that the degree of debt at graduation is related to careful planning and stringent use of borrowed money and that motivated students can graduate with significantly less debt.

A third reason that optometry school graduates seek employment is because of personal or family obligations that make it necessary to remain in a certain location or to provide financial support for a period. These obligations can be overriding if a student does not have adequate time to investigate options and identify the best opportunities. Again, time during school must be used to explore the choices that are available and to select the best available opportunity so that the graduate will not be forced to choose a less-than-desirable beginning.

Optometry school graduates seeking employment opportunities usually look to an associateship with optometrists or ophthalmologists, residencies, corporate optometry, the uniformed services, the Veterans Administration (VA), academia, and health maintenance organizations (HMOs). This chapter briefly discusses these employment options (Box 4-1).

Associateship

An associate is an employee and, as such, holds no ownership interest in the business entity for which the employee works. An associate does not share in the profits and losses but rather is salaried and may receive additional employee benefits. The ultimate responsibility for the practice belongs to the

Box 4-1 Advantages and Disadvantages of Employment

Advantages
- Stable income and employee benefits available and paid by employer (e.g., paid vacations, health insurance, malpractice insurance premiums, continuing education expenses).
- Gain experience from other practitioners, learn the "art of optometry," and increase business knowledge and skills.
- Minimal or no start-up costs and minimal or no investment required.
- Minimal management decisions required.
- The appropriate opportunity could lead to a future partnership.

Disadvantages
- Average income, limited earning potential, limited upward mobility.
- No equity acquired in a practice.
- Dictated office policies and minimal independence.
- Very few good long-term arrangements unless they lead to partnership.
- After several years of employment, employees are at risk for termination because of high salary and benefits; thus, there is poor long-term security.
- A limited scope of practice may be found in certain settings because of the volume of patients that must be seen.

employer; the associate is not responsible for its financial status. An associate may participate in management decisions only to the extent permitted by the employer and will receive only a few of the tax breaks available to persons in small businesses. Despite these limitations, associateship can be used as a stepping-stone to partnership or sole proprietorship. For many newly graduated optometrists, it has proved to be an ideal means of making the transition from an academic environment to the business world. In selecting associateship, a graduate may work for an optometrist or an ophthalmologist.

Employment by an Optometrist

Many graduates begin their practice experience as the employee of an optometrist in private practice. Often the motivation for the associateship is the hope that employer and employee will agree to form a partnership. The associateship, which is usually for 1 to 2 years, serves as a trial period during which the optometrist and the associate determine their compatibility and the feasibility of partnership (see Chapter 5).

Because the usual associate is a recent optometry school graduate with relatively little practice experience, the earnings of optometric associates, when compared with those for other types of employed optometrists, tend to be toward the bottom of the scale. Figures from surveys, such as those conducted by the American Optometric Association, reflect this (Box 4-2). These results are misleading, however. Other types of employment have a higher proportion of individuals who have been out of optometry school for more than 3 years and who are therefore higher wage earners by virtue of their years on the job. These surveys also do not recognize the long-term potential of optometric associateship, which commonly results in a partnership arrangement. Benefits complement salary and are of particular importance to associates because, if paid for by the associate, they cannot be fully deducted for tax purposes, whereas they can be deducted fully as legitimate business expenses by the employer.

If associateship is contemplated, the practice should be evaluated to determine whether it is large enough to support two optometrists. General guidelines should be used to assess practice income, growth, and number of annual examinations. The office should be large enough to accommodate another practitioner, and adequate equipment and instrumentation should be available.

The associateship allows both parties to consider and discuss the prospect of partnership. If the associateship results in the decision to form a partnership, the typical buy-in period is 5 to 7 years, which means that the associate becomes a full partner within a few years after graduating from optometry school. If the practice is maintained, it will support the new partner for the next 30 to 40 years, or until retirement is planned. If the asso-

Box 4-2 Mean Net Income for Employed Optometrists, 2000

EMPLOYER	MEAN NET INCOME
Ophthalmologists	$123,567
Multidisciplinary clinics	$102,941
Optical chains	$98,667
Optometrists	$95,412

Data from AOA: 2001 AOA economic survey. St. Louis, 2001, Author.

ciateship does not result in partnership, the associate usually leaves the practice to pursue other opportunities.

Employment by an Ophthalmologist

Increasingly, optometry school graduates are finding employment opportunities with ophthalmologists in private practice. The reason for this trend may be explained by the primary care orientation of optometry. Ophthalmologists have found that employee optometrists can provide refractive care; contact lens services; management of a wide range of ocular pathologic conditions; and specialized services, such as those needed by children, senior citizens, and people seeking low-vision rehabilitation. Employing optometrists to provide these services allows ophthalmologists to concentrate on ocular surgery and other secondary and tertiary services.

Because ophthalmologists earn, on the average, a higher mean income than optometrists do, they provide, on the average, a higher salary than that paid by optometrists (see Box 4-2). Part of the reason for this difference in remuneration is the ability of ophthalmologists to offer more benefits (e.g., moving expenses, allowances for use of an automobile, group-term life insurance, disability insurance) than optometrists.

There can be some significant drawbacks, however, to ophthalmologic associateship. The duties assigned to the associate may not be ideal. An associate who would prefer to treat ocular pathologic conditions may have to provide refractive care or perform work-ups for the surgeon rather than manage a wide variety of patients with ocular disease. For this reason, it is important to determine whether the duties of the associateship match the optometrists practice goals. Another drawback is that ophthalmologic associateship does not offer much opportunity for long-term advancement. It is rare for ophthalmologists to join into partnership with optometrists. In fact, in many states optometrists and ophthalmologists are prohibited by law from jointly forming a professional association or corporation for that purpose. Therefore, optometrists employed by ophthalmologists tend to either remain employees or leave the practice to begin or join an optometric practice.

Whether a graduate wishes to work for an optometrist or an ophthalmologist, the likelihood of finding an associateship opportunity is directly related to the effort put into the search and the graduate's ability to form a personal relationship with the potential employer before graduation. The associate-ship market is a competitive one, and students who begin early, meet potential employers, and work in their practices before graduation are the ones who graduate with opportunities awaiting them. To wait until the fourth year of optometry school to solicit by mail an invitation to interview and to have but one opportunity to make a favorable impression is to invite disappointment. If associateship is desired, the process of looking for a potential employer should begin as soon as possible, and when opportunities are found, the student should try to visit the practitioner frequently. The better the personal relationship, the more likely it will result in a successful associateship.

Residency

There are approximately 200 accredited residency positions that provide postgraduate education for optometrists. These positions may be found in a variety of practice locations, including schools and colleges of optometry, VA hospitals and outpatient clinics, Indian Health Service facilities, eye care surgery referral centers, and U.S. military posts. They offer a wide range of experiences and environments for learning, providing a year of intense clinical and educational experience in a particular area of optometry. Residency programs are currently available for training in family practice optometry, binocular vision therapy, contact lens practice, low-vision rehabilitation, pediatric care, and diagnosis and treatment of ocular disease. To apply for a residency program, the applicant must have graduated from an accredited school or college of optometry. Because there is only one residency program available for every 10 graduates, residency positions are highly competitive. It is important for applicants to take and pass parts one and two of the examination given by the National Board of Examiners in Optometry. Excellent academic records also are advisable.

Residency programs offer a concentrated clinical experience, with some time devoted to other activities, such as didactic education, research, and teaching. The range and extent of nonclinical activities varies from program to program. Residents can expect to work full days and to serve as necessary providing emergency and on-call care. Salaries for residents are standard and provide essentially subsistence level wages. Pay can be an issue for residents who must live in expensive metropolitan areas.

Optometrists who have recently completed a residency are the individuals best able to discuss a particular program's strengths and weaknesses. They should be consulted by students interested in applying for a specific residency position.

Veterans Administration

The VA was organized in 1930 and is one of the largest independent agencies within the U.S. government, operating the world's largest system of hospitals and clinics as part of its overall responsibility for the nation's veterans. The VA also plays an important role in the education of health care professionals. It is estimated that, in any given year, more than 25% of all U.S. medical and surgical residents receive training at VA hospitals.

The involvement of optometrists in VA education and patient care has a much shorter history. Optometrists were not eligible to serve in VA staff positions until 1957, and the first VA residency position for optometrists was not created until 1972. Today, opportunities may be found both for VA staff optometrists and for residency positions.

To be selected for an entry-level VA staff position, the applicant must have a Doctor of Optometry degree from an accredited school and an optometry license from one state and must pass a physical examination. These qualifications allow an optometrist to apply for an associate-grade position. A limited number of entry-level positions are available, however, and to be competitive, applicants also should have completed a residency or have experience as a practitioner. To be selected for the next level, full grade, the optometrist must have served in a residency program or served 2 years as a practitioner. There are three more levels— intermediate, senior, and chief—which require increasingly stringent qualifications. There are numerous benefits, such as health and disability insurance, paid vacations and similar entitlements, and a generous retirement plan.

There are more than 150 staff positions in the VA system, located in hospitals or outpatient clinics. Staff and clinic sizes vary from facility to facility, as do practice privileges, because the scope of practice for each practitioner is determined by the facility rather than by state law (VA facilities are subject to federal rather than state regulation). Primary care is offered to a diverse population of veterans, and there is ample opportunity to participate in research projects. VA staff optometrists commonly contribute to the professional literature and provide postgraduate education. They also contribute to the education of optometrists through VA residency programs.

There are about 50 residency positions at VA facilities, providing excellent clinical postgraduate training for young optometrists. To be eligible to apply, applicants must have graduated from an accredited school of optometry. Although not a requirement, it is highly desirable for applicants to have passed the examination given by the National Board of Examiners in Optometry. Because there are a limited number of VA residency positions, there is significant competition for these positions. The pay for VA residency positions, like all residency positions, is low. Days are full, and there are after-hours responsibilities as well. The year of training, however, enables residents to qualify for VA staff positions, to apply for positions in academic institutions, or to provide improved skills in a private practice setting.

Corporate Practice

Ophthalmic companies employ optometrists to provide services in several types of practice settings, including "next-door" or mercantile lease arrangements, as part of a trademark chain, or within a "superstore." Although the financial arrangements vary among these types of employers, optometrists in corporate settings serve as "independent contractors" rather than as employees. An independent contractor is someone who contracts to perform work by his or her own methods and without being subject to the direct control of the employer. The advantage to the corporate employer of such an arrangement is that the employer is not responsible for the negligence of the independent contractor and does not have to contribute half of the independent contractor's social security payments to the federal government. Thus, the independent contractor is liable for any liability claims arising from employment and is solely responsible for the withholding and payment of the his or her income tax and social security contributions.

The advantages to corporate practice are that there is little investment, the beginning income is usually good (see Box 4-2), and positions are readily available for new graduates. In the typical situation, the employer provides the office, staff, and equipment and uses advertising to attract a patient base. As payment, the optometrist receives all fees charged for services or a percentage of fees charged for services, with a minimum salary usually guaranteed. In rare instances, the optometrist may share in the fees received from the sale of ophthalmic materials, but typically these fees are paid solely to the corporate employer. The lease arrangement between employer and optometrist is inevitably favorable, with the optometrist typically paying a nominal fee for the rental of the office space. The lease arrangement is for a limited period, however, and may be cancelled at the option of the employer. The arrangement also may assert that the patient records are the property of the corporate employer and must remain in the office after the relationship with the optometrist has ended.

The disadvantages of corporate practice are a lack of security, limitations in the scope of practice, and a ceiling on earnings. Because an optometrist working in a corporate environment has no ownership interest, there is no long-term security. Unlike a private practitioner, at retirement there is nothing to sell to a successor practitioner. In a corporate setting, the scheduling of patients often does not permit a full scope of practice to be enjoyed, and the optometrist may not be able to develop specialized skills because so much time must be devoted to routine examination. Although the optometrist receives a minimum salary and is remunerated based on fees for services, there is a ceiling on earnings that is based on the corporate employer's profit margin. If profits get too low, the optometrist gets no further increase or is discharged so that a newer optometrist can be employed at a lower pay rate. As a consequence, the optometrist in a corporate setting does not achieve the job security or the income earned by self-employed optometrists in private practice.

New graduates often look to corporate practice as a means of obtaining practical experience while reducing the debts of professional education. Although these goals can be accomplished, employment for a period of years is required. Unfortunately, after several years it can be financially difficult for the optometrist to leave a steady income for the uncertainties of beginning a new practice or purchasing an existing practice. Regardless of the practice option chosen, debt must be incurred (to open or buy the practice), and this indebtedness may conflict with other financial needs or priorities. The longer the optometrist remains in the corporate setting, the more difficult it can become to leave.

Uniformed Services

Employment positions exist for optometrists within the U.S. Army, Air Force, Navy, and Public Health Service (PHS). The majority of these positions are in patient care, although some are purely research and some are purely administrative. Most of these positions require optometrists to be commissioned officers, but in a few positions, optometrists are civil service employees.

There are more than 400 optometrists serving in the armed forces. Optometry school graduates entering military service enter with the rank of O-3. If they enter the Army or Navy, they will serve in the Medical Service Corps; in the Air Force, they will serve in the Bioscience Corps. A limited number of optometry school graduates enter military service each year through the Health Professions Scholarship Program, which pays for 1 to 4 years of the graduate's professional school education.

Optometry officers provide patient care in multidisciplinary environments such as medical centers, community level hospitals, and clinics. Although the scope of practice varies between installations, in general it is broader (particularly with respect to the management of ocular disease and trauma) than the scope of practice traditionally seen in the civilian optometric community. For the new graduate, the patient care experience in the first few years of military service practice is usually more extensive than the experience enjoyed by contemporaries in private practice settings. Since the dependents of military active duty personnel and retirees and their dependents are eligible for care from military health care providers, the optometry officer will see patients of all ages.

More than 80 optometrists serve as officers in the PHS. The vast majority of patient care positions within the PHS are in the Indian Health Service. Most optometrists serve as commissioned officers and, like the military services, the entering rank is O-3. A few optometrists serve as civil servants. Eligible beneficiaries in the Native American patient population also include all age groups, although almost half of the beneficiaries are younger than 21 years. Many health care facilities of the uniformed services provide clinical training to optometry students, thereby allowing clinicians of the uniformed services an opportunity to teach.

Commissioned officers and civil servants receive a salary, tax-free housing, and subsistence allowances and do not share in the cost of operating a practice. In general, the patient care equipment and facilities are very good. A retirement plan, health care coverage, protection against disability, and malpractice coverage are provided. Junior officers usually have few administrative requirements related to operating the practice. All members of the uniformed services receive 30 days of paid vacation each year.

For midcareer practitioners, several opportunities exist to enter graduate degree programs or residencies, at government expense, while remaining on active duty and drawing full pay and allowances. The number and type of positions vary from time to time and between services. There also are a limited number of career-broadening assignments in administrative areas and research.

Military officers may be assigned to different facilities all over the world, allowing for the opportunity to travel to many exotic locations. Time off and funding for continuing education are generally provided to meet credentialing and state licensing requirements.

In the multidisciplinary environment of the uniformed services, commanders will nearly always be medical officers (M.D. or D.O.). In most locations, if an ophthalmologist is present, the optometrist will be part of the ophthalmologist's service. Even though relations are often cordial, when they are not, the optometrist is at a decided disadvantage. Though trained and licensed as an independent health care practitioner, the optometry officer may not be able to function as such.

Most assignments allow for a varied patient population, but in some locations the patient census consists mostly of young, healthy men. These locations are generally in training centers, where the practitioner may provide only very limited basic care to a large volume of patients each day. Because of the chronic shortage of optometrists in the uniformed services, the opportunity to provide specialty care, such as contact lenses, low-vision rehabilitation, and binocular vision therapy, may be very limited.

The salary received by both officers and civil servants is not competitive with that of most other positions available to new graduates. Also, the special pay for optometry officers is a small fraction of that paid to medical and dental officers. Although the retirement pension is very good, it is only authorized for those with at least 20 years of service.

Many officers complain of being required to perform nonpatient care duties such as administrative officer of the day, linen inventory officer, and so forth. Administrative performance is often perceived as being more important to promotion and success than is patient care. Usually, most officers of equivalent education, such as physicians and dentists, are not required to serve in such nonprofessional capacities.

Many Indian Health Service clinics are in remote locations and require extensive travel. Moving is required of military officers on a frequent basis. This obligation can cause considerable disruption in family life. Although many positions are in exotic locales, there also are a number of hardship tours, including assignments in combat areas.

Academia

Fewer than 600 full-time faculty positions exist within schools and colleges of optometry for clinical and classroom teaching and for clinical and basic research. Academicians progress through various academic ranks, beginning with instructor, assistant professor, associate professor, and culminating with professor. Promotion depends on the faculty member's contributions to teaching, scholarly activities, and service.

Accepting a faculty position requires no investment of capital and does not incur the same type of time demands found in a private practice setting. There are far fewer administrative tasks generally required of junior faculty when compared with optometrists in a private practice. Optometrists in academia receive a guaranteed salary as well as benefits such as health, disability, and malpractice insurance; vacation; and a retirement plan. Time and stipends are usually provided for attending professional conferences. Optometrists at schools and colleges of optometry have opportunities to pursue areas of special interest in an intellectual environment. In many cases income can be supplemented by offering continuing education and providing patient care outside the academic institution. Excellent job security is obtained when a faculty member achieves tenure. Eligibility for tenure occurs 7 to 10 years after being placed on a tenure track.

From an economic viewpoint, academia provides a relatively low level of remuneration for doctors of optometry. Although there is no development of equity, as is found in private practice, retirement plans are usually generous. To gain a position as a faculty member, additional professional or graduate degrees or a residency are usually required. Thus, the educator must train longer to be paid relatively less than contemporaries in other settings. Faculty members have minimal independence, and junior members have very little ability to affect academic policy. If a faculty member is on a tenure track but not awarded tenure, other employment must be sought.

Health Maintenance Organizations

HMOs provide comprehensive health maintenance and treatment services for a voluntarily enrolled group of patients who pay a periodic fixed rate for services. These patients also may pay a small copayment fee at each office visit. There are two types of HMOs: staff models and independent practice associations (IPAs).

Staff model HMOs provide services to members through their own professional staff, which is employed by the HMO. An optometrist working for a staff model HMO is usually paid a salary, with the workload being an additional consideration.

IPAs contract with a private practitioner to have that practitioner deliver health services to its members. These practitioners are usually paid either on a capitation basis or on a fee-for-service basis.

Staff model HMOs offer an immediate income with no start-up costs (see Box 4-2). Although a staff optometrist does not have to be concerned about clinic coverage for patients when the optometrist is out of the office, the daily schedule of office hours is usually beyond the optometrist's control. To compensate for the moderately attractive salary offered to optometrists, many HMOs offer a good fringe benefit package that includes paid time off for continuing education; a monetary stipend for continuing education expenses; health, life, and disability insurance; sick leave; and a retirement plan.

Staff model HMOs require minimal management time and few management decisions from the optometrist. The optometrist, as a primary care provider, usually operates as the gatekeeper of the system for all patients with vision problems. There is no limit to the age of patients seen in this setting, and with the optometrist as the entry point into the system, there is diversity in the types of cases the optometrist will encounter. It is a multidisciplinary practice environment, and the optometrist often practices side by side with the primary care physician.

As an employee, the optometrist will build up little or no equity in the practice. Depending on the organization of the HMO, medical practitioners may control the administration of the optometrist's department. Under medical control, the optometrist may not be used as the gatekeeper of the system. It also may result in the optometrist not being allowed to practice the full scope allowed by state law, seeing a restricted age of patients and being allocated a decreased amount of examination time per patient.

Conclusion

The choice of an employment option after graduation from optometry school is usually based on a decision by the graduate not to become an employer but to obtain practice experience as an employee. In making such a decision, graduates should always consider whether the employment opportunity possesses the flexibility to allow changes in career direction. Because so many graduates enter employment positions thinking that they will provide a short-term experience, it is important that the option chosen provides an opportunity to change when it is appropriate and timely to do so.

Acknowledgement

The authors of this chapter in the first edition of *Business Aspects of Optometry* were James Albright, Craig Hisaka, W. Howard McAlister, and Timothy A. Wingert.

Bibliography

American Optometric Association: *Caring for the eyes of America–a profile of the optometric profession.* St. Louis, 2002, Author.

Anonymous: Federal service optometry, part II. *AOA News* 29(1):9–10, 1990.

Anonymous: Military optometry makes problem-solving strides. *AOA News* 28(24):1,8, 1990.

Anonymous: Optometry in the Alaskan bush. *AOA News* 28(24):1,13–14, 1990.

Anonymous: Special report: federal service optometry. *AOA News* 27(23):1,3–4,13, 1989.

Berman MS: Challenges for optometric education. *J Optom Ed* 17(4):105–6, 1992.

Clausen LR: Advanced education. *J Optom Ed* 17(4):107–10, 1992.

Department of the Army: *The Medical Service Corps, the Army Medical Team.* Falls Church, Va, 1988, U.S. Government Printing Office.

Department of the Navy: *Navy Recruiting Command: Navy Medical Service Corps.* Falls Church, Va, 1988, U.S. Government Printing Office.

Grosvenor T: The clinical master of science degree. *Optom Vis Sci* 69(3):255–6, 1992.

Kaz MA: Five steps that determine your practice's true value. *Rev Optom* 132(12):33–8, 1995.

Luft H: *Health maintenance organizations: dimensions of performance.* New York, 1981, Wiley.

McAlister WH, Davidson DW: A 1988 survey of federal service optometrists. *J Am Optom Assoc* 62(7):500–3, 1992.

Newcomb RD, Marshall EC, editors: *Public health and community optometry,* ed 2, Stoneham, Mass, 1990, Butterworth.

Scerra CA: Seeking the substance of practice valuation. *Optom Economics* 5(2):42–6, 1995.

Schwartz C: Optometry and HMOs: the view from inside. *Optom Economics* 5(2):17–19, 1995.

Shipp MD, Talley DK: A 1987 survey of military optometrists: activities, roles and attitudes. *J Am Optom Assoc* 59(10):802-14, 1988.

Siemsen DW: The role of the institution. *J Optom Ed* 17(4):117-8, 1992.

Sparks BI: Military externships: recruitment friend or foe? *J Am Optom Assoc* 61(6):471-3, 1990.

Stein G: HMO–Here's what it's all about. *J Am Optom Assoc* 47(2):136-41, 1976.

U.S. Department of Health, Education and Welfare, Health Services and Mental Health Administration: *Health maintenance organizations: the concept of structure.* Washington, DC, 1972, Department of Health, Education and Welfare.

www.aoa.org. Web site for the American Optometric Association.

www.opted.org. Web site for the Association of Schools and Colleges of Optometry.

Chapter 5
Associateship

John G. Classé

"You mean there's a catch?"

"Sure there's a catch," Doc Daneeka replied. "Catch-22. Anybody who wants to get out of combat duty isn't really crazy."

There was only one catch, and that was Catch-22, which specified that a concern for one's own safety in the face of dangers that were real and immediate was the process of a rational mind. Orr was crazy and could be grounded. All he had to do was ask; and as soon as he did, he would no longer be crazy and have to fly more missions. Orr would be crazy to fly more missions and sane if he didn't, but if he was sane he had to fly them. If he flew them he was crazy and didn't have to; but if he didn't want to he was sane and had to. Yossarian was moved very deeply by the absolute simplicity of this clause of Catch-22 and let out a respectful whistle.

"That's some catch, that Catch-22," he observed.

"It's the best there is," Doc Daneeka agreed.

Joseph Heller *Catch-22*

An associate is an employee who holds no ownership interest. The usual associate—a young, just-licensed optometrist—is often looking for a permanent practice opportunity and views associateship as a means of undergoing a trial period. Employment is considered to be a stepping-stone to partnership and provides a means of measuring the good faith of both parties. Thus one of the key goals of associateship often is to determine whether a partnership is feasible.

Finding an associateship opportunity and negotiating an employment contract are not simple tasks, and they are made more difficult if the associate is an optometry student still in school. Lack of experience in negotiation and unfamiliarity with the customary terms of employment put the prospective associate at a disadvantage. For these reasons a thorough, well-written employment agreement is necessary. Of course, contracts have been based on no more information than the length of employment and the amount to be paid and have been sealed by the execution of little more than a firm handshake. Thus there is a frequently expressed attitude that written contracts are an unnecessary entanglement for salaried employees. However, such an attitude puts the associate at a significant disadvantage.

The associateship agreement is a way of expressing the conditions of employment and the financial benefits to be received by the associate. It anticipates possible eventualities and establishes the responsibilities of the parties. Negotiation of its terms forces both employer and employee to address the difficult issues that handshake agreements customarily avoid. Without written provisions, the parties may ultimately find that they have failed to agree to important aspects of the employment and that litigation is the only way to clarify a dispute.

There is a natural concern that written agreements may contain terms that are Byzantine in expression and draconian in effect. But a contract with a "Catch-22" clause can easily be avoided by parties who understand the terms to be negotiated and the limitations of personal service agreements. It is the purpose of this chapter to describe how to assess an associateship opportunity, the provisions that should be included in an employment agreement, and how to structure the contract negotiation to achieve a successful result.

Assessing Associateship Opportunities

The first step in the effort to find employment is to determine whether a practice can support another practitioner. Some of the factors deemed to be of significance are listed in Box 5-1. Among the most significant are the gross and net incomes and the growth curve of the practice.

Gross and Net Income

A major consideration in the decision to increase the number of practitioners in a practice is the practice volume. Although there is no magic number that can be used to determine whether a practice can support another practitioner, the gross income should be equal to or greater than the national mean for such practices nationwide or have the potential to equal or exceed such earnings (see Chapter 1). If the gross income is less than the national mean, a rapidly escalating growth curve is an important indicator that the practice is growing and may be able to accommodate another practitioner.

Growth Curve

A growth curve in which the gross and net incomes are increasing rapidly indicates that the practice has not reached its potential; a growth curve that is decreasing indicates a practice that is diminishing or downsized; and a stabilized growth curve may indicate that the practice has reached its maximum or that the practi-

tioner is so busy that further growth cannot be achieved without another pair of hands. Analysis of the practice will yield the answer to the "flat" growth curve. When assessing practice growth, inflation must be taken into consideration when determining the gross and net incomes so that the amount of true growth can be ascertained. The cost of living index can be used to make this calculation.

A more detailed analysis can be performed, if desired, involving the overhead expenses for the practice, laboratory costs, percent of net income being generated, percent of income from services and materials, and similar matters (see Chapter 1), with these results being compared with national norms. If the practice results differ markedly from the mean figures found nationally, determination of the reason is helpful in assessing the ability of the practice to thrive with another practitioner. Because of the cost and complexity of partnership (often the ultimate aim of an associateship), the time spent collecting and analyzing information is time well spent.

Determining an Associate's Salary

Probably the most difficult issue to resolve is the associate's salary. There is often uncertainty over whether an employer's salary will be reduced because of the extra cost of the associate. This is a legitimate concern but one that is directly tied to the productivity of the associate. If the associate merely sees patients that otherwise would have been examined by the employer, then gross income will not go up and the employer's income will inevitably go down. The key factor is the ability of the associate to see patients the employer cannot (such as overflow) or to generate new patients altogether. The associate also can generate income by providing coverage when the employer is out of the

---

Box 5-1 Factors That Indicate a Practice Can Support an Associate

- When the appointment book is consistently booked weeks in advance and the doctor must spend long hours in the office.
- When the practice population has begun to grow older, to the exclusion of a young patient base.
- When the annual number of new patients has declined to less than 20% of the patient population.
- When the doctor is so busy that it is difficult for him or her to provide a full range of services.
- When the doctor is interested in a specialty area but must spend the majority of time with primary care patients.
- When the doctor wants to reduce the time spent in the office.
- When the doctor has had a period of poor health or is currently in poor health.
- When the doctor desires to protect his or her equity in the practice by transferring part of the ownership to a younger doctor, thereby acquiring some retirement security.

office, by offering a service not provided by the employer (e.g., low vision, binocular vision, sports vision), or by providing a greater range of needed services to existing patients (e.g., Medicare, Medicaid). Because an associate is typically younger than the employer, lives in a different part of town, and shops and enjoys recreation different from the employer, it is expected that the associate will generate patients by virtue of this exposure to new people and places. This generation of patients is necessary for the associateship to be successful.

Cost of an Associate

One way of analyzing the cost of an associate is to determine the number of patients the associate must see to pay his or her own way. The answer obviously depends on how much the associate is being paid, but assuming that an associate is to be paid $50,000 annually and that the net income in the practice is one third of the gross income (which is a representative figure for well-established practices), a gross income of $150,000 must be generated for the associate to pay his or her own way. How many patients does this $150,000 gross represent? If an optometrist grosses $200 per patient (a conservative figure), 750 patients must be seen during the course of a year, or about three patients a day (for 250 working days) to generate $150,000. Actual numbers from the practice can be substituted to achieve a more accurate count, but even so, the daily patient load will not be overwhelming. Actually, because having two practitioners together causes a certain amount of expense sharing, the $150,000 gross will not only pay the associate's salary but also will generate additional income for the employer. This also is true for bonus compensation.

Bonus Income

To gauge an associate's motivation, it is often desirable to offer a bonus. For example, for every dollar more than $150,000 generated by the associate, he or she gets 25%. Thus, if the associate generates an extra $1000 of gross income per month, a bonus of $3000 is earned for the year. The associate also earns income for the employer (the difference between the percent paid the associate and the actual net profit percentage), a profit for which the employer has to do nothing. If an associate shows no interest in generating this bonus income, the employer has learned an important lesson about the associate, a lesson for which the employer has paid nothing.

Salary

Associates quite naturally rate the remuneration that is offered as either the top or one of the top factors to be considered. But economic surveys, such as those conducted by the American Optometric Association, have shown that associate income paid by an optometrist is not as high as the income paid by other types of employers (see Chapter 1). Does this mean that associateships with optometrists are less desirable than other types of employment? The answer is clearly "no" because salary is not the sole factor that should be assessed when considering an associateship with an optometrist that may lead to partnership. The smaller salary for a year of associateship, followed by a career in an optometric partnership, pales when compared to career earnings as the employee of an ophthalmologist, health maintenance organization, or optical chain. Self-employed practitioners earn substantially more than employed practitioners throughout a career; therefore, the potential of an associateship to lead to a lifetime of earnings has a much greater economic value than the immediate salary received.

Benefits

The salary earned during associateship may be affected by the cost of living at the employer's location, the amount of federal and state taxes, and the ability of a spouse to find employment and add to income. If the salary offered to an associate is insufficient, the associate should be able to document this with statistics. It may be possible for the employer to improve the associate's remuneration by offering fringe benefits (Box 5-2). The economic value of

---

Box 5-2 Examples of Fringe Benefits

- Moving expense reimbursement or allowance
- Health insurance premiums
- Malpractice insurance premiums
- Continuing education reimbursement or allowance
- Optometry license renewal fees
- Professional society dues
- Automobile use reimbursement or allowance
- Disability insurance premiums
- Group life insurance premiums
- Sick pay
- Retirement plan with employer contributions (e.g., SIMPLE IRA, 401[k])

these benefits exceeds their actual cost because the associate would not only have to generate the income necessary to pay for them but also the tax on this income. In addition, an associate who must pay for these benefits rather than receive them as part of compensation for employment will likely find that they cannot be used as tax deductions, whereas the employer may deduct the cost of associate benefits as a business expense (see Chapters 38 and 39). An associate may find that the fringe benefits are valuable enough to compensate for the lower salary, particularly if bonus income also is available.

Negotiation of the Contract

Successful resolution of the salary issue is dependent, at least in part, on the negotiations between the employer and potential associate. Because of the prohibitive expense of hiring an attorney, negotiations are conducted face to face by the individuals involved. The negotiation process is made much easier when the parties know one another well; visits to the practice by the potential associate or part-time work by the potential associate in the practice while in school are excellent ways of forming a personal relationship. There are several general rules that may be helpful to both parties in negotiating an associateship agreement, but they may be especially useful to the potential associate, who most likely has little, if any, actual negotiating experience (Box 5-3).

The main objectives of an employment contract are threefold:

- To create a written expression of the agreement between the parties
- To achieve a comprehensive description of the agreed-upon employment
- To enter into a bargained-for exchange that is fair

A contract is an agreement, upon sufficient consideration, to do or not do a particular thing. To form a contract, the following three elements must be present:

Mutual assent. This is often referred to as a "meeting of the minds"; both an offer and an acceptance are required. An offer must be definite, certain in its terms, and not illusory ("I may offer you a partnership in 12 months" is not definite and thus is not an offer). An acceptance must be absolute and unconditional; adding or changing any terms results in a counter-offer ("I accept your offer if the salary is $10,000 higher" is a counter-offer, not an acceptance).

Consideration. This is a bargained-for exchange that results in a gain or loss (employment in return for wages satisfies the requirement for consideration).

Capable parties. If a party is not capable (e.g., insane), the contract will be deemed void (not valid to either party); temporary incapacity (e.g., drunkenness) will make the contract voidable (it can be disaffirmed by one party).

A contract for services cannot be enforced by making the employee work because persons cannot be made to work against their will. However, an action for damages (economic loss) may be brought by the employer for

---

Box 5-3 Negotiation of an Associateship Agreement

Begin negotiating early. Negotiations require time and, if possible, should be begun early. The process is made easier when the parties know one another and negotiations proceed in a personal, relaxed atmosphere.

Establish negotiation goals. The goals of the negotiation should be written, in prioritized fashion, with the most important items first.

Be realistic. Unrealistic expectations can derail negotiations; young practitioners should "do their homework" and research the associateship market so that expectations—especially financial ones—are realistic.

Negotiate compromise items first. Take the list of prioritized goals and turn it upside down, then negotiate the least important items first; they are the easiest issues to compromise.

Know how to overcome an impasse. The usual stumbling block is salary. To overcome an impasse, counteroffers should be planned before the negotiations. The inclusion of fringe benefits and bonus salary may be used to make the salary offer acceptable.

Initiate the contract proposal. The first draft of the associateship contract can be prepared by the potential associate. Sample contracts are readily available and can be used to move negotiations closer to closure.

Use professional expertise. Obtaining professional advice before, during, or after the negotiations can be quite valuable to young negotiators; if such advice is available, it should be used.

breach of a personal services contract. It also makes for a poor reference.

Both verbal and written agreements are contracts. However, proof of a written contract is much easier than proof of a verbal contract. Verbal contracts also promote superficiality in negotiation and misunderstanding of contract terms. If an employer refuses to provide a written agreement, a letter of acceptance may be used to describe the necessary details of employment.

Fairness is a most important consideration; without it, one of the parties is likely to feel that the arrangement unduly favors the other and that a long-term association such as a partnership is not desirable. The important provisions of an associateship agreement that require negotiation should be compiled on a checklist (Figure 5-1). This list can structure the negotiation process and serve as the starting point for the construction of a contract. It also can serve as documentation of the agreement reached by the parties and submitted to an attorney for the drafting of the contract. The final agreement should be drafted by a competent attorney rather than by the parties themselves; the cost is relatively low and this ensures that the contract is in compliance with state law and appropriately executed.

Provisions of the Associateship Agreement

An associateship agreement is no more than an employment contract in which the associate agrees to provide specified services in return for a stated compensation. It consists of a series of clauses that define the relationship between the parties and provide for certain eventualities. It is signed by the parties so that there can be no question that each has read and understood its provisions. A well-drawn contract should discourage legal action by its succinctness and completeness; a poorly worded, vague, or incomplete contract may require a court to ascertain its meaning and effect. Both parties should keep this in mind when reviewing a proposed contract; if it is not clear, it should be made so. The time spent on revision will be worth the effort. The basic provisions of a contract include recitals, employment and duties, term, compensation, facilities, fees, insurance, illness and disability, records and files, covenant not to compete, termination, and miscellaneous provisions.

Recitals

Each contract begins with a recitation of the preliminary matters fundamental to the contractual arrangement, such as the identification of the parties, the date of agreement, and the nature of the relationship being formed.

If the employer is a professional association or corporation, S corporation, or a limited liability company, the employment relationship will be between the associate and the business entity rather than with the optometrist personally.

Employment and Duties

The contract should explain the duties expected of the associate, where the duties are to be performed, and the number of hours involved in the employment on a weekly basis. If the associate wishes to be assured of the right to perform certain duties (such as postoperative care of patients), it should be specifically mentioned in the contract. If a certain day or part of a day is to be an off day, the day should be specifically included. If evening hours are contemplated, the day and hours should be described in the contract. If there is more than one office location, the agreement should identify the days or hours spent at each location. These provisions protect both parties against arguments over what the duties of the associate will be and where and when they are to take place.

If a contract specifies that the hours per week shall be a "minimum of 40 hours," this wording permits the employer to have the associate work on an open-ended schedule. From the point of view of the associate, it would be preferable to specify a maximum number of hours per week or to list the actual hours of employment per day, with a clause that states the associate may be required to work extra hours on duties associated with the administration of the practice, after-hours coverage of patients, and promotion of the practice in the community.

Facilities

An employee is usually not expected to bring equipment or supplies to the employer's facilities. If an associate brings equipment to the practice (e.g., binocular indirect ophthalmoscope), it is best to list these items on a separate page (called a "schedule") that can be incorporated into the contract. The agreement specifies that at the termination of the agreement these items remain the property of the associate and may be removed from the practice by the associate.

It is customary for the contract to state that it is the responsibility of the employer to provide reasonable

Employer _____   Employee _____

The parties negotiating the associateship contract should reach agreement on each of the following items.

1. **Conditions of employment.** The contract should describe the employee's working conditions; special duties (e.g., post-operative care), hours (e.g., night appointments), or practice locations (if there is more than one office) should be described in the contract.

____ Duties:

____ Location of employment:

____ Days of employment:

____ Hours of employment:

2. **Term of employment.** The specific dates of the contract's beginning and ending should be listed; one year is the usual minimum term of employment.

____ Beginning date:

____ Ending date:

3. **Salary.** The total amount per year, and how it is to be paid (e.g., on the last day of each month) should be specified.

____ Annual salary:

____ How paid:

4. **Bonus income.** To provide an incentive for performance, a bonus may be offered. It is customarily based on the employee's gross income; above a specified floor amount, the employee receives a percentage of the gross income he or she generates (e.g., 25% of every dollar over $120,000). Payment may be monthly, quarterly, semiannually or annually.

____ Base amount:

____ Percentage bonus to be paid:

____ When bonus is to be paid:

5. **Employee benefits.** These benefits are tax deductible to the employer and are not taxable as income to the employee.

____ Moving expense reimbursement or allowance:

____ Health insurance premiums:

____ Malpractice insurance premiums:

____ Continuing education reimbursement or allowance:

____ Optometry license renewal:

____ Professional society dues:

____ Automobile use reimbursement or allowance:

____ Disability insurance premiums:

____ Group life insurance premiums:

6. **Paid vacation.** Customarily, an employee is entitled to 1 or 2 weeks of paid vacation after 6 months of work. If a special time of year is desired (e.g., first week in June), it should be described in the contract. Office holidays should also be listed in the contract.

____ Amount of paid vacation:

____ When it is to be taken:

____ Office holidays:

7. **Equipment provided by employee.** To prevent disagreement over the ownership of equipment purchased by the employer for use by the employee or equipment brought to the practice by the employee, a schedule (i.e., a list) should be attached to the contract, describing the equipment owned by the employee and used in the practice.

____ Equipment to be purchased by employer for use by the employee:

____ Equipment the employee is to bring to the practice:

8. **Patient names and addresses.** It is customary for the contract to specify that the names and addresses of patients seen by the employee remain the property of the employer and for the employee to have no right to the reproduction or use of these names and addresses.

____ Use of patient names and addresses:

Figure 5-1 Associateship agreement negotiation checklist.

Continued

9. **Patient records.** Patient records, even those of patients seen exclusively by the employee, customarily remain the property of the employer. If the associateship agreement terminates, however, it is appropriate for the employer to agree to provide copies for the former employee, when patients request that they be transferred.

____ Ownership of patient records:

____ Transfer of records after termination of employment:

10. **Covenant not to compete.** The parties may agree to include a covenant not to compete in the agreement. (Note: state law must be consulted to determine the enforceability of such a provision.) After termination of the contract (for whatever reason), the employee agrees not to practice within a specified time and distance from a described location. Damages (e.g., $50,000) may be described in the contract for breach of the covenant.

____ Time covenant to be in force:

____ Distance (radius) of covenant; location from which calculated:

____ Damages for breach:

11. **Termination of the contract.** The reasons for termination of the contract should be described (e.g., insolvency, death, disability, insanity, loss of license, mutual consent). It is customary for the employer to be able to terminate the contract upon the giving of adequate written notice (e.g., 2 weeks, 30, 60 or 90 days) to the employee.

____ Reasons for termination:

____ Period of notice to the employee:

12. **Disability of the parties.** The agreement should describe the obligations of the employer if the employee is permanently disabled (which must be defined). The agreement should also provide the employee with an option to purchase the practice if the employer is permanently disabled or dies; the amount to be paid (e.g., $250,000) should be specified in the contract.

____ Disability of employee:

____ Disability or death of the employer:

Figure 5-1 Cont'd.

facilities, staff, equipment, and other items necessary to the practice of optometry.

Fees

In an employer-associate relationship, fees are paid by patients to the employer, and the associate has no right to them.

Insurance

An employer may provide several types of insurance: life, disability, personal property, personal injury (worker's compensation), and professional liability (malpractice). Life, disability, and professional liability insurance are often offered as an employment benefit. Personal property coverage insures the associate's property against loss from fire, theft, or other hazard, and personal injury insurance protects the employer against claims for injury by an employee that are work-related (the employer may have private insurance coverage or worker's compensation). Some employers may require the associate to "indemnify" the employer for any professional liability claim involving the associate. This means that the associate must reimburse the employer's insurer for any money paid as damages based on an act or omission by the associate. To protect against such claims, the associate will need to take out a professional liability (malpractice) policy.

An employer also may require an associate to have liability insurance coverage of a stated amount, which is described in the contract. This clause also will require the associate to take out a professional liability (malpractice) policy.

Illness and Disability

A young associate is much more likely to be disabled than to die, but employment contracts do not usually provide disability benefits. The reason is that a non-working employee is a drain on practice income, and during the course of several months the payment of benefits with no offsetting income could jeopardize the financial stability of the practice. Disability insurance can be purchased to cover this eventuality, of course; however, it is relatively expensive, which usually means that dollars spent for disability coverage are used to provide coverage for the employer rather than the employees. The expense of this insurance is one reason that new graduates do not purchase it themselves; it also is limited as to the amount of coverage because a newly licensed optometrist receives a limited income.

Therefore, in the usual case, the associateship agreement states that if the associate is permanently disabled, the associate loses his or her job. If the associate has not taken out private disability insurance, which is the usual case, the associate's only source of income will be Social Security (see Chapter 10).

"Permanent disability" needs to be defined in the associateship agreement. It is often described as an inability to perform the duties of one's occupation for 90 consecutive days or a total of 90 days out of a 12-month period.

One other provision that may be added to an associateship agreement involves the employer. The contract may specify that, in the event of the permanent disability or death of the employer, the associate is given the first right to purchase the practice for an amount stated in the contract. This provision benefits both parties, since the employer will have a ready buyer for the practice and the associate can see the value that the employer places on such a sale.

Records and Files

Patient files (names and addresses) and examination records are owned by the employer, and it is customary for the employer to retain ownership of the records of all patients examined by the employee after the termination of the employment agreement. Even so, there are several important negotiating points that concern these records.

One issue involves the right of the associate, at the termination of the agreement, to have access to the records in the event the associate becomes involved in legal action. Another involves the right of the departed associate to make copies of the records of patients examined by the associate or to make lists of the names and addresses of the patients seen by the associate. This latter provision is rarely included in employment contracts.

The usual clause addressing these issues states that the employer will provide copies of the records of patients examined by the associate to the departed associate at the patients' request. The employer is, in fact, ethically obligated to do this. The employer also would be obligated to turn files over to attorneys or courts in the event the associate became embroiled in legal action.

Restrictive Covenant

An employment contract may include an agreement between the parties that the associate, upon conclusion of the employment, will not practice within a specified period or within a certain circumscribed area in competition with the employer. This provision, in jurisdictions where it is enforceable, allows the employer to institute legal action against the associate if there is a breach of the covenant. The remedies available to the employer include injunctive relief, which is an order from a court prohibiting the associate from continuing the competitive conduct, or liquidated damages, which is a contractually agreed upon sum that the associate must pay if found to be in violation of the covenant not to compete.

Even though a covenant not to compete may be included in an associateship agreement, it may not be enforceable. In several states the courts have refused to enforce these clauses, whereas in others, the courts will uphold them if the limits of time and place are reasonable, or will reform them to make them so.

Legal counsel should always be consulted whenever a covenant not to compete is being considered, so that all parties understand their rights and responsibilities at the termination of the contract.

Termination

Although contracts are for a stated period, there are circumstances that can intervene and terminate the agreement prematurely (e.g., death, loss of license, bankruptcy). The parties also may mutually agree to terminate the relationship, and this is so even if not expressly stated in the contract. Employment contracts should list the specific reasons for termination and avoid "catch-all" phrases that are vague and may be subjectively interpreted by the employer (e.g., "if employee fails to faithfully or diligently perform the duties of employment or discharge the provisions of this contract").

Contracts should provide for termination by either party upon the giving of notice. The period required for notice varies from contract to contract, but 30 days is the most commonly used. Severance pay may be included in the contract. One common method is to compensate the associate for any unused vacation time at the date of termination. For example, if the associate had worked for 6 months, on a pro-rata basis the associate would be entitled to 1 week of vacation (if allowed 2 weeks per year under the contract), assuming the associate had taken no vacation before termination. In this example, the associate would receive 1 week's pay as severance compensation.

An associate who is terminated with wages unpaid is usually due the wages, unless the contract provides for loss of wages when terminated for certain specified reasons (e.g., dishonesty). Although an associate cannot be forced to fulfill a personal service contract, the termination provisions of the contract should be obeyed. If the associate breaches the agreement (by failing to give notice as required), the employer may bring a legal action for any monetary damages suffered by the employer as a result of the associate's abrupt departure.

Miscellaneous Provisions

Most contracts conclude with several miscellaneous provisions that are intended to clarify the applicable law ("this contract shall be construed under and regulated by the laws of New York") and to list certain restrictions that apply to the contract. These restrictions typically prohibit changes to the contract unless they are in writing, prohibit the associate from allowing another person to fulfill the associate's duties under the contract, and declare that the written instrument is the entire contract that has been agreed to between the parties.

The contract is concluded with the "seal" of the parties, which is their signatures. The signatures can be notarized, but that is not necessary. The contract usually provides for duplicate copies to be made, so that each party has a duly signed agreement. The contract should be stored in a secure location so that it cannot be lost or destroyed.

Tax Considerations

An associate is paid an income in cash, which may be deducted as a business expense by the employer. However, there can be income other than cash that must be reported by the associate, and this income can be substantial (Box 5-4).

From the gross income of the associate, the employer will withhold certain items, such as income, Social Security, and state or local taxes.

The employer withholds income tax from wages if the wages are more than the employee's withholding allowances. In general, an employee's withholding allowances equal the number of exemptions that the employee will be entitled to in figuring annual income tax (see Chapter 40). Every new employee has to file a form W-4, *Employee's Withholding Allowance Certificate*, which is used by the employer to determine the correct withholding for the employee (Figure 5-2). The amount to be withheld for federal income taxes is based on gross wages before any other deductions are taken. Similarly, the employee must fill out a state

> **Box 5-4 Noncash Income That Associates Must Report**
>
> - Sick pay received while an associate is ill or injured is taxable, but benefits received under an accident or health insurance policy paid for by the associate are not taxable.
> - Medical insurance premiums, if paid for by an employer, are not included in income.
> - Vacation allowances are considered to be wages and are included in income.
> - Severance pay is taxable as income.
> - Moving expense allowances or reimbursements are included in gross income for the associate (but are offset by the expenses incurred); these allowances or reimbursements are not considered wages for purposes of income tax or Social Security withholding.
> - Interview expenses paid by an employer or prospective employer are considered to be income but are not subject to income tax or Social Security withholding.
> - Rewards and bonuses are considered to be income.
> - Christmas gifts, such as turkeys, or other gifts of nominal value from an employer are not considered to be income; cash, gifts certificates, or like items are considered to be income, to the extent of their cash value.
> - Educational expenses paid by an employer (such as continuing education) must be included as income.

withholding allowance certificate so that the correct state income tax deduction can be made (unless the state does not tax income). There may be a local income tax to be withheld as well (county or municipal). These deductions are reported to the employee (and the IRS) on form W-2, *Wage and Tax Statement* (Figure 5-3).

The Federal Insurance Contributions Act provides for a federal system of old age, survivors, and disability insurance. This system is financed through Social Security taxes, which are deducted from the employee's wages on a percentage basis up to a certain maximum income. A similar system exists for Medicare, which provides hospital insurance, except there is no maximum income after which there is no tax (see Chapter 40).

There are deductions that an associate may find subtracted from his or her paycheck, including contributions to a retirement plan (e.g., individual retirement account, 401(k) plan), health insurance plan, or county or municipal government for reasons related to the

Form W-4 (2002)

Purpose. Complete Form W-4 so your employer can withhold the correct Federal income tax from your pay. Because your tax situation may change, you may want to refigure your withholding each year.

Exemption from withholding. If you are exempt, complete only lines 1, 2, 3, 4, and 7 and sign the form to validate it. Your exemption for 2002 expires February 16, 2003. See Pub. 505, Tax Withholding and Estimated Tax.

Note: *You cannot claim exemption from withholding if (a) your income exceeds $750 and includes more than $250 of unearned income (e.g., interest and dividends) and (b) another person can claim you as a dependent on their tax return.*

Basic instructions. If you are not exempt, complete the **Personal Allowances Worksheet** below. The worksheets on page 2 adjust your withholding allowances based on itemized deductions, certain credits, adjustments to

income, or two-earner/two-job situations. Complete all worksheets that apply. **However, you may claim fewer (or zero) allowances.**

Head of household. Generally, you may claim head of household filing status on your tax return only if you are unmarried and pay more than 50% of the costs of keeping up a home for yourself and your dependent(s) or other qualifying individuals. See line E below.

Tax credits. You can take projected tax credits into account in figuring your allowable number of withholding allowances. Credits for child or dependent care expenses and the child tax credit may be claimed using the **Personal Allowances Worksheet** below. See **Pub. 919, How Do I Adjust My Tax Withholding?** for information on converting your other credits into withholding allowances.

Nonwage income. If you have a large amount of nonwage income, such as interest or dividends, consider making estimated tax payments using **Form 1040-ES,** Estimated Tax for Individuals. Otherwise, you may owe additional tax.

Two earners/two jobs. If you have a working spouse or more than one job, figure the total number of allowances you are entitled to claim on all jobs using worksheets from only one Form W-4. Your withholding usually will be most accurate when all allowances are claimed on the Form W-4 for the highest paying job and zero allowances are claimed on the others.

Nonresident alien. If you are a nonresident alien, see the **Instructions for Form 8233** before completing this Form W-4.

Check your withholding. After your Form W-4 takes effect, use Pub. 919 to see how the dollar amount you are having withheld compares to your projected total tax for 2002. See Pub. 919, especially if you used the **Two-Earner/Two-Job Worksheet** on page 2 and your earnings exceed $125,000 (Single) or $175,000 (Married).

Recent name change? If your name on line 1 differs from that shown on your social security card, call 1-800-772-1213 for a new social security card.

Personal Allowances Worksheet (Keep for your records.)

A Enter "1" for **yourself** if no one else can claim you as a dependent . . . . **A** _1_

B Enter "1" if: { • You are single and have only one job; or
• You are married, have only one job, and your spouse does not work; or
• Your wages from a second job or your spouse's wages (or the total of both) are $1,000 or less. } . . **B** _1_

C Enter "1" for your **spouse.** But, you may choose to enter "-0-" if you are married and have either a working spouse or more than one job. (Entering "-0-" may help you avoid having too little tax withheld.) . . . . **C** _1_

D Enter number of **dependents** (other than your spouse or yourself) you will claim on your tax return . . . . . **D** _1_

E Enter "1" if you will file as **head of household** on your tax return (see conditions under **Head of household** above) . **E** ____

F Enter "1" if you have at least $1,500 of **child or dependent care expenses** for which you plan to claim a credit . . **F** ____
(**Note:** *Do* **not** *include child support payments. See* **Pub. 503,** *Child and Dependent Care Expenses, for details.*)

G **Child Tax Credit** (including additional child tax credit):
• If your total income will be between $15,000 and $42,000 ($20,000 and $65,000 if married), enter "1" for each eligible child plus **1 additional** if you have three to five eligible children or **2 additional** if you have six or more eligible children.
• If your total income will be between $42,000 and $80,000 ($65,000 and $115,000 if married), enter "1" if you have one or two eligible children, "2" if you have three eligible children, "3" if you have four eligible children, or "4" if you have five or more eligible children. . . **G** _1_

H Add lines A through G and enter total here. **Note:** *This may be different from the number of exemptions you claim on your tax return.* ▶ **H** _5_

For accuracy, complete all worksheets that apply. {
• If you plan to **itemize or claim adjustments to income** and want to reduce your withholding, see the **Deductions and Adjustments Worksheet** on page 2.
• If you have **more than one job** or are **married and you and your spouse both work** and the combined earnings from all jobs exceed $35,000, see the **Two-Earner/Two-Job Worksheet** on page 2 to avoid having too little tax withheld.
• If **neither** of the above situations applies, **stop here** and enter the number from line H on line 5 of Form W-4 below.
}

---------------- Cut here and give Form W-4 to your employer. Keep the top part for your records. ----------------

Form **W-4**
Department of the Treasury
Internal Revenue Service

Employee's Withholding Allowance Certificate
▶ **For Privacy Act and Paperwork Reduction Act Notice, see page 2.**

OMB No. 1545-0010
2002

1 Type or print your first name and middle initial	Last name		2 Your social security number
Hardy A.	Worker		876 54 3210

Home address (number and street or rural route)
1040 Labor Lane

City or town, state, and ZIP code
Anytown, ST 12345

3 ☐ Single ☒ Married ☐ Married, but withhold at higher Single rate.
Note: *If married, but legally separated, or spouse is a nonresident alien, check the "Single" box.*

4 If your last name differs from that on your social security card, check here. You must call 1-800-772-1213 for a new card. ▶ ☐

5 Total number of allowances you are claiming (from line H above **or** from the applicable worksheet on page 2) | **5** | _5_

6 Additional amount, if any, you want withheld from each paycheck . . . . | **6** $ _0_

7 I claim exemption from withholding for 2002, and I certify that I meet **both** of the following conditions for exemption:
• Last year I had a right to a refund of **all** Federal income tax withheld because I had **no** tax liability **and**
• This year I expect a refund of **all** Federal income tax withheld because I expect to have **no** tax liability.
If you meet both conditions, write "Exempt" here . . . . ▶ | **7** |

Under penalties of perjury, I certify that I am entitled to the number of withholding allowances claimed on this certificate, or I am entitled to claim exempt status.

Employee's signature
(Form is not valid unless you sign it.) ▶ Hardy A. Worker

Date ▶ 1 Jan 2002

8 Employer's name and address (Employer: Complete lines 8 and 10 only if sending to the IRS.)
John G. O'Dee, 321 Main St., Anytown, ST 12345

9 Office code (optional)

10 Employer identification number
09 8765432

Cat. No. 10220Q

Figure 5-2 Sample W-4 form and instructions for determination of withholding.

a Control number	22222	OMB No. 1545-0008		

b Employer identification number 098765432		1 Wages, tips, other compensation $23,100	2 Federal income tax withheld $2,880

c Employer's name, address, and ZIP code Dr. John G. O'Dee 321 Main Street Anytown, ST 12345	3 Social security wages $23,100	4 Social security tax withheld $1,432

Figure 5-3 Sample W-2 form.

associate's status as a licensed professional doing business within the county or city.

The associate also may be able to claim certain business-related expenses as a tax deduction, but to do so the associate must itemize deductions on Schedule A (see Chapter 38), as part of the miscellaneous category. They will be deductible, however, only to the extent that they exceed 2% of the adjusted gross income.

Tax planning is important, even for employment opportunities, and associates should understand the applicable tax law to take full advantage of deductions and bargain for benefits.

Bibliography

Baldwin B, Christensen B, Melton J: *Rx for success*. Midwest City, Okla, 1983, Vision Publications.

Classé JG: *Legal aspects of optometry*. Boston, 1989, Butterworth.

Internal Revenue Service publication 15, *Employer's tax guide (circular E)*.

Internal Revenue Service publication 15B, *Employee's tax guide to fringe benefits*.

Internal Revenue Service publication 17, *Your federal income tax*.

Internal Revenue Service publication 334, *Tax guide for small businesses*.

Internal Revenue Service publication 520, *Scholarships and fellowships*.

Internal Revenue Service publication 552, *Recordkeeping for individuals*.

62 *American Law Reports* 3d 1014.

62 *American Law Reports* 3d 970.

62 *American Law Reports* 3d 918.

www.aoa.org. Web site for the American Optometric Association.

www.irs.ustreas.gov. Web site for the Internal Revenue Service, which contains forms and publications that can be downloaded.

Section Two

Business Organizations

Chapter 6

Individual Proprietorship

John G. Classé

No physician, insofar as he is a physician, considers his own good in what he prescribes,
but the good of his patient; for the true physician is also a ruler having the human body
as subject, and is not a mere moneymaker.

Plato *The Republic*

The practice of optometry is a business, just as the practice of medicine is a business, and the successful conduct of a business relies on the generation of a profit. The profit motive is a necessary aspect of practice; without it, the undertaking becomes one that is more properly termed a hobby. Optometrists must regard their profession as a form of business enterprise for which the production of a profit is a desired and necessary result.

As Plato points out, however, there are unique characteristics that elevate a health care professional above the level of "mere moneymaker." First, the product of a profession is the skill and judgment of its practitioners. An optometrist provides services (just as would a physician), and although an optometrist also provides materials, these are incidental to the services (in the same fashion that crutches are incidental to the services of an orthopedist).

A second consideration involves the relationship between an optometrist and the optometrist's patients, which—because of the specialized learning of the optometrist and its relationship to patients' health—requires the optometrist to adhere to certain standards and to divulge findings fully. Although spectacles and contact lenses are products that are sold in the course of business, when handled by an optometrist incidental to the performance of professional services the transaction becomes one quite apart from the mere sale of merchandise. Consequently, the motto of the marketplace—*caveat emptor* ("let the buyer beware")—has no application to optometry.

A third characteristic of the professional nature of optometry concerns the requirement that nothing be permitted to interfere with an optometrist's obligation to his or her patients. This problem most commonly involves the employment of optometrists by businesses that rely on the sale of ophthalmic goods and materials for profit. The necessity to sell goods can intrude on the optometrist-patient relationship, adversely affecting the ability of the optometrist to exercise an independent judgment (i.e., one in the patient's welfare rather than for the benefit of the business). Numerous legal decisions have cited this problem as justification for upholding statutes prohibiting the practice of optometry by corporations.

Even so, optometry remains a form of business, and its practitioners must confront the legal and tax requirements incidental to the conduct of a business. For self-employed optometrists, the most important consideration in this regard is the type of business organization the optometrist chooses for the delivery of services. For a private practitioner, this decision will have significant ramifications, affecting the income the optometrist will earn, the amount of time that must be devoted to the complexities of the business, the optometrist's exposure to liability issues, the tax accounting and reporting that must be performed, and even the choices available to the optometrist for retirement planning. The self-employed practitioner may choose one of the following four types of business organizations: individual proprietorship, professional association or corporation (PA or PC), subchapter S corporation, or limited liability company (LLC).

Although one-practitioner PAs or PCs, S corporations, and LLCs are permitted, these types of business organizations are customarily used to form partnerships. An individual proprietorship is the only type of business organization that is limited to one owner.

Individual Proprietorship

Sole proprietorship can be described as a non-incorporated business organization that is owned in its entirety by an individual. Because the proprietor and the business entity are considered one, tax is not paid by the business organization, only by the practitioner. The formalities of formation and the administrative demands of maintenance are less for sole proprietorships than for other types of business organizations, and doubtless this has been a major reason for their popularity (Box 6-1). The individual proprietorship has been the mainstay of optometry for more than a century, but events within the profession and U.S. health care have caused a slow decline in this form of practice. Statistics compiled by the American Optometric Association have shown that the percent of optometrists in solo practices has declined from more

than 70% in the 1960s to less than 50% in 2000. This trend is expected to continue, due in large part to the concomitant growth of optometrists in partnership and in salaried positions.

Professional Association or Corporation

These business organizations are artificial entities that are endowed by law with the capacity of perpetual succession, consisting of either a single individual or a collection of individuals, and are accorded a legal status that is akin to that of a person. Because ownership and management are merged in PAs and PCs, they differ from traditional corporations, but the administrative, liability, and tax issues that set corporations apart from other types of business enterprise also are found in PCs. Although PAs and PCs provide a unique shield from liability, this protection is not realized in one-optometrist practices as it would in those that are composed of two or more optometrists. Because of the complexity and expense of their operation, PAs and PCs are rarely the choice of a beginning practitioner.

Box 6-1 Advantages and Disadvantages of Individual Proprietorship

Advantages
- The formalities of organizing the individual proprietorship are minimal, as are the fees to be paid to begin practice.
- The individual proprietor may make business decisions without delay or formality and without having to confer with others.
- The individual proprietor is not subject to the legal risks inherent in business organizations composed of two or more practitioners, either for contract actions or torts.
- The individual proprietor is less encumbered with the regulatory and reporting requirements commonly demanded of other types of business organizations (especially corporations).
- The financial posture of the individual proprietorship is not dependent solely on the economic status of the practice but is judged on the personal assets of the practitioner as well.
- The dissolution or sale of an individual proprietorship is usually less complex and less difficult than that of a partnership or professional corporation.

Disadvantages
- The resources of the practice are limited to those of the individual proprietor or to the capital that can be raised by the individual proprietor, who is solely responsible for repayment.
- The individual proprietor does not enjoy the tax advantages of an incorporated practice for business-related tax deductions or the sharing of expenses that are inherent in a partnership.
- The individual proprietor is the sole source of revenue for the practice, and the absence or incapacity of the proprietor results in cessation of income.
- The individual proprietor is subject to personal liability for the obligations of the practice and for tort claims that arise out of the conduct of the practice.
- The individual proprietorship ends at the death or incapacity of the proprietor.
- The value of an individual proprietorship drops rapidly at the death or incapacity of the proprietor and thus may not be a source of significant income for the proprietor's surviving spouse.

Subchapter S Corporation

Named after the section of the Internal Revenue Code in which they are described, sub-S or S corporations offer an alternative to PAs or PCs. To become an S corporation, an optometrist must first establish a corporation, then elect sub-S status. This decision is usually made, in part, to escape the "double taxation" found in PAs and PCs. S corporations pay no income tax, being regarded as a nontaxable entity, but S corporations are still entitled to corporate tax benefits and other benefits associated with doing business as a corporation. The decision to elect sub-S status is subject to several limitations, but these do not present an obstacle to a solo optometrist. Consequently, subchapter S corporations have slowly grown in popularity among optometrists.

Limited Liability Company

In the 1990s a hybrid form of a non-incorporated business organization was recognized, blending together key advantages of both corporations and partnerships. Although first intended to be an alternative to partnership, one-person LLCs have now been authorized in all states. The formalities for organization and administration of LLCs are less than those for incorporated forms of business but distinctly more than the formalities required for individual proprietorships. Like sole proprietorships and subchapter S corporations, LLCs are not taxed as business entities, and they also provide protection from liability, although this benefit is not fully realized in one-optometrist LLCs. Primarily, they offer an alternative to subchapter S corporations because they provide the same tax advantages without incurring the administrative demands of a corporation. Because LLCs are new, few optometrists have chosen to practice as LLCs, but it can be anticipated that they will grow in popularity with time, as they seem well-suited for adoption by professionals.

Formation of the Business Organization

The type of business organization chosen determines the complexity and cost of getting it started. Legal formalities must be respected when beginning a business, and these range from minimal for sole proprietorships to significant for PAs or PCs and subchapter S corporations.

Individual proprietorship

The business does not have to be registered with the state; there is no paperwork that must be filed to form the proprietorship.

LLC

The LLC must file articles of organization with the state (usually in the county where it will be located), using a name that accurately portrays its purpose and not deceptively similar to that of any other LLC; it also will need to adopt an operating agreement (see Chapter 7).

PA or PC

The PA or PC must file articles of association or incorporation with the state (usually with the Secretary of State), comply with other statutory requirements applicable to corporations, elect a board of directors and officers, adopt bylaws, purchase a seal, issue stock, hold meetings, and document the decisions reached at these meetings as necessary—all part of beginning business operations (see Chapter 8).

Subchapter S Corporation

The requirements for incorporation in the state must be met, then the corporation must elect sub-S status within the number of days specified by state law, which necessitates additional filings with the state and the Internal Revenue Service; the business must comply with the formalities expected of corporations to begin doing business (see Chapter 8).

The cost of satisfying these requirements is greatest for corporations and least for sole proprietorships. As this cursory review illustrates, sole proprietorship is the easiest and least expensive way to begin practice and thus may be preferred by beginning practitioners starting "cold." Even with individual proprietorships, however, there are certain obligations that must be observed (Box 6-2). Much of the reporting that is required of sole proprietorships relates to tax matters. Federal and state taxation is typified by a series of deadlines, usually quarterly or annually, that must be met by the proprietorship. The most important of these reporting requirements are described in Chapter 40.

Two aspects of individual proprietorship that are of particular significance concern professional liability and tax issues.

Box 6-2 Beginning an Individual Proprietorship

- The proprietor must have a current state license, to be displayed as required by law.
- A federal tax identification number must be obtained from the Internal Revenue Service.
- A state tax identification number must be obtained from the appropriate state agency.
- A local business license is required in most communities and must be purchased by the practitioner.
- A business checking account must be opened at a bank.
- The proprietor must enroll in third-party plans such as Medicare, Medicaid, and vision and medical insurance plans.
- W-4 and other tax forms have to be completed by employees so that the appropriate withholding for federal, state, and local taxes can be determined.
- An account with a federal bank must be established so that federal withholding taxes can be deposited quarterly, as required.
- Sales or use tax forms or permits are required in states that tax ophthalmic materials.
- Necessary insurance coverage should be purchased.

Liability

The individual proprietor is legally responsible for the conduct of the practice. There are two key areas in which this legal responsibility can be applied: contractual obligations and injuries to others.

Contractual Obligations

The proprietor will customarily be the person authorized to negotiate and ratify contracts for the business, although this responsibility may be delegated to another person by creating a principal and agent relationship. Any contracts entered into by the proprietor or the agent for the benefit of the business become the personal responsibility of the proprietor, for which the proprietor's personal assets (including the assets used in the business) are at risk. The reason for this personal liability is that the proprietor typically signs such contracts as an individual, and in the event of default, the injured party may proceed against the proprietor for damages. If damages are awarded, they will be taken from the assets of the proprietor (if not covered by insurance).

Unlike partnerships and corporations, which may own assets in their own name, the title to property in an individual proprietorship must be held by a person or entity other than the proprietorship. Thus, of the basic types of business organizations, individual proprietorships create the most exposure to personal liability. However, insurance may be obtained that provides indemnification in the event of legal claims.

Injuries to Patients and Others

The law relating to personal injury is complex, but generally stated, the responsibility for injury in an individual proprietorship falls on the shoulders of the proprietor. If a person is injured on a proprietor's premises or is injured by a proprietor's act (or failure to act) and there is legal fault on the proprietor's part, then the proprietor may be held solely liable for the injury and consequent damages. Under certain circumstances, the proprietor may be legally responsible for the conduct of employees, when the conduct results in injury to a person by an employee who is acting in the line and scope of his or her duties. This responsibility results from the legal relationship of employer and employee and applies to employee optometrists, opticians, assistants, technicians, and receptionists.

Thus the liability of sole proprietors is not limited to their own acts but also can result from the acts of others performing duties on their behalf. For this reason, appropriate professional liability insurance is a necessity.

Tax Considerations

Tax reporting is the principal form of regulation to which the individual proprietor is subject. There are two basic types of tax reporting that must be observed in a sole proprietorship: that which is related to the financial status of the business and that which is related to the financial status of the individual proprietor.

Business Taxation

There are federal, state, and local tax requirements that must be observed by individual proprietorships. The profit or loss of the practice is calculated on Schedule C, and this amount is then entered on the individual proprietor's Form 1040 (see Chapter 39). Schedule C, however, is not the only federal tax form required of an individual proprietor, because periodically a proprietor must remit taxes for Social Security, Medicare, and unemployment insurance and for federal income tax withholding, including self-employment taxes (see Chapter 40). In addition to these obligations, the individual proprietor must comply with state and local (county, city) tax withholding requirements. As a result, the individual proprietor faces a constant succession of tax deadlines that must be met, or penalties will be incurred. Tax reporting requirements are among the most vexing problems facing young or inexperienced practitioners and must be understood before the business venture is started.

Individual Taxation

The income tax obligations of the proprietor are intimately tied to the profit or loss earned by the business. Although there are exemptions, personal deductions (calculated on Schedule A), and credits that affect the tax to be paid, the income earned from business exerts the greatest effect on taxation. This also is true for Social Security and Medicare taxes, which are based on the income reported on Schedule C. Individual proprietors must remit taxes periodically for income, Social Security, and Medicare to the federal government or face severe penalties for failing to do so on a timely basis. A calendar that outlines the customary deadlines for tax reporting can be found in Chapter 40.

Expense Sharing

Expense sharing is not a type of business organization; it is a way of doing business (see Chapter 2). Two individual proprietors may find that there are financial advantages to the sharing of facilities, personnel, and other expenditures, or an eventual partnership may be envisioned, and this form of practice may be used as a means of assessing the potential for such a merger. The arrangement falls short of a partnership, for neither practitioner has any ownership interest in the practice of the other; rather, it consists of two independent businesses that have found it advantageous to share certain common expenses.

In creating such a relationship, there are certain legal and administrative matters that must be considered. The most important of these involve the formal agreement between the expense sharing proprietors. An expense sharing arrangement requires a carefully drafted contract that reflects the agreement of the parties. Such a document is best prepared by an attorney. Key clauses within the contract are those describing the manner in which expenses are to be shared; how and what payments are to be made out of the joint account; how large, nonroutine expenditures are to be managed; the procedure to be used in the event the agreement is to be terminated; and a mandatory requirement that periodic review of the arrangement be conducted by the parties.

Liability in an expense-sharing arrangement is usually as follows: injuries to patients that occur in individual areas of the office (e.g., examining rooms) are the responsibility of the individual practitioner occupying that space; injuries that occur in shared areas (e.g., waiting room) are a joint responsibility. Liability for the acts or omissions of an assistant is dependent on for whom the assistant was working at the time the injury occurred. Legal responsibility for contractual obligations is similar: contracts entered into by an individual proprietor are the responsibility of the individual; joint contracts are the responsibility of all who have entered into them. Liability insurance should be purchased to provide protection against legal claims arising out of shared premises.

In expense sharing, each individual proprietor files a separate Form 1040, and the calculation of business-related expenses (including the shared costs of operations) is performed by each practitioner on Schedule C. Careful accounting of expenses will be required to ensure that proportionate deductions for expenses—as agreed to by the proprietors—are made.

Bibliography

Allergan, Inc: *Pathways in optometry.* Irvine, Calif, 1995, Author.

American Optometric Association: *Career advocate for the new practitioner.* St. Louis, 2001, Author.

American Optometric Association: *Caring for the eyes of America–a profile of the optometric profession.* St. Louis, 2002, Author.

Classé JG: *Legal aspects of optometry.* Boston, 1989, Butterworth.

Elmstrom G: *Advanced management strategies for optometrists.* Chicago, 1982, Professional Press.

Gregg J: *The business of optometric practice.* New York, 1981, Advisory Enterprises.

Internal Revenue Service publication 15, *Employer's tax guide (circular E).*

Internal Revenue Service publication 17, *Your federal income tax.*

Internal Revenue Service publication 334, *Tax guide for small businesses.*

Internal Revenue Service publication 533, *Self-employment tax.*

Internal Revenue Service publication 583, *Starting a business and keeping records.*

www.aoa.org. Web site for the American Optometric Association.

www.irs.ustreas.gov. Web site for the Internal Revenue Service, which contains forms and publications that can be downloaded.

Chapter 7
Partnerships

John G. Classé

"You'll never understand me, but I'll try once more and then we'll give it up. Listen. When a man's partner is killed he's supposed to do something about it. It doesn't make any difference what you thought of him. He was your partner and you're supposed to do something about it."

Dashiell Hammett *The Maltese Falcon*

The agreement to enter into partnership creates legal and personal obligations that are probably unmatched outside of any relationship except marriage. As the fictional detective in The Maltese Falcon, Sam Spade, points out, partners are responsible for one another and are expected to conduct themselves accordingly. The association between partners is professional, social, financial, legal, and—in its contractual sense—limited only by the death of the partners themselves.

A *partnership* may be legally defined as "an association of two or more persons to carry on as co-owners a business for profit." From this description it is apparent that there are three necessary requirements for the formulation of a partnership, described in the following:

- Two or more "persons"
- Co-ownership among these persons
- The intent to earn a profit through a mutual undertaking

Thus a partnership is an aggregate of persons rather than a separate entity. The reason for this can be found in law, which requires that partners be sued separately, as persons, rather than jointly as a partnership. Statutory law has managed to convert the status of partnerships into quasi-entities, capable of holding title to property and enjoying certain other property rights but remaining a non-entity for tax purposes and for the purposes of litigation. In fact, statutes have been adopted in all jurisdictions except Louisiana to establish the legal rights of partners and partnerships, and because the law is uniform from state to state, the statute is referred to as the *Uniform Partnership Act (UPA)*.

Although the UPA sets forth in detail the rights and responsibilities of partners, many of these provisions are qualified by the phrase "unless otherwise agreed," which permits the partners to determine the conduct of many of the partnership's internal matters. These agreements are best committed to writing. Consequently, the rights and duties of the parties are defined in a written instrument known as the *articles of partnership*, or the *partnership agreement*. Even though partners turn to attorneys, accountants, or other advisors for guidance in determining the provisions of a partnership agreement, it should be realized that there is no standard partnership agreement that will be acceptable to everyone. Partnership details that have worked for one set of practitioners may be inappropriate for another group because of differences in personalities, professional philosophies, and perhaps economic needs. When a partnership agreement is being contemplated, individuality of effort will be an important factor, and prospective partners should realize that they need to formulate their partnership agreement so that it is tailor-made for them.

Probably the most important prerequisite for a successful partnership is for the practitioners involved to have a solid understanding and appreciation of how they are going to work together. If they do not agree on such matters as attitudes toward optometric care, sharing of patient responsibilities, and financial management, their relationship is not likely to endure. Optometrists who are contemplating entering into partnership should take the time to discuss at length their partnership plans to ensure that they are compatible. A thorough discussion may ward off a union that is preordained to failure, thus avoiding the heavy financial and emotional costs of a subsequent split-up.

This discussion concentrates on partnership between an established practitioner and a new licensee. The agreement to form a partnership is usually the result of a trial period between an individual practitioner and an associate. The successful termination of this arrangement is an offer on the part of the practitioner to allow the associate to purchase half of the practice, thereby creating a partnership between the two. An associate who has spent a number of months working with a more experienced optometrist will acquire a familiarity with both the practitioner and the practice that should enable the associate to make an informed decision as to whether the associate would like to remain with the practice and eventually make it his or her own. Even if the associate feels good about the practice opportunity, there are a number of matters that must be discussed and clarified before a partnership agreement is formalized. Foremost among these is the motivation of the individual proprietor, including the factors that have led this practitioner to look to partnership; the financial obligations that the new partner will be expected to assume; and the expectations that both individuals have for the future.

Associateships provide an excellent opportunity for the prospective partners to measure one another and determine whether partnership is for them. It also allows them the time to discuss the many important issues that must be successfully agreed to before a partnership agreement can be drafted.

Characteristics of Partnership

Because of their legal status as associations of individuals, partnerships have some unique legal provisions that need to be understood by prospective partners. The most important considerations involve liability issues and the tax ramifications of partnership.

Liability of Partners

Individual proprietors are liable for their conduct and for the conduct of employees. Partners have a like obligation, for each is individually responsible for his or her conduct and collectively they are responsible for the conduct of their employees. Because each partner is considered the agent and partner of the other partners, partners have a responsibility for one another as well. This liability is referred to as *joint and several.*

Joint and several liability allows an injured party to sue one or more of the partners separately or all of them together, at the party's option. Thus partners are liable for one another's acts and may be sued individually or collectively, which increases their liability beyond that faced by the sole proprietor. The most likely types of legal actions that partners face are those based on contract and those alleging injury to others.

Because any partner with apparent authority to do so may sign a contract binding the partnership (and hence the other partners) to its provisions, partners need to carefully oversee contractual obligations. One means of limiting the opportunity for misadventure is to require the agreement of all partners whenever an expenditure in excess of a certain sum is contemplated. Another time-tested means is to require the signatures of at least two persons on partnership checks.

Injuries to others may result in liability claims, and if a partner has been negligent, not only is that partner potentially responsible but so is each of the other partners and all the partners collectively. Thus all partners may end up as defendants to a lawsuit for damages. If the injured party wins a judgment and is unable to satisfy it by proceeding against the assets of the negligent partner, the law permits the injured party to proceed against the assets of any of the other defendant partners or of the partnership if it was a defendant in the case. To protect against this eventuality, partnerships purchase a special form of professional liability insurance that covers the joint and several liability of partners.

Tax Issues

A partnership is not a taxable entity, and partnership profits (and other income and gains) are not taxed to the partnership. The partnership must report its income and file Form 1065, *US Partnership Return of Income,* which provides basic information on partnership income or losses for the year and the partners' distributive shares of that income or loss, which is reported to the partners on Schedule K-1. The partners list this income or loss on their individual Form 1040. Taxes are paid on the income reported and deductions claimed on the 1040 by each individual partner.

Partnerships are permitted to deduct certain expenses that are ordinary and necessary to the conduct of business. These deductions reduce the distributive share of partnership income that is to be allocated to the partners.

They are, in effect, borne by the partners themselves in a proportional fashion. Income to partners is usually referred to as a *draw against profits*, paid on a monthly basis and applied at the conclusion of the tax year to the partners' distributive shares of the partnership profit.

Individual partners may claim many of the same tax deductions as individual proprietors, and a working knowledge of the basics of tax law is essential.

Limited Liability Companies

Limited liability companies (LLCs) were originally established to permit two or more individuals to create a hybrid business entity that melds together the most desirable aspects of partnership and corporation. The two major advantages of LLCs involve liability issues and taxation.

The "partners" (owners) in an LLC have limited rather than joint and several liability, as in a partnership. This protection from liability in an LLC is akin to that of a professional association (PA) or corporation (PC): the business entity is responsible for liability issues, such as contract or negligence claims, rather than the partners of the LLC. For example, if a partner in an LLC is negligent, the legal claim will involve the partner and the LLC, but not the other partners. This insulation from liability for the other partners is an advantage of doing business as an LLC rather than as a partnership.

Taxwise, an LLC is treated the same as a partnership: the business entity pays no tax and merely reports income and expenses on Form 1065, just as a partnership does. The LLC's profits are allocated to the partners, with each partner receiving a Schedule K-1, which shows the income to be reported on that individual's Form 1040. Because there is no tax paid by the LLC business entity (unlike PAs or PCs), the so-called "double taxation" of both the business entity and the owner-employees is avoided by operating as an LLC rather than as PA or PC (see Chapter 8). In addition, the organization and administration of an LLC are less formal than those of a PA or PC. For example, periodic board meetings, minutes, and other formalities of operating as a corporation are not required of an LLC. However, the partners (owners) of the LLC may elect managers to run the business entity in the same manner as the directors of a PA or PC are elected by the shareholders to run the PA or PC. The owners also may choose to operate like a partnership, with each owner having an equal say in the management of the practice.

Even though the business entity in a multiple-owner LLC is treated as a partnership by the Internal Revenue Service, the LLC may elect to be treated as a corporation. Tax Form 8832 must be completed and submitted to the Internal Revenue Service, with the corporate income tax treatment box checked.

Although an LLC must have *articles of organization* and file them with the state, much as a PA or PC does, it is not required by law to have a written *operating agreement*, like articles of partnership. Even so, an operating agreement is clearly needed to clarify issues related to the organization and administration of the LLC and to ensure that the partners understand and agree to the many issues related to the conduct of the business. Therefore, negotiating a partnership created by the formation of an LLC will entail discussion of the same issues required for negotiating a traditional partnership. The operating agreement for the LLC that results from these negotiations will in many ways resemble the articles of partnership drafted to form a traditional partnership. The operation of the LLC, however, will not be controlled by the UPA, and state laws that regulate the administration of LLCs have few provisions that relate to the types of issues described in the UPA. To provide clarity, practitioners seeking to create a two or more owner LLC should negotiate and reduce to writing the same issues as those encountered by practitioners seeking to do business in the more traditional manner, as a partnership.

Although a subchapter S corporation resembles an LLC in that it insulates "partners" (shareholders) from liability and is not taxable as a business entity, it must be formed and operated as a corporation and thus is not considered here (see Chapter 8).

Negotiating a Partnership Agreement

Discussion of the details of partnership will vary between individuals, but there are common subjects that all prospective partners will need to consider, including the following:
- Philosophy of the practice
- Capital contributions
- Partnership income
- Partnership expenses
- Partnership benefits
- Transfer of partnership interests

Each of these matters needs to be debated and decided, for they constitute the bedrock on which a partnership agreement will be constructed.

Philosophy of Practice

There are two basic philosophies that can be used by a partnership. The first approach requires all patients to be the patients of the partnership and not of any particular partner. Scheduling of patients is based on which practitioner is available, and all patient records are merged without regard to which practitioner was responsible for an individual patient's care. Advantages to this approach are that all partners will acquire experience with each patient and the patient load can be divided as equitably as possible between each of the partners. A disadvantage is that each practitioner will have less continuing personal contact with a single patient. Also, if any of the partners offers specialized services that the others do not, this approach to patient care will be unfeasible since the patient load cannot be as easily divided.

The second approach is merely to continue with separate responsibilities for individual patients, which is complemented by the expanded opportunities for coverage and peer consultation that partnership offers. A patient's regular appointments will be scheduled with one partner, whereas emergencies or other occasions can be covered by the partner who is available at the time. Patient records are coded according to the partner responsible for them. Advantages of this system include ongoing personal contact with individual patients and an easy means of separating the patient pool. Disadvantages include inequitable patient loads between partners and inability to provide certain services (if the only partner who offers them is unavailable).

Capital Contributions

When a partnership is formed, it is customary to create a partnership account and to contribute capital toward this account, which is used to pay the expenses of the practice. In addition, the partners may contribute property, real or personal, to the partnership, and such contributions also serve as capital for the benefit of the partnership. A careful record of the capital contributions of the partners will have to be made at the time the partnership is formed, and each year the partners' basis in the property will have to be determined (by a tax attorney or accountant).

At the termination of the partnership as a result of the withdrawal, retirement, death, or disability of a partner, the partner's interest in the partnership will have to be liquidated. Payments in liquidation, to the extent that they are made in exchange for the partner's interest in the partnership property, are treated as distributions subject to income taxation. When a distribution or withdrawal of property is made, the withdrawing partner will have to consider the tax ramifications.

Partnership Income

A key subject of negotiations is how the partnership income will be divided. Decision making does not concern merely the division of profits but goes much deeper, beginning with the determination of what income will be shared with the partnership and what is to be considered personal income.

One approach is to designate all optometry income, however earned, as partnership income; thus, income from teaching, writing, and outside consulting activities would be designated as going to the partnership and not to an individual partner.

Another approach is to designate only the income generated within the partnership and recorded in the partnership's books as partnership income. Earnings outside the practice belong exclusively to the individual receiving them, and the other partners do not share in this income.

Partnership Expenses

Partners must determine which expenditures are to be borne by the partnership and which are to be personal. Although the usual and customary expenses (e.g., rent, utilities, employee salaries) are clearly partnership expenses, items such as automobile expenses, professional liability premiums, professional society dues, purchases of texts and subscriptions to journals, and travel to and attendance at professional meetings and educational seminars will create differences of opinion (as will expenditures for entertainment expenses).

Partnerships vary in their attitudes toward these items: some pay them through the partnership because they feel that these expenses are for the benefit of the partnership as a whole; others exclude some or all of them from the joint books because they believe that the partners should be free to spend as much or as little on the items as they wish without generating concern over the possible inequity of individual spending levels.

In general, common items such as insurance premiums, licensure renewal fees, subscriptions to journals, and professional society dues can be paid by the partnership without inequity, whereas automobile ownership and expenses, professional meeting and educational program costs, and expenses related to entertainment are personal items that are best left to each partner. Some partnerships entitle each partner to a stated dollar amount of expense for the common items, with any additional expenses greater than this amount being paid by the partner who has incurred them.

As to continuing education meetings, an alternative approach is to entitle each partner to a stated number of days of absence each year to attend educational and professional programs. The partnership will then pay for all expenses incurred at the meetings, using as a rationale the belief that, over a period of years, these expenses will be more or less equal.

Partnership Benefits

Entitlement to partnership benefits is a complex issue that partners must address and agree to; foremost among the issue of benefits is whether the partnership will establish a retirement fund (e.g., Keogh plan). The decision to establish such a fund will require a lawyer's expertise and an accountant's assistance.

Any benefit that the partnership contemplates, even one as seemingly straightforward as vacation time, must be agreed to by the partners. Some of these issues can be difficult to decide: for example, if a partner is disabled, what benefits will be provided and for how long? If the partnership wishes to purchase disability insurance, this is a related issue that must be discussed and an agreement reached.

Transfer of Partnership Interests

The formation, maintenance, and dissolution of the partnership must be discussed and agreed to by the partners before the partnership is formed. There are two key questions that need to be answered: how does the junior partner acquire his or her interest at the start of the partnership and how does the senior partner sell his or her remaining partnership interest at the end of the partnership? The closely associated issue of income for the partners influences the answers to these questions, particularly during the building phase of the partnership, when the junior partner is "buying in" to the practice.

Although dissolution of the partnership seems to be a poor choice of subject matter when first entering into a partnership arrangement, it is a problem that must be settled before the partnership begins because all partnerships are limited to the lives of the partners and will end. A partnership between an established practitioner and a new licensee creates unique financial difficulties for the junior partner. Among these difficulties is the problem of how to compensate the senior partner at withdrawal or retirement. The death of a partner poses a different problem—whether to use life insurance to purchase the interest of the deceased partner requires consideration.

Similarly, there are difficulties involved in determining the procedure and compensation for a partner who is disabled and for the liquidation of the partnership itself. Again, a thorough understanding of the issues by the partners and a well-written partnership agreement will be required.

Partners' Income

Of the factors influencing the decision to enter into partnership, probably the most important issue is the sharing of partners' income. There are two questions that need to be answered: how should income be shared during the period the junior partner is acquiring his or her partnership interest and how should partnership income be divided once parity of ownership is achieved? The answers to these questions will vary from partnership to partnership, but there are general guidelines that may be used to formulate solutions to the complex problems posed by these two questions.

How Is the Junior Partner's Income Determined?

The issue of income is tied to how the junior partner is going to pay for his or her partnership interest. The usual arrangement is one in which the junior partner acquires an equal ownership interest during a period of years (typically 4 to 8) (e.g., 10% per year for a 5 year buy-in period to acquire a 50% interest). The amount to be paid by the junior partner for this partnership interest must be negotiated by the parties and is dependent on the value of the practice. (The valuation of practices is discussed in Chapter 3.)

The first issue to be considered is whether the junior partner will need to pay money "up front" to demonstrate his or her commitment to the partnership. Senior partners may feel that the younger practitioner will have greater motivation if a "down payment" is required (usually obtained through a bank loan). The partnership agreement stipulates that this sum may be forfeited if the junior partner breaches the agreement and withdraws from the partnership before equal ownership has been realized, with the forfeited money being considered as liquidated damages. (For example, for a 5 year buy-in the agreement may state that the junior partner forfeits 100% of the down payment if he or she withdraws in the first year of partnership, 80% in the second year, 60% in the third year, and so on until the sixth year, when the junior partner is an equal partner.) If the junior practitioner has significant debt, the payment of such an amount may impose economic hardship or it may be difficult to obtain a bank loan because of the indebtedness. In such cases, the senior partner may decide to forego the payment of money "up front" because it may be counterproductive.

Of course, it may be possible for the junior partner to borrow the purchase price from a bank or another creditor and to pay the senior partner a lump sum for the partnership interest. This alternative is rarely used, however, because financing may be impossible to obtain and the tax bill for the senior partner is typically much larger than if payment is made to the senior partner in smaller amounts during the course of years.

If the senior partner self-finances the buy-in, the payment of the balance due by the junior partner can be direct or indirect. A direct payment occurs when the junior partner earns an income from the practice and pays part of this income to the senior partner. The federal government is a partial beneficiary of this type of arrangement, since the money is taxed when it is earned by the junior partner and taxed again when it is received by the senior partner. For this reason, indirect payment is often preferred.

An indirect payment is made when the junior partner receives as compensation from the practice less money than the junior partner actually generates. If the junior partner accepts a lesser amount than is actually earned, the difference between what was earned and what was paid becomes, in effect, a payment to the senior partner. For example, if the junior partner generates $80,000 of income in the first year of the partnership but is paid $60,000, the $20,000 difference is the junior partner's contribution toward the purchase price. This differential is usually expressed in the junior partner's monthly salary, which is significantly less than the senior partner's salary during the first year, but which decreases in difference during the course of years required for the young doctor to become an equal partner (i.e., 5 to 7-years). At the end of this period the junior partner will have contributed the amount agreed to for purchase of his or her partnership interest, and the salaries for the partners—like their ownership interests—will be equal.

The same type of division may be used with the profit earned by the partnership at the end of the year (after all salaries and expenses of the partnership have been paid): the senior partner gets a larger share (usually expressed on a percent basis) than the junior partner, with the difference becoming less during the course of years until a 50-50 division of profit is realized. For example, if the partnership generated $200,000 of profit for the year, with $190,000 paid out to the partners as a monthly "draw" (i.e., salary), there would be $10,000 of profit remaining to be distrib-

uted. If it had been agreed that the distribution of this profit for the year would be 60-40, the senior partner would receive $6000 and the junior partner $4000. This division of profit could continue unequally for as long as is necessary to allow the junior partner to contribute the amount owed for his or her equal ownership interest in the practice.

This strategy is used to keep the senior partner from experiencing a drop in income during the early years of the partnership. Although the junior partner is paid less income for the same amount of work, he or she also receives a percentage of ownership of the practice. At the conclusion of the buy-in period, each partner owns equal shares of the practice, and they are drawing equal incomes. Furthermore, the practice should have doubled in size (about 6 years is required on average).

How Should Partners Split Income? There are two basic methods used to divide income: percentage and productivity. They can be combined to create a third method that is an amalgam of the two.

The percentage method requires the partners to divide partnership income based on some predetermined, fixed ratio. This method offers a group incentive: all partners will prosper as long as the partnership generates sufficient income, regardless of which partner actually performs the work. Thus competition is minimized between partners, but conflicts can be created if there are in fact widely disparate contributions to income.

The productivity method compensates each partner in direct proportion to the amount that partner has contributed: the common measure of each contribution is the amount credited to each partner in the partnership books. This method is self-adjusting in that if a partner works less, the partner receives less income. But it can create competition between partners for patients and tends to reward income-producing activities at the expense of less measurable contributions to patient flow. It also requires careful bookkeeping.

Commonly a combination of the two methods is used to distribute income equitably. The simplest procedure is to divide half of the practice income among the partners on the basis of percentage and the other half on the basis of productivity. Variations on this approach are common. This method rewards both group participation and individual contributions and may be resorted to as a compromise.

Eventually, every partnership must end. The hoped-for conclusion occurs when one of the partners retires, at which time the retiring optometrist's remaining partnership interest must be sold to the other partner (or partners) or to another buyer.

How Is a Senior Partner's Interest Paid For at Retirement or Withdrawal? The problem of the senior partner's remaining interest in the partnership is one that many beginning partnerships ignore altogether. If possible, it should be solved at the outset of the relationship.

The difficulty is how to determine the fair value of the remaining interest (usually 50%) at a future date that may not be known with any degree of exactness. Of course, if a specific date is known, it makes planning easier. The further the date is in the future, the more speculative the price and hence the greater the reluctance of the partners to set a specific amount. For the junior partner this is a serious problem, for in several years' time his or her efforts on behalf of the partnership will have made it far more valuable, thus placing the junior partner in the position of having to pay for the benefits of his or her own labors.

The usual solution is to set a value that is somewhat flexible, either through the use of a price that can be adjusted annually according to the economic fortunes of the practice or through the use of a formula that has been deemed acceptable by the partners. Whichever method is used, the benefit to the partners is obvious: financial planning is made easier for both. The senior partner knows that even if he or she dies unexpectedly the partnership interest will be sold for a fair price; the junior partner knows the terms of the sale and can plan for this eventuality.

The purchase of the senior partner's interest must be planned for by the junior partner, who may not want to purchase it himself or herself, rather preferring that another practitioner assume the former senior partner's position. This may, in fact, be accomplished through an associateship that blossoms into partnership or through a direct substitution of partners. The customary provision is to give the remaining partner the right of first refusal on the purchase of the retiring or withdrawing partner's interest; if the junior partner does not want a new partner, he or she exercises the right and purchases the remaining portion of the practice. This right of first refusal is usually coupled with a right on the part of the remaining partner to approve or reject a potential buyer. Failure to settle on an acceptable substitute within a reasonable period automatically requires the remaining partner to make the purchase.

Restrictive Covenants

Partnership agreements often include covenants not to compete, which are intended to preserve the partnership's patient base in the event one of the partners leaves the practice. These covenants specify that, in the event one of the partners leaves the partnership, he or she agrees not to practice within a circumscribed distance from the practice for a specified period. In a few states these provisions are not enforced by the courts, and a withdrawing partner cannot be legally constrained from setting up a new practice in violation of the covenant. In most states, however, covenants not to compete in partnership agreements are enforceable, and the partnership may obtain an order from the court restraining the partner from violating the time and distance requirements of the covenant. In some states, the courts enforce the covenant even if it goes beyond reasonable bounds of time and distance by reforming the restrictions to make them reasonable. Another remedy available to the partnership is to ask for the payment of liquidated damages, which may be specified in the partnership agreement as an amount the departing partner agrees to pay should he or she violate the covenant not to compete. The damages must bear a reasonable relation to the injury suffered by the partnership to be enforceable.

The covenant also can prohibit the withdrawing partner from soliciting or hiring any employees of the partnership for a period or from using a name, title, or phonetically similar name or title to that used by the partnership.

Patient Records

The partners need to determine the disposition of patient records when a partner withdraws or the partnership is dissolved. These provisions may vary between partnerships and often are dependent on the history of the partnership. For a partnership formed by merger of two or more practices, the agreement may state that the records belonging to each partner before execution of the partnership agreement remain the property of each partner and that all new records of patients seen subsequent to formation of the partnership will be divided based on the choice of practitioner made by individual patients when notified of the dissolution of the partnership.

In a senior-junior partnership, the agreement may specify that a withdrawing junior partner has no right to the records of patients seen during the partnership, but that copies will be provided to the withdrawing partner at the request of individual patients.

The partners also may specify that a withdrawing partner cannot make a list (or electronic copies) of the names and addresses of patients seen by that partner during the partnership and that such information remains the property of the partnership.

Whenever contractual arrangements as complex as these are being contemplated, professional assistance is required. When searching for an attorney or an accountant, it is best to find someone with specialized knowledge and experience. To locate a knowledgeable professional, it is best to ask practitioners who have used the services of attorneys or accountants for practice sales or for drafting associateship or partnership agreements. If a high degree of satisfaction with the skills of the attorney or accountant is expressed, an interview can be scheduled. The time and effort spent to locate a professional with specialized knowledge will be worthwhile.

Buy-Sell Life Insurance

Partners may want to consider the use of life insurance policies to fund the purchase of a deceased partner's interest. The insurance proceeds are used to purchase the deceased partner's share of the partnership from his or her heirs, thus ensuring that they will receive prompt payment for the agreed upon value. There are two types of partnership buy-sell arrangements that can be funded by life insurance: entity-purchase plans and cross-purchase plans.

Entity-Purchase Plans. Such an arrangement requires the partnership to buy out and the deceased partner's estate to sell the partnership interest held by the deceased for the value of a life insurance policy. The funding insurance is owned and paid for by the partnership and made payable to it. Advantages and disadvantages of the entity-purchase method include the following:

- Funding is simple since partnership funds are used directly to purchase the policies.
- If the ages of the partners vary widely—for example, 30 and 60 years—payment of premiums by the partnership equalizes the cost of premium payments, which is helpful to the junior partner since the premiums for the senior partner will be more costly.
- If life insurance proceeds are paid to the partnership, it affects the basis of the surviving partners in the partnership, an important tax consideration when these partners sell their interest at withdrawal or retirement.

Cross-Purchase Plans. In this type of agreement, each partner agrees that at death the partner's share of the partnership will be sold to the surviving partners, usually in pro rata amounts. This arrangement obligates each partner to purchase life insurance payable to himself or herself on the life of each of the partners. If a

partner dies, the surviving partners will have the funds required to discharge their duties under the purchase arrangement. Advantages and disadvantages to cross-purchase insurance plans include the following:

- In a small partnership (two or three partners), this arrangement is simple; in a large partnership, the cost and administration are burdensome.
- Payment by a surviving partner increases the partner's basis in the partnership more than with an entity-purchase plan, thus making cross-purchase plans advantageous for tax purposes when the surviving partner retires or withdraws from the partnership.
- If the ages of the partners vary considerably, there will be an inequity in the premiums paid, with the junior partner paying greater amounts to insure the older partners.

An important limitation of buy-sell arrangements is that the insurance policy can place an artificial value on a deceased partner's share in the partnership. This amount may not conform to the true value of the partnership interest at the time of death because the practice may have grown during the course of years while the life insurance death proceeds did not. Furthermore, the partner to whose estate the proceeds are paid shares in the cost of the premiums. Thus the partner's estate receives an amount that was purchased with the deceased's own income, which is no more than any insured who takes out an insurance policy would expect to receive. Buy-sell arrangements, while offering a measure of security, may not be appropriate for practitioners who would prefer to buy the life insurance as individuals and leave the practice purchase to some other alternative to be described in the purchase agreement.

Disability of Partners

Disability insurance provisions in a partnership agreement customarily are written to protect the partnership rather than to provide a source of income for a disabled partner. The problem of disability payments and sick pay is a troublesome one that must be thoroughly addressed by the partners and described in the partnership agreement.

Disability insurance may be purchased by the partnership or partners to protect against loss of income should a partner become permanently disabled. If disability insurance is contemplated, when drafting the partnership agreement the definition of disability should be at least as strict as the one used in the disability policy that is purchased. In this event the partnership avoids the financially disastrous possibility that a partner will be disabled enough to be bought out of the partnership but yet not sufficiently disabled to require the insurance company to pay off on its policy to the partnership of the individual partner who has paid the premiums.

Private disability insurance coverage is usually purchased for this purpose; the selection of a particular policy requires an understanding of the key provisions of disability insurance (see Chapter 10).

Partnership Agreements

To ensure compatibility and to provide time for negotiation of the partnership provisions, a period of associateship should proceed the formation of a senior-junior partnership. The potential partners must negotiate the complex matters that constitute the business basis for their relationship, and the more time they have to discuss these issues frankly and comprehensively, the easier it will be to reduce their agreement to a written document. Completeness is a desirable goal, for if the partnership agreement is unclear or silent, legal action may have to be resorted to because the law provides remedies in the event the agreement is breached by either of the parties. It should be noted that the courts will not force a party who has contracted to provide personal services to continue to provide these services against the party's will; the party may be held liable for damages (payment of money) but the party cannot be forced to remain at work. Thus a partner who decides to leave cannot be held involuntarily by the partnership agreement.

Disagreements between partners may be resolved by the UPA, which is applied in the event the partnership agreement is silent or unclear or unenforceable (or the Limited Liability Company Act, if applicable). For this reason, the task of drafting the partnership agreement should be left to a knowledgeable attorney.

Bibliography

Allergan, Inc: *Pathways in optometry.* Irvine, Calif, 1995, Author.

American Optometric Association: *Career advocate for the new practitioner.* St. Louis, 2001, Author.

American Optometric Association: *Caring for the eyes of America—a profile of the optometric profession.* St. Louis, 2002, Author.

Classé JG: *Legal aspects of optometry.* Boston, 1989, Butterworth.

Elmstrom G: *Advanced management strategies for optometrists.* Chicago, 1982, Professional Press.

Gregg J: *The business of optometric practice.* New York, 1981, Advisory Enterprises.

Internal Revenue Service publication 15, *Employer's tax guide (circular E).*

Internal Revenue Service publication 334, *Tax guide for small businesses.*

Internal Revenue Service publication 533, *Self-employment tax.*

Internal Revenue Service publication 541, *Tax information on partnerships.*

Internal Revenue Service publication 535, *Business expenses.*

Internal Revenue Service publication 560, *Retirement plans for small businesses.*

Internal Revenue Service publication 3402, *Tax issues for limited liability companies.*

Milkie G: *Partnerships and professional corporations.* St. Louis, 1972, Optometric Development Enterprises.

Can we ever have too much of a good thing?
Miguel de Cervantes *Don Quixote de la Mancha*

The right of professionals to enjoy the benefits of that artificial offspring of business law, the corporation, has traveled an arduous and uphill path to reach its present status. However, corporations composed of professionals have become an accepted means of doing business and have permitted professionals to enjoy tax advantages unique to this form of business enterprise. For a few decades, they were the preferred choice of professionals in all aspects of health care, but professional associations (PAs) or corporations (PCs) have always enjoyed more popularity in medicine than in optometry. Probably the major reason for the incorporation of fewer than 10% of optometric practices today can be attributed to the independent-minded optometrists, who have been the backbone of optometry throughout its history. Whereas physicians have tended to form groups, optometrists traditionally have done just the opposite, although this trend is changing. The formalities necessary to form a corporation, the technical obligations required to maintain it, and the complicated financial transactions that must be performed to realize favorable tax advantages have mitigated against widespread acceptance within optometry. Also, federal tax laws have been changed to elevate the tax benefits available to non-incorporated, self-employed practitioners, and—when combined with new forms of business organization (such as limited liability companies [LLCs])—these events have decreased the allure of corporations. Even so, the unique characteristics found in corporations make them a good choice for some practitioners.

Characteristics of Corporations

A corporation is an artificial creature of the law that is endowed with certain characteristics. Among the most important is the right of perpetual succession, which allows the corporation to continue despite the withdrawal, disability, or death of those who comprise its ownership or are employed by it to perform services. Unlike individual proprietorships, which end with the retirement or death of the proprietor, and partnerships, which likewise must be dissolved when the partners end their association with one another, corporations may continue for as long as it is profitable for them to do so.

Another important general characteristic of corporations is the separation of ownership and management. In a sole proprietorship the individual owner has sole authority over how the practice is run; in a partnership the same result is obtained because ownership and management are merged in the partners, who direct among themselves the conduct of the practice; in a corporation, ownership and management may be separated so that the owners will not have any direct responsibility for or any direct authority over the manner in which the practice is managed. In PAs and PCs, however, this advantage is not fully realized.

Ownership of a corporation is indicated through the purchase of shares of stock. The stock is issued by the corporation for a face value, and afterwards its value is set by the law of supply and demand; the more profitable the corporation, the more valuable the stock. The stock is freely transferable, although in a PA or PC there are certain restrictions for its sale established by state law. The primary restriction limits ownership of stock in PAs or PCs to certain licensees who are eligible to incorporate. Many states do not permit licensed professionals who are in different disciplines to join together in ownership of a common professional services corporation. In these states, optometrists would be barred by law from forming a PA or PC with ophthalmologists.

Because a corporation is recognized as a separate entity by the law, it possesses several of the rights normally accorded only to persons. Among these rights are the ability to own property in its own name, sue or be sued, and claim tax advantages that are separate and apart from those accorded to individuals. This status as an artificial being is one of the most meaningful characteristics of a corporation.

Liability for the debts of the corporation is limited to the corporation itself. If the corporation defaults on a loan, the creditor must proceed against the assets owned by the corporation and not against the assets of the stockholders or employees of the corporation. If the corporation enters into bankruptcy, the owners of the corporation are not responsible for more than their respective shares of ownership, which means that their personal assets cannot be invaded to satisfy the indebtedness of the corporation.

The tax advantages available to corporations have traditionally been cited as the primary reason for professionals to incorporate. The sheltering of income through pension and profit-sharing plans, the purchase of life and health insurance through the corporation, the more effective management of business-related expenses, and the use of voluntary death benefit plans are all distinguishing features of incorporated practice. However, the tax advantages held by corporations have been significantly reduced by changes in federal tax law (see Chapter 33).

Professional Associations and Corporations

Several characteristics distinguish both PAs and PCs (Box 8-1). Although there are technical legal distinctions between the two, in practical effect there is so little difference that the two terms are used synonymously here. Because the corporation is a separate business entity, those dealing with a corporation must be notified that it is the form of business organization being used. Thus professionals who are incorporated are required to place PA or PC (depending on whether the state law authorizes the formation of an association or a corporation) behind the name of their organization.

The decision to incorporate is primarily financial in nature, although there are personal issues that also must be considered. For the majority of optometrists, the decision to incorporate centers around the amount of money that may be set aside for retirement through the tax shelters available to self-employed individuals. With the growing similarity between incorporated and non-incorporated retirement plans, however, the advantages of incorporation have been greatly reduced.

The decision to incorporate requires thoughtful deliberation and astute financial advice from a competent financial counselor because of the formalities that must be observed in incorporated practices, the costs that must be borne to fund incorporated retirement plans for eligible employees, and the tax liability that corporations can incur for profits not paid out for expenses or benefits.

Organization

Although the original laws recognizing PAs and PCs required two or three persons to form the corporation, most states today permit one person to serve as the incorporator, thus making it possible for an individual proprietor to incorporate. To establish a PA or PC, certain legal formalities must be observed, which are set out in the state code. Typically, a set of documents known as the *articles of association* or *articles of incorporation* must be filed with the office of the Secretary of State in the state capital. These articles describe the type of profession that is to be practiced, list the names and addresses of the stockholders of the corporation or association (and of the officers in some states), contain an averral that all incorporators are licensed to practice the profession in the state, and identify the regulatory board to which the incorporators are subject. A fee is charged for filing the papers. This is only the start of the formation process (Box 8-2).

Ownership of the corporation vests in the shareholders, who must meet to elect a board of directors. The board is responsible for the long-term management of the corporation and not surprisingly is composed of the shareholders. The daily management of the PA or PC is left to the officers, who are elected by the board of directors. In many states the officers and directors do not have to be licensed professionals, although the shareholders (owners) do. If there is only one incorporator, this individual may become the sole director of the corporation, but non–health care professionals can serve as officers. In some states the sole incorporator may be required to be the president of the corporation, but non–health care professionals can serve in the other officer positions. The officers perform the short-term decision making and conduct the scheduled meetings and other formalities necessary to doing business as a corporation.

Box 8-1 Characteristics of Professional Associations and Corporations

Mode of Organization

One or more persons who perform professional services may form a PA or PC to practice a profession. The articles of association or incorporation will describe the profession to be practiced, define the identities of corporate shareholders and directors, and specify that each of the stockholders and directors is duly licensed to practice the profession. PA or PC must be placed after the corporate name, which may have to contain the name of one or more of the shareholders or other designations.

Scope of Services

The association or corporation may be organized only for the purpose of rendering one type of professional service (in many states) and may render its services only through its officers and employees, who shall be duly authorized to render the services.

Professional Liability

Employees of the association or corporation are responsible for any liability arising out of personal services rendered by the employees, but no employee will be personally liable in any tort for any act in which he or she did not personally participate. A director, officer, or employee of a PA or PC will not be liable in contract for any contract executed on behalf of the association or corporation within the limits of his or her actual authority.

Restrictions on Ownership

Only persons licensed to perform the services for which the association or corporation was formed may hold membership interest or be shareholders, and shares of stock in the corporation or membership interests in the association may not be transferred or sold except to persons so licensed. The personal representative or estate of a deceased member or shareholder may continue to hold the deceased individual's share for a reasonable period after death but may not participate in decisions concerning the rendering of personal services. The articles of association or incorporation may contain restrictions on the transfer of shares of membership interests and for the redemption or purchase of the shares or membership interests by the corporation, association, or its owners.

Termination of Employment

If an officer, shareholder, director, or employee of the association or corporation becomes legally disqualified to render professional services, he or she must sever, within a reasonable period, all employment with or financial interest in the association or corporation. Severance pay or other compensation for past services may be authorized by the association or corporation at termination of employment.

Annual Statements

The PA or PC may be required to file at the anniversary date of incorporation a statement with the secretary of state that lists the identities of all members, shareholders, directors, officers, and employees.

Liability Issues

There are two types of liability claims that are of significance to incorporated practitioners: those that arise out of a contract and those that are a result of personal injury.

Contractual Claims. Because a PA or PC may contract in its own name, it is customary for officers authorized to execute contracts on behalf of the corporation to do so in their official capacity. The officer's signature binds the corporation, which is solely responsible for any breach or failure to comply with contract terms that results in damages to the contracting party. If damages must be paid, they must come from the assets (or the insurance) held by the corporation. Neither the officers nor the shareholders will be held liable. If the corporation fails, the loss to the shareholders will be the money invested by them in the business enterprise. Their personal assets will not be vulnerable unless they were obligors as individuals along with the corporation (i.e., signed the contract personally). Thus a corporation affords some protection from contractual liability that an individual proprietorship and a partnership cannot. (LLCs also provide this type of shelter from contract liability claims.)

Liability Claims. If an employee of a corporation injures a person or property, and the employee is held

---

Box 8-2 Formation of a Professional Association or Corporation

- The association or corporation must comply with all state requirements for its formation.
- The association or corporation must secure its own federal and state tax identification numbers.
- The name of the association or corporation must be used on office doors, professional listings, telephone listings, invoices, checks, business cards, and other documents.
- All contracts, leases, deeds, and other legal documents must be signed in the name of the association or corporation.
- Ownership of business assets must be transferred to the association or corporation.
- Insurance policies taken out by the association or corporation must be in its name.
- Bank accounts must be opened for the association or corporation.
- A corporate seal and stock book must be obtained and an issuance of stock made.
- A corporate minutes book must be maintained and the articles of incorporation, bylaws, and other significant documents kept with it.
- Organizational meetings should be recorded in the minutes book, particularly election of the board of directors and officers, adoption of bylaws, establishment of annual dates for shareholders' and directors' meetings, adoption of employment contracts, determination of salaries for employees, adoption of retirement plans, and similar matters.
- Meetings of the board of directors and shareholders must be held, at least annually.
- Contracts for employment must be adopted and signed by employees.
- Buy-sell agreements for the death, disability, or withdrawal of stockholders must be drafted, adopted, and signed.
- Provisions for the timely payment of federal and state taxes must be made.

---

to have been legally at fault, not only is the employee responsible for the resultant damages but the employer also may be held liable if the employee was acting within the line and scope of the employee's duties at the time of the injury. In this respect the liability of a corporation is no different from that of any other type of business organization. As with contracts, the liability of the corporation is limited to the extent of its assets. PAs or PCs, however, may purchase liability insurance for indemnification in the event of such claims, and in the usual case the damages are paid by the insurance that is purchased by the corporation for the protection of its employees. If the insurance coverage is adequate to pay the claim, cor-

porate employees are shielded at least to this extent in the incorporated practice. Of course, if the negligent employee is the optometrist in a one-person PA or PC, the optometrist is personally liable and so is the corporation. In an individual proprietorship, the owner optometrist is similarly liable; in a partnership, the partners are liable both individually and as a group (Table 8-1).

Trade Names

One key consideration when forming a corporation is the use of a trade name (e.g., "Southern Eyecare Center"). The right to use a trade name is regulated by

---

Table 8-1 Liabilities of Business Organizations

	INDIVIDUAL PROPRIETORSHIP	PARTNERSHIPS	LLCs	PAs OR PCs	S CORPORATIONS
Contracts	The optometrist is liable	Partners are jointly liable	The LLC is liable	The PA or PC is liable	The S corporation is liable
Negligence by the optometrist	The optometrist is liable	Partners are jointly liable	The LLC is liable	The PA or PC is liable	The S corporation is liable
Negligence by a non-optometrist employee	The optometrist is liable	Partners are jointly liable	The LLC is liable	The PA or PC is liable	The S corporation is liable

LLC, limited liability company; *PA*, professional association; *PC*, professional corporation.

state statute, and states may lawfully prohibit the use of trade names by optometrists. When a trade name is used, it is usually necessary for the name of the practitioners (or practitioner) to be listed along with it. This requirement is intended to put the public on notice as to the identity of the practitioner performing services under the guise of a trade name. Failure to observe the legal requirements established by state law for use of a trade name can subject the optometrist to discipline by the state board of optometry.

Tax Considerations

The PA or PC is treated as a separate tax entity, which results in both advantages and disadvantages. The tax rate for a professional service corporation is considerably more than rates for individual practitioners. And although the federal tax rates for corporations are based on income–ranging from 15% (for net income of up to $50,000) to 39% (for net income from $100,000 to $335,000)–PAs and PCs must pay a flat 35% tax on net income. Since both the corporation and the employee-optometrist are subject to income taxation, it may be considered disadvantageous that a "double tax" can be imposed on an incorporated practitioner. But the tax deductions permitted to PAs or PCs usually enable taxable income to be reduced to zero or to a minimal amount, so that the PA or PC pays no or little tax, leaving the employee-optometrist's salary as the major item subject to income taxation.

The distribution of corporate income takes the form of salary (or bonuses) or dividends. Dividends are a distribution of any profit remaining after the costs and expenses of running the corporation have been paid. Since dividends are not tax deductible and the salaries paid to employees are a major deduction for any business, the preferable distribution of corporate income is as a salary. Salaries paid to corporate employees (and particularly to optometrist-owners) must be reasonable; income that is in excess of what is considered reasonable may be treated as a dividend by the Internal Revenue Service (IRS) and may be denied as a deduction for the corporation. Therefore, determining the reasonableness of salaries is an important consideration for PAs and PCs.

If the salaries paid by the corporation have reached the maximum level of reasonableness, it may not be feasible to distribute further income. In this event the profits may be retained in the corporation. To prevent using the corporation as a shield against taxation, the IRS imposes an accumulated earnings tax, which is 34%. This serves as an incentive to use earnings to purchase benefits for employees or for tax-deferred retirement plans.

Corporations must file a tax return even if the corporation has no taxable income. The federal income tax form for corporations is Form 1120, *US Corporation Income Tax Return*. Corporations also are required to make estimated payments of income and Social Security tax. Estimated tax payments must be deposited with an authorized depository of a Federal Reserve Bank. The due date of deposits and the number of installments depend on the earnings of the corporation (see Chapter 40).

Employees of a corporation are paid a salary, and the corporation is responsible for the proper withholding of taxes. Employees will receive an annual summary of salary and withholding on the W-2 form issued by the corporation. The employee reports this income on the employee's Form 1040 and attaches the W-2 to it.

Subchapter S Corporations

A newly formed corporation may elect to be taxed under subchapter S of the tax code. The election to obtain S corporation status has traditionally been less popular than the formation of PAs and PCs. The decision, when made, is primarily motivated by a desire to escape the double taxation found in the corporate earnings structure. S corporations pay no income tax, like a partnership or LLC. However, the S corporation is still entitled to corporate tax benefits, such as contributions to retirement plans, premiums paid for insurance coverage, and other tax-deductible items used by PAs or PCs.

The S corporation also enjoys other advantages, including elimination of the problem of accumulated earnings tax, the controversy over whether compensation to employees is a salary or a dividend, and the difficulty of determining whether compensation is reasonable.

To elect subchapter S status, a corporation must meet certain requirements. The most important are the following:

- The election must be unanimous among the shareholders.
- The election must be made during the first month of the tax year (or in the month preceding).
- There must be no more than 75 shareholders; partnerships or corporations cannot serve as shareholders.
- Not more than 20% of corporate income can be passive investment income (e.g., from royalties, rents, dividends).

One major problem with these corporations has been the technical requirements necessary to maintain subchapter S status, which, if lost through some unintended act, could have consequential and undesirable tax ramifications for shareholders. Compliance with state and IRS requirements is essential for this reason.

Optometrists who have formed S corporations may participate in tax-deferred retirement plans, such as Keogh defined benefit and defined contribution plans, and thus may enjoy the same tax advantages as other self-employed optometrists. In some circumstances, these business entities may provide an advantage, such as when used as the form of business for an optical dispensary. Because shareholders do not have to be licensees (as in a PA or PC), an optometrist may share ownership with another professional (such as an optician) or nonprofessional (such as a spouse). The decision to qualify for subchapter S status is one that should be made only after careful discussion with a tax advisor. Once formed, care should be taken to comply with technical requirements necessary to maintain an S corporation.

Bibliography

Allergan, Inc: *Pathways in optometry.* Irvine, Calif, 1995, Author.

Classé JG: *Legal aspects of optometry.* Boston, 1989, Butterworth.

Empey v. United States, 406 F.2d 157 (10th Cir. 1959).

Friedman v. Rogers, 440 US 1, 99 S.Ct. 887 (1979).

Gregg J: *The business of optometric practice.* New York, 1981, Advisory Enterprises.

Internal Revenue Service publication 15, *Employer's tax guide (circular E).*

Internal Revenue Service publication 17, *Your federal income tax.*

Internal Revenue Service publication 334, *Tax guide for small businesses.*

Internal Revenue Service publication 542, *Tax information on corporations.*

Internal Revenue Service publication 560, *Retirement plans for small businesses.*

Internal Revenue Service publication 589, *Tax information on subchapter S corporations.*

Internal Revenue Service publication 3402, *Tax issues for limited liability companies.*

Kurzner v. United States, 413 F. 2d 97(5th Cir. 1969).

Milkie G: *Partnerships and professional corporations.* St. Louis, 1972, Optometric Development Enterprises.

O'Neill v. United States, 410 F.2d 888(6th Cir. 1969).

Section Three

Insurance

Chapter 9

Life Insurance

John G. Classé

Down went the owners—greedy men whom hope of gain allured;
Oh, dry the starting tear, for they were heavily insured.
Sir William Gilbert *The "Babs" Ballads*

Life insurance is an essential part of both professional and personal planning. Creditors will insist on life insurance as a prerequisite for business loans; partners may want to insure their lives so that, if one partner dies, there will be ready money to purchase the deceased partner's share of the partnership; and an optometrist will want to provide some security for his or her family in the event of premature death. Life insurance is indispensable in today's complex society, and most optometrists will be forced to purchase some form of life insurance (if they have not done so already) as a matter of personal or business necessity.

Although life insurance offers a range of costs to suit most pocketbooks and has many options to choose from, selecting the right policy with the most cost-efficient coverage remains a difficult chore for many professionals. To make this important choice, it is necessary to understand the basic types of policies and how they may best be used.

Life insurance may be defined as "that kind of insurance in which the risk contemplated is the death of the particular person; upon which event (if it occurs within a prescribed term, or, according to the contract, whenever it occurs) the insurer agrees to pay a stipulated sum to the legal representatives of such person, or to a third person having an insurable interest in the life of such person."

Despite its name, life insurance is purchased to pay a death benefit. The cost of this benefit depends in part on the type of company that issues the policy.

Life Insurance Companies

Life insurance–although sold to provide guaranteed protection over long periods–is provided without an insurer knowing at the time of granting the policy exactly how much the costs of providing the insurance will be. There are two basic approaches taken by insurers to solving this problem.

Types of Policies

Under one approach, companies sell *participating* policies, which means that, as the actual costs of providing the insurance become known, they are shared with the policyholders. If the premiums charged for insurance coverage prove to be more than is actually needed, portions are returned annually in the form of policy dividends.

Under the other approach, stock life insurance companies sell *nonparticipating* policies. If the premiums charged to policyholders prove to be more than are actually needed, the company has a profit; if the premiums instead prove to be inadequate, the company suffers a loss. In neither case does the policyholder share in the gain or loss. The premiums for participating policies are more than those for corresponding nonparticipating policies, but the dividends paid by participating companies give policyholders a choice of several extra options (to be discussed) that tend to compensate for the increased cost.

Types of Insurance Companies

There are two types of insurance companies: stock companies and mutual companies. *Stock companies* are owned by stockholders; they finance the company's operation and assume the risks and responsibilities of ownership and management. Most stock companies issue only nonparticipating policies; a few also issue participating policies. *Mutual companies* have no stockholders. Management is directed through a board, which is elected by the policyholders for whose benefit the company is operated. Nearly all mutual companies issue only participating policies; a few also issue policies on a nonparticipating basis, but the owners of these policies have no voice in the company management.

Types of Insurance Sold

In 2000, life insurance policies comprised 23.6% of net insurance premiums written, but the nearly $130 million paid for these policies was significantly less than the more than $330 million paid for annuities, which constituted 55.4% of premiums for that year. By comparison, policies for accident and health insurance only amounted to 17.9% of premiums, or $98 million (Table 9-1).

Types of Life Insurance

There are two types of life insurance: term and permanent.

Term Life Insurance

Each type of insurance has its own particular distinctions, but term insurance differs from the others by offering temporary rather than life-long coverage. Premiums for term policies also differ from those of whole life and universal life because term policies periodically jump in cost every few years, as the policyholder becomes older. However, term insurance is much cheaper—at least initially—than the other types of life insurance. Term insurance exists for a stated period, usually 1 or 5 years. The premium is fixed for the term

of the policy, and at the expiration of the policy term, the insurance coverage expires. The policyholder may choose to renew the policy for another term, but the premium for the new term will be more because the policyholder will be older. The premium will rise at each renewal, but the renewal option is not usually offered past age 65. For an additional premium charge, the policyholder may obtain an option to renew that cannot be cancelled by the insurance company, no matter what the policyholder's state of health. A term policy also can be converted to permanent insurance if this option is paid for by an additional premium. The policyholder then has the right to convert the policy without a physical examination whenever he or she desires to do so.

Since term coverage is straight insurance, it is cheaper than any other type, at least for the short run. However, over a lengthy period of years, term coverage actually costs more than permanent insurance, and it is limited by the inability to be renewed past a certain age (65 or 70 years). Because of its initial low cost, term is often the choice of young persons purchasing their first insurance or young married persons looking for maximum protection. Term also offers other advantages, including the following: it can be purchased for mortgage protection; it can be used for practice buy-sell agreements; it can be used to protect the unpaid balance of a practice purchase agreement; and it can be used to supplement permanent insurance. Whenever there is a short-term insurance need that must be satisfied, term insurance usually is given first consideration.

Permanent Life Insurance

Permanent insurance offers coverage "for a person's whole life." The premiums are paid in equal install-

Table 9-1 Insurance Industry Premiums, 2000

TYPE OF INSURANCE	NET PREMIUMS WRITTEN	PERCENT OF TOTAL
Ordinary life (individual)	$102,375,792	18.7
Group life	$27,067,644	4.9
Annuities (individual)	$140,188,340	25.6
Annuities (group)	$163,634,253	29.8
Accident and health (individual)	$29,277,679	5.3
Accident and health (group)	$69,294,875	12.6
Other types	$16,369,442	3
Total	$548,208,025	100

Data from A.M. Best, Inc., Oldwick, NJ, 2002. Available on line at ambest.com.

ments, but the length of time that installments must be paid can vary.

Whole Life Policies. This type of insurance offers coverage throughout the life of the insured. There are three types of policies:

An *ordinary life* policy requires the payment of a set premium for the policyholder's entire life. The premiums are divided into the following two parts: protection and investment. The protection is provided by term insurance; the investment is provided by cash value, or savings, that accumulates above the cost of the term insurance. During the first few years of a policy, most of the premium is devoted to the cost of providing insurance and little is used for investment. Gradually, as the cash value increases, a proportionally greater and greater part of the premium is used for investment, further adding to the cash value of the policy. As a result, after a period of years the annual increase in cash value (including dividends) can exceed the cost of the premium. This gradual rise in cash value is usually free of income taxation. The cash value can be borrowed—at rates that are established at the time the policy is taken out and that are quite reasonable—and it can be collected whenever the policy is cashed in. Tax is paid only on the amount that exceeds the total premiums paid, less dividends. Therefore, an ordinary life policy can be used as a form of investment.

- A *limited payment life* policy, as the name implies, requires premium payments for a limited period, either for a certain number of years or until a certain age is attained. Premiums are more than those for ordinary life because of the shortened period for premium payments, but the cash value escalates at a higher rate than would the cash value of a comparable ordinary life policy. Otherwise, it is similar to an ordinary life policy.
- A *variable life* policy offers investment-oriented "whole life" insurance coverage, with a minimum death benefit and fixed premiums and also provides an investment return based on a portfolio of securities that usually includes stocks, bonds, mutual funds, and money market funds. The value of the policy at the death of the insured is primarily dependent on the return of the investments rather than the death benefit.

Universal Life Policies. This type of insurance policy is intended to improve the investment opportunities of permanent insurance. The policy combines renewable term insurance with a cash-value account resembling a money market fund; either element of this policy can be adjusted, thus allowing the policyholder to change the amount of insurance coverage and the investment yield as needed. The investment return on these policies is greater than that of whole life policies (except for variable life), which permits the policyholder to accumulate greater cash value (but there are minimum levels of insurance coverage that must be maintained to enjoy tax-free withdrawals). As in a whole life policy, all earnings of the cash-value account are tax sheltered: no income tax is paid until more money is withdrawn than has been put into the policy. As the cash value increases, money can be withdrawn at no cost to meet major expenses. The cash value also can be used to pay the policy premiums, thereby making the policy self-funding.

Universal life policyholders get an annual statement summarizing their insurance protection and cash value; the interest rate that is being paid on the investment portion; and how much of their money has gone for insurance, investment, and company fees. (Universal life companies charge a fee for management.) These disclosures were a major innovation for life insurance.

Survivorship universal life policies cover two policyholders, and the value of the policy is paid at the death of the second person. The premiums for this type of policy are much lower than those for whole life policies. *Variable universal life* policies also may be purchased. As the cash value increases, the money can be invested in stocks, bonds, or mutual funds, but there is no guaranteed minimum interest rate, as with a regular universal life policy.

Riders

There are five commonly used riders that can be purchased to supplement a whole life insurance policy:

Mortgage protection. A decreasing term insurance policy can be added to the basic policy, providing the homeowner with insurance protection for the mortgage balance. Actually, the benefits are paid to the policy beneficiary directly and may be used to pay the mortgage if the beneficiary desires to do so, but this is not mandatory. The money can be applied as the beneficiary sees fit.

Insurability protection. A young policyholder can acquire the right to purchase additional insurance at specific intervals, even if the health of the policyholder is poor and without the necessity for a physical examination, thereby guaranteeing that additional insurance can be acquired at stated times to supplement the basic policy. These riders usually limit the option to add such insurance to persons age 40 or younger, so that a 30-year-old policyholder would be able to exercise the option to purchase the additional insurance at stated intervals during a 10-year period.

Family income protection. A monthly income can be provided to the policyholder's family should the policyholder die within a stated period. The monthly benefits are paid for a certain period, and then the face amount of the ordinary life policy is paid out to the beneficiary in a lump sum or as an option of some kind. This rider is actually a form of decreasing term insurance, but the premium is less expensive when it is purchased as a rider to a basic insurance policy.

Accidental death protection. A policy's face amount will be doubled in the event of accidental death if this rider is purchased by the policyholder. Some policies will triple the face amount if death occurs while traveling on a common carrier (e.g., plane, train, bus).

Disability protection. A policyholder who is disabled for 6 months or longer can protect the basic life insurance policy by providing for payment of the policy premiums during the period of disability. If the policyholder is totally and permanently disabled, the insurance premiums will be paid by the insurer rather than waived. The cash value of the life insurance policy continues to grow in amount, even though the disabled policyholder is contributing nothing. If the disability is temporary but lasts for more than 6 months, the waiver of premium payments is retroactive to the beginning of the disability and lasts as long as the disability does. These disability benefits are available only for policyholders younger than 60 or 65 years (depending on the age limit allowed by the insurance company issuing the policy).

Whether to add these riders to an individual policy depends on the needs of the individual and the cost of the added coverage. Therefore, the decision to purchase a rider is a matter of personal judgment.

Payment Options

There are several options available to a policyholder or policy beneficiary as to how the policy proceeds are to be received:

Lump sum. The entire face value of the policy is paid out to the policy beneficiary, whether a term, whole life, or universal life policy.

Fixed period. The face value of the policy is paid out in equal installments, usually monthly, for a stated number of years. Since part of the insurance policy principal is being held by the insurance company, the company agrees to pay a stated amount of interest on this principal. Thus payments made to the beneficiary include both principal and interest. Payments are made whether the policy is term, whole life, or universal life.

Fixed income. The face value of the policy is paid out in equal installments that are fixed until the proceeds of the policy are depleted. Since part of the policy principal is being held by the insurance company, interest also will be paid to the beneficiary.

Interest income. The face value of the policy may be retained by the insurance company, with payments to the beneficiary consisting of interest only, with the amount of interest to be specified by the policy. This provision is used to prevent creditors from obtaining any rights in the insurance proceeds received by a beneficiary (often called a "spendthrift clause" because it prevents a beneficiary from dissipating the insurance principal and keeps it out of the hands of the beneficiary's creditors as well).

Life income. The beneficiary may receive periodic payment for as long as the beneficiary lives, with the size of the payments depending on the face value of the insurance policy and the life expectancy of the beneficiary. Such an option is much like an annuity.

The settlement option that is most appropriate depends on the nature of the policyholder's estate plan and the needs of the policyholder's survivors. Since the various options may present a difficult choice to the beneficiaries, the decision as to which payment option is the most appropriate is usually made during the lifetime of the policyholder.

Annuities

The cash value of a whole life policy can be converted into an annuity. This in fact provides a life (rather than a death) benefit from a life insurance policy. There are various types of annuities from which to choose:

Single premium immediate annuities are purchased in a lump sum with the policy cash value, and benefits begin immediately. The annuity pays a certain amount each month to the policyholder for the remainder of the policyholder's life. This is the simplest type of annuity, called a *straight life* immediate annuity, and it has the highest monthly benefits. *Life with period certain* annuities guarantee payment for a minimum number of years, and if the policyholder dies before the minimum period has elapsed, the beneficiary receives the annuity proceeds for the remainder of the period. Because payments can extend for a period longer than the life expectancy of one person, monthly benefits are lower than those for straight life annuities. *Period certain* annuities are not tied to the death of the policyholder and may be purchased for periods of 5 to 20 years. *Joint and survivor* annuities are similar and provide payments throughout the life of two spouses. Full payments are made as long as both individuals are alive, and at the death of one, the payments are reduced in amount (usually by 50%), but continue until the death of the second spouse.

Single premium deferred annuities are purchased in one payment and increase in value at a reasonable rate of interest (and at a guaranteed minimum) until such time as the annuity is scheduled to begin paying benefits to the policyholder (called an "annuitant"). The interest accrued by the annuity is tax deferred, and the annuity can increase substantially in value by retirement, when payments to the annuitant are scheduled to begin (and the annuitant should be in a lower tax bracket). Usually, a loan is taken out of the insurance policy cash value to purchase the annuity. Only part of the annuity benefits are taxable as income because after-tax dollars were used to pay for the insurance premiums for the policy. Furthermore, the loan used to purchase the annuity is not income and hence is not taxable to the purchaser. The annuity also protects the death benefits of the insurance policy from which the cash was borrowed. For example, if $20,000 is borrowed from a whole life policy and a single premium deferred annuity is purchased, the face value of the annuity–$20,000–becomes payable as a death benefit and makes up for the deficit.

In addition, annuities can be used strictly as retirement funds. These annuities are investments into which money is paid, invested, and allowed to grow on a tax-deferred basis (see Chapter 33). Withdrawal without penalty may begin after $59\frac{1}{2}$ years and before $70\frac{1}{2}$ years. Fixed annuities pay a fixed interest rate, usually with a guaranteed minimum return. Variable annuities allow the investor to select the investment fund and determine the return. The annuity beneficiary receives the fund at the death of the policyholder.

Uses of Life Insurance

Life insurance can be used to achieve the following three important goals: protection, funding, and investment. All three of these uses of life insurance may occur during the professional life of an optometrist. Although protection is the most common reason for obtaining life insurance, particularly among married persons, the capacity for funding that life insurance offers in an optometric partnership, along with its use as a fringe benefit or an inducement to join a practice, should not be overlooked. The use of buy-sell agreements (or stockholder cross-purchase arrangements) in partnerships also is worthy of consideration. The purchase of insurance for investment purposes is the least used, but universal life policies do offer a return that provides a semi-compulsory investment plan.

When considering the uses of insurance, the following three basic questions must be answered:
• What kinds of insurance coverage are needed?
• When should they be purchased?
• How much of each is necessary?
Although there are no set answers that can be applied to everyone, professionals are linked through common insurance problems that are part of a professional career. From school to retirement, there is a commonality to life insurance needs that can be used to suggest some general answers to the three questions posed.

Studenthood

Most professionally oriented individuals have their first contact with life insurance during their college years. Few have a clear understanding of life insurance and its uses or whether they are getting a good deal, but many purchase it anyway. The insurance acquired is usually term insurance, bought either as a group policy or as individual coverage. Term policies provide a lot more coverage for the same insurance dollar paid compared with whole life and for this reason can satisfy the following two pressing needs: an instant estate in the event of death and less cost, which translates into more money for living expenses, the costs of education, and other financial obligations.

The decision to obtain insurance depends on the personal circumstances of the individual: a married person would have more need than would a single person and a married person with children would have even more need. Term insurance can provide adequate protection against untimely death, whatever the status of the policyholder, and can even be converted into permanent insurance at a later time if a convertible term policy is purchased. Flexibility to meet changing insurance needs is always a desirable aspect of any insurance policy. Convertible term coverage offered by a stock company allows the policyholder to convert later to whole life and to participate in any dividends earned by the company (which usually more than make up for the greater expense of the mutual company policies).

What is a realistic amount of coverage for these early years? The answer lies in the individual circumstances of the purchaser; if single, the purchaser may only need to insure any debts and the expenses connected with death; if married, the purchaser may wish to insure not only any indebtedness but also the living expenses needed by his or her survivors (a commonly cited figure is 4 to 5 years' worth of income). Economics no doubt plays a role in the amount of insurance that can be secured; whatever the amount, the best buy at this stage is a term policy.

Early Career

For most young practitioners, the beginning years coincide with plans to purchase a home, get married, and have a family–decisions that have significant insurance ramifications. These are the years in which financial obligations incurred during the optometrist's professional education must be repaid as well, further adding to the financial burden. Despite these expenses, the early years of practice are the optimal time to initiate a permanent insurance program because as the practitioner gets older, the cost of insurance increases. Permanent insurance is useful to a professional for the following two reasons: the loan value is a source of low-interest cash and the policy provides ready cash for estate taxes and administrative costs at the time of death. However, the cost of permanent insurance is more than the cost of term coverage.

Policy premiums for permanent insurance vary from insurer to insurer, but some policy dividends and cash values may be so poor as to make the lowest-premium policy anything but a bargain. Caution must be exercised when comparison shopping for insurance; the size, assets, longevity, and reputation of an insurer must be given just as much consideration as the cost of the insurance.

If convertible term coverage already has been purchased, then a policyholder may convert it to permanent insurance but should be careful to convert to coverage that is affordable. Some term coverage can be retained to keep overall coverage at an acceptable level, and a decreasing term rider can be added to permanent insurance to protect the mortgage balance on a home.

Still another alternative is to purchase universal life insurance. Premiums are substantial at the start of the policy but can be paid out of the cash value in later years. It is the utility of universal life for financial needs that arise later in life that makes it worth considering from the beginning. Whatever type of insurance is selected, the coverage chosen should be part of a planned insurance program rather than purchased piecemeal.

Mid-Career

At this stage the young practitioner has traded in the financial obligations of the early professional years for new ones, the most common being the costs of educating children and the initiation of an investment program. Since the earnings of a mid-career optometrist should have escalated significantly throughout the years, tax considerations have become very important, as have the permanent life insurance policies begun several years earlier.

Throughout the years the cash value of these policies will have grown, and this money can be borrowed and put to use. One obvious use is to defray the cost of insurance coverage: to pay the premium on existing permanent insurance policies or purchase new coverage (called minimum deposit insurance). The interest on such an insurance loan is tax deductible (if for business purposes) when the premiums of the permanent insurance policy were paid with unborrowed money for at least 4 of the first 7 years the policy was in force. Although the interest on insurance policy loans is relatively modest and the amount borrowed must be deducted from the policy value should death occur, the cash value of permanent insurance is a resource that can be tapped to meet the financial exigencies of mid-career. A universal life policy is especially good in this regard. However, it is not advisable to plunge this borrowed cash into speculative ventures. To do so could upset an otherwise carefully constructed insurance program. Rather, it is preferable to maximize the return from the investment and to minimize the risk to be incurred. One type of investment that meets these requirements is the single premium deferred annuity, which provides a guaranteed return.

Whenever cash is borrowed from an existing insurance policy, the loan does not have to be repaid, only the annual interest. The interest can be deducted completely if the loan is used for business purposes. If cash is taken from a universal life policy, there is no interest charged and no tax ramifications unless the amount withdrawn is more than has been paid into the policy.

Late Career

With advancing age there is usually some relief from debt: children's education, mortgages, and most major purchases have been nearly or completely paid. Over the years, insurance coverage has been increased to the necessary levels and cash values of permanent insurance have been used to supplement retirement plans. This permanent insurance coverage has probably been strengthened by continued usage of some term coverage, bought through a group plan or as an individual policy or rider. As a person approaches age 60, however, the cost of term coverage becomes rather expensive, and a decision as to whether to continue term insurance inevitably must be made. After the policyholder turns 65 years old, term insurance usually will no longer be sold by the insurer. Premium money may be better put to use if added to an annuity or other investment vehicle that the practitioner has initiated.

Since the optometrist's income has risen while expenses presumably have lessened, participation in some kind of investment program in which income is tax deferred becomes a must. Individual retirement accounts, Keogh plans, 401(k) plans, or professional corporation pension or profit-sharing plans are the most likely alternatives. No matter what investment plan is used, the purpose is to defer taxes on income until after retirement, when a lower income tax bracket usually prevails. As these programs grow, reliance on life insurance lessens; eventually, the point is reached at which the optometrist must decide whether to drop the whole life insurance policies.

The decision and manner in which to end a permanent insurance policy are significant matters that call for professional consultation. As an estate grows, so does the tax liability that arises at the time of transfer. Permanent insurance may have to be retained to ensure adequate cash to pay estate taxes at death; it may constitute an important part of an overall estate plan, such as the conversion of a paid-up insurance policy into an annuity. These are considerations that have their beginnings back in early or mid-career and that are most easily resolved when clear planning and unbroken execution lead to an anticipated conclusion late in the optometrist's professional life. Since retirement is an anticipated goal of most professionals, the retirement income to be enjoyed by the optometrist is of paramount importance. A well-planned life insurance program can add significantly to the realization of this goal.

In establishing a well-planned life insurance program, the optometrist should be careful to consult competent insurance agents. The selection of the appropriate agent, like the selection of the appropriate insurance, must be undertaken with deliberation and caution.

Tax Issues

Life insurance proceeds paid as the result of the death of the insured are exempt from income taxation. Therefore, the beneficiary of life insurance proceeds pays no income tax on the amount received. There is one exception to this rule, which arises when a life insurance policy is sold or exchanged for a valuable consideration. For example, a partner or a stockholder in private practice who purchases a life insurance policy from the partnership or corporation could incur an income tax liability when the policy proceeds are paid out. A tax advisor should be consulted before initiating this type of purchase.

Even though life insurance proceeds are exempt from income taxation, they are not necessarily exempt from estate taxation. If the proceeds are payable to the estate of the insured, such proceeds are taxable to the estate. If the insured has retained "incidents of ownership" in the policy (rights to control the policy), even though the insured's spouse is the beneficiary, the face value of the policy can be included in the taxable estate of the insured and hence subject to estate tax. Incidents of ownership include such matters as the right to borrow against the insurance policy, change the beneficiary, assign the policy, and cash in the policy. To avoid estate taxation of life insurance proceeds, the insured must relinquish all rights in the policy to someone else (usually the insured's spouse). Such a transfer is rarely a taxable event in itself, although a gift tax can be incurred if the policy has sufficient cash value. The transfer is a permanent event, one that removes the insured's rights in the policy forever. If the policy is given to the insured's spouse and the spouse dies before the insured, then the spouse's estate incurs the estate tax on the insurance proceeds at death (see Chapter 42).

Bibliography

American Council of Life Insurance: *Life insurance fact book.* New York, 2000, Author.

American Council of Life Insurance: *Understanding your life insurance*. New York, 2001, Author.

Brosterman R, Adams K: *The complete estate planning guide*. New York, 1990, Mentor.

Classé JG: *Legal aspects of optometry*. Boston, 1989, Butterworth.

Internal Revenue Service publication 560, *Retirement plans for small businesses*.

www.consumersunion.org. Web site for the organization that publishes *Consumer Reports*.

www.iii.org. Web site for the Insurance Information Institute.

www.naic.org. Web site for the National Association of Insurance Commissioners, including its research library listings.

www.ultimateinsurancelinks.com. Links to insurance industry Web sites.

Chapter 10

Disability Insurance

John G. Classé

The world breaks us all. Afterwards, some are stronger at the broken places.
Ernest Hemingway *A Farewell to Arms*

Disability is a distinct and sobering possibility when analyzed statistically. There is a 90% probability that one in three men 25 years old will be disabled for at least 3 months before reaching age 95; a 92% probability that one in four men 40 years old will be disabled for at least 3 months before reaching age 65; and a 91% probability that one in five men 50 years old will be disabled for at least 3 months before reaching age 65 (Table 10-1). Professional men (and women) are not exempt from these rather surprising odds, even at a relatively young age (Box 10-1).

The risk of disability is not the sole statistic that creates concern; the likelihood that disability will be long term also is significant. For example, of 24-year-olds who are disabled, only 44% will recover and 46% will still be disabled after 5 years. This genuine risk has to be considered when entering into practice (Table 10-2).

Before purchasing disability coverage, however, a practitioner must understand the types of disability insurance that are available.

Types of Disability Insurance

There are three principal sources of disability insurance that can be used by an optometrist: government plans, occupational plans, and private plans.

Government Plans

Among the major providers of disability protection are federal and state governments. Benefits can be obtained from any of the following five programs: Social Security, worker's compensation, sickness disability, veteran's disability, and GI insurance. For the individual who qualifies, these plans will be an important source of financial support while disabled. However, the amounts usually paid by these plans compare unfavorably with the benefits payable under occupational or private plans.

Occupational Plans

A common source of disability insurance for optometrists is the job-related plan, which can come from contractual disability compensation plans, self-employed retirement plans, profit-sharing plans, pension plans, or group health insurance plans.

Contractual disability compensation plans. These plans may be included in partnership agreements to allow a disabled partner to receive disability income for a stated period, often as a percentage of the base salary the partner was earning before being disabled. Benefits usually decrease on a percentage basis during the term of disability, so that after a number of months the partner's disability income is reduced to zero. An employer may voluntarily pay a disabled employee disability income or may supplement disability payments made by the government, but in the absence of some contractual obligation (which is rare), payments are made at the generosity of the employer and can be terminated at any time.

Self-employed retirement plans. These plans may be used by a disabled individual who qualifies to provide income during the period of disability. The retirement act for the self-employed (called ERISA) permits such withdrawals to be made without penalty. Of course, doing so initiates the gradual depletion

Table 10-1 Mortality Versus Disability for Men

	NUMBER OF MEN IN GROUP					
	1	2	3	4	5	6
AGE (YEARS)	**PROBABILITY OF AT LEAST ONE DEATH BEFORE AGE 65**					
25	30%	51%	66%	76%	83%	88%
30	29%	50%	65%	75%	82%	88%
35	29%	49%	63%	74%	81%	87%
40	27%	47%	62%	72%	80%	85%
45	26%	45%	59%	70%	78%	83%
50	23%	41%	55%	65%	73%	80%
	1	2	3	4	5	6
AGE (YEARS)	**PROBABILITY OF AT LEAST ONE LONG-TERM DISABILITY BEFORE AGE 65***					
25	53.7%	78.6%	90.1%	95.4%	97.9%	99.0%
30	52.2%	77.1%	89.1%	94.8%	97.5%	98.8%
35	50.3%	75.3%	87.7%	93.9%	97.0%	98.5%
40	47.7%	72.7%	85.7%	92.5%	96.1%	98.0%
45	44.3%	69.0%	82.7%	90.4%	94.6%	97.0%
50	39.4%	63.2%	77.7%	86.5%	91.8%	95.0%

Data from Commissioner's Mortality Table, 1958; Commissioner's Disability Table, 1964. Available online at www.xxxx.org.
*Disability lasting 90 or more days.

of the individual's retirement fund, a course of action that should not be undertaken without necessity.

Profit-sharing plans. These plans are often an important fringe benefit. Qualified plans can include provisions for disability income, with benefits payable either periodically or as a lump sum.

Pension plans. These plans may provide for payment of retirement funds in the event of total and permanent disability, but there can be major differences in the benefits to be paid out, depending on how closely related the retirement and disability provisions are. Some plans determine the amount of disability benefits to be paid in accordance with the pension rights that have vested before the time of the disability; others reduce benefits if disability payments are received through Social Security or other government plans; and the best plans clearly separate retirement and disability income so that both can be received.

Group health insurance plans. These plans may not only offer the usual medical, surgical, and hospital care but also may include provisions for disability. Plan benefits are typically expressed as a percentage of salary, with the percentage declining over the term of the disability to some minimum. An alternative form of payment is a strict percentage of salary, payable for a term of years or until age 65. The funding of these plans has significant tax ramifications that must be understood by both employer and employee.

Box 10-1 Probability of Long-Term Disability*

AGE (YEARS)	PROBABILITY OF DISABILITY
25	44%
30	42%
35	41%
40	39%
45	36%
50	33%
55	27%

Data from Society of Actuaries, 1985. Available online at www.xxxx.org.
*90 days or more before age 65.

Although government and occupational plans are important to disability protection, most optometrists

Table 10-2 Probability of Continuing Disability after 5 Years

AGE (YEARS) AT ONSET OF DISABILITY	RECOVERED	DIED	STILL DISABLED
24	44.1%	9.7%	46.2%
35	34.0%	12.4%	53.7%
45	21.5%	19.9%	58.6%
55	11.8%	28.5%	59.7%

Data from Society of Actuaries, 1985. Available online at www.soa.org.

find it necessary to obtain supplemental coverage through private sources, especially optometrists who are early in their careers and have little or no occupational coverage.

Private Plans

Private insurance is a difficult problem for practitioners because the possibility of disability cannot be ignored, but insurance coverage is expensive. In considering the purchase of disability insurance, the following five basic questions can be used to determine the suitability of a disability policy:
- How long must the disability last before the insurance begins?
- How long does the disability coverage continue?
- What type of disability is covered?
- What is the maximum benefit under the policy?
- What is the cost of the policy?

How Long Must the Disability Last Before the Insurance Begins? The period before benefits begin is called the *elimination period*; the longer this period is, the cheaper the policy will be. Of course, a lengthy elimination period may mean no income at a time when money is sorely needed, and so the economic advantages and disadvantages of a policy's elimination period must be given careful consideration.

How Long Does the Disability Coverage Continue? The benefit payment period may be a year, 5 years, or until age 70; the longer the period during which benefits will be received, the greater the value of the policy (and the greater its expense). Rarely do policies pay for benefits for life (except for disabilities due to accident). The definition of disability under the policy plays a key role in determining whether full benefits will be received. Some policies require that the disabled individual be confined to home to qualify for payments; others may pay only partial benefits (or none at all) if

the individual can work at any occupation. A recurrent disability (one that occurs again) is a potentially troublesome problem for both the insured and insurer; whether a policy awards full compensation for recurrent disability should be ascertained.

What Type of Disability Is Covered? How a policy defines disability establishes the value of coverage. Disability is best described as being "an inability to perform the duties of one's regular occupation"; some policies may define disability as being unable to perform one's own occupation for 2 years, and after that period, the definition changes to "any reasonable occupation that one is suited for by education, training, and experience." An alternative definition is "an inability to work at any gainful occupation for which one might be considered reasonably fitted by education or training," and an even broader definition is "an inability to work at any occupation." The less specific the definition, the less likely that the insured will be able to draw full benefits for an extended period.

Certain conditions may be excluded from the definition (such as pregnancy) or be excluded from coverage if they did not originate after the insurance began. For this reason, the best policies cover illness that manifests itself before the policy is issued (rather than illness that originates after the policy has been taken out). Another aspect of the definition that is important is the type of disability being covered: whether it is total, partial, or both has a significant influence on the value of benefits. In addition, a policy that offers an incentive to return to work can provide for the cost of rehabilitation programs that speed recovery. Also, a policy that includes residual benefits will pay partial benefits in the event the policyholder is able to return to work part time. However, years of part-time benefits are likely to be eroded severely by inflation; fortunately, some policies raise the earnings limit periodically and thus defray the effects of inflation. Cost-of-living adjustments also can be included to adjust policy benefits upward annually, but they are an expensive addition to a basic policy.

What Is the Maximum Benefit Under the Policy?

The benefit paid to a disabled practitioner is based on the income of the practitioner before taking out the policy. Income tax returns are used to determine the practitioner's income for purposes of establishing the benefit. The benefit to be paid is usually expressed as a percent of the practitioner's income, with 50% to 60% being customary. For example, an optometrist earning $100,000 who takes out a policy providing a 60% benefit would receive $60,000 per year if totally disabled as defined in the policy.

Beginning optometrists without a record of earnings may obtain coverage based on the first year's salary offered by an employer. For self-employed optometrists starting a practice or an optometrist purchasing a practice, projections by the insurer may be used to determine benefits to be paid in the event of disability. However, the disability income levels offered by such policies are soon inadequate, requiring that new income limits and premiums be established.

When a policy is taken out, the disability benefits are based on the income of the optometrist at the time of application. If income increases and the optometrist wishes to increase the benefit, the policy provisions will determine how this can be done. Some policies specify a level benefit, which means that the optometrist will have to apply for another policy. Because the optometrist will be older, and the benefit higher, the cost of the policy obviously will be affected. Other policies may permit periodic increases in the benefit, based on increases in the optometrist's income. If the optometrist chooses to increase the benefit, the premium cost also will increase.

What Is the Cost of the Policy?

The foregoing considerations are of obvious importance when discussing cost because the policies with better benefits will cost more than less-comprehensive competitors. In addition, there are costs that are not as obvious as the premium to be paid. For example, if the cancellation clause permits, an insurer may be able to cancel the policy, refuse to renew it, or increase the premium by a substantial margin. Thus, one of the most expensive types of policies is one that is "guaranteed renewable and non-cancelable"; no matter what the state of the policyholder's health, the insurer cannot cancel the policy or alter the premium (although premiums may systematically increase at stated ages).

A "guaranteed renewable" policy is cancelable, but the policyholder can renew the policy, even though there is a risk that the insurer may raise the premium for the policyholder's risk class. The worst policies are those that are "optionally renewable"; they only require the insurer to keep the policy in force until the next premium is due to be paid. The benefits to be paid in the event of disability may be substantially raised by the insurer even during the period of guaranteed renewability, thus increasing the premium cost. Also, the policy may contain a provision that does not waive the payment of premiums during the period of disability, thereby reducing the value of the benefits actually received.

Disability policy coverage is more expensive for age-matched women than for men. The reason is that although women make up 11% of disability insurance policyholders in the United States, they file about 85% of all disability claims.

Sources of Disability Income

The obvious use of any type of disability insurance is to supply income during an extended period of sickness or injury. Since disability income can arise from any or all three types of insurance—governmental, occupational, or private—it is necessary to understand the interrelation of these three sources of disability benefits and how they can be used to maximum advantage.

The first step in planning the use of disability insurance is to assess the income that would be needed should serious and debilitating illness or injury occur. During the period of disability, certain expenses could be expected to decline: travel, entertainment, clothing, charitable contributions, and other non-necessary budget items. Taxes also would be reduced. At the same time, medical expenses could be expected to increase. Careful planning—such as waiver of premium riders on life insurance—can reduce some expenses. However, some contingencies cannot be totally anticipated. For instance, a working spouse may find it necessary to work less or to give up working altogether to care for a disabled mate. Although individual needs may differ, the actual amount required to sustain a family during a period of disability for the breadwinner may be less than two thirds of the family's predisability income.

Once the amount of income necessary to support the family is determined, the next step is to identify the sources of disability income that can be relied on, particularly during the first year of disability. These sources include accounts receivable, Social Security, disability insurance (occupational or private), cash reserve, and personal investments.

Accounts Receivable

For optometrists in private practice who operate on other than a cash-only basis–which is the overwhelming majority–some income can be expected during the first 3 months of disability (or perhaps even longer) because of patient fees that are due and have not been received. Of course, some of this income will be needed to cover the costs of office overhead (unless office overhead insurance is purchased). The cost of operating the office during this period, including hiring a temporary stand-in, and the income that can be anticipated from collecting receivables should be analyzed.

Social Security

The following two major hurdles must be cleared before Social Security benefits for disability can be secured: the disabled optometrist must prove that the disability will last for more than a year (or will result in death) and a 5-month waiting period must elapse before benefits begin to be paid during the sixth month of sickness or injury. If an optometrist-employee is injured on the job and has a worker's compensation claim pending, the Social Security benefits may be reduced or payment delayed. Once begun, however, Social Security benefits continue for as long as the disability. Unfortunately, the benefits are relatively meager.

Disability Insurance

Since Social Security benefits require a 5-month waiting period and accounts receivable can probably provide only about 3 months (if that) of income, there is an obvious need for some form of insurance protection during these first few months. Occupational disability plans often fulfill this function: partnership agreements and pension and profit-sharing plans are used to provide income to a disabled partner or shareholder, typically on a decreasing basis as the disability persists over an extended period. Since there are other practitioners available to cover for the disabled partner or shareholder, the optometrist's practice continues to operate. However, the solo practitioner is often faced with the twin problems of no occupational insurance and no one to cover the practice but may be able to

plan for these eventualities through the purchase of personal insurance.

The following two policies could be used to alleviate this situation: one, with a 90-day elimination period, could pick up after accounts receivable has ended and could provide needed income until Social Security benefits begin and the other, with a 6-month or 1-year elimination period (which would make it considerably cheaper), could restore income to needed levels in the event a long-term disability is incurred. During the 3- to 9-month period that only one insurance policy is paying benefits, it might be necessary for the optometrist to supplement income with money withdrawn from a cash reserve.

Cash Reserve

The purpose of a planned-for and adequately funded cash reserve is to provide ready cash for eventualities such as disability. If not enough income is realized during the first few months after sickness or injury, this fund may have to be used so that other sources of revenue (such as investments, retirement accounts, and prized assets) will not have to be liquidated.

Personal Investments

If no other source of income is available, investments may have to be used; such a move should be a last resort because the result is an invasion of the optometrist's retirement plan. In many instances, the sale of investments will not incur significant taxation since the disabled optometrist's tax bracket will doubtless be low. Money market funds should be sold with great caution because of early withdrawal penalties for certificates of deposit that are cashed before maturity, and it might be difficult to reinvest in a fund after recovery from the disability. For a sole proprietor who has initiated an individual retirement account or Keogh plan, withdrawals made before retirement as a result of disability are not subject to penalty and neither are similar withdrawals made from corporate retirement plans. Of course, reducing the amount of money set aside for retirement may have rather significant consequences as the years pass.

When income is not sufficient to meet anticipated expenses, an income gap can arise that must be filled from some source. Planning for such an eventuality requires care and is commonly a long-term proposition. Analogous to these personal considerations is the equally difficult problem of how to keep a practice open and running when the primary source of income—the optometrist—is no longer able to work. The most vulnerable practitioner is the sole proprietor.

The Disabled Practice

Since optometry is widely composed of individual practitioners, the specter of disability is an ominous one for many members of the profession. If an optometrist in solo practice becomes disabled, the ability of the practice to generate new income is likewise disabled. Yet, to keep the practice running, there are overhead expenses that must be paid. No private disability insurance policy offers the payment of overhead expenses as a benefit. This form of indemnification can only be obtained though the purchase of office overhead insurance.

If the disability of the optometrist is short term—lasting but a few months—the optometrist will want to keep the practice open to collect any accounts receivable and to render any services that can be offered. Most optometrists would consider the financial burden of doing so as much an obligation to their patients and employees as an economic necessity. Of course, if the accounts receivable are substantial (and collectable), they may not only be able to keep the office doors open but also be able to provide some income for the disabled optometrist.

Many practitioners prefer not to allow substantial accounts receivables to accumulate, which can make the cost of maintaining the practice during disability prohibitive even though office personnel are reduced to a minimum. One way to generate new income is to have a substitute practitioner, an eventuality for which plans can be made. However, the substitute may not be able to produce enough income to pay both the office overhead and the substitute's salary, and office overhead insurance does not provide for a substitute's salary. For the individual practitioner, the longer the disability lasts, the smaller an asset the practice becomes. A long-term disability (which the optometrist knows will last for years) will most likely result in an effort to sell the practice because the longer the practice goes unattended, the fewer are the number of patients who will remain loyal, with a corresponding diminution in the value of the practice.

Office Overhead Insurance

One type of private disability coverage is office overhead insurance. It is a limited form of insurance that reimburses a disabled practitioner for fixed expenses that are normal and customary to the practitioner's practice and office. To qualify for benefits, the practitioner must be totally disabled—the definition of which will be found in the policy—and satisfy the elimination period (usually half or an entire month). The benefits are limited to the actual overhead expenses incurred by the practice, for which the doctor will be reimbursed up to 100% (or to the policy limits).

Office overhead expenses are rent, electricity, heat, water, laundry, employees' salaries, and similar costs of operation. Excluded are the practitioner's salary (or any other remuneration payable to the disabled practitioner); substitute fees; and cost of frames, lenses, instruments, or equipment. The expenses that will be paid are only those that are actually incurred; if the office staff becomes reduced and overhead is thereby cut, the insurance only compensates the disabled practitioner for the expenses required to maintain the reduced staff and overhead. Benefits are payable for a stated period and may or may not be retroactive to the first day of disability, depending on the policy (18 months to 2 years is customary). Like disability policies, there are several provisions that should be examined, including the right to cancel, waiver of policy premiums during disability, option to convert the policy into disability insurance, and extended benefits in the event of death.

Riders

Disability policies vary in cost because of the presence or absence of various riders. Most of the available riders have been discussed in the preceding sections, but some of the more important ones include the following:

Disability period. Some plans offer extended benefits (payable for life or until age 65 or 70) for both accidental disability and disability resulting from sickness.

Recurrent disability. The most liberal policies will consider a recurring disability to be a new disability (thereby extending the period of benefits) after a relatively brief period of recovery.

Residual benefits. Partial benefits may be offered to a practitioner who can return to work part time, with guaranteed escalation in the annual earnings limit so that the total loss of insurance benefits is delayed.

Right to renew. The best policy is one that is guaranteed renewable and non-cancelable.

Cost-of-living adjustment. Since inflation erodes income, some policies offer annual adjustments to the benefits being paid to the disabled policyholder.

Limited exclusions. The fewer the exclusions (for illness or accident), the more comprehensive the policy.

Waiver of premium. In the event of total disability lasting for a stated period of months, the premiums for the disability insurance policy will be waived for the remainder of the period for which benefits are payable.

Although cost is a major consideration when evaluating a policy, it is the overall package of benefits for a particular cost that must be assessed before deciding that one particular policy is a better buy than another.

Tax Issues

The disability income that a self-employed practitioner receives as the result of insurance coverage purchased with the practitioner's money is not taxable as income because it is considered to be compensation for injury. The premiums paid for the insurance are not deductible.

If disability benefits are received as the result of an employer-purchased plan, the tax considerations are somewhat more complicated, and an accountant's advice will be needed. Any premiums paid by an employer for an employee's disability insurance policy may be deducted as a business expense; the premiums are not considered to be income for the employee.

Disability insurance will have more appeal for solo practitioners, older optometrists (who are more at risk to be disabled), and practices for which the tax considerations are favorable. However, because the likelihood of long-term disability is a statistically significant one, this form of insurance will deserve consideration at one time or another by virtually all optometrists.

Bibliography

Brosterman R, Davis K: *The complete estate planning guide.* New York, 1990, Mentor.

Classé JG: *Legal aspects of optometry.* Boston, 1989, Butterworth.

Department of Health and Human Services, Social Security Administration: *Social Security: understanding the benefits.* Washington, DC 2002, U.S. Government Printing Office.

Elmstrom G: *Advanced management for optometrists.* Chicago, 1982, Professional Press.

www.consumerreports.org. Web site for *Consumer Reports,* which contains online reports of insurance products.

www.insure.com. Web site for Standard and Poor's insurance company profiles and ratings.

www.pueblo.gsa.org. Web site for Federal Citizen Information Center, which has many federal government publications online.

Chapter 11

Professional Liability Insurance and Risk Management

John G. Classé and Lawrence S. Thal

The die is cast.

Jean-Paul Sartre *Les Jeux Sont Faits*

The potential professional liability issues that can befall a private practitioner can involve the practitioner's person (malpractice, defamation), employees (vicarious liability, worker's compensation, embezzlement), ophthalmic materials (product liability), office and equipment (premises liability), or casualty loss (fire, burglary, theft, or other perils). With so much at stake, and the cost of professional liability insurance relatively low, it is little wonder that practice-related insurance has become a high priority for most optometrists. Unfortunately, both the cost of professional insurance and the number and likelihood of claims have escalated throughout the past few decades. The trend toward increased exposure is expected to rise in the years to come, as optometrists increase the number of patients for whom primary eye care is provided. For this reason, adequate professional liability coverage has become a necessity for all practitioners.

Types of Coverage

Since the potential for loss touches on so many areas of optometric practice, professional liability insurance policies must protect against a wide array of risks. For purposes of this discussion, insurance coverage will be divided into the following four categories: personal liability insurance, worker's compensation, fire insurance, and other property insurance.

Personal Liability Insurance

An optometrist can be personally liable for injuries to patients that arise out of acts of negligence (mal-

practice, breach of contract); injury to character (defamation); damages from lenses, frames, drugs, and solutions (product liability); injuries that occur on the premises (premises liability); or the negligence of employees (vicarious liability). Indemnification can be obtained for each of these potential sources of liability.

Malpractice insurance pays for all costs of a legal defense and for any judgments or settlements arising out of a malpractice claim or a claim of breach of contract (up to the policy limits). Policies usually do not require the approval of the doctor before a settlement becomes legally binding, so an optometrist who wishes to insist on his or her day in court must ensure that the policy requires the practitioner's approval before any settlement of a claim can be made. Malpractice coverage also includes claims involving employees who are acting in the line and scope of their duties, which means that technicians, assistants, and receptionists are provided with protection. Professional employees, such as other optometrists or opticians, may be added to a policy for little cost. Partners—who are legally liable for one another's negligence—can indemnify themselves against "joint and several liability" through the purchase of appropriate liability coverage. The employees of professional associations or corporations or limited liability companies can obtain coverage through a policy taken out by the corporation or company.

Defamation insurance provides all legal fees and pays all judgments and settlements (up to the limits of the policy) for any injury to the reputation of another person that arises out of the optometrist's professional activities. The defendant doctor's approval usually is not necessary for the settlement of a claim. The persons covered under a standard policy typically include employees.

Product liability insurance indemnifies the optometrist (to the stated policy limits) against any claim arising out of a defect in a lens or frame or defective drug or solution that results in damage to a patient's person or property; the optometrist's approval usually is not necessary for the settlement of a claim.

Premises liability insurance protects (to the policy limits) against any claims by a patient that result from injury while in the optometrist's office or on the office premises. These claims include injuries from equipment as well as injuries from falls, shocks, and similar mishaps.

The forgoing are considered part of the basic coverage required for private practice. Additional coverage can be obtained to insure against the following eventualities:

- Automobiles used to conduct business can be insured against accident claims arising out of the negligence of an employee driver
- Fire loss to leased or rented premises resulting from the negligence of an optometrist or office employees also can be covered
- Injuries to employees that occur while the employees are acting in the line and scope of their duties can be covered

The last eventuality is of particular importance, since insurance coverage for employee injuries will have to be purchased if the optometrist's practice is not covered by state worker's compensation laws.

Worker's Compensation

Worker's compensation laws were enacted to provide benefits for employees injured in on-the-job accidents or by occupational diseases and to limit the liability of employers for legal claims based on these accidents or diseases. Employees are guaranteed a "benefit certain" for their injuries or illnesses, which is paid for by the insurance purchased by the employer. In return, the employer is protected by the "exclusive remedy" provisions of these laws, which prevent employees for suing the employer for damages in court.

State law determines whether an employer must participate in worker's compensation. The key factor in making this determination is the number of employees that work for an employer; this number varies from state to state. For example, in Alabama an employer with more than four employees–full time or part time–must have worker's compensation coverage.

Generally, an employer can cover worker's compensation liability in the following five ways :

- Purchase insurance from an approved commercial worker's compensation carrier
- If commercial insurance carriers will not provide insurance, the employer may purchase insurance through the state's "assigned risk pool"
- Obtain coverage through a group self-insurance fund
- Provide self-insurance, if the employer is qualified to do so
- Purchase an approved alternative worker's compensation policy from an authorized insurance carrier

Most optometrists who participate in worker's compensation plans choose to purchase insurance from an approved commercial worker's compensation carrier.

Employers with fewer than the requisite number of employees may elect to participate in a state's worker's compensation, usually by applying to that state's worker's compensation agency. This usually requires little more than the filling out of a form. The employer may later withdraw from the plan if the employer chooses to do so.

Professional liability insurance policies usually do not include compensation for on-the-job injuries suffered by employees (unless it is added as optional coverage), making it essential that coverage from a commercial carrier be purchased if the employer does not elect to apply for coverage under the worker's compensation law. This coverage will increase the cost of the insurance policy, but probably will be less costly than payments to a worker's compensation plan. The benefits that may be claimed by injured or ill workers under worker's compensation are limited by state law. Worker's compensation benefits paid to the employees of an employer will increase the insurance premiums paid by the employer in the future.

Fire Insurance

Although liability insurance can protect against negligence that causes fire loss, to be fully indemnified for loss of instrumentation, equipment, records, furniture, supplies, and other items damaged by fire, an optometrist must acquire fire insurance. There are two fire insurance problems that an optometrist faces when leased office space is occupied: adequate insurance for all property located within the office and adequate insurance for the building in which the office is located. Unless the optometrist owns the building, the only problem that can be solved directly is the first, by adequately insuring all the personal property used in the practice. However, there is still the worry that the structure within which the office is located may not be adequately insured. The best way to obviate this problem is to be certain that the office lease contains a clause requiring the lessor to insure the building adequately.

As for the insurance itself, insurance companies usually require that a building be insured to a prescribed minimum of its value, often 80%, for full benefits to be paid in the event of its loss. As long as the 80% minimum is adhered to, a full 100% of any fire loss will be paid by the insurer, no matter whether the loss is partial or total. But if the insurance on the building falls to less than 80% of its value (which it can easily do if fire insurance policies are not adjusted for structure appreciation each year), the insurer is no longer obliged to pay 100% of the claim, reducing its liability in proportion to the percent of underinsurance. This can hinder repairs of partially damaged areas by the lessor and seriously impair an optometrist's ability to keep a damaged office functioning.

The same considerations are involved in the optometrist's leased office space. The lessee optometrist must act as a co-insurer with the lessor and acquire fire insurance for all property located within the office, with such insurance amounting to a minimum of 80% of the property's value. Failure to do so will result in only partial insurance coverage, just as with damage to the building. Again, yearly review of fire insurance coverage is a must because new equipment additions can substantially boost a practice's property value.

Documentation of purchased items should be accomplished in the following two ways: all sales receipts and check stubs should be retained and stored for safekeeping, and photodocumentation of all new office contents should be performed routinely. Proof of loss is a burden that rests solely on the policyholder, and the contractual requirements to document loss under most fire insurance policies are considerable.

The money received for a claim can either be used to restore an item or to purchase a new one. Restoration costs will be paid in full by the insurer, but insurance checks for totally damaged items may not be adequate to purchase a brand new replacement. That is because an item's *cost value* is considered to be the fair market value of the item at the time of loss, which means that an instrument or piece of equipment that is several years old will be reduced in value according to its age. To obtain a new item, *replacement value* insurance must be obtained. However, replacement value coverage is more expensive than cost value coverage.

Interrupted business losses—those losses incurred by virtue of the disruption of the practice from the fire—also can be included in a policy, but proof of loss can again be a substantial burden for the policyholder.

Other Property Insurance

Besides premises liability and medical premises insurance (which pays for reasonable medical expenses incurred by persons injured on the premises, regardless of fault), optional property coverage that can be obtained includes loss from burglary and embezzlement.

Professional equipment, furniture, and office equipment can be insured against loss on a replacement cost basis, which means that in the event of loss, new items will be paid for in full, as long as the policy limits reflect the current replacement cost value. Improvements and alterations of an office (such as paneling, fixtures, and similar changes) also can be insured on a replacement cost basis.

Loss from burglary, theft, and robbery can be protected against through the purchase of federally sponsored crime insurance.

Loss from embezzlement can be a shock for an unsuspecting optometrist, but the traditional method of protecting against employee stealing—by taking out a bond on employees who handle money—is generally distasteful to an office staff. Fortunately, insurance providing for bonding of necessary employees can be purchased without the stigma that actual bonding confers. However, proof of economic loss can be difficult to obtain, making reimbursement for embezzled amounts often less than the actual losses sustained.

Other property insurance available to optometrists includes the following:
• Transit coverage can be obtained for equipment while it is away from the office at another location or while it is in transit
• Personal effects of the optometrist, staff, and patients can be insured against loss by perils such as fire, theft, and burglary
• Office records can be insured for the costs of reproduction
• Owner, landlord, and tenant liability offers protection against claims that arise from an optometrist's ownership or operation of a building
Multiperil insurance is a package policy that provides coverage for fire, burglary, theft, office contents, professional equipment, general liability, and other perils; comprehensive coverage under such a package can sometimes be cheaper than purchases of individual policies for various contingencies.

Extent of Coverage

A major decision facing any practitioner is how much protection to acquire. Fortunately, professional liability insurance for optometrists is relatively cheap. A practitioner can easily afford not only basic coverage but also "umbrella" coverage, which extends the personal liability provisions of the basic policy. Umbrella coverage also extends the amount of protection beyond that found in a standard policy, usually to $1 million. The cost of this extended coverage is typically less than 1% of the average optometrist's net income. In addition, extra coverage may be obtained at discounted cost, such that an extra million dollars of coverage costs significantly less than the first million dollars of coverage.

Coverage is typically written to include the insurance provided per person and per occurrence. For example, a $1 million/$3 million policy would indicate that the policy limits are $1 million per person and $3 million for the event. Therefore, if an optometrist defamed three persons at once, each person would be covered for up to $1 million dollars in damages, and the total amount of coverage for all claims stemming from the event would be $3 million.

Policy coverage pays for an attorney to represent the optometrist, but the attorney in fact represents the insurer. Insurance attorneys typically handle many liability claims and are experienced in liability law, but an optometrist may choose to hire personal counsel to work with the insurance lawyer and represent the optometrist's interests in the case. In such an event, the optometrist is solely responsible for payment of the personal lawyer's fees.

Type of Policy

Professional liability exposure can continue for a period of years after the optometrist has changed policies or retired from practice. Thus there is a risk that a lawsuit will be filed after the insurance coverage has ended, leaving the optometrist's personal assets at risk. This period of vulnerability after policy premiums are no longer being paid is known as the *risk tail*, and coverage should be acquired to protect the optometrist during this period.

With an *occurrence* type policy, all errors and omissions are covered, provided the incident occurred during the policy period, even if the claim is made after the policy has been terminated. This means that an act of negligence, committed during the period that occurrence policy premiums were being paid, is covered even if the claim is brought after the policy has been terminated and another policy purchased (or all coverage ended).

Under the more common *claims-made* form of policy, the optometrist is covered as long as premiums are being paid, but coverage ends after the policy is terminated. The insured usually has the right to purchase an *extended reporting endorsement* or *nonpracticing policy* within a stated period after terminating the basic policy, and this additional coverage is intended to cover against the risk tail. With such an endorsement policy, an optometrist is insured for a liability claim brought after basic coverage has ended; without it, there is no insurance coverage.

The following are points to consider when choosing the type of policy for private practice:

- Although an occurrence type of policy does not require the purchase of additional risk tail protection, it is more expensive than the claims-made policy, may have less broad coverage, and thus may be a less desirable choice
- The right to purchase risk tail coverage should be guaranteed in the claims-made policy, irrespective of whether the policy is terminated by the insurer or the policyholder and regardless of the reason for termination
- The cost of the extended reporting endorsement for the risk tail should be stated in the claims-made policy, either as a specific amount or a definite percentage of the basic policy

Malpractice Claim Reporting Requirements

In 1986 the federal government enacted the Health Quality Improvement Act, which was intended to address rising concerns over medical malpractice litigation and the quality of medical care. This law established the National Practitioner Data Bank (NPDB) and set as its goal the improvement of health care by doing the following:

- Encouraging state licensing boards, hospitals, professional societies, and other health care entities to identify and discipline practitioners who engage in unprofessional behavior
- Restricting the ability of incompetent practitioners to move from state to state without disclosing past malpractice payments or other adverse actions against them (e.g., loss of license, hospital privileges, professional society membership, or participation in Medicare or Medicaid)

The NPDB began collecting and disseminating information in 1990, as part of the Department of Health and Human Services. It acts as an "alert" system, assisting boards in the review of health care practitioners' professional credentials. Reports must be submitted to the NPDB in the following two instances: when an insurer makes a malpractice payment in response to a claim against a practitioner and when a hospital or other health care entity, state licensing board, or professional society takes an adverse action against a practitioner.

This information is available to state licensing boards, hospitals, professional associations, and other entities that license, hire, or grant privileges or membership to health care practitioners. Because of the use of this information by state boards, it should be realized that settlement of a liability claim can lead to disciplinary action. Individual practitioners may query the NPDB to determine whether personal disciplinary information is in the data bank and whether the information is correct.

Tax Issues

Liability insurance coverage is a necessary aspect of the practice of optometry, and as such it is a necessary business expense for tax purposes. An optometrist may claim a tax deduction for the liability insurance premium, whether it is for basic or optional coverage.

Should an optometrist be unfortunate enough to have to file an insurance claim under any policy providing property coverage, the reimbursement to the optometrist by the insurer is not taxable. In the event the insurance payment is less than the fair market value of the property at the time of the loss, the optometrist can claim a tax deduction for the amount of the loss in excess of the insurance proceeds (see Chapter 38).

If an optometrist is a defendant in a professional liability lawsuit and the optometrist decides to hire a personal attorney, the cost of this additional counsel can be deducted. Any judgment that an optometrist is ordered to pay that is in excess of the optometrist's insurance coverage also would qualify as a deduction.

Risk Management

Professional liability insurance is necessary protection against the risk of a liability claim. The need to manage risk is an integral part of health care and is as important to the practitioner in private practice as to the clinician within an institutional setting. Through the use of appropriate communication, testing, and treatment, the risk of injury to patients may be minimized; by providing adequate documentation of care, the details of management may be preserved. Only by attending to both aspects of care—appropriate testing and adequate documentation—can it be said that risk is truly managed.

Risk management, when properly applied, results in optimum patient care. One beneficial effect of proper care is a reduced likelihood of malpractice litigation. Professional liability has become a serious concern for medicine, reflected in the sizable malpractice insurance premiums that physicians must pay. Premiums are a reflection of liability risk and may be used to determine the exposure of various specialties to malpractice claims. Although the risk of litigation in ophthalmology is about average for all medical specialties, ophthalmologists pay about 3% to 5% of gross income for professional liability coverage. In comparison, the risk in optometry is much less, resulting in significantly lower expenditures for premiums, less than 1% of net income for coverage comparable to that obtained by ophthalmologists.

Although laws defining the scope of practice for optometrists vary from state to state, there is no differentiation in premium costs based on whether optometrists are permitted to prescribe therapeutic drugs or are limited to the prescription of diagnostic drugs only. The reason may be found in the types of liability claims brought against optometrists (Box 11-1). Most claims for substantial damages allege failure to diagnose disease rather than errors of treatment; the most important claims involve failure to diagnose open-angle glaucoma, retinal detachment, and tumors affecting the visual system. Because of the pre-eminence of these diseases, about three fourths of claims alleging misdiagnosis of disease involve the posterior segment of the eye. For the anterior segment, injuries to the cornea are the most important. Contact lenses are a significant contributor to corneal injury; 40% to 50% of all malpractice claims involve contact lens practice. The great majority of these claims are for minor damages, and a minority of claims involve bacterial or herpetic infection of the cornea. Ocular injury from shattered spectacle lenses is another cause of malpractice claims; the usual allegation is that polycarbonate plastic should have been prescribed rather than a less impact-resistant lens material. Injury from the adverse effects of ophthalmic drugs is a rare cause of litigation involving optometrists.

Proof of Malpractice

To apply risk management to the practice of optometry, the legal elements of malpractice must be understood. Malpractice is more properly termed *medical*

Box 11-1 One Hundred Optometric Malpractice Claims Involving Optometrists	
MISDIAGNOSIS OF INTRAOCULAR DISEASE	**58% OF CLAIMS**
Open-angle glaucoma	20 claims
Retinal detachment	17 claims
Tumors	
Intraocular	6 claims
Brain	8 claims
Diabetic retinopathy	4 claims
Histoplasmosis	1 claim
Toxoplasmosis	1 claim
Temporal arteritis	1 claim
MISDIAGNOSIS OF ANTERIOR SEGMENT DISEASE	**11% OF CLAIMS**
Corneal disease	6 claims
Ocular foreign bodies	3 claims
Tumors of the anterior adnexa	1 claim
Iritis	1 claim
INJURIES FROM OPHTHALMIC MATERIALS	**21% OF CLAIMS**
Contact lenses	
Complications of lens-related corneal abrasions	7 claims
Misdiagnosis of corneal disease	3 claims
Failure to obtain informed consent	1 claim
Spectacles	
Failure to prescribe polycarbonate plastic lenses	7 claims
Defective sports-frame design	3 claims
IMPROPER CO-MANAGEMENT	**5% OF CLAIMS**
Complications of cataract surgery	2 claims
Complications of refractive surgery	3 claims
INJURIES FROM OPHTHALMIC DRUGS	**3% OF CLAIMS**
Adverse effects of diagnostic agents (angle closure)	3 claims
MISDIAGNOSIS OF BINOCULAR VISION ANOMALIES	**2% OF CLAIMS**
Failure to treat amblyopia	2 claims

Classé JG: Standards of practice for primary eyecare. *Columbus, Ohio, 1998, Anadem.*

negligence it is a civil action brought by an injured party seeking compensation (money). A professional liability claim requires the injured party (the plaintiff) to offer the following to establish proof of negligence:
- The doctor-patient relationship existed
- The defendant practitioner did not act reasonably; the defendant's conduct is measured against the "*standard of care*," which is the conduct that is deemed to be reasonable under the circumstances by members of the profession
- There was actual physical injury to the patient (e.g., loss of visual acuity, visual field, or ocular motility)
- There was a legal link between the act (or failure to act) of the practitioner and the injury suffered by the patient; this link is termed *proximate cause*

All four elements must be supported by the preponderance of the evidence, which is provided through expert testimony. Expert witnesses explain technical information and offer opinions concerning the standard of care. If misdiagnosis or improper treatment of ocular disease is at issue, an ophthalmologist may be deemed competent to offer expert testimony. Thus, an optometrist may be held to a medical standard of care with respect to the diagnosis and treatment of eye disease.

Standards of Care in Clinical Practice

Risk management is based on an understanding of clinical standards of care and stringent observance of them. Because of the importance of proper diagnosis, the procedural aspects of care receive the greatest emphasis: what to ask during the history, which tests to perform, when to periodically re-evaluate the patient, and when to refer to another practitioner. Because adherence to standards of care must be established to avoid liability, proper documentation of communications, test results, and recall and referral appointments are essential. Examples of standards of care and of documentation are provided for the areas of practice which are most likely to produce a negligence claim: misdiagnosis of ocular disease, use of ophthalmic drugs, and the prescribing of contact lenses and spectacles.

Diagnosis of Ocular Disease

The three diseases most likely to result in allegations of misdiagnosis are open-angle glaucoma, retinal detachment, and tumors affecting the visual system. The most common reason for errors of diagnosis is failure to dilate the pupil. Clearly, the most important step to limit the risk of misdiagnosis is to develop a protocol for the use of pupillary dilation. Examination of the fundus should include both the retinal periphery and the posterior pole and should entail the use of the appropriate instrumentation (e.g., 60, 78 or 90 D fundus lenses, direct and binocular indirect ophthalmoscopes). Communication of findings and planned follow-up also are significant aspects of care and should not be neglected.

Open-angle Glaucoma. Failure to diagnose open-angle glaucoma often has been linked with failure to perform tonometry; however, a significant number of glaucoma suspects will have applanation intraocular pressures (IOPs) that are normotensive, and patients with low-tension glaucoma will possess IOPs in the mid- to low teens. Although tonometry is a test that should be performed liberally, without regard to the age of the patient, it will not detect glaucoma suspects who are normotensive. Although the effect of open-angle glaucoma is to diminish the field of vision, few practitioners perform a sensitive test of the visual field unless there is clinical justification for it. A screening test, such as confrontation fields, is often used as part of the general examination, but this test will not reveal diminution of the visual field until the disease has reached an advanced stage. For these reasons, examination of the optic nerve head is often the most crucial aspect of diagnosis. Assessment through a dilated pupil–with the advantage of stereopsis offered by fundus biomicroscopy–may offer the best opportunity to detect disease, for often one eye will precede the other in degree of involvement. Distinct or subtle differences in the cupping of the neu-

roretinal rim may provide the clue that leads to further testing and to differential diagnosis.

If a patient is a glaucoma suspect, a sensitive test of the visual field must be performed, which requires the use of perimetry at threshold. This obligation extends to ocular hypertensive patients, who have about a 10% risk of developing the disease. Periodic reassessment of intraocular pressures and visual fields must be performed, which creates a long-term obligation for management. The risk of disease and the rationale for testing must be explained to the patient and documented in the record of care.

Retinal Detachment. There is a timeliness to the diagnosis of retinal detachment that, if not observed, can lead to significant loss of vision. Therefore, patients who are symptomatic for retinal detachment– blurred vision, seeing sparks or lights, reduced visual field–must receive a timely dilated fundus examination and a thorough assessment of the retina. Both the periphery and the posterior pole must be examined; failure to perform a dilated fundus examination will inevitably be construed as negligence. Prompt referral is necessary if a detachment is found.

Patients who are at risk for retinal detachment also should receive a dilated fundus examination. These patients include individuals with the following:
- Significant myopia
- Aphakia or pseudophakia
- YAG capsulotomy
- Open-angle glaucoma and significant myopia that is treated with miotic drugs
- Lattice degeneration
- Proliferative retinopathy (e.g., proliferative diabetic retinopathy, sickle cell hemoglobinopathy, branch retinal vein occlusion)
- Nonpenetrating trauma to the eye
- Retinal detachment in the fellow eye

Patients with acute onset symptomatic posterior vitreous detachment (PVD) also must receive a timely, thorough evaluation of the ocular fundus. Between 8% and 15% of patients with symptomatic PVD will have suffered a retinal tear, and approximately one third of these patients will experience a retinal detachment. The retinal break may not be apparent at the time of examination; a partial PVD may produce a retinal tear afterwards, when there is complete separation of the vitreous. Even if the results of the initial assessment are negative, the patient must be re-examined 4 to 8 weeks later because the risk of retinal detachment remains significant, especially for aphakic patients. The patient must be warned of the symptoms of detachment and instructed to return for assessment immediately if they occur. These communications should be carefully documented in the patient's record.

Tumors. Intraocular tumor is an exceedingly rare disease, but if a tumor produces symptoms, misdiagnosis caused by failure to perform a dilated fundus examination may result in litigation. Even tumors as rare as malignant melanoma, retinoblastoma, and von Hippel–Lindau have been the source of malpractice claims. Failure to examine the peripheral retina in symptomatic patients is considered to be a breach of the standard of care.

Silent intraocular tumors pose a genuine diagnostic challenge to practitioners. The most troublesome situation is in asymptomatic first-presenting patient: does the standard of care require a dilated fundus examination and evaluation of the peripheral retina of these patients? The growing medical orientation of the standard of care is moving inexorably in that direction, as indicated by recent litigation. Therefore, it is wise to include a dilated fundus examination as part of the general assessment of "routine" first-presenting patients.

Misdiagnosis of external tumors, such as basal cell and squamous cell carcinoma, also can be construed as negligence. Questionable lesions of the adnexa should be referred for biopsy and, when appropriate, for surgical removal. Patients with visual field loss indicative of intracranial neoplasms must likewise receive referral for definitive diagnosis. For patients with a suspicious history (e.g., headaches, neurologic symptoms) or findings (e.g., decreased acuity, papilledema), perimetry is indicated. Tumors can threaten life as well as vision, and optometrists must remain vigilant for these rare but potentially devastating diseases.

Use of Ophthalmic Drugs

Although the adverse effects of drug use are a liability issue for ophthalmologists, they are a rare source of litigation for optometrists. In fact, considering the importance of the diagnosis of intraocular disease, failure to use a mydriatic drug (to obtain pupillary dilation) is a much more likely source of litigation than an adverse effect of drug use (e.g., acute angle closure). All drugs have side effects, however, and ophthalmic drugs are no exception. For convenience of discussion, drugs are categorized as diagnostic or therapeutic.

Diagnostic Drugs. The most commonly used drugs are anesthetic and mydriatic agents. Anesthetic agents should not be applied copiously to a cornea with a compromised epithelium; a permanent corneal opacity may result. Mydriatic agents should not be administered without first assessing the anterior chamber angle. If the angle is anatomically narrow and has the potential to precipitate an angle closure during pupillary dilation, the patient must be warned of this risk, and an informed consent to proceed must be obtained (Figure 11-1). Provisions also must be made for management of the angle closure should it occur. Patients who have undergone pupillary dilation during general examination should be advised that blurred vision and photophobia will persist for several hours and that caution is needed while operating a motor vehicle or performing other potentially hazardous tasks. The same warning must be given to patients who have received cycloplegia. In some instances (e.g., uncorrected hyperopes with significant refractive error), it is prudent to have a third party transport the patient during the period that acuity is reduced.

Therapeutic Drugs. Litigation from therapeutic drug use most often involves topical steroids. Adverse side effects of long-term use include cataracts and open-angle glaucoma. Patients who must undergo a long-term regimen of use must be warned of side effects and monitored with sufficient frequency to detect these effects if they occur. Prescriptions should specify the number of permissible refills. If no refills are permitted, the prescription should contain language to this effect.

A second source of litigation is the use of systemic steroids, which often have significant side effects. These drugs should not be used unless it can be ascertained that a topical route of administration would not be adequate. Warnings of expected side effects should be given and documented.

Drugs used for the treatment of open-angle glaucoma also can produce the following undesirable side effects: β-blockers can significantly affect individuals with uncompensated congestive heart failure or chronic obstructive pulmonary disease; miotic agents may precipitate a retinal detachment in patients who are significantly myopic; and systemic carbonic anhydrase inhibitors may cause adverse effects ranging from kidney stones to aplastic anemia. Patients must receive adequate warnings of drug side effects and must be examined periodically to ensure that injurious effects have not occurred. In all cases, ophthalmic drug use must be adequately documented in the patient's record of care.

EXAMPLE INFORMED CONSENT DOCUMENT FOR DILATION OF THE PUPIL WHEN A PATIENT HAS A NARROW ANTERIOR CHAMBER ANGLE

Dilation of the pupil is a common diagnostic procedure used by optometrists to better examine the interior of the eye. It allows a more thorough examination by making the field of view wider and by permitting the doctor to see more of the inside of the eye. Being able to examine the inside of the eye is essential to determining that your eye is healthy.

To dilate the pupil, eye drops must be administered. They require roughly half an hour to take effect. Once your pupils are dilated, it is common to be sensitive to light, a symptom that is usually alleviated by sunglasses. If you do not have any sunglasses, a disposable pair will be provided for you. Another common symptom is blurred vision, especially at near. It will require about 4-6 hours for your vision to return to normal. During this time you must exercise caution when walking down steps, driving a vehicle, operating dangerous machinery, or performing other tasks that may present a risk of injury. If you have any special transportation needs, please let us know so that they can be arranged prior to dilation.

In about 2% of people there is a possible complication of dilation of the pupil; it has been determined that you fall into this category. You must understand this complication before you give your consent to have this procedure performed.

The doctor's examination has revealed that there is a possibility of elevating the pressure inside your eye when dilation is performed. The medical term for this eventuality is "angle closure glaucoma". Because of this possibility, once your eye is dilated and the interior of the eye has been examined, the pressure will be checked again. Should it become elevated, it will be necessary to lower the pressure by administering eyedrops and oral medication. Afterwards, it may be necessary to refer you to an eye surgeon for treatment with a laser to prevent further occurrences of this kind.

Because of the structure of your eyes, it is possible for an angle closure to occur at some other time, when the symptoms may not be recognized and treatment may not be immediately provided. Such an eventuality could seriously affect your vision. Therefore, there is a benefit to you in having dilation perfomed today and in allowing this complication, if it occurs, to be diagnosed and treated immediately.

The decision to undergo dilation is yours. You may choose not to have dilation performed, but because of your history, symptoms, or examination findings, the doctor recommends that dilation of the pupil be used today to examine your eye for disease. If you have any questions concerning the procedure, please ask them so that we may answer them. Then please sign your name in the appropriate place below to signify your decision.

☐ I understand the risks and benefits of pupillary dilation and I consent to have the procedure performed.

☐ The risks and benefits of pupillary dilation have been adequately explained to me and I understand them, but I do not wish to undergo the procedure.

_____   _____
Date   Signature of Patient

Figure 11-1 Sample informed consent agreement for dilation of the pupil when there is a risk of angle closure.

Contact Lenses

Risk management in contact lens practice is most easily described by type of lens modality: daily wear or extended wear. Although the risk of significant complication is greater for patients fitted with extended wear lenses, the much larger number of individuals wearing daily wear lenses causes more legal claims to be brought by these patients. Because of the greater likelihood of complications found in extended wear—estimated to be 4 to 15 times that for daily wear—patients must be informed of the risks, and a structured program of care should be devised. Written agreements are used to satisfy informed consent requirements and to describe management, which should obligate patients to return at stated periods for follow-up (Figure 11-2). Agreements may be tailored to meet the needs of the

University Optometric Group
908 19th Street South
Birmingham, AL 35294
(205) 934-5161

Fitting Agreement for Extended Wear (Overnight) Contact Lenses

Extended wear (overnight) contact lenses present both patient and doctor with special obligations and requirements. To ensure successful lens wear, a specially designed program of fitting, lens care, and followup evaluation has been designed for you. To receive the benefits of this program, however, you must adhere to recommended lens care and wear procedures and must return as required for periodic progress evaluations. The details of our program are explained in the paragraphs that follow.

Eligibility

Extended wear contact lenses are available only to patients who have received an eye health examination at University Optometric Group during the past 12 months and who have no obvious contraindications to wear. The use of overnight lenses is not for everyone, and your doctor will advise you concerning the suitability of extended wear lenses for you. Because it is not always possible to determine in advance of lens wear whether you will enjoy a successful response to overnight use of lenses, frequent examination is necessary at the beginning of wear. Various personal, physiological and environmental factors may necessitate a change in the recommended wearing schedule or even termination of extended wear. These factors include, but are not limited to:

- Inability or unwillingness to return for followup care
- Inability or unwillingness to follow instructions for lens care and maintenance
- Poor lens hygiene
- Manual dexterity problems that prevent periodic lens removal and cleaning
- Severe emotional stress
- Use of certain medications
- Dryness of the eye
- Ocular allergic response

If you suspect that these or other factors may affect your ability to wear overnight lenses successfully, please discuss your concerns with the doctor before initiating the lens fitting process.

All patients must have a pair of spectacles which can be worn in place of contact lenses as needed.

Contact Lens Fitting

Your doctor will perform a careful fitting and lens evaluation which will include the following:

- Assessment of any contraindications to lens wear
- Examination of external eye and tear film
- Measurements for the fit of lenses
- Placement of trial lenses in the eye
- Determination of appropriate lens power and design
- Evaluation of ocular response to trial lens wear

You will have an opportunity to wear trial lenses and to assess the sharpness of your vision through them. If after this evaluation it is determined that you do not wish to wear overnight lenses, you will be charged a fee of $35 for the fitting and examination.

If you decide to wear overnight lenses, you will be charged an additional fee for lenses, solutions needed for cleaning and disinfection, training in lens insertion and removal, education in lens cleaning and maintenance procedures, and for progress evaluations that are part of the fitting period. The total cost is dependent upon the type of lenses selected for you, the solutions needed for maintenance, and the number of progress evaluations. We will be happy to review these costs with you at the time of payment.

Progress Evaluations

Evaluation of lens wear is a necessary aspect of the proper care of patients using overnight lenses. Complications can occur rapidly, and periodic examination is needed to safeguard eye health and prevent injury. For these reasons, progress evaluations will be scheduled for:

- 24 hours after beginning overnight wear
- 3 days after beginning overnight wear
- 10 days after beginning overnight wear
- 4 weeks after beginning overnight wear

The initial schedule for your progress evaluations is as follows:

Examination	Date/Time
24 hour	_____
3 days	_____
10 days	_____
4 weeks	_____

Figure 11-2 Sample informed consent agreement for overnight wear of contact lenses.

Additional examinations may be necessary, depending upon your response to overnight wear.

It is important for the health of your eyes that you return as required for examination, follow the recommended wearing schedule, and clean and disinfect your lenses as directed. Failure to fulfill these obligations may result in termination of lens wear.

Wear of Lenses

You have been fitted with the following type and brand of extended wear contact lenses:

Type	Manufacturer/Brand
Gas permeable	_____
Soft	_____
Disposable	_____

As with any other medical device, the use of extended wear contact lenses is not without risk. This risk is higher than for daily wear lenses (lenses that are not worn overnight). A small but significant percentage of individuals wearing extended wear lenses develop potentially serious complications that can lead to permanent eye injury and vision loss.

Therefore, it is important that you recognize the symptoms of potentially serious complications of wear, which include the following:

- **Decreased (blurry) vision**
- **Eye pain or irritation**
- **Redness of the eye**
- **Watering or discharge**
- **Sensitivity to light**

If you experience any of these symptoms, you should immediately remove your lenses, call the clinic, and schedule an appointment. Do not delay in calling for an appointment and do not resume lens wear until advised to do so by your doctor.

A proper wearing schedule is essential to reducing the risk of complications. Although extended wear lenses are intended to be worn overnight, the US Food and Drug Administration has issued an advisory letter recommending that lenses be worn continuously for no more than 6 nights. After wear for the period recommended by your doctor, lenses are to be left off one night and cleaned and disinfected before wear is resumed.

You are advised to wear your lenses no more than _____ nights continuously. After removal, the lens must be properly cleaned, disinfected, and stored overnight.

Lens Care

Proper care of lenses is necessary for successful wear, proper vision, good eye health and normal lens life. You will be instructed in the proper methods of lens care and handling and provided with the proper solutions and materials for the cleaning, disinfection and storage of extended wear (overnight) lenses.

You should not hesitate to ask your doctor or a staff assistant about lens care and maintenance, and you should become familiar with the lens care products listed below, for they have been prescribed specifically for your eyes and lenses. **You should never change or substitute brands without first checking with your doctor.** The use of improper solutions may result in eye irritation or lens damage.

The following products have been selected for use with your lenses:

Lens cleaner _____

Lens disinfectant _____

Soaking solution _____

Rinsing solution _____

Wetting solution _____

Eyedrops _____

If a lens accumulates deposits which cannot be removed, it must be replaced. Lens life is unpredictable, and frequent replacements may be necessary. The cost of replacing damaged lenses is $_____ per lens during the period this agreement is in effect. Lost lenses may be replaced for this same fee.

A successful lens fit cannot be guaranteed, despite the best efforts of your doctor and full compliance on your part with all requirements for lens wear and care. If a change of lens type is required, a fee of $_____ per lens will be charged. If the decision is made to terminate extended lens wear, you will be eligible for a refund of $ _____ per lens if the lenses are returned within _____ days of beginning wear.

Disposable Lenses

Disposable lenses are a type of extended wear (overnight) lens used to reduce the likelihood of certain ocular complications of contact lens wear. If disposable lenses are prescribed for you, they must be removed and discarded in accordance with the schedule that has been advised. As with other types of extended

Figure 11-2, Cont'd

Continued

wear lenses, continuous wear is limited to no more than 6 nights. After a night without wear, a new set of lenses is placed in the eye. Disposable lenses should not be used after being taken out of the eye, but if a lens is accidentally or deliberately removed, it should not be reused without first being cleaned and disinfected.

Your wearing schedule is listed below:

Remove lenses after _____ days of wear.

Do not wear lenses for 24 hours.

Replacement lenses can be worn for _____ days.

If no problems are encountered, repeat the above schedule for _____ weeks, after which time you will be scheduled to return for a progress evaluation and a new supply of lenses.

Because disposable lenses cannot be inspected by the doctor prior to dispensing, you should examine each lens prior to insertion in the eye. Defective lenses should be discarded or brought to the clinic for inspection. Lenses should be removed immediately if significant symptoms occur, such as blurred vision, pain, redness, ocular discharge, or sensitivity to light, and an appointment should be scheduled with your doctor.

Contact Lens Prescriptions

Until your doctor has had an opportunity to fit you with lenses and evaluate the response of your eyes to lens wear, the prescription for your contact lenses cannot be determined. For that reason, a contact lens prescription cannot be provided until the conclusion of the fitting period, which is generally about a month after lens wear has begun.

The contact lens prescription provided by your doctor will describe the exact lens parameters needed to ensure that, if it becomes necessary, you can obtain these same lenses from another practitioner. The prescription will be valid for a period of time which may range from 3 months to one year, depending upon the type of lenses you received. Patients who are fitted with disposable or planned replacement lenses usually require the shorter periods of time, because lenses may be modified at progress evaluations. There is no fee for providing you with a copy of your prescription.

Patient Responsibility

Please read carefully the five paragraphs that follow, for they constitute your obligations as a contact lens patient of University Optometric Group.

I understand that my cooperation and compliance is vital to my success with extended wear (overnight) contact lenses.

I have been instructed in the proper methods of lens care and handling. I understand the importance of adhering to proper lens care procedures and the need for periodic progress evaluations. I agree to follow the recommended wearing schedule and to keep scheduled appointments. I agree to follow my doctor's advice for the safe wear of lenses as indicated on this form and in my record of care. I will notify my doctor or University Optometric Group immediately if any eye or vision problems occur.

I understand that extended wear (overnight) contact lenses have many benefits but, as with any other drug or device, they are not without risks. I have been told that the risk of complications with extended wear (overnight) lenses is greater than for daily wear lenses. I have also been told that a small percentage of wearers develop serious complications, including conditions that can cause permanent eye injury and vision loss. For this reason, I agree to follow the advice and instructions provided by my doctor. I will remove my lenses and seek care immediately if I experience eye pain, redness, discharge, sensitivity to light, or decreased vision.

I have been told the nature, purpose, and benefits of extended wear (overnight) contact lenses. I know that there are feasible alternatives, including daily wear contact lenses and spectacles, available to me. I understand that I may not be able to wear extended wear (overnight) lenses successfully and that lens wear may have to be terminated. I know that I may ask any questions I wish concerning my lenses or the policies of University Optometric Group prior to the ordering of lenses.

By my signature I acknowledge that I have read, understood and received a copy of this fitting agreement. I agree to adhere to the policies, fees, and clinical requirements of University Optometric Group's **Fitting Agreement for Extended Wear (Overnight) Contact Lenses.**

_____

Signature of Patient

_____

Signature of Parent or Guardian

_____   _____

Date   Witness (initials)

Figure 11-2, Cont'd

mode of wear: daily wear, extended wear, disposable wear, or monovision for presbyopia. An important component of any fitting agreement is the contact lens prescription. The practitioner's policy for release of the prescription—which must be in accordance with the provisions of state law—should be made clear to the patient before the fitting. When a prescription is released to the patient, it should contain all the information necessary to allow the patient to obtain the lenses fitted.

Liability issues vary somewhat, based on the type of lens prescribed.

Daily Wear Lenses. The six major areas of litigation involving daily wear lenses, requiring the application of risk management, are the following:

- Fitting patients with nonapproved lenses or solutions or using approved lenses or solutions in a nonapproved manner (e.g., allowing disposable wear lenses to be cleaned overnight and reused)
- Inadequate disclosure of the limitations of monovision wear
- Failing to verify lens parameters before dispensing lenses to patients
- Negligence by a contact lens technician
- Misdiagnosis or inadequate management of contact lens–related corneal abrasions or infections
- Failing to periodically evaluate the ocular health (external and internal) of contact lens patients

The most important considerations are the management of contact lens–related abrasions and the periodic evaluation of the ocular health of contact lens wearers. If neglected, they create the best opportunity for significant injury and large damages.

Extended Wear Lenses. In addition to the problems enumerated for daily wear lenses, the following special considerations apply to patients fitted with extended wear lenses:

- Improper selection of patients for extended wear (e.g., patients with dry eye)
- Inadequate instruction given to patients (e.g., failing to inform patients of proper methods of lens disinfection and maintenance)
- Improper wearing schedule (e.g., recommending continuous wear beyond 6 nights without clinical justification)
- Improper management of contact lens–related complications (e.g., corneal abrasions that evolve into ulcerative keratitis)
- Inadequate monitoring of ocular health

A special concern is found in disposable lens wear. Because several months' supply of lenses are dispensed

to patients at one time, the customary obligation of inspecting and verifying lenses before dispensing cannot be fulfilled. The patient must be informed of this deviation from usual practice and instructed to return immediately for re-evaluation if acute problems arise after insertion of lenses (e.g., pain, redness, decreased acuity, discharge). This information should be included in the informed consent agreement.

Spectacle Lenses and Frames

Legal claims involving spectacles are brought because a lens or frame breaks, causing ocular injury. Spectacles are prescribed based on the primary purpose for which they will be used: dress wear, occupational or industrial use, or for athletic competition or sporting activities. Protection from injury is always a consideration regardless of the type of use, but whenever protection becomes a key clinical concern, the lens material of choice must be polycarbonate plastic. Patients for whom ocular protection is of importance constitute a sizable group of individuals, including the following:

Monocular persons

Athletes

Individuals whose occupation may place them at special risk for ocular injury (e.g., law enforcement officers)

Children

Persons with corneas that have been compromised by surgery (e.g., aphakia, penetrating keratoplasty, radial keratotomy)

Dress eyewear may be inadequate to protect patients from injury; industrial strength frames or athletic frames may be necessary, with polycarbonate lenses. If secondary use (such as occasional participation in athletic events) poses a significant risk of injury, patients must be advised of the need for protective eyewear, and the proper lenses and frames must be prescribed.

All lenses and frames prescribed for occupational or industrial use ("safety glasses") must meet specific federal standards for impact resistance. Eyewear must be inspected before it is dispensed to ensure that it meets these standards, which include a minimum lens thickness requirement (3 mm, regardless of lens material) and a "Z-87" logo for the frame.

Frames prescribed for athletic use—particularly for the racquet sports—should meet the requirements of American Society for Testing and Materials standard F803. Polycarbonate lenses are mandatory. The same type of frames should be prescribed for persons involved in contact sports such as baseball, basketball, and football.

Important Information About Your Glasses

Before you select the frames and lenses for your glasses, there are several things we need to consider. It is important that you describe to us the kinds of activities that you plan to undertake while wearing your glasses. If you will be wearing glasses at work, we need to know if there is a risk of injury to you from flying objects that could strike a lens and break it. If your job requires the use of safety glasses, you must tell us because special frames and lenses must be ordered. If you plan to wear your glasses while playing sports, please let us know so that we can help you select frames and lenses that will not create a risk of injury. In fact, if you participate in any activities that could potentially cause eye injury, you need to describe these activities to us so that we can advise you. Although no glasses are unbreakable, there are important differences between lenses and frames that make some glasses more protective when compared to others. We are here to help you choose the glasses that best satisfy your needs.

Lenses

A very important part of selecting your glasses is the choice of lens material. There are several different materials to choose from, and each has advantages and disadvantages, which are described below.

Glass—reasonably resistant to scratching and, as a photochromic lens, has good ability to darken in sunlight; in high prescriptions glass can be heavy; glass lenses may not withstand impact well.

Plastic—scratches more easily than glass, but lighter, especially in high prescriptions; can change darker in sunlight, and makes excellent sunwear; impact resistance is similar to glass.

High index plastic—used for high prescriptions because lenses are thinner and much lighter than other materials; withstands impact a little better than regular plastic; good for sunglasses.

Polycarbonate plastic—a high index material that is very impact resistant, which makes it the best choice for ocular protection; scratches more readily than glass but like other plastic materials is light and thus appropriate for high prescriptions; makes good non-prescription sunglasses too.

Frames

Another important consideration is the frame you select for your glasses. It should fit properly, be comfortable, and complement your appearance. It should also be safe. There are three basic categories of frames from which to choose.

Dress—these are the frames worn for everyday activities that do not pose a risk of injury; the great majority of frames serve this purpose, being suitable for wear at home, at work, and during play.

Safety—some frames have been specially designed to provide protection in the workplace; they can be identified by a "Z-87" logo on the frame; lenses for these frames must be of a certain thickness and have a special design in order for them to meet the requirements for "safety glasses".

Sports—eyewear for high risk activities such as racquetball, squash, baseball, basketball, and football must meet special design standards and be made of polycarbonate plastic; frames must meet the standards of "ASTM F-803" to provide optimum protection.

Making Your Choice

Please consider carefully your needs for both frames and lenses. Based on these needs, we will be pleased to advise and assist you in the selection of the eyewear most suitable for you, which will be marked below.

LENS MATERIAL	☐ Glass	☐ Plastic	☐ High Index	☐ Polycarbonate
FRAMES	☐ Dress	☐ Safety	☐ Sports	
SPECIAL ORDERS	☐ Antiscratch	☐ Antireflective	☐ Photochromic	☐ Sunglasses

_____   _____

Verified By   Date

Figure 11-3 Sample information sheet for ophthalmic materials.

In the dispensary, patients should be informed of the difference between lens materials and frame types, and the choice of eyewear should be documented (Figure 11-3).

Recordkeeping and Documentation

Even though care is provided in accordance with recognized standards, the defense of a legal claim may be impaired because the practitioner's record does not adequately describe the care rendered. There are two aspects to proper risk management: the use of an appropriate method of recordkeeping and the diligent documentation of test results, important communications, and treatment plans.

Problem-Oriented Records

To obtain efficient, clear, and thorough recordkeeping, a problem-oriented system should be used. Problem-oriented recordkeeping, whether applied to written or electronic records, achieves effective risk management and is the preferred method for optometrists (see Chapter 28). Risk management through documentation is most importantly directed at descriptions of findings, informed consent, and follow-up appointments.

Description of Findings. When recording examination findings, the optometrist should use descriptive terminology. Rather than empty terms such as "normal," "unremarkable," and "WNL" ("within normal limits"), language describing the practitioner's observations should be used (e.g., the optic nerve may be recorded as "C/D .3/.4, margins distinct, no pallor, NRRI" [neuroretinal rim intact]). Of particular importance are the findings of ophthalmoscopy and the slit lamp examination; in addition, the details of testing should be recorded (e.g., instruments used, drugs administered). All aspects of the eye health assessment should be accorded this descriptive documentation, which constitutes a most important part of the defense of a malpractice claim.

Informed Consent. The obligation to provide informed consent arises in many aspects of practice; examples include contact lens fittings, dilation of a narrow anterior chamber angle, and prescribing of drugs for treatment. To ensure that the appropriate information is conveyed and to preserve a written record of the patient's consent, printed forms are often used. These forms expedite the process of adhering to

informed consent requirements, provide excellent evidence should a legal dispute arise, and are a necessary part of clinical practice.

Follow-up Appointments and Referrals. If patients require follow-up visits, a definite recall appointment should be scheduled, even if the date is remote (e.g., 3 to 6 months in the future). The patient should be contacted by mail or telephone (or both) just before the appointment date and reminded of the examination. If referral is necessary, a practitioner should be chosen and contacted, and a definite appointment should be scheduled. The date of the appointment should be noted in the patient's record. If practical, a letter should be sent to the practitioner to whom the patient is being referred, describing the reason for the referral and requesting notification if the patient does not keep the appointment.

Maintaining well-organized records is one of the most important steps that clinicians can take to manage risk. The importance of proper recordkeeping and documentation as necessary components of risk management cannot be overemphasized.

Bibliography

Alexander LJ: *Primary care of the posterior segment*, ed 2. East Norwalk, Conn, 1994, Appleton & Lange.

Bettman JW: A review of 412 claims in ophthalmology. *Int Ophthalmol Clin* 20(4):131-42, 1980.

Bettman JW: Seven hundred medicolegal cases in ophthalmology. *Ophthalmology* 97:1379-84, 1990.

Classé JG: A review of 50 malpractice claims. *J Am Optom Assoc* 60:694-706, 1989.

Classé JG: *Legal aspects of optometry.* Boston, 1989, Butterworth.

Classé JG: The eye-opening case of *Keir v United States*. *J Am Optom Assoc* 60:471-6, 1989.

Classé JG: Medicolegal aspects of glaucoma. In Lewis TL, Fingeret M, editors: *Primary care of the glaucomas.* Norwalk, Conn, 1993, Appleton & Lange.

Classé JG: *Standards of practice for primary eyecare.* Columbus, Ohio, 1998, Anadem.

Classé JG, Harris MG: Medicolegal complications of contact lens wear. In J Silbert, editor: *Anterior segment complications of contact lens wear*, ed 2, Boston, 2000, Butterworth-Heinemann.

Davis MD: Natural history of retinal breaks without detachment. *Arch Ophthalmol* 92:183-94, 1974.

Elmstrom G: *Advanced management for optometrists.* Chicago, 1982, Professional Press.

Harris MG, Dister RE: Informed consent for extended wear patients. *Optom Clin* 1(4):33-50, 1991.

Lindner B: Acute posterior vitreous detachment and its retinal complications. *Acta Ophthalmol* 87(suppl 1):1-108, 1977.

Poggio EC, Glynn RJ, Schein OD, et al: The incidence of ulcerative keratitis among users of daily wear and extended wear contact lenses. *N Engl J Med* 321:779-83, 1989.

Schein OD, Glynn RJ, Poggio EC, et al: The relative risk of ulcerative keratitis among users of daily-wear and extended wear contact lenses: a case study. *N Engl J Med* 321:773-8, 1989.

Tasman W: Posterior vitreous detachment and peripheral retinal breaks. *Trans Am Acad Ophthalmol Otolaryngol* 72:217-24, 1968.

www.npdb-hipdb.com. Web site for the National Practitioner Data Bank.

Chapter *12*

Personal Insurance

John G. Classé

Protection is not a principle, but an expedient.
Benjamin Disraeli *Speech before the House of Commons, March 17, 1845*

A discussion of insurance would not be complete without some mention of the personal coverage that each individual requires to protect three very important aspects of life: health, home, and transportation.

Health Insurance

Before 1965, when Medicare was authorized by the U.S. Congress, health insurance provided lifetime care that was guaranteed to be renewable. Today, however, most policies terminate at age 65, when Medicare benefits begin, which means that the average optometrist will need a health care plan for about four decades (ages 25 to 65).

Health insurance is a highly preferred benefit of employment, but employed optometrists may find themselves limited by the plan that is offered by the employer. Extra or more inclusive provisions, if they can be added, must be paid for by the employee.

Self-employed optometrists have the following two concerns: health insurance as a benefit for employees and personal coverage for the optometrist and his or her family. In choosing a personal plan, the optometrist may be able to enroll in a health maintenance organization or preferred provider organization or may opt for basic medical coverage under Blue Cross/Blue Shield or similar providers.

The most basic coverage is a *major medical* policy, which is intended to defray the cost of catastrophic illness, a financially devastating eventuality for the uninsured. The following are two key aspects of major medical coverage: there is an annual deductible, which the insured must pay before the major medical coverage applies, and medical expenses that qualify under the plan and that exceed the deductible will be paid by the insurer up to a stated percentage, usually 80%. In addition, some plans will pay 100% of eligible expenses once a certain level is reached.

Hospital indemnity insurance is a supplemental insurance plan that can be used to provide protection for hospital expenses, and it can be added to pre-existing major medical or other health insurance. Benefits are typically paid directly to the recipient, beginning with the first day of hospitalization, and pay for as much as a year of continuous confinement. Benefits are often increased for a limited period if intensive care is required. There are limitations to such policies (60 and 65 being the customary ages beyond which no insurance can be obtained), and there are several important exclusions that are usually present in the policy (e.g., suicide, pregnancy, nursing home services, or pre-existing conditions).

Health insurance is usually available to employees of self-employed optometrists. Often, coverage is purchased at group rates, through organizations such as the American Optometric Association.

Individual coverage is more expensive, and cost, benefits, complexity, and other factors determine which coverage is appropriate for a given practitioner or family.

Plans that provide maternity leave are usually desirable; although a self-employed practitioner can choose a health insurance plan that provides appropriate coverage, an employed optometrist is limited to the plan provided by the employer. There is no legal requirement that an employer offer a health plan to employees, but if an employer opts to do so it must comply with the federal Employee Retirement Income Security Act (ERISA), as well as state requirements that often mandate maternity and prenatal care (unless the employer is self-insured). In many states these laws require that health care plans include minimum maternity stays. When an employer is self-insured, the plan is not governed by state laws but only by ERISA. These ERISA-controlled plans have been affected by the federal Health Insurance Portability and Accountability Act (HIPAA), which specifically addresses maternity leave.

HIPAA was enacted to provide health care coverage when changing employment. However, HIPAA only applies to employer-sponsored group health insurance plans. If a pregnant employed optometrist changes jobs, because of HIPAA the new employer's group health insurance plan cannot deny coverage (by citing a "pre-existing condition"). But an employee changing from one individual health plan to another individual health plan or from a group plan to an individual plan might not get prenatal or maternity coverage at all, might have to endure a "waiting period" (period before the new plan becomes effective), or may have to buy expensive individual coverage.

A self-insured employer that offers group health benefits, if it includes maternity coverage, cannot exclude a new employee's pregnancy under a "pre-existing condition" clause. However, there can be a waiting period before coverage begins, even for employees eligible for insurance coverage under HIPAA.

A federal law known as COBRA (Consolidated Omnibus Budget Reconciliation Act) allows qualified workers, their spouses, and their dependent children to maintain insurance coverage when it might otherwise be cut off. Under COBRA, if an employee voluntarily leaves a job or is terminated for any reason other than "gross misconduct," the employee is guaranteed the right to continue the former employer's group plan for individual or family health insurance, for up to 18 months, at the employee's expense. However, individual plans–those purchased individually rather than through work or an association–are not subject to COBRA law. In addition, employers are not required to offer COBRA unless they have at least 20 employees.

If maternity leave is offered by an employer, plan requirements must conform to the federal Pregnancy Discrimination Act (PDA). The PDA requires that women affected by pregnancy be treated in the same manner as other employees with similar abilities or limitations. The Federal Maternity Leave Act requires employers to permit 12 weeks of unpaid leave for the birth and care of a newborn, but the law only applies to employees who have at least a year of employment and to large employers (more than 50 employees).

Homeowner's Insurance

There are three types of homeowner's insurance: mortgage insurance; personal liability insurance; and dwelling, unscheduled personal property, and living expense insurance. Mortgage insurance is usually purchased as a decreasing term rider on a permanent insurance policy, but it can be purchased separately. Personal liability insurance and dwelling, unscheduled personal property, and living expense insurance both can be included within a standard homeowner's policy.

Mortgage insurance. This type of insurance protects a spouse against the eventuality that, with the insured's death, the spouse will no longer have the income to meet the mortgage payments. Mortgage insurance pays the mortgage balance in the event the insured dies, thus ensuring that the home will be unencumbered (see Chapter 9).

Personal liability insurance. Coverage provides an insured with protection against legal liability for any nonvehicular accidents that might occur on the insured's property. The usual type of eventuality is a "slip and fall" injury.

Dwelling, unscheduled personal property, and living expense insurance. This type of insurance covers a number of perils that involve an insured's home. It protects the dwelling against fire, lightning, and other catastrophe, to the policy limits; in addition, extended coverage against hail, windstorm, explosion, riot, falling trees, or crashing cars can be obtained. Coverage also can be provided for the theft or loss of personal items. As an adjunct to such coverage the insured needs to keep the receipts of all major purchases or take photographs of these items in the house or apartment. (An inventory also is a good idea.) The preferred type of coverage is called "replacement value" (rather than "cash value") because it allows replacement of the damaged or destroyed item with one of the same kind and quality, to the limits of the policy. "Extended Replacement" coverage will pay above the policy limits, if necessary.

The owner of items of special value (e.g., jewelry, art, antiques) should check with the insurer to make sure that those items are covered. If there is a homeowner's policy, the personal goods in the home may be insured for a percentage of insurance on the dwelling (between 50% and 70%), but this coverage may not be sufficient for extreme valuable items (discussed infra).

In the event that a home is damaged and made unfit for habitation, living expense insurance provides coverage for the period that the insured and his or her family are forced to live outside the home while it is being repaired, but the extent of these payments is limited to a percentage of dwelling coverage (usually 20%).

To these basic homeowner's provisions there may be added a fourth type of coverage: "scheduled" property. All standard homeowner's policies will limit financial reimbursement for the loss of certain items, such as jewelry, silverware, works of art, antiques, and similar things of value. To insure this property, the individual items (e.g., a wedding ring, silver flatware, or original paintings) will have to be valued separately, or "scheduled," on the policy. The item will be protected for the scheduled value in the event of theft, loss, or destruction. Of course, the premium cost escalates when there is increased insurance coverage, and the policyholder will have to weigh this added cost and the risk of loss before deciding whether to schedule such items. In addition, before purchasing a home-owner's policy, care should be taken to ensure that it meets the policyholder's needs.

Vehicle Insurance

An optometrist must adequately insure any vehicle that is used in a private practice, especially if employees are permitted to drive it. A personal vehicle also deserves adequate insurance coverage. The types of coverage are established by state law and usually include liability, collision, comprehensive, medical payments, and uninsured motorist coverage.

Liability insurance. This type of coverage provides protection if the insured (or other insureds) cause an accident that results in personal injury, property damage, or both. The insurance company will defend the policyholder in court and pay all judgments against the policyholder up to the policy limit. The policy limit is expressed as a ratio, such as $100,000/$300,000; this example means that coverage extends up to $100,000 per claimant and up to an aggregate total of $300,000 for all claimants involved in the accident.

Collision insurance. This type of coverage reimburses the insured for damage done to the insured's vehicle (less a deductible), even if the insured is at fault.

Comprehensive insurance. This type of insurance protects an insured vehicle against virtually all hazards (e.g., fire, vandalism, hail, theft) except collision. Deductible coverage is probably the best form in which to purchase this coverage.

Medical payment insurance. This type of insurance covers the expenses that the insured and passengers incur if

injured in an accident—even the ambulance bill—no matter who is responsible for the accident. These benefits are limited in amount.

Uninsured motorist insurance. This type of coverage protects the insured against personal injury caused by a motorist who has no insurance. It also provides coverage in the event of a hit-and-run accident that results in personal injury caused by an uninsured or unidentified motorist. In some states this coverage can be added to the insurance of an underinsured motorist whose coverage is inadequate to pay for the insured's personal injuries.

An optometrist should not neglect personal insurance needs in favor of those for the practice. Premium costs can be controlled by a knowledgeable purchaser. Higher deductibles for liability coverage and lower collision and comprehensive coverage for older vehicles of reduced value can assist in decreasing premiums. Medical payments coverage will not be necessary if the insured also has health insurance. In addition, discounts may be offered by insurers, usually for the following:

- Low-mileage use of the vehicle
- Safety features (e.g., airbags, anti-lock brakes)
- Anti-theft devices (e.g., alarms, wheel-locking systems, window identification systems)
- Safe driving records and passage of approved driver's education courses
- Good grades achieved by students

Insurers should be asked about discounts for vehicle coverage, especially for younger drivers for whom premiums tend to be high.

Uses

Since individual needs and circumstances vary, trying to predict the insurance coverage appropriate for all persons would be an impossible undertaking. Therefore, only the most common use of personal insurance is described.

Health Insurance

Health insurance in general, and major medical coverage in particular, is most commonly purchased through a group plan because of the reduced cost. The best policies are those that provide virtually unlimited maximums and are offered by large, stable companies. If coverage other than major medical is desired, care should be exercised. Certain limited policies—such as those paying benefits only for certain diseases (cancer, for example)—may be duplicative and unnecessary. Probably the biggest decision in this regard comes when the optometrist has reached 65 and is eligible for Medicare; extra insurance may be purchased to "plug the gaps" in Medicare coverage.

Homeowner's Insurance

Homeowner's insurance should be reviewed annually to ensure that the policy limits are adequate, particularly in the event there is a total loss. Since the premiums are paid as part of the monthly mortgage, it is easy to forget about policy details. Property appreciation and inflation make such an omission a serious mistake.

Familiarity with the homeowner's policy also is necessary to understand the type of eventualities for which there is coverage, the applicable deductibles, and the maximum coverage for each type of loss. Of particular interest are the types of casualty discussed previously: mortgage protection; personal liability; dwelling, unscheduled personal property, and living expense coverage; and scheduled property insurance.

Casualty and theft losses not covered by insurance are deductible only to the extent that they exceed 10% of the individual's adjusted gross income in the year of loss, which means that only a very limited deduction is possible. This fact makes adequate insurance protection more important than ever.

Vehicle Insurance

Most individuals have their first exposure to insurance when they insure an automobile, and during the course of years, the ownership of automobiles (or other vehicles) will result in the contribution of many thousands of dollars for insurance protection. Nevertheless, because of the risk of loss, automobile insurance is an absolute necessity, including uninsured motorist coverage, which is optional in some states.

A long-term proposition such as vehicle insurance requires selectivity on the part of the individual seeking coverage. Insurers vary tremendously in terms of coverage offered, cost, renewability, and reputation, and policies should be selected with great care. Vehicle policies generally fall into one of the following two categories:

Family policies. Insurance protection exists whether the insured is driving his or her vehicle, a vehicle belonging to someone else, or a rented one. These policies also extend protection to members of the household when they drive an insured vehicle and to others who drive the vehicle with permission. Additional coverage may protect members of the household when they drive someone else's vehicle.

Special policies. Insurance protection is offered as a package at rates less than those of family policies. Benefits automatically include medical payment coverage, death benefits, and uninsured motorist coverage. The addition of comprehensive or collision insurance brings with it personal property coverage and towing coverage. Special policies usually do not pay for injuries that are covered by other insurance.

Family policies that are not markedly more expensive than special policies should be given preference because they will provide some coverage that special policies cannot. Another consideration is how the coverage is purchased: if all casualty insurance—automobile, homeowners, practice—is purchased from one insurance company, the optometrist with a valid claim has a little more leverage to exert than he or she would otherwise.

Tax Issues

Self-employed optometrists may deduct the premiums paid for health insurance coverage for themselves, their spouses, and dependents (see Chapter 38). In addition, the health insurance premiums purchased by an optometrist for the benefit of employees are deductible as a business expense.

There is no deduction permitted for insurance premiums paid for an individual's private vehicle insurance. Premiums for business vehicles may be deducted as a necessary business expense. The extent of the deduction depends on the extent of the vehicle's use for business purposes (see Chapter 39).

A homeowner cannot deduct the cost of the premiums paid for homeowner's insurance. Uninsured casualty losses may be deducted to the extent they exceed 10% of the homeowner's adjusted gross income and if they are not compensable by insurance.

Bibliography

Classé JG: *Legal aspects of optometry.* Boston, 1989, Butterworth.

Consumer Reports: *Annual automobile rating guide.* Available at: *www.consumerreports.org.*

Elmstrom G: *Advanced management for optometrists.* Chicago, 1982, Professional.

Internal Revenue Service publication 17, *Your federal income tax.*

Internal Revenue Service publication 969, *Medical savings accounts.*

Newcomb RD, Marshall EC, editors: *Public health and community optometry,* ed 2. Stoneham, Mass, 1990, Butterworth.

www.iii.org. Web site for the Insurance Information Institute.

www.insure.com. Web site for Standard and Poor's profiles and ratings of insurance companies.

www.pueblo.gsa.gov. Web site for the Federal Consumer Information Center, which provides information on insurance.

Section Four

Starting a Practice

Chapter *13*

Principles of Negotiation

Lawrence S. Thal

We arg'ed the thing at breakfast, we arg'ed the thing at tea,
And the more we arg'ed the question, the more we didn't agree.
William Carleton *Farm Ballads*

Whereas many authorities believe that good negotiators are born that way or that negotiation is a skill best learned through experience, successful negotiators are almost always those individuals who are best prepared–best prepared with information regarding their own position and the position of the person(s) with whom they are negotiating. This chapter discusses the process of negotiation to help optometrists prepare for a successful negotiating experience, whether it be for a lease, associateship or partnership, purchase of a practice, purchase or sale of equipment, or other opportunity.

Negotiation is a process in which two or more participants attempt to reach a joint decision on matters of common concern in situations in which they are in actual or potential disagreement or conflict. The quality of a negotiated agreement is measured by the extent to which it meets the interests of all parties concerned. Inherent in this process is the need to determine accurately what those interests are, for both parties. It often has been proved that the negotiation that provides a clear winner in the short run provides no winners in the long run. The early "winner" often ends up a loser because the other party has realized that the agreement is unfair.

Conversely, in a "win-win" negotiation, both parties are motivated to abide by their agreements, thereby avoiding conflicts and problems. Negotiation is primarily an exercise in problem solving, an exercise in which the process identifies and exploits opportunities for joint gain.

Competitive tactics, such as threats or demands, undermine a negotiator's credibility and prevent the attainment of a mutually beneficial outcome. Cooperative tactics, on the other hand, include reasonable offers, fair and just arguments, and concessions designed to encourage reciprocity. The use of cooperative tactics is based on the premise that behavior that is fair, reasonable, and accommodating is more likely to encourage a similar response. Although the rationale for using cooperative tactics is an expectation that the other party will reciprocate, the weakness of this strategy is its vulnerability to exploitation by a negotiator who does not match a cooperative negotiator's concessions. Cooperative tactics also require an exchange of information between the negotiators and a responsiveness by the negotiators to each other's interests and needs. Each negotiator must assess the willingness of the other to be cooperative; if this willingness is not present, the offering of concessions or compromise should be curtailed.

Negotiations should adhere to the following steps:

- Fact-finding
- Planning and preparation
- Establishment of an initial relationship with the other side
- Initial proposals
- Exchange of information
- Narrowing of differences
- Closure and implementation

Each of these steps is described briefly, as applied to negotiation by optometrists.

Fact-Finding

The optometrist seeking to negotiate an agreement should attempt to obtain useful information regarding the other negotiator. Does this person enjoy a good reputation? Does the person have a past history of legal conflicts or problems? If there were problems, what were their nature and outcome? If the person is an optometrist, what have previous relationships with other optometrists been like? What do other associates (present and past) or other tenants have to say about the person? This type of fact-finding is aimed at determining whether the individual is someone with whom one wishes to negotiate at all.

If this is a lease negotiation, what are the market rents? What are other tenants paying, and what are the terms of their leases? What do other tenants say about the landlord's willingness to honor the terms of the lease? What is the vacancy rate now, and what has it been in the past? What mortgages exist, and what is the financial condition of the owner?

If this is a partnership, what has been the negotiator's relationship with other partners, employers, or associates? What are the revenues of the practice now, and what does a pro forma analysis reveal for the future?

If this is the sale of a practice, have there been other attempts to sell it? What was the outcome of those negotiations? What are the seller's plans: to remain in the area or to move away after the sale? What is the seller's reputation in the community? Is the practice growing? Is it economically sound? The answers to these questions, as well as to questions considering the future economic prospects of the practice, will dictate whether negotiation should be undertaken.

The negotiator with the greater knowledge of the subject matter to be negotiated is in the more advantageous position by far. Fact-finding, however, is not limited to the period before the negotiations begin. Fact-finding continues throughout the negotiations because, to the extent that one side learns of the other side's needs and concerns, it becomes more likely that a compromise can be structured creatively to satisfy everyone's goals.

In Chapter 17, the preparation of pro forma economic analysis is discussed. Such an analysis is essential in determining a "bottom line" in the negotiation process. Too often leases are entered into because the negotiator rationalizes that "it was the best I could find" or "all the leases are at that rate," regardless of what the economic projection might have shown.

Part of the fact-finding process should be devoted to considering what sources of influence, leverage, or power one party holds over the other. Each party's alternatives to a negotiated agreement and their relative needs to reach an agreement are the most important factors in determining bargaining power.

Planning and Preparation

This part of the negotiation process involves preparing a strategy, developing goals, and anticipating argu-

ments from the other negotiator. It involves the preparation of arguments and demonstrations (e.g., graphs, charts, economic projections) that justify an offer or show why concessions requested by the other negotiator can or cannot be met.

The willingness to show why certain positions are taken and others are rejected further contributes to a cooperative approach and helps to avoid antagonism and mistrust. Anticipating the other negotiator's position and arguments helps improve preparation and may even reveal areas in which more fact-finding is necessary. This part of the process must determine—at a minimum—the specific goals, terms, and conditions necessary for the negotiation to be a success.

Establishing an Initial Relationship with the Other Side

In using a cooperative strategy to achieve an agreement that is fair and just to both parties, it is necessary to develop a relationship with the other negotiator that is characterized by goodwill and trust. The first phase of negotiation sets the initial tone of the relationship between the parties and may establish the character of the relationship for the remainder of the negotiation. This phase of the negotiation process may include information gathering and disclosure and exchange of initial proposals, and, to some degree, it sets the foundation for later phases.

It is usually advantageous to be the first to present an initial draft agreement or written offer. That act often establishes the first position, from which offers of compromise will be made. Once a draft agreement is offered, it should be possible to determine which issues are contentious. Sometimes it is best to negotiate the least contentious issues first to build rapport and trust between the parties before tackling the most difficult topics. On the other hand, should the parties get through the most contentious issues first, it is unlikely that negotiations will break down over less controversial provisions, thereby jeopardizing the agreements already reached. However, negotiators should avoid the tendency to allow animosity resulting from contentious bargaining on major issues to overflow into negotiations on issues that are less important.

Some negotiators believe that there is a decided advantage to negotiate on one's own premises or in one's own surroundings, and some empirical research seems to confirm that negotiators who bargain on their own territory are likely to increase both their assertiveness and the chances of a favorable negotiation outcome. However, "home" advantage means only as much as the negotiator permits it to mean. Negotiations, like sporting events, cannot always take place in the negotiator's own surroundings, and neutral sites (as diplomats often seek in Geneva or Helsinki) are not always practical. Even if a negotiator feels more comfortable and less likely to lose confidence in familiar surroundings, that seeming advantage may be offset by other factors. For example, if documents are needed to refute a certain contention, one is expected to access them immediately when negotiating in his or her own office. The documents would not necessarily be available in the other negotiator's office; this delay can allow more time for preparation.

In this phase of the negotiation process, it is desirable to create an atmosphere in which negotiators attempt to maximize joint gains by first creating a psychological state characterized by mutual trust, a shared desire to achieve joint gains, and open and honest communication.

Initial Proposals

The first proposal in a negotiation, if credible and convincing, usually becomes the focal point from which further bargaining proceeds. It should be thoughtfully and carefully considered before presentation. Justification for this initial proposal should be presented to validate its credibility and to limit the extent of further negotiation.

It is a mistake, when presenting an offer, to imply that it is the final offer or that the other side must "take it or leave it." Such an attitude destroys the negotiation process, is rarely credible, and demonstrates an attitude completely unfavorable to maximizing joint gains.

An initial proposal should be moderate enough to communicate to the other party that the negotiator is trying to be reasonable in establishing a cooperative bargaining relationship. On the other hand, the initial proposal must contain enough of a cushion to allow the negotiator to make concessions so that he or she does not appear intractable in later phases of the negotiation. Early cooperation facilitates the development of trust and a mutually beneficial and amicable relationship.

Exchange of Information

No other aspect of negotiation is as important as the exchange of information between negotiators. Negotiation can be viewed as a process in which each negotiator learns enough about what the other party needs and wants in order to propose an agreement that is acceptable to both sides. A full and accurate exchange of information allows both parties to participate in the creation of compromises and solutions. Even though providing information to the other negotiator can be risky to one's bargaining position, it dramatically enhances the ability of the negotiator to reach a fair and just compromise. The expectation is that both parties will exchange concessions in the same spirit that they trade information.

Any information that assists in determining the other side's requirements, abilities, or expectations is useful. For example, when leasing an office, it is valuable to learn the terms and conditions of the lease agreements held by other tenants. Knowledge regarding the building owner's costs, renewal rates, vacancy history, financial condition, and related matters can be obtained independently, before negotiations begin. This information can be expanded during the negotiations themselves.

The most effective way to gather information is to ask questions. Even the most direct question ("What will it take to resolve this issue?") can be helpful. Less direct and open-ended questions often yield more information. Different forms of questioning should be attempted to determine which will elicit the most information. Specific questions work best, however, when the questioner's information needs are well defined.

Silence is an overlooked information-gathering technique. Obviously, it is difficult to gain information when one is doing all the talking. However, there are ethical and legal considerations involved with failing to disclose material facts. Such concealment could be fraudulent. It is important to be truthful in responses because the other negotiator relies on the information provided as a basis for agreements.

Narrowing of Differences

This phase involves the bargaining or "haggling" part of the negotiation process. Even while narrowing down the differences in their positions, negotiators continue to gather information. Awarding concessions is an affirmative step. It is taken to elicit cooperation and to receive concessions in return; it is not an indication that the negotiator is losing. Human nature is such that individuals tend to cooperate with those who cooperate in return. Therefore, the willingness to offer concessions should not be viewed as a weakness in the negotiation process. Sometimes it is best to indicate flexibility on an issue before offering a specific concession, since once a concession is offered, it usually cannot be withdrawn easily.

If fatigue, irritability, or anger during this phase of negotiations threatens the success of the negotiation process, it is advisable to take a recess and resume negotiations at a later time. Often a break will allow one side or the other to develop a compromise. For example, if a lease agreement hinges on the insistence of the owner that the prospective tenant pay $2300-per-month for 7 years, when, during the first 2 years, the prospective tenant can only pay $1600, an impasse is obviously reached. During a break in the negotiations, the prospective tenant can calculate a counter offer (based on his or her knowledge or with assistance from someone who has that knowledge) that would provide the owner exactly the same total rent in today's dollars and yet meet the prospective tenant's financial expectations. Such a counter offer might entail the use of graduated payments during the 7 years, starting with $1600 per month in the first year and increasing each year so that during the 7-year period a $2300 per month average is obtained.

Occasionally it may appear that negotiations are breaking down entirely. It is better to allow this to happen than to enter into a completely unfavorable agreement. Sometimes a more creative approach may be able to salvage the negotiations. A perfect example of creativity in the case of a practice sale is to consider purchase on the basis of an earn-out (conditional sale price) versus a fixed price. This provides flexibility and yet preserves the financial expectations of both parties. The use of expert advice or a mediator might help. Options are limited only by the creativity of the negotiator.

Closure and Implementation

When it appears that the parties have reached an agreement, all the elements agreed on should be repeated in summary form to ensure that there has been mutual understanding and that a "meeting of the minds" has resulted on each issue. It may be advisable to reduce the agreement to a written summary at this time. At a minimum, a letter summarizing the terms agreed on should be prepared the next day. This summary or letter can be used as the basis for a formal written contract.

Typically, one of the negotiators volunteers to have an attorney draft the written agreement. It is often to one's advantage to have one's own attorney do this, rather than the other negotiator's attorney; the language used will not be necessarily the same from attorney to attorney.

Additionally, minor details not specifically negotiated are often identified in this first draft. It is important that each party review the written contract carefully to ensure that it clearly and correctly describes each and every point. Each party will expect the other side to abide by the contract's provisions, and the contract will be used to settle any disagreements or questions arising after it has been signed.

Conclusion

Negotiation is a vital skill that every optometrist will be required to demonstrate periodically during a professional career. The most important phase of the negotiation process is the gathering of information, which is used to prepare for negotiations and to justify the offering of compromise positions when negotiations have reached an impasse. The underlying principle that should guide negotiators is one of fairness, which is usually attained through compromise by both parties. If an agreement is not fair, it usually will fail—with the complications and difficulties that are attendant to such failure. Therefore, negotiators should enter into discussions having obtained the necessary information, with "win-win" alternatives prepared for presentation. They should be willing to propose compromises that will obtain a successful result for both parties.

Bibliography

Cleary PJ: *The negotiation handbook.* Armonk, NY, 2001, M.E. Sharpe.

Gifford DG: *Legal negotiation, theory and applications.* St. Paul, Minn, 1989, West Publishing.

Gulliver PH: *Disputes and negotiations: a cross-cultural perspective.* New York, 1979, Academic.

Lewicki RJ: *Negotiation,* ed 3. Boston, 1999, Irwin/McGraw-Hill.

Lewicki RJ: *Essentials of negotiation,* ed 2. Boston, 2001, Irwin/McGraw-Hill.

Martindale DA: Territorial dominance behavior in dyadic verbal interaction. *Proceedings of the 79th Annual Convention of the American Psychological Association* 6(1):305-6, 1971.

Rubin J, Brown B: *The social psychology of bargaining and negotiation.* New York, 1964, Academic.

Thal L: The practice sale: getting to the bottom line. *Optom Management* 10(6):66-7, 1986.

Chapter 14

Deciding Where to Practice

Craig Hisaka and John G. Classé

"Would you tell me, please, which way I ought to go from here?"

"That depends a good deal on where you want to get to," said the Cheshire Cat.

"I don't much care where—" said Alice.

"Then it doesn't matter which way you go," said the Cat.

Lewis Carroll *Alice in Wonderland*

How does an optometrist decide where to practice? Many choices and options exist, in terms of the type of practice and its location. Is a private group practice in the downtown of a major city–specializing in contact lenses–preferable or would a solo, small-town family practice in the rural countryside be more appealing? Would the practice of low vision hospital-based optometry be rewarding or would a teaching career in a pediatric clinic be of more interest? Practice opportunities exist from Guam to Alaska, from England to Japan. With so many areas of the world available in which to live and work, the decision on where to locate requires serious thought and study. It also requires goal setting. If an optometrist cannot identify the type of practice and community that is preferred, attempting to determine a location will be an exercise in frustration. In choosing a place to practice, individual values and lifestyle, the part of the country in which one has lived, and the personal and professional goals of the person are all factors that affect the decision.

This chapter provides guidance intended to focus thoughts on how to select the ideal community. The aim is to help optometrists (and students) determine what they desire in terms of livability of a community, assess the practice potential of the area, and decide whether the economy of the area can support the type of practice desired. The answers to these questions constitute the components of a *feasibility study* (Box 14-1). This chapter helps one to understand the analysis process through the presentation of information on livability, economics, and practice potential.

Finding "Value" in a Location

The assessment of "value" in determining livability will be the most significant issue in deciding where to practice. Is it important that there be local access to hunting, boating, five-star restaurants, live theater, mountain climbing, golf, professional sports, or symphony performances? Would the slower pace of a rural community be preferable? Is it critical that family members live close by? Are the presence of crowds, air pollution, crime, and traffic jams bothersome? If a practitioner loves the community in which the practitioner works, this attitude will be reflected to patients and staff. Similarly, if a practitioner enjoys living in a locale, the practitioner will want to become an integral part of local society and will give to the community more than just optometric care. Most patients enjoy seeing their doctor participate in local and civic activities. Today, so much information is available, that with an investment of time and effort, a community can be thoroughly evaluated for livability. There are numerous books and magazines that address the livability of communities. For example, *Places Rated Almanac* is a guide to finding the best places to live in America. The book ranks and compares 337 metropolitan areas for climate, housing, health, crime, transportation, education, the arts, recreation, and economic outlook. A visit to the local bookstore or library or a search of the Internet will provide access to many other references that examine livability factors of communities. If an optometrist has selected a particular state, information should be sought that has been published specific to that state. For example, if an optometrist were

Box 14-1 Components of a Feasibility Study

A feasibilty study of an area should do the following:
- Identify a target patient base for the area and determine how best to serve it
- Recognize current and potential competition in the area's eye care market
- Assess the financial risks involved in pursuing the objective of establishing a practice
- Establish the financial resources needed to begin the practice
- Determine whether the practice can differentiate itself from other practices in the area, based on available resources and capabilities

interested in California, it would be helpful to review the book *California, Where to Live and Work*. The book provides essential information on topics such as affordable housing, ratings of schools, climate, cultural information, and fastest-growing job areas. The local Chamber of Commerce can be very helpful with information regarding livability. A letter requesting information regarding livability is usually answered with many pamphlets, fliers, and general information regarding the benefits of living and working in the community. A sample letter to a Chamber of Commerce is easy to write and requires little time (Figure 14-1). The addresses of Chambers of Commerce can be found in the *World Wide Chamber of Commerce Directory*. Optometrists should be cautious about the literature that is received, however, since each Chamber of Commerce is in the business of promoting its community. The advertising that is received may be biased.

Once the decision has been narrowed to three to six communities, it is highly advisable to plan a trip to each community. These trips inevitably will include communities that appeared great on paper but that may not accommodate the optometrist's priorities. On a first visit to a community, an initial impression of the city and area will be formed. If a poor first impression is obtained, the optometrist should continue to the next community. The optometrist should plan to spend at least one full day in communities that give a positive first impression.

Figure 14-2 provides a necessary guideline to assist in the proper assessment of a community. The optometrist should begin by thinking about what is valued in a community. The directions for the exercise are printed at the top of the form. The form should be filled in as directed with an "H," "M," or "L" to indicate whether the item is of high, moderate, or low importance. The exercise helps determine what is of priority

Chamber of Commerce
Main Street
Anytown, CA

To Whom it May Concern:

Would you please send me information about _____? I am interested in the economic profile, housing, weather, education and recreation. Helpful information would include major employers, population statistics for 1990 and 2000, ethnic breakdown and income levels (per capita, median household).

I would also like information about the current eyecare providers in your city. If possible, please send me a photocopy of the yellow pages that list optometrists, ophthalmologists and opticians for the area.

Thank you very much for your help. If you have any questions, please let me know.

Figure 14-1 Sample letter to a Chamber of Commerce requesting information about a community's economy, livability, and optometric practice potential.

WHAT YOU WANT A COMMUNITY TO OFFER

DIRECTIONS: For each item below, think about its relative importance or value to you. Place an (H) for high importance, (M) for moderate importance, or (L) for low importance next to each item.

____	Clean water	____	Small chance of radon gas
____	Low crime rate	____	Commuting time
____	Clean air	____	Low unemployment rate
____	Many doctors	____	Local amusements
____	Availability of hospitals	____	Proximity to a big airport
____	Strong state government	____	Near places of worship
____	Cost of medical care	____	National forests or parks
____	Low income taxes	____	Chance of natural disasters
____	Low property taxes	____	Sunny weather
____	Housing appreciation	____	Close to relatives
____	Recession insulation	____	Quality restaurants
____	Inexpensive cost of living	____	Near a big city
____	Strong local income growth	____	Low housing prices
____	Future job growth	____	Public transportation
____	Low sales tax	____	Museums nearby
____	Cheap car insurance	____	Major league sports teams
____	Good public schools	____	Local symphony orchestras
____	Conservationists' rating	____	Major zoos or aquariums
____	Civic involvement	____	Amtrak service
____	Near lakes, oceans	____	Skiing close by
____	Close to colleges	____	Minor-league sport teams
____	Potential state tax rise	____	Near golf courses

Figure 14-2 Rating scale to determine the personal "value" of a community.

to a given optometrist in a community. The "high importance" elements should be used as a reference and guide when analyzing communities. A spouse or other significant advisor also should perform this exercise, so that all persons affected by the decision can analyze and discuss answers among themselves.

Assessing the Past and Present Economic Pictures of a Community

When most new businesses begin (or if a business expands), an economic study is performed to determine whether the community can support the business. For example, if McDonalds or Pizza Hut decided to place a restaurant in a city, the area involved would be critically and analytically studied with respect to population, employment statistics, retail sales, and many other factors. An optometrist's practice plans likewise should include an economic study to help ensure that the community can support another practice.

To perform such an evaluation, a market study needs to be performed. Information must be collected

regarding population, growth rate, new building permits, per capita income, median household income, eye care providers, and ethnic and age analyses (Figure 14-3).

A thorough comparison of communities regarding demographic and economic characteristics will be of great assistance in selecting a practice location. Economic characteristics include factors such as population changes, number of households, educational attainment, income and poverty, civilian labor force, housing units, new building permits, and municipal financial revenues and expenditures. An excellent source of information for statistics related to an area's economy can be found in the *Rand McNally Commercial Atlas and Marketing Guide*. The atlas is one of the best resources for economic data, population demographics and estimates, and city ratings.

The atlas is an excellent reference for statistics and interpretation of business data. It includes many categories, including the following:
- Buying power index
- Drug store sales
- Effective buying income

Date _____

Market analysis for_____
                              City,   State
City population   1990_____ 2000_____

County population 1990_____ 2000_____

City population forecast for 2000_____

City growth rate_____%; County growth rate_____%

New building permits_____

* * * * * * * * *

Per capita income_____ Median household income_____

Persons in poverty_____ Total households_____

* * * * * * * * *

Three major employers:

   1._____ Employing_____

   2._____ Employing_____

   3._____ Employing_____

Unemployment rate:_____

* * * * * * * * *

Optometrists in city_____ Ophthalmologists in city_____

Opticians in city_____ Optical chains in city_____

* * * * * * * * *

Ethnic analysis: Asian/Pac. island_____   Black_____

Amer. Indian_____   Hispanic_____   Spanish origin_____

White_____

Age analysis

| Under 5_____ | 6-17_____ |
| 18-64_____ | >64_____ |

Figure 14–3 Research form for information collected during a feasibility study.

- Estimated population
- Food store sales
- Per capita income
- Shopping goods sales
- Zip code sectional areas

Another source of information is the *Census Catalog and Guide*. This book, published by the U.S. Department of Commerce's Bureau of the Census, is a resource for reports, computer tapes, maps, micro-fiche, online access, and floppy disks. The information available is in areas of business, construction, housing, manufacturing, population, transportation, and related subjects.

If new major national stores have recently moved into an area, it is likely that they have conducted significant economic studies. One predominant new business can greatly impact a community's population, tax base, housing, and business climate. Conversely, the loss of a vital business can have a deleterious effect on a community.

Determining the Optometric Practice Potential for an Area

One key aspect of the study of an area is to determine whether there is a need for additional optometrists. Opening a practice in an area highly saturated with eye care providers may lead to slow practice growth and development. Box 14-2 provides a current evaluation of the distribution of optometrists, including areas that are saturated and areas that have need for additional optometrists. A thorough study of an area's current eye care providers, the types of services provided, and the vision care needs of the population will enable the optometrist to make an intelligent assessment. Key questions to ask during this assessment include the following:

- Can the community support another eye care provider?
- Does the community makeup support practice goals?

Box 14-2 U.S. Optometrist Demographics, 1997

AREA	LICENSED OPTOMETRISTS PER 100,000 PERSONS	AREA	LICENSED OPTOMETRISTS PER 100,000 PERSONS
		Georgia	9.3
Northeast	**12.2**	Maryland	9.0
New England	14.6	North Carolina	10.5
Connecticut	12.9	South Carolina	9.2
Maine	15.1	Virginia	11.7
Massachusetts	15.9	West Virginia	12.3
New Hampshire	12.8	**East South Central**	**11.4**
Rhode Island	16.2	Alabama	10.2
Vermont	11.6	Kentucky	11.4
Mid-Atlantic	11.3	Mississippi	8.3
New Jersey	11.8	Tennessee	14.0
New York	9.5	**West South Central**	**10.2**
Pennsylvania	13.8	Arkansas	12.1
		Louisiana	8.1
Midwest	**13.1**	Oklahoma	16.1
East North Central	12.7	Texas	9.3
Illinois	13.7		
Indiana	14.3	**West**	**13.1**
Michigan	10.7	Mountain	12.4
Ohio	12.8	Arizona	9.8
Wisconsin	12.6	Colorado	14.5
West North Central	13.8	Idaho	15.2
Iowa	14.3	Montana	20.2
Kansas	15.5	Nevada	9.6
Minnesota	11.4	New Mexico	12.5
Missouri	12.4	Utah	9.9
Nebraska	15.4	Wyoming	17.6
North Dakota	24.8	Pacific	13.4
South Dakota	19.0	Alaska	13.8
		California	13.0
South		Hawaii	17.5
South Atlantic	10.5	Oregon	15.6
Delaware	8.9	Washington	13.5
District of Columbia	12.6	**U.S. Total**	**12.0**
Florida	11.4		

Sources: Project Hope National Census of Optometrists, 1997; American Optometric Association, St. Louis. Reprinted with permission.

- What are the referral patterns of professionals in the area?
- Does state law allow adequate use of therapeutic pharmaceutical agents?

To find answers to these questions, the optometrist needs to analyze the practice potential of a community. A key consideration is the optometrist-to-population ratio in a community. These ratios serve as guidelines to estimate the economic viability of an area. When individual communities are studied, it may be found that a community with 10,000 people has five optometrists. However, the community may be able to support an additional optometrist who offers a particular specialty. Furthermore, the community may have a true drawing population of 80,000 people.

Conversely, a community of 48,000 people may have only one or two eye care providers. The statistics suggest that the community could easily support an additional optometrist. However, the community may have a per capita income so low, with so many people below poverty level, that an additional optometrist would have a difficult time supporting a practice.

The rule of thumb for optometrist-to-population ratio varies from 1:4000 to 1:6000 in rural areas to 1:25,000 to 1:45,000 in urban areas (see Chapter 3). Optometrist-to-population ratios should be used as a guide only, and too much weight should not be given to these ratios when reaching a decision. If the buying population of the community can be accurately determined, the ratios may be more applicable. If city populations alone are used as a guide, without considering drawing areas, it may be difficult to find a community that needs an optometrist.

How does a researcher find out how many active optometrists are practicing in an area? The best way is to review the Yellow Pages listings. Because of the high cost of Yellow Pages advertising, most optometrists who have retired or relocated will not continue a listing in the Yellow Pages. A copy of the Yellow Pages for a community may be obtained from the local telephone company. It also is important to review the listings of ophthalmologists and opticians. (The Yellow Pages also will be of help when calling for information regarding schools, churches, real estate, shopping areas, and similar community resources.)

The *Blue Book of Optometrists* provides a comprehensive list of optometrists, by city and state, throughout the United States, Canada, and Puerto Rico. The *Blue Book* also lists retired optometrists and optometrists who are in education or research, in active military service, and in health maintenance organizations.

These optometrists should not be figured into practice potential ratios. A companion reference may be found in the *Red Book for Ophthalmologists*.

A second rule of thumb that has been applied throughout the years is to have one optometrist to every three dentists. The reason for this ratio is that, in most cases, people visit a dentist about three times for every one visit to an optometrist. A third rule of thumb suggests that there should be one optometrist for every three to four physicians in a community.

Another fact to explore in relation to practice potential is the vision care needs of the population. It should be determined whether the community primarily consists of elderly patients, who would require treatment for pathologic conditions and low vision services, or of a young adult population, with children who would require contact lens and pediatric services. A community profile that analyzes age categories will provide helpful information regarding the vision care needs of the population. The local Chamber of Commerce usually has available Census information that lists age, sex, income, and ethnic categories.

Practice potential information can be obtained through local optical laboratories. Laboratory representatives cover particular geographic areas and can serve as excellent sources of information for practice opportunities. Many laboratories have toll-free telephone numbers.

Opportunities for practice potential can be found through state and national placement efforts. The membership services department of the American Optometric Association (AOA) can be contacted for placement information. The AOA Practice Resource Network is a computerized service established to help AOA member doctors of optometry and fourth-year optometry student members find mutually satisfying practice opportunities. This service provides a national listing of optometrists seeking employees, partners, and purchasers. In addition, many state optometric associations offer placement services.

When a selected community is visited, it is important to try to talk to as many professionals as possible about the need for optometric services, the economy of the area, and its livability. It also is useful to talk with other health care providers (e.g., school nurses, pharmacists, physicians) about the community.

When assessing a community, local optometrists should be contacted by mail or telephone regarding potential practice opportunities. A well-written letter expressing interest in the community and asking about practice opportunities may be favorably received by an optometrist looking for an associate or potential buyer. Office visits to optometrists are usually well worth the effort; an associateship, partnership, or purchase option may develop from the encounter.

Locating an Office

Once a community has been chosen, the next step is to determine the location of the office. Of course, if a practice is being purchased, the location is part of the overall evaluation of the proposed sale. However, for a graduate looking to begin a practice, the location of the office is an important consideration. In fact, it is a key part of achieving financial success.

The same sources that were consulted when deciding on a community can be used to evaluate potential locations for a practice. The U.S. Economic Census for an area can be found at a city's Chamber of Commerce. City records can provide information of new developments in business and residential areas. Future trends about a community and patterns of population can be obtained from real estate associations, utility companies, public libraries, planning boards, school district administrators, and marketing departments of colleges. These data will be essential in guiding the decision-making process. A beginning optometrist should discuss future plans with representatives from all the foregoing organizations. The *Rand McNally Commercial Atlas and Marketing Guide* should be consulted for demographic information. A personal diary should be kept of important contacts and events during the information-gathering process.

The most important consideration in selecting an office site is visibility. If an office is readily visible to the public, there will be a positive effect on patient flow. In some communities, it may be preferable to locate in a medical complex with other health care providers. In this situation, the presence of patients in the building (and hopefully the referral of some of these patients by other tenants) will assist in building a patient base. In some high-visibility locations, such as malls and shopping areas, the cost of office space is expensive. Financial projections need to be carefully made to ensure that such a location is economically viable.

If an office is to be built or remodeled, a contractor will be needed. Determining the right person to do the job is essential. Discussions should be held with tenants, builders, and developers to obtain answers to the following questions:
- Who are the best commercial builders?

- Why is a particular builder considered to be preferable?
- Has the builder experienced legal difficulties or conflicts with clients?
- How long has the builder been in business?
- Where are some of the builder's offices located?

There should be a consistent pattern of behavior and usually a consensus of opinion about the better individuals in the building industry, especially in smaller communities.

Because practices are often open in the evenings to accommodate the schedules of working families, a well-lighted and safe location may be an important priority. It also is an advantage to be near a major thoroughfare and recognizable buildings, especially when a staff member has to give directions to the patients regarding the location of the office. Accessibility is a very important consideration when choosing an office location. Adequate parking is a key part of ensuring accessibility.

In most cases, the selection of an office location will be based on the input received from the business people in the community. In particular, dentists seem to understand the economics and business aspects of their profession and community. Initially, the new optometrist has to rely on and trust the opinion of others. If adequate effort has been placed on the collection of information from knowledgeable sources, the choice of location will be a good one.

Putting It All Together

To begin the process of determining a practice location, practice goals must be established. To evaluate potential practice locations, information should be requested from different communities. A determination of what is valued in a community should be made. A feasibility analysis should be completed for each community that is being considered. The most promising communities should then be rated for practice potential, economics, and livability (Figure 14-4).

Finding the ideal community in which to practice is an exciting yet demanding endeavor. Planning, travel, and analysis are necessary. To find the time needed to perform an adequate assessment, the process should begin early in optometry school. School holidays and summer vacations are the ideal times to plan community and practice visitations. The earlier the process can be initiated, the better the assessment that can be performed and, hopefully, the better the outcome that can be realized.

Community Analysis_____

COMMUNITY	1	2	3	4	5
Practice Potential Index					
O.D./population ratio	☐	☐	☐	☐	☐
Vision care needs	☐	☐	☐	☐	☐
Types of practices	☐	☐	☐	☐	☐
Attitude of professionals in the community	☐	☐	☐	☐	☐
Number of physicians	☐	☐	☐	☐	☐
Opinions of optical labs	☐	☐	☐	☐	☐
TOTAL					
Economic Index					
Employment statistics	☐	☐	☐	☐	☐
Retail sales	☐	☐	☐	☐	☐
Population growth rate	☐	☐	☐	☐	☐
Community buying power	☐	☐	☐	☐	☐
Amount of new building	☐	☐	☐	☐	☐
Rate of bank deposit	☐	☐	☐	☐	☐
Business starts	☐	☐	☐	☐	☐
TOTAL					
Livability Index					
Housing and neighborhood	☐	☐	☐	☐	☐
Schools	☐	☐	☐	☐	☐
Churches	☐	☐	☐	☐	☐
Cultural and recreational	☐	☐	☐	☐	☐
Shopping areas	☐	☐	☐	☐	☐
Community organizations	☐	☐	☐	☐	☐
Climate	☐	☐	☐	☐	☐
Your impression of the area	☐	☐	☐	☐	☐
TOTAL					
GRAND TOTAL	☐	☐	☐	☐	☐

INSTRUCTIONS: Use a scale of 1 point for the lowest value to 5 points for the highest value for each of the factors listed above. When completed, the total points for each index can be added together to determine the most desirable community.

Figure 14-4 Worksheet to rate and analyze different communities.

Acknowledgement

The authors of this chapter in the first edition of *Business Aspects of Optometry* were David L. Park, James Albright, and Craig Hisaka.

Bibliography

American Automobile Association: *AAA tourbook.* Heathrow, Fla, 1996, Author. Also available at: *www.aaa.com.*

American Business Directories: *Optometrists, the 1999 directory.* Omaha, Neb, 1999, Author.

Barreto H: *California, where to live and work.* New York, 1989, Prima Publications and Communications.

Blue book of optometrists, ed 49. New York, 2001, Jobson.

Boyer R, Savageau D: *Places rated almanac: your guide to finding the best places to live in America.* New York, 1997, Prentice Hall.

Census catalog and guide. Washington, DC, 2001. U.S. Department of Commerce, U.S. Bureau of the Census. Also available at: *www.census.gov.index.html.*

Commercial atlas and marketing guide, ed 130. Skokie, Ill, 1999, Rand McNally.

Statistical abstract of the United States: the national data book, ed 121. Washington, DC, 2001, U.S. Department of Commerce, U.S. Bureau of the Census. Also available at: *www.ntis.gov.*

US Small Business Administration: *Marketing strategies for growing businesses.* Washington, DC, 2001, U.S. Small Business Administration. Business plans and the step-by-step construction of them are described online at: *www.sba.gov/library/pubs.html.*

Worldwide Chamber of Commerce directory. Loveland, Colo, 1996, Worldwide Chamber of Commerce Directory Inc.

www.sba.gov. Web site for the Small Business Administration.

Chapter 15

Practice Financing

Gary L. Moss

Between two evils, I always pick the one I never tried before.
Mae West *Klondike Annie*

For most optometry school graduates, the initial encounter with financing a business venture is the creation of a business plan to either start or buy into a practice. Once identified, the steps of the business plan will guide the strategy used to create practice goals, make financial projections, organize the office, identify target markets, and obtain required resources and financing. A business plan should anticipate and answer basic questions (Box 15-1) that will be asked by potential creditors from whom the graduate seeks funding.

Proper financing is an integral part of the success of every optometric business. Understanding the basic financial concepts and methods used by lending institutions is fundamental to obtaining favorable financing. Money is necessary to start a new practice, to purchase part or all of an existing practice, or to obtain working capital to expand an operating practice. It is an unfortunate situation when a new practice with great potential fails because it was undercapitalized. This chapter identifies fundamental components in the financing process and describes basic financial situations a graduate encounters, types of loans available, sources of funds, seller financing, and standards used to evaluate applicant credit worthiness.

Determining Financing Need

Projections of income, expenses, potential profit, and financing requirements are, as a rule, required by nearly all lending institutions. A good understanding of financial or accounting statements can benefit an optometrist by facilitating this undertaking. The three primary financial statements are:
- Income statement (profit and loss statement)
- Balance sheet
- Cash-flow statement

Each of these three tools has a different purpose and can be used to help assess the financial implications of the business plan for the practice.

Income Statement

The income statement, also referred to as the profit and loss statement, shows the profit that a practice produces in a given period, usually a year. Income statements are based on the accrual method of accounting. In this method, income is recorded when earned rather than received, and expenses are recorded when incurred rather than paid. The income statement shows just how profitable a practice is and is represented by the following formula:

$$\text{Income} - \text{Expenses} = \text{Net profit}$$

Five areas are reported in the income statement:
- Revenue generated from the sale of products and from services (income)
- Costs of acquiring products and inventory that have been sold (cost of goods sold)
- Operating expenses (fixed and variable expenses)
- Financing costs (credit interest and principal)
- Tax payments (taxes paid)

An example income statement may be found in Chapter 41.

Balance Sheet

The balance sheet offers a glimpse of a practice's financial health at any given point by reporting the cumulative result of all previous decisions that influenced the finances and operations of the practice to that time. It shows the assets owned by the practice, the debt obligations owed, and the equity (net worth) the owner has

---

Box 15-1 Business Plan Questions to Answer When Requesting Financing

- Have all expenses associated with location, patient demographics, rent, laboratory costs, and fixed and variable office overhead been explained and justified?
- Have projected revenue and expenses been realistically estimated?
- Is the business plan achievable and practical to implement? Has the business plan been reviewed by advisors?
- Has a marketing plan that satisfies practice objectives been given an adequate budget allocation?
- Does the borrower have a favorable credit history?
- Are emergency funds available for slow periods?
- What is the amount of the loan, and what collateral will secure the loan? How much equity or personal funding is the borrower investing?
- Is there an outside guarantor who is willing to secure the loan?

---

invested in the practice. The balance sheet is represented by the following formula:

Liabilities (debt) + Owner's equity (net worth) = Assets

An example balance sheet may be found in Chapter 41.

Cash-Flow Statement

This statement reveals the sources and uses of practice income for any given period. It is the definitive account of cash-flow status because it is generated using the cash basis method of accounting. In this method, income is reported when received and expenses are reported when paid. Non-cash expenses such as depreciation, credits, or uncollectable debts are not included. An example cash-flow statement may be found in Chapter 41.

The amount of capital required will vary with the type of practice situation. New offices require equipment, inventory rental deposit, and sufficient working capital funds to operate until the practice becomes self-supporting. The purchase of an existing practice usually requires a substantial down payment, ranging from 10% to 25% of the purchase price, and adequate working capital for operations and payments to the seller for financing. These payments should be included in the monthly projected operating budget.

It is necessary to accurately determine the amount of money that will be needed from a creditor. If funds are inadequate, the creditor may not be willing to extend the amount borrowed or modify the terms of the loan. To support insufficient start-up capital, most optometrists incur long-term debt rather than sell equity in the practice. Long-term debt is paid with interest, usually over a period of more than 5 years; it gives the creditor neither ownership interest nor control during the practice.

Increased expenses, a slowdown in patient visits or payments, or rapid office expansion may create a shortage of working capital. The classic resolution is the use of medium- to long-term credit. New or additional debt should only be obtained, however, if cash-flow projections show that the loan will generate sufficient profits to pay the debt.

Financial Forecasting

The projected performance of a practice is used by loan officers to substantiate the worthiness of giving a loan. Projected data come from proforma financial statements (see Chapter 17) that are used to answer the following questions:

- How profitable can this practice be given the likely level of revenue and associated operating expense?
- What determines the optimal amount and type of financing, either debt or equity?
- Will the practice have sufficient cash flow, and how is it to be used?

Potential practice profit can be forecast by making the following calculation:

Make realistic sales projections based on recent past performance.

Subtract the anticipated cost of goods sold and operating expenses to obtain the operating profit of the practice or earnings before interest and tax.

Deduct the amount of interest to be paid on anticipated outstanding loans to acquire and operate the practice.

Deduct the estimated amount of taxes that will be owed. The result will be the net profit (or loss).

An example of this calculation may be found in Chapter 3.

Liquidity measures the ability of a practice to pay off current debt obligations through adequate working capital. A way of measuring liquidity is to calculate financial ratios. The *current ratio* is a measure of cash, accounts receivable, and inventory (collectively referred to as *current assets*) that is divided by the amount of short-term debt, or *current liabilities*, as shown in the following equation:

$$\frac{\text{Current assets}}{\text{Current liabilities}} = \text{Current ratio}$$

This ratio should be at least 2 to 1 to be considered adequate. Another related ratio that indicates a practice's liquidity is the *debt-to-asset ratio*, which measures the total amount of debt as a percentage of tangible assets.

Capital financing of a practice is accomplished through either of two means. The first is *equity capital*, which may be external (financing from the initial investment an optometrist makes in a practice) or internal (financing generated from practice operations that is reinvested into the practice, not paid out as salary or profit). The second means is through the *loan* process (assumption of debt capital).

Loan Categories

Financing available to optometrists generally falls into the following categories:

Long-term capital: an arrangement in which repayment extends for more than 5 years. Long-term loans are repaid from earnings. This type of loan is usually required when purchasing a practice or when a practice is unable to meet the obligations of an intermediate-term loan.

Intermediate-term capital: an arrangement in which repayment must be made over 2 to 5 years. These loans also are repaid from earnings.

Short-term capital: an arrangement in which repayment usually takes no longer than 1 year.

Short-term loans are used to finance the purchase of a new piece of equipment or a large quantity of inventory, with repayment expected from the use of the equipment or the sale of goods.

Banks may make a loan based on the borrower's reputation, usually for a small amount and for a short term, as an unsecured loan. Collateral is not required, and the bank relies on the borrower's good credit rating. Credit cards and lines of credit are examples of unsecured loans. A secured loan requires the borrower to possess an asset ("collateral") that can be taken or sold by the bank if the borrower cannot repay the loan. The bank requires the collateral as protection for its depositors against the risk that the loan will fail.

There are many factors in the loan process for which the borrower has no control. Recession, fluctuating interest rates, and changes in bank regulations can interfere with an optometrist's ability to obtain financing.

Determining Credit Worthiness

When an optometrist applies for a loan, the creditor will ask two major questions. The first is: What is the likelihood that the borrower will default on the loan? To answer this question, the creditor will want to ascertain how risky the loan is and assess the borrower's ability to repay. Creditors will find answers by analyzing the practice's profit and loss statement, balance sheet, and cash-flow summary. Loan institutions often request all data about both business and personal income, including expenses and equity. For start-up offices, comparisons to industry data can be obtained from *Annual Statement Studies* (Philadelphia, Robert Morris Associates). If the borrower is purchasing an existing practice, financial information about the practice will be requested as part of the loan proposal.

The creditor's second question is: What is the borrower's credit history, as obtained from a credit report? To answer this question, the creditor will investigate the borrower's prior ability to repay debt. Any late payments, even from years earlier, will require proper explanation to the lending company. A poor credit repayment history will severely affect the ability to obtain funds. An excellent credit rating will not guarantee a loan but will help significantly in the total process of obtaining funds.

Before a lending agency will advance money, the institution must be satisfied with the borrower's answers to the questions listed in Box 15-2.

To determine whether a borrower's business is credit worthy, satisfactory financial data will be necessary. Loan institutions want to make loans to businesses that are solvent, earning profits, and expanding. The two fundamental financial documents used to ascertain those positions are the income statement and the balance sheet. The income statement is a primary measure of profits and losses, and the balance sheet is a fundamental gauge for assets and liabilities. The bank usually will request the profit and loss statements and balance sheets of an office for at least 5 years preceding the loan. If these documents are not available, tax returns are substituted. A consecutive sequence of these two statements over a period is the primary means for measuring financial balance and development capacity.

Evaluating a Loan Applicant

After a borrower has furnished the required data, the next phase in the borrowing process is the evaluation of the application by the bank's loan officer. Most lending agencies consider similar factors when determining whether to award or decline a loan, based on what has come to be known as the *5 Cs of credit*:
• Borrower's character
• Borrower's capacity to repay the loan
• Amount of capital invested by the borrower
• Current economic and industry conditions
• Amount of collateral used to secure the loan
Additional factors that will influence the decision to grant or withhold a loan are based on the borrower's previous history of debt payment, previous business experience and employment history, the ratio of the borrower's debt to net worth, and the practice's past financial performance.

In reviewing loan documents, the banker will be particularly interested in the following:

Fixed assets. What is the fair market value of the major equipment and furnishings? What are the depreciation values? Fair market value appraisals by qualified appraisers for banks often will need to be obtained. Qualified appraisers for ophthalmic equipment often can be hired from companies involved in selling ophthalmic equipment. The loan institution will inform the borrower of its requirements for an appraisal. A second type of appraisal involves the

calculation of *book value*. The book value of equipment is determined by subtracting the amount of depreciation claimed from the original cost of the equipment. Depreciation tables can be used to determine an item's book value.

Accounts receivable. Are accounts receivable part of the sale and value of the practice? Are the accounts receivable low in value because many patients are behind in payments? What is the percentage of accounts receivable that is being collected? The lending institution must be asked to state its policy for loans that include accounts receivable. If funds are not available for the payment of accounts receivable, the purchase agreement must be negotiated with the seller so that the accounts receivable are not part of the sale.

Inventory. Are frames and supplies current? Is a large part of the inventory on consignment (held for sale rather than purchased)? Is the inventory turnover similar to that of other offices? Many lending institutions prefer not to support a portion of a loan that is backed with inventory as collateral. The reason is that inventory used as collateral is difficult to liquidate by a creditor in case of foreclosure.

General business information. Are the books and records up-to-date? What are the salaries? Have the taxes been paid? What is the number of employees? Does the office provide insurance? These and similar questions will customarily be posed by the creditor.

Obtaining a Loan

The quantity of funds needed by a borrower depends on the objectives for use of the capital. Determining the amount of money required for equipment, furnishings, supplies, construction, expansion, or buy-out is easy. Equipment companies, architects, and builders will eagerly supply cost calculations. On the other hand, the amount of working capital that is needed depends on the projection of income and expenses.

In general, most lending agencies will provide loans that can be secured by collateral. *Collateral* is the offering of a form of security or guarantee that a loan will be repaid. When a loan cannot be justified by financial statements alone, a pledge of security from either the borrower or a third party may enable the borrower to secure the loan. If the borrower defaults, the collateral can be used by the creditor to offset any deficit. A borrower may offer the bank collateral in many different forms. Each lending institution has certain collateral that it will accept. Some of the common types of collateral are listed in Box 15-3.

Box 15-3 Different Types of Collateral That May Be Offered When Applying for a Loan

- Borrower's signature: required for a line of credit or a signature loan.
- Endorsers: other people sign the note as endorsers to improve the borrower's credit. The endorsers are liable for the loan if the borrower fails to make payments.
- Chattel mortgages: if equipment (e.g., a visual-field instrument) is purchased, the bank may file for a security interest in the equipment (which permits the creditor to sell the equipment to satisfy the amount still due if the borrower defaults on the loan).
- Real estate: an excellent and preferred type of collateral. If the borrower is willing to assume the risk of using real estate as collateral, the bank is usually more willing to provide a loan.
- Accounts receivable: can sometimes be used as collateral. Banks count on the optometrist's patients paying their bills, and a good report of the borrower's accounts receivable performance is necessary to use this asset as collateral. It may be possible to borrow up to 50% of current (fewer than 30 days) receivables.
- Savings accounts: can be assigned to the bank to serve as collateral.
- Life insurance: cash value in a life insurance policy can serve as collateral. In such an arrangement, the policy is assigned to the bank (the bank has the first right to death proceeds to satisfy the loan due).
- Stocks and bonds: may serve as collateral if they are marketable. Up to 75% of the value of the stocks and bonds may be eligible to be borrowed.

It can be difficult to obtain a loan for working capital that involves no collateral. A borrower may need to contact various lending agencies about a *line of credit* to obtain money for operating expenses. A line of credit is an agreement from a creditor to supply funds, up to a certain stated maximum, for use by the borrower. After the line of credit is established, the borrower can draw against it when needed. The borrower incurs no obligation to repay the loan until money is actually withdrawn. The amount of money needed to start an optometric practice can be roughly calculated by using Box 15-4. For the type of analysis required for a loan proposal, see the example in Chapter 16.

Sources of Funding

Financing is available from a variety of sources, including both commercial and government lenders. These sources include the following:

Banks. Full-service banks are the most visible lenders and make the largest number and variety of loans. Bankers look for borrowers with business experience, excellent credit records, and good ability to repay the loan.

Commercial financial companies. These companies are similar to banks, and many offer the same types of loans and terms as banks. Commercial financial companies often provide loans based on the borrower's collateral rather than on the office's past history. Finance company loans sometimes exceed the net worth of the borrower, a situation that is undesirable to most banks.

Life insurance companies. A whole life insurance policy can be used to provide business cash when the owner borrows on the policy. Repayment to most insurance companies is made with interest, in the same manner as standard loans from banks.

Consumer finance companies. These companies are high-risk lenders that charge higher interest rates than banks for similar types of loans. They typically supply personal loans for any personal need, including money for a small business.

Savings institutions. These businesses specialize in real estate financing. They often make loans on commercial, industrial, and personal residences.

Box 15-4 Estimating Start-up Expenses for a Practice*

- Equipment and inventory to be purchased
- Renovations and leasehold improvements
- Furniture and signage
- Stationery and printing expenses
- Accountant and attorney fees, permits, and licenses
- Initial marketing program
- Malpractice, disability, and office insurance coverage
- Rental (first and last month's, security deposit)
- Personal living expenses (e.g., rent, food, utilities, insurance) for 6 months
- Miscellaneous (for unforeseen expenses)

*The estimated costs of these items, when added together, permit the borrower to determine roughly the cash needed to start up an office.

Small Business Administration (SBA). The SBA guarantees bank loans (85% of the amount borrowed, up to $150,000, and 75% of the amount borrowed that is more than $150,000) to small businesses and makes a limited number of direct loans to small businesses.

Small business investment companies. These companies are privately owned venture capital firms eligible for federal loans that are used to invest in or lend to small businesses.

Minority enterprise small business investment companies. These companies serve small businesses in which at least 51% of the company is owned by socially or economically disadvantaged Americans.

Farmers Home Administration (FHA). The FHA guarantees bank loans to nonfarming businesses in rural areas. It does not make direct loans but will guarantee up to 90% of a bank loan to a qualifying applicant.

Credit unions. These institutions offer loans at rates competitive with other conventional lenders.

Finance and leasing companies. These companies may offer financing as part of a leasing arrangement for equipment or other items.

Friends and family. Relatives often will be willing to make small loans to young practitioners. This type of loan is very convenient and easily obtained (often at low interest), but it can be potentially quite stressful for the family involved.

Trade creditors. These companies may offer short-term accounts-payable deferments or give installment loans on equipment. They typically require a chattel mortgage (inventory or other types of moveable property are pledged as collateral).

Internet based. America's Business Funding Directory (*www.businessfinance.com*) and Intuit's *Quicken Business Cash Finder* (*www.cashfinder.com*) are both free resources available to small business owners.

Additional sources of loans may be available to individual borrowers; the effort to locate funding is worth the investment of time. As a profession, optometry has a very good credit-worthy record, and this will benefit optometry school graduates seeking financing.

Loan Restrictions

When looking for a creditor, the borrower may have to search to find the best match. Some lenders base loans on debt ratio, whereas others may look at collateral. The following three facts should be understood when facing the formidable task of obtaining funds from a borrower:

- An established office with a good record of operations has a better chance of obtaining a loan than an office started "cold."
- Some personal equity capital investment is a virtual requirement to receive any type of additional creditor loan.
- The more collateral or security the borrower is willing to give, the easier it will be to obtain financing.

In general, a financially sound practice will incur few limitations on a loan. A new practice started "cold" or a practitioner who is a poor credit risk can expect to incur greater restrictions and limitations in the loan agreement. Limitations include requirements intended to protect the creditor's investment and usually involve the following:

- Type of collateral
- Repayment terms (length of time and interest amount)
- Periodic reporting (required reporting by the borrower)

Restrictions are found in a loan agreement in the section known as *covenants*; these obligations can be either positive or negative. Negative covenants are things the borrower cannot do without approval from the lender. An example of a negative covenant is the inability of the borrower to take on additional debt without the lender's approval. Positive covenants include things the borrower must do. For example, the borrower may be obligated to maintain a minimum net working capital under the terms of the loan.

A borrower should keep in mind that all terms are negotiable, and being prepared to negotiate various terms is an important part of the loan process. A borrower should not be afraid to be assertive when protecting personal interests. For this reason, it is a good practice to obtain and review the loan documents in advance before closing.

Seller Financing

One popular method for transferring the ownership of a practice has been the use of financing by the selling optometrist. Seller financing can be primary or secondary and involve the use of mortgages. A mortgage is the purchase of property in which the buyer is given the title to the property, even though the purchase is financed by a loan from a creditor. The creditor may be able to take title to the property, however, if the buyer does not repay the loan. The creditor also may sell the property to obtain the amount due.

Box 15-5 Advantages and Disadvantages of Seller Financing

Advantages

To the buyer

1. The buyer usually needs to provide less money to purchase the practice:
   - The buyer often saves money, with minimal closing costs and no points.
   - The buyer may be able to negotiate a lower down payment from the seller than the payment required by a bank (which is typically 20%).
   - The buyer has more control over costs, such as appraisals, inspections, and reports.
2. Financing keeps a selling practitioner more active in the practice (to keep the practitioner's investment secure). The selling practitioner has a vested interest in the success of the new owner and wants the new practitioner to succeed.
3. The buyer may be able to negotiate a lower interest rate than through a commercial loan.
4. Seller financing may be the only means to purchase a practice if banks are unwilling to provide capital to a new practitioner who has high debt and minimal collateral.

To the seller

1. Since there will be principal and interest paid over a period of years, this money will add to the seller's retirement living expenses.
2. The tax consequences will be lessened if the practice is purchased over time.

Disadvantages

To the buyer

1. This method of financing may entail more years of repayment than other methods and thus would ultimately cost more.

To the seller

1. The seller does not receive a large sum of money as a down payment that can be invested.
2. If the repayment plan fails, the seller may be required to take over the practice.

An example of *primary seller financing* may be found in the following practice sale agreement. The buyer agrees to purchase the practice for $150,000 and makes a 20% down payment ($30,000) to the seller. The seller is willing to finance the balance of $120,000 and gives a mortgage to the buyer for that amount.

An example of *secondary seller financing* may be found in the following example. The buyer agrees to buy the practice for $150,000 and borrows $50,000 from a bank for a down payment. The balance of $100,000 is financed by the seller, who gives a second mortgage. In this arrangement, the bank holds the first mortgage of $50,000 and the seller holds the second mortgage for the remaining balance. There are advantages to both buyer and seller in this arrangement, and some of the advantages and disadvantages are listed in Box 15-5.

Because of the difficulty in obtaining financing, creative methods for the transfer of practice ownership have been devised. In the situation in which a prospective buyer is unable to obtain the full financing necessary to purchase a practice, the seller's willingness to finance part of the purchase price often will enable the transfer of ownership to take place.

Conclusion

The information in this chapter provides an introduction to the fundamentals of financing an optometric practice. In Chapter 16, the details of business loans are discussed, and an example of a loan proposal is presented. This proposal includes a projected profit and loss statement, a projected income statement, and a sample business plan.

Acknowledgement

The authors of this chapter in the first edition of *Business Aspects of Optometry* were David L. Park, Craig Hisaka, and Gary Moss.

Bibliography

American Academy of Family Physicians: *On your own: starting a medical practice from the ground up*. Table of contents available online at:

http://www.aafp.org/newpractice/toc_regular.html.

Dean J: *Practice finance, your questions answered*, ed 2. New York, 1998, Radcliffe Medical.

Fischer A: Financing options help stem declining revenues. *Admin Eyecare* 7(4):50-2, 1998.

Greene J: Wanted: deep pockets (starting a medical practice is a costly endeavor). *Hospitals Health Networks* 71(7):87, 1997.

Keene D: *2000 Financial planning of a medical practice.* Alpharetta, Ga, 2000, Robert D. Keene.

Messinger S, Stevenson P: Practice financing strategies should match investors' objectives. *Healthcare Finan Management* 53(5):72-4, 1999.

Parkyn T: Getting the start-up loan you need. *Optom Management* (Suppl) 33(3):12-6, 1998.

Perry K: Are fortitude and cash all you need to open a solo practice? *Med Economics* 78(7):162, 2001.

Vaughan J, Wise J: How to choose the right capitalization option. *Healthcare Finan Management* 50(12):72-3, 1996.

www.centersite.com/mba/mbalinks.html. Web site that offers a large list of small business resources accessible through the Internet.

Chapter 16

Obtaining a Business Loan

John G. Classé

Hold fast to dreams
For if dreams die
Life is a broken winged bird
That cannot fly.
Langston Hughes *The World Tomorrow*

The traditional means of delivering optometric services—sole proprietorship—requires offices to be equipped with an array of up-to-date instruments, inventories of frames and contact lenses, and tasteful fixtures and furnishings, which places a heavy financial burden on practitioners seeking to practice in the time-honored way. In addition, there are operating costs that must be met (e.g., rent, taxes, utilities, and salaries), which means that the graduate seeking entry into private practice must obtain financing to be able to afford the start-up costs of such a practice.

In the usual case, financing must be acquired both for capital assets and operating expenses. Thus the creditor may be required to loan more money than there will be collateral to serve as security, which necessitates careful planning and meticulous preparation on the part of the borrower because the creditor will have to be convinced that the risk is minimal to make such a partially unsecured loan. To ensure that the risk is low, the creditor will dictate the terms of the agreement and will protect the interest in the collateral. This chapter discusses the conventional devices used by creditors to secure loans and to protect collateral in the event of default on the part of the borrower. It also describes the preparation of a loan proposal intended to secure the necessary financing.

Fundamentals of Financing

The usual source of loans for the initiation of a practice is a full-service bank, although there are numerous other alternatives (see Chapter 15). The most basic aspects of bank financing involve the method of repayment and the type of interest. Borrowing money involves not only the act of obtaining the loan but also the repayment of principal and interest. Although there are number of methods used for the repayment of loans and for the computation of interest, this discussion is limited to the usual techniques used by banks.

Banks rely on the following two principal methods for the repayment of loans:
- *Renewable short-term notes:* instruments that acknowledge the loaning of money for relatively brief periods (usually 90 days), with provisions for renewal at the option of the lender. At the close of any 90-day period, the lender can demand payment of the balance due—in full.
- *Installment notes:* instruments that provide for the periodic repayment of a stated sum at regular intervals, such as monthly payments, usually over 3 to 5 years.

Either of two types of interest rates—simple or add-on—may be applied to short-term loans:
- *Simple interest.* This rate applies a fixed percentage to the amount borrowed for a stated period. An example that illustrates how the interest is computed is found in Box 16-1. Simple interest is one of the most advantageous ways to borrow money. Should the borrower decide to pay off the loan early, there is no prepayment penalty because the interest is *prorated* for the actual number of days that the money has been borrowed. However, renewable 90-day notes are subject to fluctuating interest rates based on the prime lending rate during any 90-day period. Rates may be set at the start of the 90-day period or change each time the prime rate goes up or

Box 16-1 Sample Simple Interest Loan

If $10,000 is borrowed at 10% simple interest on a renewable 90-day note, what would be the interest payable at the end of 90 days?

Amount borrowed	$10,000
Interest rate	× 10%
Total interest if the note was held for a year	$1000
Interest for one-fourth of a year	$250

If the note is due in 90 days without renewal, the total amount that has to be repaid is $10,250.

From Classé JG: Legal aspects of optometry. Stoneham, MA, 1989, Butterworth.

down. In the latter case, the rate may change many times during the course of the life of the note. Simple interest short-term bank loans are a preferred means of borrowing money to purchase equipment and start a practice.

- *Add-on interest.* This method of determining interest is the more costly of the two rates. It is called add-on because the interest is computed on the amount borrowed, without proration, and added to the principal. This total is then repaid in installments during the course of the loan, which is usually 3, 4, or 5 years. An example that illustrates the method of determining repayment is found in Box 16-2. Add-on interest is commonly encountered in installment loans, such as those used for the financing of automobiles and boats. If a borrower decides to prepay (i.e., pay before maturity) an installment loan, the interest is *shortrated* rather than prorated. Shortrating

Box 16-2 Sample Add-On Interest Loan

If $10,000 was borrowed at 10% add-on interest for a period of 3 years, what would be the total cost to the borrower?

Multiply $10,000	$10,000
By 10%	× 10
Yearly interest	$ 1000
Multiply by 3 years	×3
Finance charge	$ 3000
Add principal	+10,000
Total amount financed	$13,000
Divide by 36 months	÷ 36
Monthly payments	$ 361.11

From Classé JG: Legal aspects of optometry. Stoneham, MA, 1989, Butterworth.

means that the if the borrower pays off the loan early, the lender will charge a fee for administrative expenses and profit. Normally this fee is governed by the Rule of 78, which is a standard formula for figuring the interest due (Box 16-3). A borrower should always inquire into the shortrate charge with add-on interest before borrowing money, if the borrower believes there is a possibility that the loan could be repaid early. Early repayment of an add-on loan usually is not advantageous if the interest is shortrated. The reason is that the interest charge is heavily weighed toward the start of the loan (Box 16-4).

Usual banking custom is to use simple interest notes for relatively small amounts and for short periods, if based on the borrower's signature. Although an unsecured simple interest note often can be obtained for various personal needs, the financing of equipment and the start-up of a practice will necessitate the use of the equipment (and other collateral) to provide security for the loan.

Add-on interest is used for longer-term financing involving periodic payments and is normally secured by the automobile, equipment, or other collateral that is financed. Of course, the personal endorsement of the borrower also is obtained.

The burden is on the borrower to determine the type of financing that is being offered and whether the rate and terms of the loan are favorable and competitive for the market.

Box 16-3 Calculation of Interest Under the "Rule of 78"

How is $1000 in interest computed over a 12-month period under the "Rule of 78?"

The 12-month period is summed as follows:
$12 + 11 + 10 + 9 + 8 + 7 + 6 + 5 + 4 + 3 + 2 + 1 = 78$

The interest is computed as follows:

First month	12/78 = $153.84
Second month	11/78 = $141.02
Third month	10/78 = $128.20
Fourth month	9/78 = $115.38
Fifth month	8/78 = $102.56
Sixth month	7/78 = $ 89.74
Total	$730.74

Therefore, 73% of the interest due is paid in the first 6 months, leaving $270 of interest to be paid in the last 6 months.

From Classé JG: Legal aspects of optometry. Stoneham, MA, 1989, Butterworth.

Box 16-4 Short-Rated Interest Under the "Rule of 78"

3-YEAR NOTE	4-YEAR NOTE	5-YEAR NOTE
50% of interest in first year	43% of interest in first year	36% of interest in first year
33% of interest in second year	29% of interest in second year	28% of interest in second year
17% of interest in third year	18% of interest in third year	18% of interest in third year
	9% of interest in fourth year	12% of interest in fourth year
		6% of interest in fifth year

From Classé JG: Legal aspects of optometry. Stoneham, MA, 1989, Butterworth.

Basic Provisions of a Bank Loan Agreement

Although individual bank agreements may differ somewhat in their terms, there is a commonality to these contracts that permits some generalizations to be made. The basic provisions of loan agreements invariably include the amount to be borrowed and the terms of the loan, the interest type and rate, collateral requirements, limitations on additional indebtedness, the repayment provisions, and an acceleration clause.

Amount and Terms

Any creditor will have loan limits that will not be exceeded without good cause and will have established loan repayment terms that vary with the purpose of the loan and the amount borrowed. For example, most automobile loans are for 3 to 4 years; most practice loans are for 5 to 7 years. There will be an upper limit on the amount loaned that can be used for nontangible items; the more conservative the bank, the lower the amount allowed for these expenses (e.g., working capital).

Interest Rate

If the loan is for simple interest, it is likely that the agreement will specify a short-term renewable note. In this event the interest charge will probably fluctuate in accordance with changes in the prime interest rate; the only variable will be the frequency with which the rate changes. Some banks specify a floating rate that changes whenever the prime rate rises or falls, whereas others set the rate at the renewal of the note (e.g., quarterly).

If the loan is for add-on interest, the rate usually is set at the start of the loan and does not change thereafter; add-on rates are customarily found on installment notes. If add-on interest is used in conjunction with a renewable short-term note, the rate can be changed at each renewal.

Collateral Requirements

There are two customary collateral requirements in practice loans: a purchase money security interest in the equipment (and other tangibles) and a life insurance policy that is assigned to the bank.

A security interest is created when the borrower and creditor adhere to the following procedures:

- The creditor and borrower must agree, in writing, to the formation of the security interest, which is done through the execution (signing) of a security agreement.
- The creditor must make the loan, and the borrower must acquire the property.
- The creditor must file a financing statement, which is a document putting the public on notice that the creditor has a financial interest in the property.

The filing requirement is necessary to protect the creditor from subsequent creditors; if the borrower fails to repay the loan, the creditors will have to fight among themselves for whatever assets remain, and the creditor who has filed the earliest security interest will prevail over the others. For this reason, there is considerable emphasis placed on security interests by creditors. The bank usually will require the borrower to assign a life insurance policy to the bank that is sufficient to cover the loan balance in the event of the death of the borrower. An *assignment* is a transfer of a contractual right or benefit, which operates to extinguish the right for the one making the transfer and establish the right exclusively for the benefit of the one to whom it is transferred. Many banks require the borrower to assign the rights to a life insurance policy to the bank, placing the bank before any other beneficiary in terms of payment in the event the borrower dies unexpectedly, before the loan is repaid.

The borrower will be asked to execute an assignment agreement and will have to surrender the policy to the bank, which will hold it as long as the loan is outstanding. When the loan is repaid, the assignment will be extinguished and the policy will be returned to the borrower. In addition to the life insurance policy, the bank may require the borrower to maintain other types of insurance coverage. These requirements obligate the practitioner to purchase property and professional liability insurance sufficient to indemnify the bank in the event of the loss of the collateral. Of course, the bank may require additional collateral, a cosigner, or other such items as it deems necessary to protect its security adequately.

Limitation on Additional Indebtedness

To prevent borrowers from overextending themselves, some banks limit the ability of borrowers to obtain additional loans from other creditors. The limitation is usually expressed as a cash limit, not to be exceeded without the prior approval of the bank. These limits do not apply to consumer purchases or debts incurred during the course of everyday practice activities.

Repayment Provisions

Repayment provisions vary widely from bank to bank and with the type of note and interest charged. Installment notes specify a stated payment per month for the period of the note. The monthly payment does not change during the repayment period, which is usually for 3 to 5 years, but may be longer. Short-term renewable notes offer the bank more options. These loans are described as being for a period of years (usually 5 to 7) but are actually renewable at the option of the bank, at stated intervals that are specified in the loan agreement. Renewable periods may be as brief as 90 days or may be for as long as a term of years. Notes retain a degree of flexibility that enables the bank to adjust the repayment schedule as necessary to accommodate the borrower's ability to pay. Some notes specify interest repayment only during the first year of the loan, then amortize the principal and interest over a period of several years thereafter. Other notes allow the borrower to pay less during the first years of the repayment period.

Regardless of the type of note or repayment schedule, the bank will require the borrower to submit periodic financial statements so that the status of the borrower's practice can be assessed.

Acceleration Clause

Any note will contain a so-called acceleration clause, which permits the bank to demand the full amount of the loan due and payable in the event the borrower fails to comply with the provisions of the agreement. This provision affords the bank some protection in the event the borrower cannot make the required payments because it allows the bank to claim its collateral and proceed as necessary to collect the full amount outstanding. These clauses are a standard aspect of any financial agreement and can only be enforced by the creditor if there is some default on the part of the borrower.

Loan agreements are complex and comprehensive documents that typically involve the transfer of large sums of money. A potential borrower who is not knowledgeable in financial affairs would be well advised to secure professional counsel before entering into any long-term financial arrangements with a creditor.

The Loan Proposal

The loan proposal, which is used to secure funding for the operation of the practice, is a key element of the practice plan (Figure 16-1). Starting a practice, buying a practice, or acquiring a partnership interest in a practice requires financial investment. The amount of money needed can be many thousands of dollars. A creditor is required to provide financial support. Part of the amount borrowed will be unsecured—unprotected by assets that a creditor can sell if the borrower fails—which motivates the creditor to review the borrower's status meticulously. The loan proposal is used to create confidence in the borrower's financial acumen, justify the amount being borrowed, and provide monetary projections against which the borrower's progress can be measured. It requires a considerable amount of time to prepare. Generally, there are three phases of the proposal process: research, drafting the proposal, and presentation.

Research

This is the key component of preparing a loan proposal. The value of the proposal is directly related to the accuracy of the information in it. Reliable figures should be used for calculations. For example, repayment of educational loans is a financial burden that most new graduates must consider. The amount of each monthly payment, and when payments will begin, can be accurately determined, and so can the cost of leasing an office; purchasing insurance; or paying for water, gas, and electricity. The effort taken to secure accurate information will repay itself many times, for the value of the loan proposal as a true measuring rod for financial success will be far greater if reliable information is used. The creditor may doubt the validity of the proposal if many projections are obviously inaccurate, creating a less supportive attitude.

LOAN PROPOSAL

Purpose
To acquire capital to establish an optometric practice in southeast Townsville.

Proposal
The location of the practice will be in southeast Townsville on Vision Ease Road. At present the ratio of optometrists to population in the Townsville area is 1:16,000. The preferred ratio for an optometrist in a similar area is 1:5,000 to 1:8,000. Enclosed is a map of the Townsville city school system with the vision care providers marked in. Although there are numerous dentists and pharmacies in the southeast area, there is no vision care provider at present. The closest provider is at least 8 miles away from the proposed site. As the southeast area is an affluent and rapidly growing area of Townsville that will need vision care services, I feel that with adequate capital I can provide the vision care needed.

Office Lease
I have negotiated an office lease at the proposed location. The lease is for 5 years with an option to renew for another 5 years. A copy of the lease is enclosed.

Insurance Coverage
I have been approved to purchase a term life insurance policy in the amount of $40,000 to pay off the loan from the bank should I die before the loan is repaid. In addition, I have acquired an umbrella liability policy to cover malpractice, other types of liability claims, and property loss by fire or other casualty. A list of these policies, the insurers, and the premium costs is enclosed.

Financial Status
A financial statement is enclosed. At present, my only significant debts are an educational loan, which totals $28,366, and automobile loans with this bank, (in my name and my spouse's name), which total $17,322.
I have also enclosed our federal income tax return for the past year.

Capital Needed
I need a loan of $40,000 to establish my practice. Of this amount, $3,700 will be unsecured. The remainder will be used to purchase equipment for which a purchase money security interest may be obtained by the bank.

Financial Summary
A year-by-year summary of my projected income and expenses for the 6 years needed to repay the loan is enclosed. My spouse has been offered employment in Townsville. My spouse's income is included in the projections for each year.

Year	Projected income	Projected expenses
1	$98,200	$137,200
2	121,500	117,262
3	146,000	141,656
4	171,750	168,274
5	198,750	196,566
6	227,000	223,775

[a] For year 1, projected income and expenses are itemized in Schedule A, projected professional and personal expenses are itemized in Schedule C, and a spreadsheet of monthly projected income and expenses is outlined in Schedule D.

[b] For years 2–6, projected income and expenses are itemized in Schedule B.

Alternative Plan for Financial Supplementation
If practice revenues do not meet projections, it may become necessary to supplement practice income with outside employment. I have investigated the opportunities available to me in the Townsville area for part-time employment outside the practice. I anticipate that these opportunities will be available in the first year after I open my practice. There are three potential sources at this time:
• Employment with an ophthalmologist in northwest Townsville. I would provide low vision services.
• Instructor at Townsville State Community College. I would teach biology, which was my undergraduate major.
• Eye care provider at Bigtime Correctional Facility, which is located 30 miles from Townsville.

Summary
The projections of income and expenses used in this proposal are based on conservative national estimates. They represent reasonable goals for overhead and generated income. Based on these projections, the practice begins to generate a profit after 6 months and for the entire year incurs a loss of only $1,470. Profit in the second year should be sufficient to permit income use for practice improvements, anticipated increases in the cost of living, and for a greater doctor's draw. After the sixth year, the loan will be retired.

Schedule A: Projected Income and Expenses for Year 1
Expenses

Purchase of equipment and modification of office	$44,155
Operating expenses for office (see Schedule C)	58,050
Loan cost	-0-
Taxes (income, Social Security)	2,041
Doctor's draw	35,000
Total	$137,200

Assets and income

Cash on hand	-0-
Projected practice income	
(250 days at $150 gross per approximately	
1.54 patients per day)	$56,200
Spouse's income	42,000
Total	$98,200
Net	-40,000
Loan amount needed	$40,000

Figure 16-1 Sample Loan Proposal. Personal information, such as a financial statement, resumé, and list of credit and character references, is not included.

Continued

Schedule B: Projected Income and Expenses for Years 2 through 6

Year 2		Year 3	
Expenses		*Expenses*	
Operating expenses for office	$61,062	Operating expenses for office	$71,256
Bank loan repayment	11,400	Bank loan repayment	11,400
Taxes	4,800	Taxes	9,000
Doctor's draw	35,000	Doctor's draw	40,000
Practice improvement	5,000	Practice improvement	10,000
Total	$117,262	Total	$141,656
Assets and income		*Assets and income*	
Projected practice income		Projected practice income	
(250 days at $155 gross per approximately		250 days at $160 gross per approximately	
2.0 patients per day)	$77,500	2.5 patients per day)	$100,000
Spouse's income	44,000	Spouse's income	46,000
Total	$121,500	Total	$146,000
Net	$4,238	Net	$4,344
Year 4		Year 5	
Expenses		*Expenses*	
Operating expenses for office	$80,874	Operating expenses for office	$91,166
Bank loan repayment	11,400	Bank loan repayment	11,400
Taxes	16,000	Taxes	24,000
Doctor's draw	45,000	Doctor's draw	50,000
Practice improvement	15,000	Practice improvement	20,000
Total	$168,274	Total	$198,566
Assets and income		*Assets and income*	
Projected practice income		Projected practice income	
(250 days at $165 gross per approximately		(250 days st $170 gross per approximately	
3.0 patients per day)	$123,750	3.5 patients per day)	$148,750
Spouse's income	48,000	Spouse's income	50,000
Total	$171,750	Total	$198,750
Net	$3,476	Net	$2,184
Year 6			
Expenses			
Operating expenses for office	$101,375		
Bank loan repayment	11,400		
Taxes	31,000		
Doctor's draw	60,000		
Practice improvement	20,000		
Total	$223,775		
Assets and income			
Projected practice income			
(250 days at $175 gross per approximately			
4.0 patients per day)	$175,000		
Spouse's income	52,000		
Total	$227,000		
Net	$3,225		

Figure 16–1, Cont'd.

However, the biggest failing of insufficient research is that the predictive value of the proposal is lost and it serves only as a justification for funding. Ideally, the loan proposal should continue to be used after funding has been secured and the practice plan initiated, as part of the effort to measure success toward financial goals. It should be constantly updated and revised to reflect the evolving situation in the practice. In such a role, it fulfills the short-term goal orientation that is so necessary to a successful outcome.

Drafting the Proposal

The loan proposal requires a stepwise approach: first, all items that are to be purchased–equipment, furni-

ture, real estate, computer, inventory of frames–need to be valued; second, other key expenditures, such as loans, taxes, leases, utilities, and so forth need to be determined; third, projections need to be calculated–on a month-by-month basis for the first year and annually thereafter for the remaining years of the loan repayment period (which generally is 4 to 6 years); fourth, practice income projections need to be calculated; and fifth, the "bottom line"–the profit or loss to be realized–needs to be determined, month by month for the first year and annually for all subsequent years.

Step One: Valuing Purchases. The fair market value should be determined for all items that must be purchased. The cost of a phoropter, sofa, computer, or

Schedule C: Projections of Professional and Personal Expenses for Year 1

Operating Expenses for the Practice		Personal Living Expenses	
Office lease	$10,800	Apartment rent	$7,400
Laboratory costs	16,860	Automobile loans (2 cars)	6,064
Employee salary and benefits	15,000	Educational loans	3,600
Utilities	2,700	Automobile insurance (2 cars)	1,276
Telephone and facsimile costs	1,200	Health insurance (paid by spouse's employer)	-0-
Computer	1,690	Utilities (electricity, water, telephone)	2,160
Drugs, supplies, and postage	1,200	Subsistence	6,800
Repairs to office and equipment	500	Clothing allowance	1,200
Automobile expenses	600	Automobile operating expenses	700
Continuing education, professional dues, and licenses	2,000	Miscellaneous personal expenses	2,000
Umbrella liability insurance coverage	1,000		
Life insurance (decreasing term policy)	700		
Employee taxes	1,450		
Self-employment tax	-0-		
Legal and accounting fees	1,000		
Announcement for opening of office	550		
Total	**$58,050**	**Total**	**$30,000**

Schedule D: Projected Income and Expenses for First Year in Practice

Month	1	2	3	4	5	6	7	8	9	10	11	12	
Patients per day	1.0	1.1	1.2	1.3	1.4	1.5	1.6	1.7	1.8	1.9	2.0	2.1	
Income per patient	$150	$150	$150	$150	$150	$150	$150	$150	$150	$150	$150	$150	
TOTAL	$3000	$3300	$3600	$3900	$4200	$4500	$4800	$5100	$5400	$5700	$6100	$6500	$56200
Expenses													
Laboratory costs	$900	$990	$1080	$1170	$1260	$1350	$1440	$1530	$1620	$1710	$1860	$1950	$16860
Office lease	$900	$900	$900	$900	$900	$900	$900	$900	$900	$900	$900	$900	$10800
Employee salary and taxes	$1370	$1370	$1370	$1370	$1370	$1370	$1370	$1370	$1370	$1370	$1370	$1370	$16450
Utilities	$325	$325	$325	$325	$325	$325	$325	$325	$325	$325	$325	$325	$3900
Insurance	$141	$141	$141	$141	$141	$141	$141	$141	$141	$141	$141	$141	$1700
Other	$695	$695	$695	$695	$695	$695	$695	$695	$695	$695	$695	$695	$8340
TOTAL	$4331	$4421	$4511	$4601	$4691	$4781	$4871	$4961	$5051	$5141	$5231	$5321	$58050
Net Income													
Net loss or profit	-$1331	-$1121	-$911	-$701	-$491	-$281	$71	$139	$349	$559	$869	$1179	
Cumulative loss or profit	-$1331	-$2252	-$3163	-$3864	-$4355	-$4636	-$4565	-$4426	-$4077	-$3518	-$2649	-$1470	

Figure 16–1 Cont'd.

any other item can be reasonably ascertained; if an inventory of frames is needed, its value will have been negotiated; for all items of purchase, an accurate determination of value should be obtained.

Step Two: Valuing Key Expenditures. One important goal of the loan proposal is comprehensiveness; it should seek to include all costs that can reasonably be expected to arise during the projected period of years. Key expenditures that should be considered include both personal and business expenses (Table 16-1).

The more complete the list, the more accurate the determination of the total cost of operating the practice. These expenditures should be calculated for each month of the first year of practice and for each year thereafter until the loan repayment has been satisfied. These expenditures, taken with the cost of purchases, constitute the "overhead" of the practice. It is important that, for a new practice, the overhead not be too high. The higher the overhead, the larger the number of patients that must be seen to break even or show a profit. If the overhead is so high that the loan proposal projects the practice will operate at a deficit for years before patient flow can generate a profit, it is likely that the loan proposal will be rejected. Therefore, overhead always should be kept to a reasonable level, and extravagant expenditures should be discarded. Expensive items—such as an automated perimeter or an edging laboratory—may not be feasible for a plan to start a practice "cold." The "bottom line" should be scrutinized carefully. Creditors do not like to fund operations that seem to require a lengthy period before generating a profit.

Step Three: Drafting Projections. Once all information on expenditures has been compiled, it is organized in a spreadsheet format. The first year projections are arranged month by month; for the subsequent years, a sum of monthly expenditures is used. Projecting overhead costs for these subsequent years is an art; cost of living increases should be added to each year to approximate the rise in costs that can be anticipated.

Step Four: Projecting Income. Perhaps the most difficult aspect of creating a loan proposal is the projection of expected income, especially for a new practice. If there are other practitioners who have recently opened a practice, it may be possible to obtain information based on their experience. If there is no source of recent information, it may be useful to provide projections so that they describe the number of patients

Table 16-1 List of Key Expenditures

Personal Expenses
Rent or mortgage payment
Utilities (heat, light, air conditioning, water)
Clothing and grooming
Telephone
Subsistence (groceries, restaurants)
Automobile expenses (insurance, gas, repairs)
Health care (not reimbursed by insurance)
Taxes (personal, property, home)
Interest expenses (credit cards, personal loans, home loans)
Charitable contributions
Nonreimbursed employee business expenses
Contributions to a retirement plan (IRA)
Child care or education costs

Professional Expenses
Office lease
Staff salaries
Staff benefits (health insurance, contributions to a retirement plan)
Payroll tax (income, Social Security/Medicare, unemployment insurance)
Business property tax (equipment, furnishings)
Office utilities (heat, light, air conditioning, water)
Repairs and maintenance fees (equipment)
Answering service
Janitorial service
Postage
Health insurance premiums
Life insurance premiums
Property and casualty insurance premiums (including workers' compensation)
Professional liability (malpractice) insurance premiums
Office supplies
Computer supplies
Income taxes
Social Security taxes
Debt service for professional loans (bank loan)
Repayment of educational loans
Contributions to a business-related retirement plan (IRA, Keogh Plan, 401 [k])
Continuing education
Travel, meals and entertainment
Licensure fee
Membership in professional organizations
Legal and accounting fees

needed to pay the overhead or to generate a certain profit level. For the first year projections, the number of patients seen daily should be determined and a specific gross income attributed to each. Local practitioners can be consulted to determine the reasonable amount of income that can be expected per type of patient. Eye health examinations generate different amounts of income than do contact lens assessments or binocular vision evaluations. The number of expected patients for each service, and the projected income for each, must be calculated. If a practice has been purchased, it is much easier to make income projections. It should be remembered, however, that some loss of patient base–approximately 10% to 15%–can be expected during the first year. The number of new patients needed to eliminate this potential deficit should be determined and used as a goal.

Step Five: Calculation of the "Bottom Line." The income and overhead for each month of the first year are used to determine whether there will be a profit or loss. For a new practice, it is not unusual for the first several months to produce a deficit rather than a profit. However, the anticipated income should be such that, within the year, a monthly profit can reasonably be expected. Creditors will not finance a practice that requires years to be self-supporting. The "bottom line" calculations are the goals against which the practice's actual performance are to be measured. If they are inaccurate, they can be adjusted to reflect the actual financial circumstances of the practice and a new set of goals thereby created.

Once the loan proposal has been calculated, it must be typed up and supporting documents must be added. The proposal should begin with a statement of purpose, which summarizes the financial goals of the borrower. Documents that may be attached to the loan proposal include the following:

- A personal financial statement
- The income tax return for the past year
- A copy of the office lease (if available)
- An insurance list describing policies and premium costs

Presentation

The presentation of the proposal to the creditor should be planned, and answers to anticipated questions should be rehearsed. Professional attire should be worn for the occasion. If accepted, the usual means of financing is a line of credit, against which the borrower may draw as the need for money arises. Since creditors do not like to extend lines of credit beyond those originally agreed on, the amount of credit secured should be adequate for the practice's financial obligations. Of course, interest is charged on the amount actually withdrawn for use.

Conclusion

The loan proposal is the financial heart of the practice plan. To make the plan viable, the loan proposal must contain accurate information, attainable goals, and reasonable projections and must be capable of modification to meet the changing circumstances that are an inevitable part of practice.

Bibliography

Allergan, Inc. *Pathways in optometry.* Irvine, Calif, 1995, Author.

American Optometric Association. *Career advocate for the new practitioner.* St. Louis, 2001, Author.

Classé JG. *Legal aspects of optometry.* Boston, 1989, Butterworth.

Gregg J. *The business of optometric practice.* White Plains, NY, 1984, Advisory Enterprises.

www.businessfinances.com. A sizable business funding directory, accessible online.

www.sba.gov. Web site for the U.S. Small Business Administration; it provides a step-by-step approach to the formulation of a business plan.

Chapter 17

Understanding Office Leases

Lawrence S. Thal

Why so large cost, having so short a lease,
Dost thou upon thy fading mansion spend?
William Shakespeare *Sonnets*

The signing of a lease can represent the largest financial transaction ever made by a prospective tenant. The lease agreement is legally binding and can be enforced on the parties involved. Even though a lease should be reviewed by competent advisors or legal counsel, it is unusual for counsel to actively negotiate its terms; that burden inevitably falls on the prospective tenant. For this reason, a prospective tenant should be aware of the common terms and the usual pitfalls associated with leases. This chapter reviews many of the problems that are encountered when attempting to negotiate a lease for a professional office.

The person who occupies property owned by another is called a *lessee*. Negotiation of the lease agreement with the owner–the *lessor*–might be limited to the presentation of a contract by the owner, accompanied by the following language: "Enclosed please find your standard lease form. You should sign where indicated, initial each page, and return at your earliest convenience."

This language may be the first introduction the tenant has to the lease, and even though the term standard might seem to imply some degree of conformity or regularity, the only standard aspects of an individual lease are the matters that it addresses. There is not one customary way to address these matters, and they should be fully negotiated and understood by the tenant.

A *lease* is a contract binding its signatories to its terms, and the tenant should assume, at the inception of the relationship, that all terms are fully enforceable. There are many pitfalls for the novice tenant, and even what is perceived to be the fairest of leases may contain provisions that can lead to disastrous financial consequences. Therefore, it is important to obtain competent advice before executing a contract such as a lease.

A shrewd attorney for the tenant could write a lease allowing the tenant to delay or offset rent payments for myriad reasons–even reasons beyond the landlord's control. A landlord's attorney could be equally shrewd in writing a lease with complicated clauses that provide for rapid and unfair rent increases. The object of any negotiation, however, should be to reach a contract that is fair, equitable, and easily understood.

Often it is perceived that certain landlords–such as shopping center owners–are inflexible and powerful and that, as a result, all tenants sign the same lease. Prospective tenants should not overlook the fact that they are the ones with the power to sign or not sign a lease. Printed lease forms are sometimes meant to epitomize inflexibility or to emphasize the power of the landlord. Tenants should not be fooled by how impressively worded the lease is or by how large the law firm is that supposedly drafted the lease. Concessions can always be awarded by a landlord.

Negotiating for Concessions

It can easily be 2 to 3 months after the lease agreement has been signed before the first patient walks through the door. During this period, without the benefit of patient income, the optometrist will be paying for alterations, instruments, office furniture, and similar items. To offset these expenditures, the practitioner should not be afraid to ask the landlord for help in the form of concessions. Possible concessions in the lease agreement include the following:

- Out-and-out reduction in the rent for the full term of the lease (especially if the rent appears excessive considering the space and location)

- A few months of free rent to help the optometrist reduce overhead expenditures while alterations are being performed on the premises or equipment is being delivered and installed
- Payment by the landlord for all or part of the alterations or improvements to the office
- A "step-up" lease, in which rent is paid at a reduced rate for the first 6 to 12 months and gradually increased to the full rate over time

In some cases, the landlord might refuse to make any concessions. If the office space is highly desirable and the market for office space is very limited, the prospective tenant might have to be comforted by the knowledge that previous tenants have worked successfully under such leases. In such a case, it is appropriate to check with the other tenants. If the landlord has dealt reasonably and fairly with them, there is a good likelihood that the prospective tenant will not encounter any extraordinary difficulties. The landlord has a reputation to protect, and if tenants have been treated unfairly in the past, it will suffer. In addition, a high turnover rate will drive up the landlord's costs of doing business.

Selecting Competent Counsel

The tenant should solicit recommendations for real estate attorneys from other health care professionals in the area. Successful professionals are likely to have identified and hired the best attorneys and accountants because physicians, dentists, and other health care providers usually demand good advice and are willing to pay for it. The prospective tenant should not hesitate to schedule an interview with an attorney to obtain information about the attorney's background, philosophy of practice, fees, and experience with real estate. There is normally no charge for this initial interview. The attorney will value the opportunity to discuss matters of mutual interest with a prospective long-term client.

Location

The same type of investigation of local demographic information should be conducted to determine the best locations in which to seek an office. Real estate agents, the staff of the local planning commission, or the local Chamber of Commerce can provide demographic data. Practice sites should be prominent and readily visible to the public. In addition, the office location should be easily accessible—near public transportation and with adequate parking available.

If an office is highly visible (e.g., next to a bank or across from the post office), the practice will become known immediately. Being in the local "professional building" or in an area with other professional offices is excellent. It is worth some extra cost to obtain a good, visible location; the additional expenditure will be returned many times over. It also is important to obtain adequate space. The consistent rise in net income due to such a practice site usually will compensate for the higher cost of the lease.

Specific Contract Clauses

Several specific clauses of the lease agreement are of particular importance. These clauses include identification of the parties, property description, term, rent, tenant mix, assignment, maintenance, warning before eviction, leasehold improvements, broker's fee, exculpation, warranty to practice, and security deposit.

Parties

The parties to the contract must be identified; these are the parties who will be expected to comply with the lease's terms and conditions.

Property Description

The lease should clearly define the property to be rented. If the property is free-standing, it is relatively easy to describe the premises for which maintenance will be performed, taxes assessed, and insurance provided. This description is not as clear when the premises are part of an office complex or shopping center that includes parking facilities, elevators, and other common areas. In these cases, tenants normally pay a percentage of the taxes, insurance, or maintenance that is assessed on the whole building. The percentage to be paid should be negotiated based on the square footage occupied, rent amount, anticipated use of parking and other common areas, and type of business conducted.

Term and Renewal

For a credit-worthy tenant who is successful in a business endeavor, a long lease term can be beneficial to both the tenant and the landlord. Conversely, a long-term lease can be disastrous for the optometrist who is less successful. Even though adequate investigation, planning, and market research should minimize that risk, it is always possible for unexpected events to adversely affect anticipated revenues.

Many landlords will not be anxious to lease to an optometrist who wants only a 3-year term. A 5-year term can be more acceptable, even for a new practice. For an already established practice with anticipated revenue based on historical performance, a 10-year lease can be more reasonable. In any case, the optometrist should negotiate for renewal options to be included in the lease. These options are exercised at the discretion of the tenant, and they extend the lease period for a stated number of years. The rent to be paid during the new term should be calculated on a pre-agreed basis.

Whatever the term of the lease, the tenant should request a provision that allows the tenant to stay month-to-month at the prevailing rental charge when the lease expires. Another useful provision is one that provides for possible practice growth by requesting first refusal on adjoining or other space in the building if it becomes available.

Rent

Leases are often characterized as being either "net leases" or "gross leases." A *net lease* implies that the tenant will pay the landlord rent that includes the "net" cost of all taxes, insurance, and maintenance expenses (i.e., the tenant pays these in addition to rent). A *gross lease* implies that the landlord pays the expenses for taxes, insurance, and maintenance out of the rent proceeds. A fully negotiated lease should be a compromise between these extremes.

Even though some practitioners live in communities that have experimented with various artificial methods of controlling residential rents, those that advocate such foolishness live in a fantasy world—one where new buildings will be constructed and improved with no regard to profit and where conventional lenders will provide construction loans solely because of their sense of social responsibility. Conversely—and realistically—a fair rent should be determined from the marketplace, which is to say by demand and availability. It is a mistake, however, for the optometrist to use market factors as the only determinant of rent. A pro-forma analysis will indicate the maximum rent that will not unreasonably drain the resources of a practice (Figure 17-1). A landlord also should be motivated to ensure that rents are fair and affordable to tenants because a contract to the contrary is an invitation to early vacancy, cessation of rents, and possible litigation.

Most net leases establish a base or fixed rent (often called minimum rent), and additional amounts are added to reimburse the building owner for operating costs, which can include taxes, insurance, and common-area maintenance (e.g., landscaping, janitorial services, elevator maintenance, parking lot resurfacing, common-area lighting). In shopping centers a percentage rent can be used; this provides a bonus to the owners of the shopping center based on the tenant's success.

The tenant should attempt to negotiate "caps"—maximums on the reimbursement of operating costs—or, at a minimum, the tenant should expect a guarantee that the total expenses reimbursed to the landlord by all tenants will not exceed 100% of the actual costs incurred. Optometrists who do not wish landlords to perform advertising on their behalf should exclude assessments for advertising. When advertising is to be performed by the landlord, copies of the advertisements should be submitted to the optometrist for approval and to ensure that they conform to applicable state laws.

Even though percentage rents provide some protection to landlords from inflation, a rent based on the number of examinations performed or eyeglasses dispensed might be disagreeable to the optometrist. The negotiation of rent is a business matter, but many optometrists have difficulty reaching business decisions without some regard to practice morals or professional ethics. The decision to pay percentage rents is an individual one, and, if it is agreed to, the amount to be paid should be negotiated based on the rents paid by other tenants. A percentage rent requires that monthly accounts of income or profit and loss statements be provided to the landlord. It can be preferable to pay a higher base or fixed rent instead of entering into such an arrangement.

If percentage rents are paid, a fair percentage must be considered in relation to the total amount that the optometrist can budget for rent. A pro-forma analysis should identify the maximum available rent the optometrist can pay. Even a 2% percentage rent could increase payment over a fixed rent amount by many thousands of dollars. For example, the tenant would have to pay $4000 if the percentage rent applied to all of a $200,000 gross income, but would only pay $2000 if it was limited to gross income in excess of $100,000.

There are other factors that should also be considered, including rental per square foot per year, automatic rent increases, and steps-up in rent.

Rental per Square Foot per Year

The tenant should determine whether the "per-square-foot" cost is in line with what is being charged for comparable offices in the vicinity. The tenant should attempt to have the cost-per-square-foot figure applied only to the office's actual floor space and should try to

---

Bay View Optometry

Drs. Jones and Smith, Optometrists

Pro Forma Estimate of Income and Expenses

Estimated revenue from professional services	$312,000	
Estimated revenue from materials	290,000	
Estimated refunds	(2,000)	
TOTAL REVENUE		$600,000
Estimated variable expenses (lab fees, frames, contact lenses)	$205,000 (34.2%)	
Estimated fixed expenses (% of total revenue)		
Salary (payroll)	116,000 (19.3%)	
Employee benefits	10,000 (1.7%)	
Maximum rent	**40,000 (6.7%)**	
Insurance	5,000 (0.8%)	
Bank charges	3,000 (0.5%)	
Postage	3,000 (0.5%)	
Travel and entertainment	2,000 (0.3%)	
Continuing education (professional development)	2,000 (0.3%)	
Repairs	4,000 (0.7%)	
Dues and subscriptions	2,000 (0.3%)	
Licenses	1,000 (0.2%)	
Office supplies	6,000 (1.0%)	
Telephone	7,000 (1.2%)	
Utilities	4,000 (0.7%)	
Contributions	1,000 (0.2%)	
Professional fees (CPA)	4,000 (0.7%)	
Marketing	8,000 (1.3%)	
Property tax (equipment and furnishings)	2,000 (0.3%)	
TOTAL EXPENSES		$425,000 (70.8%)
MINIMUM NET INCOME		$175,000 (29.2%)

Figure 17-1 In this example, Drs. Jones and Smith have determined that the minimum net annual income needed to meet their needs is $175,000. To satisfy this goal, the maximum rent allowance is $40,000. Regardless of what the landlord may feel the market rent may be, rent in excess of $40,000 the first year will put Jones and Smith in a deficit. It would be far more beneficial for both landlord and tenant to structure a rent that ensures both are successful. This may mean a rent that escalates during the initial term of the lease rather than a rent that is held constant.

avoid payment of a prorated share of the building's common footage, such as halls and lobbies. Economic surveys of established practices that have been performed by the American Optometric Association have indicated that rent cost nationally averages nearly 7% of gross earnings. This percentage is similar to that found in other professions.

Automatic Increases

Many leases permit a landlord to raise the rent to allow for rises in property taxes, maintenance costs, or the cost-of-living index. If such a clause must be accepted, the tenant should attempt to limit the annual increment to a maximum fixed percentage. Late charges should be clearly stated. If a landlord expects to recover a penalty for any rent payments made late, the amount of the penalty and the date by which the penalty would be incurred need to be carefully described.

Step-Up Rents

When negotiating rents, it can be advantageous to start off a lease term with a low rent that increases over time—hopefully as income also increases. Most accountants should be able to determine an equitable rent structure. For example, if a landlord is asking for $1000 a month for a 4-year term, the tenant can offer $700 a month for the first year, $900 a month for the second year, and $1230 a month for the last 2 years. (Assuming a 6% interest rate, this proposal nets the landlord exactly the same amount as $1000 a month during the 4 years.)

The attractiveness of many community shopping centers as lease premises lies in the presence of a nationally known anchor tenant: a large department store or supermarket that attracts consumers. Should one of these tenants vacate the shopping center, the optometrist could experience a dramatic loss in revenue, making monthly rent payments a hardship. Thus, it certainly would be fair to negotiate a clause that allows for reduced rental payments during the period which such major tenant vacancies persist.

It also is reasonable to restrict landlords so they may not offer leases or subleases to competitors (other optometrists or opticians) in the part of the facility that is under the landlord's control.

What should a tenant do if the landlord wants to raise the rent by a tremendous amount at the termination of the current lease? It is difficult to protect against this event except through automatic renewal options that can be asserted by the tenant at stipulated periods. In the absence of such an option, it is probably best to open negotiations for a new lease early (e.g., 4 to 6 months before the lease expires) to prevent this from happening. Another strategy is to ask other tenants about the past history of the landlord before signing the original lease. Has the landlord been reasonable? Have rent increases been reasonable?

Tenant Mix

Landlords can claim that they entered into a lease with individuals who met specific criteria or with careful consideration of tenant mix. Even though some restrictions are appropriate to protect the landlord against the assignment of leases to undesirable tenants, absolute restrictions are unfair. Absolute restrictions on assignment might even prohibit an optometrist from selling the practice.

Assignment

Although many leases prohibit a tenant from assigning or subletting a lease, a prospective tenant needs to weigh these provisions carefully. Without such a right, an optometrist or the optometrist's heirs might be responsible for lease payments even in the case of death, disability, or lack of economic success. In planning for such an event, the optometrist will want to ensure that the lease could be assigned to another party or perhaps be terminated altogether. In the case of death or disability, it should be possible to terminate the lease when the appropriate notice is given (e.g., 90 days).

The landlord can insist that approval be obtained if the tenant wishes to move before the conclusion of the lease term and to turn the premises over to another tenant. If the landlord insists on reserving the right to veto any proposed subtenant, the following compromise should be suggested: "The tenant shall not sublet without the landlord's consent, which consent shall not be withheld unreasonably." Another proposal is for the optometrist to ask for an automatic end to the lease within 90 days (or within another reasonable period) after a disabling accident or illness has been suffered, the optometrist has been called for military duty, or the optometrist has died. A clause also should be sought that guarantees that a practitioner who buys the practice has the right to continue under the terms of the lease.

It also should be clear what the tenant's rights are when title to the property being leased reverts to the owner of a mortgage. The lease should clearly state that the rights of a tenant are not subordinated to the interests of a mortgage lender (called a mortgagee). This clause would prevent a lender from evicting tenants in the case of a mortgage foreclosure, a situation in which a transfer of ownership is effected from the original landlord to a mortgage lender.

Both parties to a lease should have the right to terminate or cancel the lease should the other significantly default on lease provisions. A reasonable period in which to remedy such a default should be provided.

Some leases obligate a tenant to keep paying rent for the full term even if the building is severely damaged by fire or other casualty or if an essential facility like air conditioning breaks down and the landlord fails to repair it. The lease should allow the tenant to terminate the agreement under such circumstances without penalty or to pay a reduced rent.

Maintenance

Typically, the landlord would like to repair nothing, whereas the tenant would like the landlord to repair everything. Absent other concessions, a fair agreement is somewhere between these two extremes. A possible fair agreement would have the building owner liable for all repairs to the building exterior, including roof and exterior glass, as well as mechanical systems such as central heating and air conditioning, whereas the tenant would be responsible for repairs to plumbing, the electrical system, interior painting, carpeting, and so forth. Maintenance provisions are subject to negotiation, and results can vary considerably, depending on the amount of rent paid and the length of the lease term.

Insurance on the building is normally carried by the owner; it is required by the building's mortgagee. The owner, likewise, should have the burden of rebuilding in the case of destruction by fire or other casualty. The tenant should be properly insured for the replacement of interior leasehold improvements, furniture, equipment, and supplies.

Maintenance of the exterior affects building appearance; thus, standards for exterior signage should be established. A professional tenant such as an optometrist should be protected from the garish signs of a retail store or amusement area next door. In fact, the optometrist can request protection from such a tenant being allowed in the same building. Examples of such restrictions include prohibitions on pawn shops, massage parlors, sex paraphernalia shops, bars, or exotic dancing establishments.

Responsibility for exterior painting and maintenance of sidewalks or parking areas should be covered in the lease. A tenant might be compensated for maintenance violations by a landlord through fair rent reductions, providing that the tenant has appropriately notified the owner of the violation and that adequate time has been given for the defaults to be cured.

Warning Before Eviction

A tenant should ensure that eviction will not result the first time a house rule (e.g., "objectionable conduct") is broken. The tenant should ask to be given written notice when in violation of a rule and to be allowed an opportunity to correct the error. A flat "no" should be given to any clause that says breaking a rule renders the tenant not only liable to be evicted but also responsi-

ble for the payment of the rent for the balance of the lease. If clauses such as these cannot be stricken from the lease in their entirety, then "objectionable conduct" (or other terms) must be clearly defined.

Leasehold Improvements

Seldom will office space vacated by one tenant be acceptable to another without renovation. The payment of office renovation costs needs to be negotiated, not only in terms of how the costs are to be borne, the extent of the renovations, and the period involved for them to be performed, but also in terms of the effect of the costs on the rent to be paid by the tenant during the lease term. Options for payment should be considered.

When an owner is highly dependent on full occupancy or when office space has had a long vacancy, a prospective tenant might be able to negotiate for the landlord to pay the renovation costs or—if the tenant pays the costs—for the landlord to provide a period of free or reduced rent. When office space is in high demand and rents are fair, it might be unreasonable to expect concessions of this type.

It can be strategically advantageous for a tenant to offer a higher rent than requested if, in return, the owner agrees to absorb the cost of renovations. When owners agree to perform renovations for a tenant, provisions should be included in the lease for monetary damages resulting from construction delays.

The landlord might agree to adhere to a tenant's specifications at the landlord's expense if the office needs painting, partitioning, or structural changes to suit the tenant's practice. If not, the tenant can suggest that an improvement allowance be rewarded as a rent rebate.

Alterations and repairs usually should not be initiated until the term of the lease begins. If the office is vacant, written permission should be obtained to start the modifications immediately. Customarily, the tenant is obligated to pay for services (e.g., electricity, water, gas) once alterations have begun. The tenant should try not to accept any clause requiring the premises to be restored to their original condition. The cost of re-creating a bare rectangle can be expensive. Also, improvements are assets to the landlord and should not have to be removed.

Broker's Fee

A broker's fee is usually due in leasing transactions and is generally payable by the landlord. In a sublease situation, the existing tenant pays the fee. The lease should identify any brokers involved and should clearly establish who is responsible for the broker's fee.

Exculpation

An exculpation clause limits the liability of a landlord to the interest in the property itself. The clause frees the landlord from legal responsibility for certain acts–committed by the tenant–that cause injury to persons on the property. It is not unusual for an owner to attempt to limit personal liability in this way.

Warranty to Practice

The tenant should be sure to include a clause stating that if local zoning laws forbid the practice of optometry on the premises or the operation of a business, the lease is null and void.

Security Deposit

The prepayment of 1 to 2 months of rent will earn the landlord money as long as the deposit is held. Unless local law so requires, the landlord will not offer to pay interest on the deposit. The tenant can ask for payment of the interest on the deposit held by the landlord.

Other Terms

In shopping plazas, leases often state that all tenants must maintain the same hours (e.g., 9 AM to 9 PM 6 days per week). A professional tenant usually can have this provision changed, and the change should be written into the lease.

The parking privileges available to staff and patients should be specified. The lease agreement should be examined to determine whether there are any additional costs for parking. The rules and regulations of the landlord regarding availability of parking during the hours the practice is to be open should be checked. Ideally, there should be seven to eight parking spaces for each professional in a building. If the practitioner and the staff do not use the spaces, a minimum of four to five spaces might be adequate.

The tenant should be sure that there are specific rights to erect customary signs–both inside and outside the building–and that these rights are contained in the lease.

Conclusion

When considering the rental of office space, other tenants should always be consulted to determine the integrity of a landlord. The law of supply and demand governs a tenant's bargaining position. That bargaining strength depends on how badly the tenant wants the space and how much the tenant is willing to pay for it. If there are two or three other prospective locations and time is not of the essence, a tenant is in a better position to bargain.

In the low-to-moderate rental field, the demand for space usually exceeds the supply. In more expensive areas, the reverse is true. Being a professional is in a tenant's favor when bargaining. Landlords would prefer to have a professional as a tenant, and a young professional should not be afraid to ask the landlord for changes and concessions.

Lease provisions can be looked at this way: A tenant is unlikely to get every clause requested in every instance. However, a prospective tenant can be sure that provisions favoring the tenant won't appear in the landlord's standard contract and that the landlord will not bring up such provisions unless asked to do so. How much compromise a landlord allows will depend on how desirable the space seems and how likely it is that a prospective tenant can find other suitable space in the locality.

From the landlord's viewpoint, professionals are good tenants. They usually pay their rent on time and do not often cause problems; they add prestige to the building and typically sign long-term contracts. These facts should not be forgotten by a young optometrist seeking to negotiate even that very first lease arrangement.

Acknowledgement

The authors of this chapter in the first edition of *Business Aspects of Optometry* were Lawrence S. Thal and Harry Kaplan.

Bibliography

American Optometric Association: *Caring for the eyes of America–a profile of the optometric profession.* St. Louis, 2002, Author.

Classé JG: *Legal aspects of optometry.* Boston, 1989, Butterworth.

Cotton H: *Medical practice management.* Oradell, NJ, 1977, Medical Economics.

Dean M, Nicholas F, Caplan R: *Commercial real property lease practice.* Berkeley, Calif, 1976, California Continuing Education of the Bar.

Dean M, Turner W: *Commercial real property lease practice* (update). Berkeley, Calif, 1992, California Continuing Education of the Bar.

Elmstrom G: *Advanced management for optometrists.* Chicago, 1974, Professional Press.

Sachs L: *The professional practice problem solver.* Englewood Cliffs, NJ, 1991, Prentice-Hall.

www.pueblo.gsa.gov. Web site for the Federal Citizen Information Center.

Chapter 18
Office Design

David Kirschen and John Crane

Let us see these handsome houses where the wealthy nobles dwell.
Alfred, Lord Tennyson *Locksley Hall*

The purpose of this chapter is to stimulate ideas about the key elements involved in office design. This discussion is not meant to serve as an exhaustive review, but rather as a resource for the new practitioner who is buying or redesigning an office for the first time.

The general public often forms an impression of a doctor's competence by the physical appearance of the exterior and interior of the office. As patients visit the office, their perception of the thoroughness of the examination can be strongly influenced by the interior décor and patient flow. These impressions can exert a significant effect on future visits and on referrals of new patients. For this reason, it is important for the practitioner to become knowledgeable in the areas of office design and patient flow, decoration, and some aspects of remodeling and construction.

Most optometrists will need the services of qualified professionals in the building trades to complete an office remodeling project. Finding the right people can be the biggest challenge. Architects, designers, contractors, and decorators should be chosen in the same manner as any advisor—by reputation in the community and by a trusted referral if possible. An interview to discuss the scope of the project, the cost, and the time involved should assist in making an intelligent selection. It is always wise to thoroughly check the references of any advisors and, if possible, to obtain firsthand knowledge of the quality and promptness of their work. Specific questions to ask include the following: "Was the cost estimate on target?" "Was the work completed on time?" "Were you satisfied with the work?"

The location of a practice contributes to the image it projects to the public. For example, an optometric practice located in a medical building will project an image of excellence in medical care, but not necessarily one in which designer eyewear would be available. On the other hand, an optometric office located in a mall projects an image of retail sales, in which products are important and "eye care" is incidental. An optometry office in a stand-alone building or in a strip center could project either or both images depending on the design, signage, lighting, and a host of other factors.

The practitioner's ability to fashion the exterior of an office depends largely on where the practice is located. In the case of a freestanding building, much can be done to positively influence the exterior, including the use of extensive landscaping, signage, and lighting (Figure 18-1). When the practice is located in a professional building or a shopping mall, these options might not be under the optometrist's direct control. However, design options might be agreed on at the time a lease is negotiated.

It is important to develop an efficient floor plan so that practitioners and staff can work effectively and efficiently. There are basically two alternatives when designing a floor plan:
- The patients are placed in examination rooms and the doctor moves between rooms.
- The doctor is placed in a room and the patients are moved to him or her.

The following describes several considerations involving patients, doctors, and staff that must be considered when designing an efficient floor plan (this is by no means an exhaustive list):
- Minimize the number of steps traveled each day by the staff
- Provide for wheelchair access
- Check-in and check-out areas should be separated

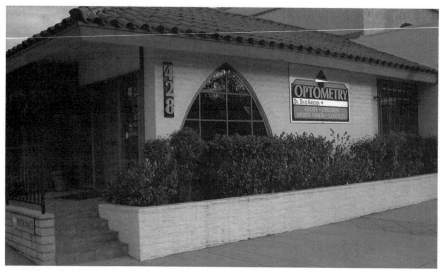

Figure 18-1 The 3-D signage, landscaping, and lighting give the exterior of this building a modern appearance. (Courtesy Dr. David Kirschen, Brea, Calif; picture by L. Ernie Carrillo.)

- Create "holding places" for patients waiting for dilation or contact lens services or patients wanting to speak to staff about personal financial matters
- Avoid bottlenecks in patient flow

The best time to consider the floor plan is when selecting a new office location. Sometimes a practitioner might be the first tenant in an open space and can have the luxury of constructing interior walls to suit the needs of the practice. In other cases, interior walls are usually in place and might have to be used "as is" for economical reasons. An established practitioner might wish to remove walls and add new walls to improve the floor plan and office flow.

It is extremely valuable to visit as many practices as possible before designing a new office or making major revisions. Photographs should be taken, if allowed, along with plenty of notes and a sketch of the floor plan. Actual measurements of existing rooms can give a better understanding of space requirements. Many eye care management journals feature photographs of and stories about office designs, and these can stimulate ideas.

Design of the Optometric Office

Office design is a very specialized field and, at times, professional advice is invaluable. A description of how the office is to be perceived by patients will provide very valuable information to design professionals. For example, is the office to convey a professional, upscale atmosphere or a homey, laid-back, comfortable atmosphere? Whatever the theme, it should be carried throughout each room in the office. The designer then can offer advice consistent with the tone that the practitioner wants to set in the office and offer design suggestions for each room, consistent with that theme.

There are three types of design services available. This first is from a professional design consultant who specializes in optometric offices. After hearing the practitioner's comments and evaluating the office space, these designers offer a number of services for a fee. They usually offer a "turn key" service, including design services, building contractors, furniture and displays, paint and carpet service, and so forth. Alternatively, they may offer design services only, and the practitioner will have to hire the necessary workers to make the plan happen.

The second kind of design service is from frame display companies. They will visit the office and help design (or redesign) the optical area. They understand patient flow, lighting, color coordination, and optical displays and furniture. Some companies charge a fee for the design service, which often includes computer-scale drawings of the floor plan and color 3-D renderings of the final layout.

The third kind of design service also is from frame display companies. Some offer a free floor plan design for an office. They generally speak with the practitioner on the telephone to assess needs and often will ask for photographs and a dimensional layout of the office as it currently exists. They then create a computer scale drawing of the new design for review, which sometimes includes 3-D renderings. This free service is offered in the hopes of earning future business, such as new frame displays and furniture.

Because optometry is such a specialized field and the particular needs of optometric offices are not generally known, this chapter covers key ideas to consider on a room-by-room basis. Not every office will have all the rooms listed, but this list hopefully will stimulate ideas both for present needs and future planning.

Vestibule or Lobby

A pleasant first impression is created when the front entrance to a building opens into a lobby or even a small vestibule. This area generally serves as a weather buffer to prevent shocks of cold, heat, or rain from entering the reception area of the office (Figure 18-2). Lobby space also can serve as a convenient area for patients waiting for transportation. Tile makes an excellent floor covering for this space, and replaceable mats provide a surface to absorb dirt and moisture.

Reception Area

The reception area should immediately welcome visitors in comfort (Figure 18-3). This area is commonly called a *waiting room*, but this term has a negative connotation because patients wait in a waiting room and no one likes to wait. A *reception area* is a place where patients are received. Something as simple as the name given to a room can help set the tone in the office. The

reception room should be kept very clean and be remodeled at least every 5 years.

The size of the reception area is dictated by the method of scheduling appointments and the number of patients who will be there at one time. Because pupillary dilation is now a standard procedure, a sizable reception area might be needed if dilated patients must be seated there. A secondary, inner room also can serve as a "holding" area, reducing the number of people who must be accommodated in the reception room and decreasing the size of the area needed. The reception area also must accommodate the family members or friends who might accompany the patient. The seating in the reception area should be visible to the receptionist from the business office desk or counter. In small offices, the receptionist can have a desk, rather than a built-in counter, in the reception area.

Anything that can make the reception room unique and special is desirable, if it is done in good taste. Considerations such as an aquarium, well-cared for plants, unusual windows with attractive exterior views, or a fireplace can set the practice apart from others and can become a form of internal marketing. Other unique ideas that can be incorporated into a reception room include bookcases with large print and regular print reading materials; a TV and VCR with cable news and weather stations or videotapes on eye care topics or children's cartoons; a display of antique eyewear; or

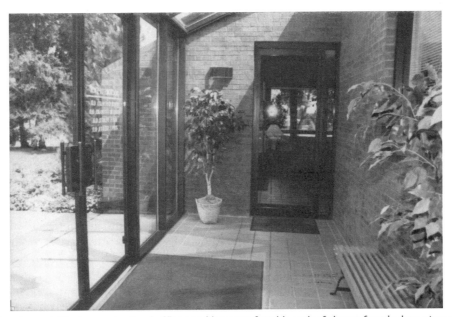

Figure 18-2 This entrance lobby to a professional office provides a comfortable and safe haven from inclement weather. (Courtesy Gailmard Eye Center, Munster, Ind.)

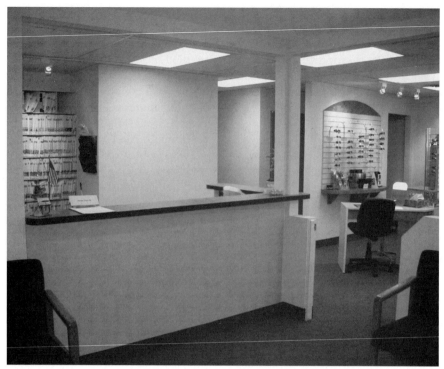

Figure 18-3 Reception area with an open appearance that is easily visible to the receptionist in the business office. It also provides easy access to the frame selection area through a door. (Courtesy Dr. David Kirschen, Brea, Calif; picture by L. Ernie Carrillo.)

a refreshment bar that might offer coffee, tea, or soft drinks. It is desirable to have a restroom available for patients immediately adjacent to the reception area so that office staff members do not have to be interrupted by patients seeking toilet facilities.

The choice of seating is a very important consideration and must provide durability while offering comfort and safety for handicapped and elderly patients. Single seating is preferable to couches, since strangers may not like to sit together. Lighting should be adequate for comfortable reading and should remind patients of the important relationship between good lighting and sharp acuity. A coat rack or closet is a nice addition and should be located in view of the receptionist. A bulletin board for announcements to patients is a useful accessory. A special corner or other built-in environment can be reserved for children, with a table and chairs as well as toys and children's reading materials (Figure 18-4); such an area demonstrates that the practice welcomes children. The reception room should provide a clear path from the front entrance doors to the receptionist's desk. A tile or vinyl floor covering makes a practical walkway to the front desk, while the rest of the reception area can be carpeted.

Some offices combine the reception area with the frame display area. In this way, patients who are waiting to be seen can "browse the optical" and get ideas for their spectacle purchases. This arrangement also offers an excellent opportunity for patient education and internal marketing.

Business Office

The business area, as the name implies, is where the business of the office is handled (Figure 18-5). This area should be easily accessible to patients and give the image of being open and available. An adjacent door to the reception room can provide for security and privacy. It works well if the check-in and check-out areas are kept separate. One area should be used for patients checking in, and the other for patients paying bills or making future appointments. It is important that patients have privacy when making such arrangements and that office procedures respect the confidentiality of patient information in accordance with the provisions of federal law (see Chapter 28). Care should be given to the location of telephones so the receptionist can view the reception room and still have some privacy for phone calls.

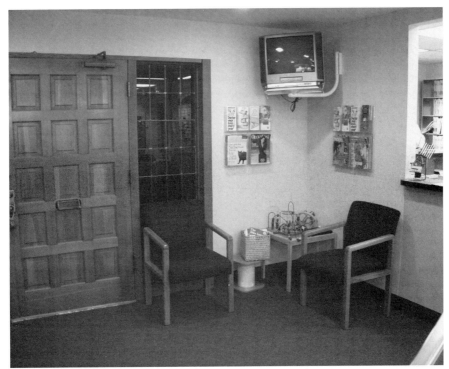

Figure 18-4 An area for children, located in the right corner of the reception room. It contains age-appropriate toys and reading material and a TV/VCR for entertainment. (Courtesy Dr. David Kirschen, Brea, Calif; picture by L. Ernie Carrillo.)

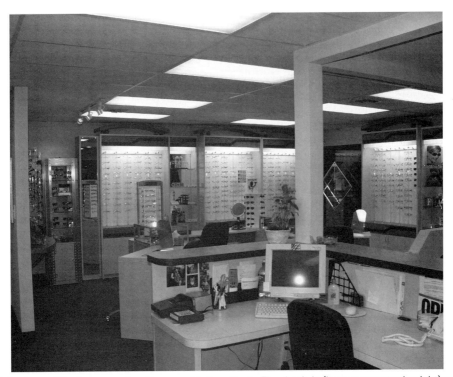

Figure 18-5 This business office is open and easily accessible to patients. The check-in (long counter to the right) and check-out (smaller counter to left of post) areas are separated, and the office has a good view of the frame selection area for security. (Courtesy Dr. David Kirschen, Brea, Calif; picture by L. Ernie Carrillo.)

The business office usually contains file cabinets or shelving units for current patient files. It might be necessary to install an additional remote filing area when the number of files exceeds the front office capacity. A system to purge older files must be devised for patients who have not returned in a certain number of years. Countertops and cabinets should be provided to allow for storage of office supplies.

The typical office equipment located in the business area includes a telephone, typewriter, computer and printer, fax machine, credit card device, and photocopier. Wall-mounted shelving units can provide an excellent visual display of contact lens solutions and other eye care supplies. Having such displays near the front desk and available at the time of final billing will result in convenience purchases. The telephone system generally can incorporate an intercom to the other rooms in the office and can even be used as a light-signaling system. An additional light-signal panel can be mounted in the business area to show which examination rooms are occupied by individual staff members. In smaller offices, it is convenient if the business office permits a view of the examination rooms. This method can be more efficient than light-signaling systems because the receptionist can simply look to see whether doors are open or closed to determine when the examination room is available for the next patient.

The business area, along with most of the office, will typically be carpeted and have a suspended ceiling; both factors help absorb sound and provide a nicer working environment. A short-weave, commercial-grade carpet is best, allowing for easy cleaning and for office chairs and stools to roll easily. The color and texture chosen should not show traffic patterns and soil. Fluorescent lighting, within the suspended ceiling, is most often used in offices because it is cool and cost-efficient. Various grid covers or lenses are available for fluorescent fixtures. The use of spotlights provides additional light where needed for emphasis and can add style to the office.

Administrative Area

It might be desirable in larger office spaces to have an additional business area that is not accessible or visible to patients. This area allows behind-the-scenes work by office staff—including the numerous billing and mailing activities that are part of a successful practice. Such activities can include the preparation and mailing of statements, recall notices, service agreement reminders, and other direct mail pieces. Additionally, this room can be used for receiving deliveries and mail and can provide a private area for the telephone activities of the staff, including calls to patients about past due accounts and the use of telephone marketing techniques. This room can have a conference table as well as an additional computer, telephone, postage meter, and photocopier.

Data Collection Room

The data collection room is used for preliminary testing, usually by an optometric technician (Figure 18-6). In some practices, it can be used as a special procedures room for procedures such as visual fields and retinal photography. A smaller examination room with a minimum size of 10 × 12 feet could serve this purpose. It may be desirable to have more than one data collection room, since the use of many instruments requires testing for significant periods. It is not likely that a practice will duplicate some of the computerized automated instruments that are necessary for data collection, so it might be preferable to conduct the automated tests in the first room and then move the patient to the second room for the remainder of the tests. This opens the first room for the next patient. A sink is useful in the data collection room so that technicians can wash their hands and contact lenses can be removed and reinserted. There are various instrument delivery tables available, ranging from automated rotating tables to individually adjusting tables for each instrument. Thought should be given to the tests that will be performed in this room so that room size and other aspects of design can be planned. For example, light switches should be easily reachable by a technician seated at the instrument. If the room is to be used for visual acuity, the placement of mirrors or other devices to measure acuity should be considered. Box 18-1 lists typical procedures that could be performed in a data collection room.

Examination Room

Multiple examination rooms should be considered for all but the smallest practices. Various methods for making the examination room more efficient include the refractive duo concept, in which the patient end of the room is wider than the end of the room where the target is projected. Often, two rooms can be designed so that they are adjacent to one another. Mirrored examination rooms have become very popular, however, and provide a nicer look than long, narrow lanes.

A room as small as 8 × 12 feet can be made acceptable for refractive distances of 20 feet with the use of

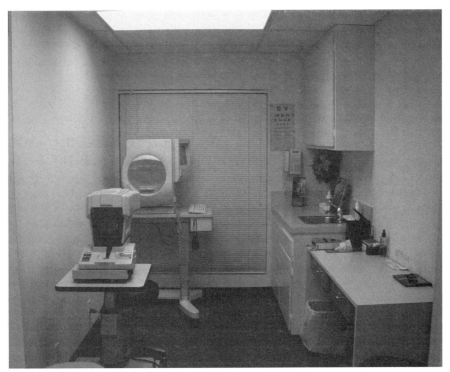

Figure 18-6 Data collection room that contains visual field unit and autorefractor despite its small size (6 × 10 feet). The table can be used for preliminary testing and the sink area for contact lens insertion and removal. (Courtesy Dr. David Kirschen, Brea, Calif; picture by L. Ernie Carrillo.)

refractive mirrors. These mirrors can be set up in a very effective manner and should not be regarded as too difficult or too confusing. If space permits, an ideal examination room might be 10 feet wide and 20 feet long. These dimensions provide a large, open feeling and offer plenty of room for chair-side technicians and visitors who might accompany the patient. It should be noted, however, that the examination chair will be at least 2 feet from the back wall of the room and that the refractive distance consequently will be close to 18 feet. The acuity chart can be adjusted to compensate for this test distance.

Examination rooms should be designed specifically for use by a right-handed or left-handed practitioner, and individual preferences should be taken into consideration (Figure 18-7). It is important to have a sink near the examination chair so that hands can be washed and solutions and contact lenses can be handled. An excellent concept is the use of the refraction desk, which serves as a writing surface and storage area near the sink and vanity. Handheld diagnostic instruments are placed in recharging wells within this refraction desk, and an inclined drawer stores the trial lens tray. Placement of a manual chart projector on the

refraction desk allows easy operation by the practitioner, especially if a small rearview mirror is incorporated so that the practitioner does not have to turn around to see the chart. Remote-control devices allow

Box 18-1 Procedures for Data Collection Rooms

- Case history
- Visual acuity (far and near)
- Noncontact tonometry
- Autorefraction
- Keratometry
- Lensometry
- Telebinocular visual skills
- Visual field testing
- Retinal photography
- Color vision
- Stereopsis
- Blood pressure measurement
- Corneal topography

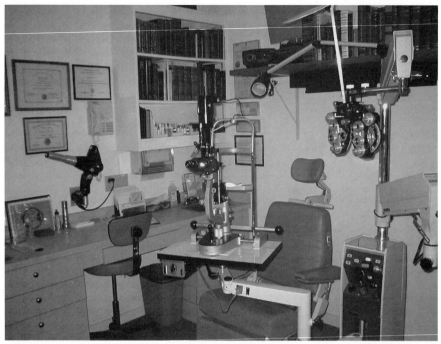

Figure 18-7 Examination room equipped with appropriate instrumentation and containing the doctor's library. Efficient design allows for storage of drugs and a large writing surface. There also are numerous visual aids to facilitate communication with patients. (Courtesy Dr. Larry Thal, Kensington, Calif.)

the projector to be mounted at the appropriate place in the room. The refraction desk can be wired electrically to control wall outlets so that various instruments can be controlled from the refraction desk. The room lights can be dimmed or turned off by controls on the refraction desk if they are prewired. It is somewhat complex to use a dimmer on fluorescent light fixtures, so it might be more practical to turn them off and use the reading light on the instrument stand as the only light for low illumination.

A clean, professional look is desirable for examination and treatment rooms, although some decoration is needed to prevent a too-sterile look. Subdued and textured wall coverings, tasteful art work, or a display of professional certificates are some decorating possibilities. Windows are not desirable in the examination room because of the need for lighting control, but if they already exist in the room, they can be covered with blinds or drapes. Some practitioners use windows as an adjunct to trial frame testing at a far distance.

Contact Lens Room

A special area reserved for contact lens fitting is a must for most practices (Figure 18-8). The contact lens area can serve as a laboratory and an inventory room that is only accessible to staff members, or it can include a dispensing and patient education room that would be used to instruct patients in contact lens use. As a laboratory, this room should have counters with convenient electrical outlets for instruments such as a radiuscope, lensometer, shadowscope, and microscope. A modification unit and sink also should be located in this room. With increased use of disposable contact lenses, larger areas are needed to store inventories. Having most lenses in stock is regarded by some practitioners as a significant practice asset, although the trend toward doctor-controlled shipment from the manufacturer directly to the patient may reduce this need.

Special dispensing counters with built-in sinks, tissue dispensers, and individual mirrors create an excellent environment for multiple- or single-patient training by the technician. Other considerations for this room include a dedicated video recorder and television for educational tapes about contact lenses and storage for educational brochures and fitting agreement forms.

Optical Dispensary

A large area within the office should be devoted to frame displays and optical dispensing since this area usually produces the largest portion of a practice's

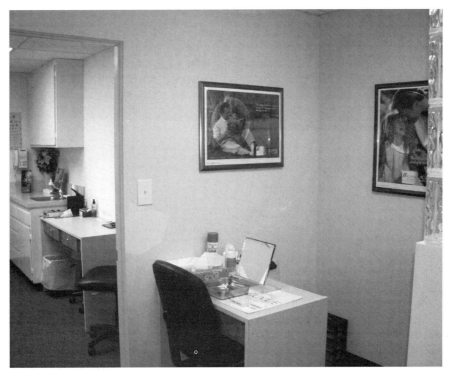

Figure 18-8 Contact lens room (right), stocked with necessary solutions for lens care; the technician can be seated opposite the patient when instruction or training is needed. (Courtesy Dr. David Kirschen, Brea, Calif; picture by L. Ernie Carrillo.)

income (Figure 18-9). A small dispensary is 200 square feet or smaller; a medium to large traditional dispensary is 500 to 1000 square feet; and a super-optical dispensary runs from 2000 to 3000 square feet. Wall space is typically used to mount frame display units or glass shelves for frames. Windows are desirable if sunlight can be controlled. Professional designers can be of great help in designing and furnishing this more retail-like area. Companies that manufacture and sell optical displays are eager to assist the doctor in choosing a theme for the dispensary and recommending the displays and furnishings that will achieve the look.

A lens design center can be incorporated into the dispensary. This center directs attention to ophthalmic lenses and optional lens features before frames are selected. A video frame-viewing center is another concept that can be included. These computer-assisted frame-display systems take a digital picture of the patients' face and electronically superimpose frames of different sizes, colors, and shapes on the picture. This gives the patient an opportunity to see what he or she will look like with frames that are not in stock. A special area or individual booths for delivering and adjusting glasses should be considered because they provide some privacy and reserve the use of dispensing tables

for frame selection purposes. Special sections showcasing frames for men, women, and children are fairly standard, but special areas for designer eyewear, sports eyewear, and brand name sunglasses are more unique (Figure 18-10). Lighting deserves special planning to highlight displays and make skin tones most attractive. Track lights work well for dramatic highlights but might need to be supplemented with fluorescent light and daylight. Indirect lighting—reflected off ceilings or walls—can be quite pleasing. Skylights are a popular architectural detail.

Many practices provide an entrance to the optical dispensary that is separate from the entrance to the professional practice. This feature allows a separate identity for the dispensary and allows more aggressive marketing than a practitioner might be comfortable with if it were strictly part of the practice. A separate entrance can prove quite functional for patients stopping in to pick up eyewear or to have glasses adjusted.

Optical Laboratory

The optical laboratory can range from a small repair center to a full-service laboratory with finishing and surfacing equipment (Figure 18-11). Square footage

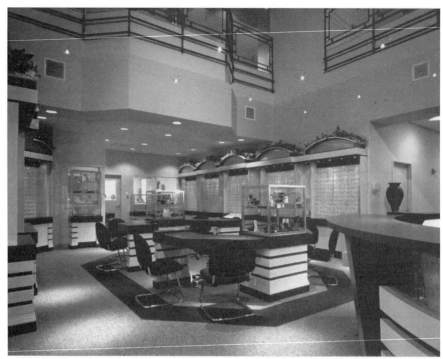

Figure 18-9 This optical dispensary's carpet accents and glass displays imply that high-quality materials are offered and that there is careful attention to detail. (Courtesy Eye Designs, Collegeville, Penn.)

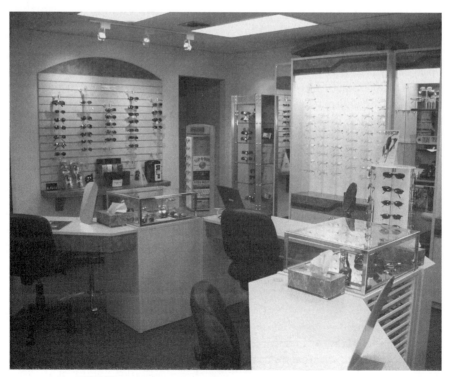

Figure 18-10 Lens design center (far left wall) within an optical dispensary that is used for discussion of lens material options with patients. Stand-alone cases (in rear) can be used to highlight specialty items such as sunglasses or sports frames. (Courtesy Dr. David Kirschen, Brea, Calif; picture by L. Ernie Carrillo.)

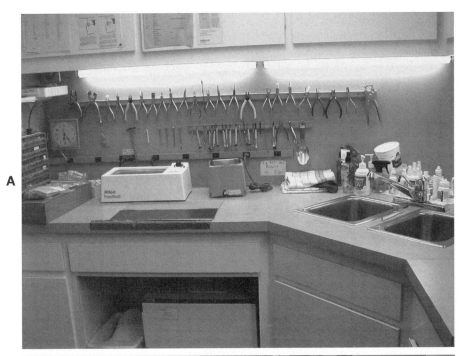

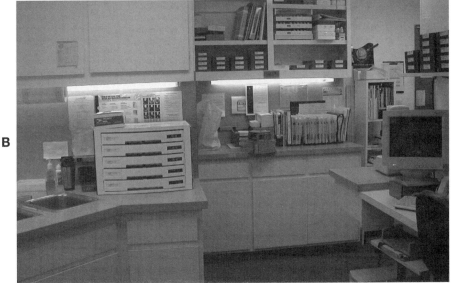

Figure 18-11 **A,** The portion of the optical laboratory used for frame adjustment and repairs; tools hang on a magnetic strip and thus are out of the way of the frame warmer and ultrasonic cleaner. **B,** The area used for verification of ophthalmic materials. (Courtesy Dr. David Kirschen, Brea, Calif; picture by L. Ernie Carrillo.)

can range from a minimal 60 to 80 square feet up to 1000 square feet for a large laboratory.

Attention should be given to the special requirements of water supply and waste drains, electrical outlets and voltage supply, and good lighting and sound control.

The laboratory design should be based on the logical flow of the steps in the lens fabrication process.

Ample counters at a 36-inch height for standing are needed, and base cabinets and wall cabinets provide important storage. If certain tasks require seating, the use of a barstool is effective, but an opening must be left between cabinets as a knee/leg hole. Certain services, such as computerized lens design, might need a special section of the counter at a desk height of 30 inches.

Special care must be taken in the tinting area to provide for adequate air ventilation, such as the installation of an exhaust hood. The walls and floor of this area will inevitably have dye splashed on them and, for that reason, can warrant special protection.

Practitioner's Private Office

It is recommended that practitioners have a private office that can be used for conducting the business aspects of managing a practice (Figure 18-12). It must be remembered that business administration is a vital component of successful practice and that not all of the optometrist's time is spent examining patients. As the owner of a small business, the practitioner must have a space to perform paperwork and meet with staff members and business associates. If space is limited, an area within an examination room can be fitted with a desk and chairs and serve as the practitioner's office.

Conference Room

A luxury in most large offices is the use of a dedicated conference room (Figure 18-13). This room can have a long conference table that accommodates all staff members. The room can include an area for a slide or overhead projector, as well as special felt-tip marker boards. The inclusion of a conference room will encourage regular and more productive staff meetings.

Staff Lounge

If space permits, a staff lounge or lunchroom is a nice addition to the office. This room can provide a lunch table, sink, refrigerator, microwave oven, telephone, and perhaps a television. If space is limited, the staff lounge can double as a conference room for staff meetings and industry presentations to staff.

Storage Rooms

Most practitioners, like homeowners, will agree that one can never have too much storage space. Unfortunately, with the high cost of commercial real estate, revenue-producing activities must take precedence. In planning an office, practitioners should consider the need for convenient storage of previous patients' records, office financial records and invoices, patient educational brochures, contact lens solutions, extra displays for the dispensary, office supplies and stationery, cleaning supplies, and maintenance tools.

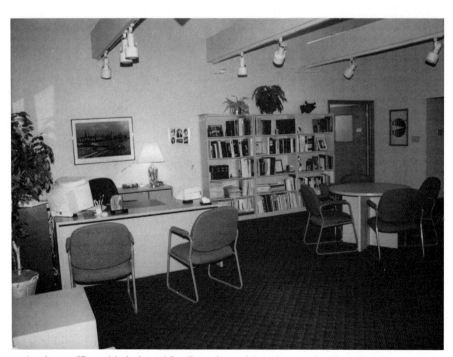

Figure 18-12 Doctor's private office, with desk used for discussions with patients and table and chairs to accommodate several persons. (Courtesy Gailmard Eye Center, Munster, Ind.)

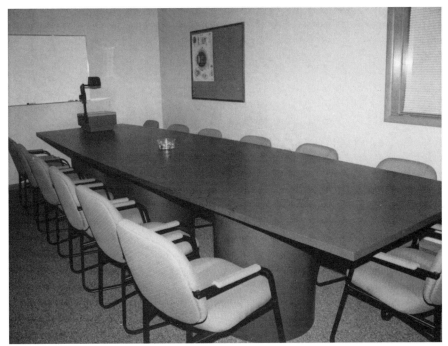

Figure 18-13 Conference room used for staff meetings and education. (Courtesy Gailmard Eye Center, Munster, Ind.)

Office Size

The space requirements needed for an office will depend on numerous factors, but in general, a small office is defined as needing less than 1000 square feet (Box 18-2), a moderate-sized office from 1000 to 2500 square feet (Box 18-3), and a large office as much as 6000 square feet (or more) (Box 18-4). The individual room sizes may vary depending on individual needs, but these figures provide approximate indications of the space needed for small, moderate, and large practices.

Building and Remodeling

It is strongly recommended that the practitioner meet with an architect or designer as early as possible to ade-

quately plan for any remodeling or new office construction. Most towns and cities have building codes and zoning ordinances, and it is best to check with the town's building inspectors before performing any construction, no matter how minor.

Parking plays a vitally important role in how an office is perceived by the public. Businesses that have easily accessible parking will have a better chance of reaching a high level of success. One must anticipate growth in the planning of any office and that includes

---

Box 18-2 Room Requirements for a Small Office

- Reception room: 12 × 15 = 180 square feet
- Business office: 10 × 12 = 120 square feet
- Examination room: 10 × 12 = 120 square feet
- Laboratory: 6 × 12 = 72 square feet
- Dispensary: 10 × 20 = 200 square feet
- Hallway and bathroom: 100 square feet

Total = 792 square feet

Box 18-3 Room Requirements for a Moderate Office

- Reception room: 10 × 20 = 200 square feet
- Business office: 10 × 15 = 150 square feet
- Data collection room: 10 × 12 = 120 square feet
- Examination room: 10 × 14 = 140 square feet
- Second examination room: 10 × 14 = 140 square feet
- Contact lens room: 10 × 18 = 180 square feet
- Finishing laboratory: 14 × 18 = 252 square feet
- Dispensary: 20 × 30 = 600 square feet
- Private office: 12 × 12 = 144 square feet
- Hallways, storage, and 2 bathrooms: 300 square feet

Total = 2226 square feet

Box 18-4   Room Requirements for a Large Office

- Lobby: 6 × 12 = 72 square feet
- Reception room: 20 × 25 = 500 square feet
- Business office: 15 × 20 = 300 square feet
- Administrative area: 12 × 14 = 168 square feet
- Office manager's office: 10 × 12 = 120 square feet
- Two Data collection rooms: 10 × 12 = 120 × 2 = 240 square feet
- Four Examination rooms: 10 × 20 = 200 × 4 = 800 square feet; or
- Six Examination rooms: 10 × 14 = 140 × 6 = 840 square feet
- Contact lens laboratory: 8 × 20 = 160 square feet
- Patient education room: 12 × 16 = 192 square feet
- Dispensary: 30 × 60 = 1800 square feet
- Finishing laboratory: 20 × 20 = 400 square feet
- Private office: 10 × 20 = 200 square feet
- Staff lounge: 10 × 20 = 200 square feet
- Hallways, storage, and 3 bathrooms: 600 square feet

Total = 5752 to 5792 square feet

adequate parking. Doctors' offices typically have a sizable allotment for parking if there is a controlling city ordinance (usually based on square footage, such as 1 space per 100 square feet).

Special considerations for wiring exist when remodeling or planning new construction. Planning must include wiring for burglar alarm systems, telephone systems, computer systems, Internet access, light-signal systems, stereo music systems, and intercoms. When working with architects and designers, the best way to approach planning meetings is with a written list of the special needs of the office. Designers can help recommend some aspects of construction, such as size requirements; lighting, heating and air conditioning needs; plumbing and electrical specifications, and so on, but they must know individual needs, which are very specific to optometry.

Conclusion

It is customary, after plans are drawn, to accept bids by contractors. An architect can serve as a construction manager—a person who generally serves as an advisor—and can eliminate the need for a general contractor. With the use of a construction manager, subcontracts with individual specialty contractors such as plumbers and electricians can be made directly, possibly saving some of the administrative fees for a general contrac-

tor. With this arrangement, the practitioner is the general contractor. It should be noted, however, that a general contractor may be quite necessary for a busy practitioner who might not have time to coordinate and supervise all of the contract work. Many general contractors also serve as designers and can provide a complete "turn key" job.

Regardless of the specific approach taken, it should be expected that construction will take longer and cost more than the amount originally anticipated.

Acknowledgement

The authors of this chapter in the first edition of *Business Aspects of Optometry* were Neil B. Gailmard and John Rumpakis.

Bibliography

Baldwin BL, Christensen B, Melton T: *Rx for success.* Midwest City, Okla, 1983, Vision Publications.

Bennett H: Not your typical doc in a box. *Rev Optom* 138(3):53-4,56, 2001.

Bennett I: *Management for the eye care practitioner.* Boston, 1993, Butterworth-Heinemann.

Bethke W: A new way to look at your sign. *Rev Ophthalmol* 6(9):58-61, 1999.

Bostick DB: Dispensary relocation: creating separate retail and clinical environments. *Optom Today* 1(4):19, 1993.

Bursett L, Nguyen K, Bleything WB: Your reception area: what do patients want? *Optom Economics* 7(3):25-9, 1997.

Cousounis H: A design for the times revives a fading practice. *Rev Optom* 135(7):33-4, 1998.

D'Addono B: Five offices where form meets function. Here's what designers like to see when they work on an office. *Rev Optom* 131(10):45-6,48, 1994.

D'Addono B: Keep your patients out of each other's space. *Rev Optom* 132(3):37-8,43-4, 1995.

D'Addono B: Don't let the roof cave in on your dream project. *Rev Optom* 133(9):33-6, 1996.

D'Addono B: Make your office user friendly ... for you. *Optician* 133(8):51-4, 1996.

D'Addono B: Optical illusions: live large in a small office. *Rev Optom* 134(9):61-2,64, 1997.

D'Addono B: Go with the flow and your practice will grow. *Rev Optom* 135(3):51-9, 1998.

D'Addono B: Maintaining production during construction. *Rev Optom* 135(11):39-40,42, 1998.

D'Addono B: This redesign fits, without the glitz. *Rev Optom* 135(9):41-3, 1998.

Del Pizzo N: Blueprints: success by design. *20/20* 21(9): 59-60,62, 1994.

Harvey D: Window of opportunity. *Optom Management* 31(11):69-71, 1996.

Kreda SH: Design of the times. *Optom Management* 31(2): 44-6, 1996.

Kreda SH: Moving on up: how to convert new office space into an optimum optometric setting. *Optom Management* 32(6):43, 1997.

Kreda SH: Big plans for a small office. *Optom Management* 34(12):45, 1999.

Kreda SH: Are you practicing in a bowling alley? *Optom Management* 35(9):43, 2000.

Kreda SH: Room for one more. *Optom Management* 35(12):56-7, 2000.

Lee J: How to see more patients—and more of your family. *Rev Optom* 137(9):69-77, 2000.

Lyon I: The professional touch: window displays. *Optician* 217(5701):20-1, 1999.

Lyon I: Small, but perfectly formed. *Optician* 217(5697):47-8, 1999.

McDermott GK: Solve your parking problem. *Rev Ophthalmol* 6(9):62-4,66, 1999.

McKercher TP: Efficiency by design. *Admin Eyecare* 10(1):30-2, 2001.

McNelis K, Franciscus C: Make your optical more child-friendly. *Rev Ophthalmol* 7(7):100-1, 2000.

Murphy J: Sprucin' up the old salt mine. *Rev Optom* 137(3):53-5, 2000.

Petersma J: How I opened cold on $20,000. *Optom Management* 32(6):14-9, 1997.

Press LJ: Building a new office: it's not the impossible dream. *Optom Management* 33(5):33-40, 1998.

Russell B: Dynamic frame displays. *Optical Prism* 15(3):22-40, 1997.

Smith A: Optimum lighting systems for offices. *Optician* 216(5678):34-6, 1998.

Smith A: Lighting for optometric and ophthalmic practices. *Optican* 217(5690):34-7, 1999.

Whitby G, Brogan R: Diary of a new practice: part 7. Six months on. *Optician* 211(5548):30-1, 1996.

Wrench J: Practice design in today's market place. *Optom Today* 3(4):38, 1995.

www.optometric.com. Online version of *Optometric Management* magazine.

www.revoptom.com. Online version of *Review of Optometry* magazine.

Chapter 19

Instrumentation and Equipment

John G. Classé

It is the Age of Machinery, in every outward and inward sense of the word.
Thomas Carlyle *Critical and Miscellaneous Essays*

Optometry is a profession that requires the use of sophisticated (and often expensive) instrumentation and equipment. The use of this technology involves all aspects of care, from diagnostic evaluation of patients to fabrication of eyewear to billing for services. Involvement in the purchase of instruments and equipment is an inevitable part of the practice of optometry and one of the most costly in terms of financial investment.

For optometry school graduates, purchasing decisions are an important step in the process of beginning a practice. The selection of instrumentation and equipment is a major consideration in opening a new practice, which must be equipped completely. When purchasing a practice, existing instrumentation and equipment often needs to be replaced. The selection of equipment is a large, never-ending task; even well-established practitioners find it necessary to periodically replace or update clinical instruments, office furnishings, and business equipment. Choosing the right supplier is a crucial part of making this investment successfully. As in selecting any professional advisor, referrals from trusted sources (such as fellow optometrists) are an excellent guide. The purchaser always should allow for time to compare prices and service among sellers. An excellent way to compare different brands of instruments, and the dealers who sell and service them, is by attending the exhibit hall at major eye care seminars and conventions. The purchase of equipment is an expensive investment, one with significant legal ramifications that should be understood before entering into a purchase agreement.

Legal Considerations When Purchasing Instruments and Equipment

There is a tendency on the part of new graduates to assume a rather cavalier attitude toward the agreements used for the purchase of equipment. This is due, in part, to the circumstances of the usual purchase: the buyer places an order, which the seller promises to deliver at a time that is often several weeks or months in the future; the buyer signs what is not much more than a list of agreed-upon items; and no money actually changes hands. Although equipment purchase agreements would not seem to be in the same category as practice purchase agreements—which require lawyers, accountants, a bank loan, and usually a period of hard bargaining—nothing could be further from the truth. As with agreements to purchase a practice, equipment purchase agreements are contracts that are formal, binding, and enforceable.

These agreements cannot be voided merely because of some unforeseen circumstance such as the disability of the buyer or the failure of the buyer to obtain an optometry license as expected. Under these circumstances, the buyer will either have to pay damages to the seller or try to sell the equipment to another buyer. The damages incurred by the seller may be relatively small if another buyer can be quickly found, or they may be rather consequential if the equipment must be warehoused, transported, and resold at a loss. In either event, the buyer's breach of the agreement creates liability for the expenses incurred.

The only way to void a purchase agreement is to place a clause in the agreement that specifies the contract will not be binding should a certain described event occur; an example circumstance would be failure to obtain an optometry license. Even though a clause stating that the purchase agreement would be void if the buyer failed to receive a license would be legal and enforceable, it is unlikely that the seller would agree to it. Contingency clauses are not in a seller's best interest, and they are not included in equipment purchase agreements for that reason. There are important issues other than the contract that must be understood when purchasing instrumentation and equipment. Other primary considerations include budgeting for instrument purchases, financing, the use of leasing rather than buying, tax issues, and selecting the appropriate equipment.

Budgeting for Purchases

A budget should be determined for the capital investment of a practice, since it is very easy to add excessively to the list of needed instruments. A rule of thumb for opening a new practice is to buy only what is needed to provide competent professional care. When the practice is economically sound, it is a wise strategy to reinvest income into the practice in the form of additional and more automated instrumentation. A rule of thumb is to allocate 2% to 5% of net income every year to this fund. Each practitioner should develop a list of instruments that identifies and prioritizes the items needed in the practice. As funds are available, the desired items can be purchased.

There is a market for good used equipment, when it functions well and looks good. Buying directly from another practitioner or a reliable equipment dealer will allow substantial savings when compared with the cost of new equipment. An equipment vendor has the advantage of cleaning, servicing, and recalibrating instruments and possibly even applying a new paint finish. It is always wise to inquire about warranties, which may not be offered with some used equipment. Instruments with advanced electronics can be very difficult and expensive to service. Equipment maintenance should be performed on a regular basis according to the manufacturer's guidelines. This maintenance may simply involve regular cleaning, which is important for accurate operation. Staff members should be trained to clean instruments daily, since lenses and mirrors can be damaged if cleaned improperly and instruments can be broken if mishandled.

Financing the Purchase

Buying new professional instruments often involves financing. There are several options available to the purchaser, but the usual choices made by optometrists are bank loans and financing through the equipment dealer. Another option is leasing rather than buying. In many cases, the time savings achieved by the use of the new instrumentation or the additional fees generated by use of the instrumentation may offset its cost. For example, an autoperimeter with threshold capability is an expensive device, costing several thousands of dollars. If an optometrist's practice requires the frequent use of autoperimetry—for the management of patients with glaucoma—the income generated by the device could more than pay for the cost of its purchase. When contemplating the purchase of equipment, thought should be given to the capacity of the device to add to services and generate income. This consideration is particularly important for optometry school graduates seeking to start a new practice. For new practices, it is essential to keep overhead expenses—the fixed expenses that must be paid every month—as low as possible.

Another important issue related to equipment purchased with a loan is that the equipment serves as collateral for the loan. In such cases the creditor retains a security interest in the equipment. In the event the borrower defaults on the loan (cannot pay the creditor), the security interest allows the creditor to take possession of the collateral and sell it in an attempt to minimize financial loss. If the collateral cannot be sold for the amount that is owed, the creditor may be able to have other assets of the borrower seized and sold in an attempt to collect the difference. Even worse, if the creditor becomes insolvent, those to whom the creditor is indebted may be able to seize and sell the equipment themselves. This unlikely event can occur if the security interest signed by the buyer is not actually with the seller but rather with the creditor of the seller.

To avoid misfortune, new graduates should negotiate with dealers that have acquired a good reputation over a period and not fall prey to impulses or succumb to the allure of cut-rate prices. Buyers always should obtain competent legal advice before entering into any contract that involves the expenditure of a considerable amount of money or requires years of obligation to repay.

Leasing Ophthalmic Equipment

When considering the acquisition of ophthalmic equipment, the buyer should consider whether it is

---

Box 19-1 Leasing of Ophthalmic Instruments and Equipment

Advantages
- One hundred percent financing of the equipment.
- No down payment.
- One hundred percent of the lease cost may be deducted.
- After the term of the lease, the equipment does not have to be purchased; instead, a new lease for new equipment can be arranged.
- The financing charge for the lease period does not change, and so fluctuating interest rates do not affect the amount due.

Disadvantages
- Most new practices do not earn enough income to justify the tax advantages of the full lease deduction.
- The cost of a lease is greater than the cost of purchasing the same equipment; at the end of the lease period a payment will have to be made (usually 10% to 15% of the equipment's fair market value) to obtain title to it.
- The depreciation deduction is claimed by the leasing company.
- The equipment must be kept for the full term of the lease. The only exceptions are if the equipment is upgraded or if equipment of greater value is obtained. If the equipment is returned because of a default in payments, it can be sold and any deficit in what is owed can be collected from the defaulting practitioner.
- The lease agreement will probably require the practitioner to pay for insurance on the equipment; the practitioner also may be required to pay for all repairs (although this will depend on the warranty received from the equipment seller or manufacturer).

---

more advantageous to lease the equipment than to buy it (Box 19-1). Although leasing is generally more expensive than financing through a bank (or purchasing equipment outright), the use of leasing can allow a practitioner to use savings for the purchase of another asset (such as a home). Although it is not technically the same as financing, there is a built-in interest rate in a lease (which usually does not fluctuate over the period of the lease). This financing cost is generally higher with leases than with bank loans. The main advantage of leasing is that a lease usually does not require a down payment or affect a line of credit that may be established at a bank. Leases from different companies should be examined and compared in detail. The term (length) of the lease is for a period of years and is very difficult to change after the lease has begun.

At the end of the lease term, the equipment may be returned to the leasing company or purchased for an agreed-upon amount. The amount paid will depend on the lease agreement but is usually the used market value of the equipment or 10% to 15% of the equipment's fair market value. The purchase option will affect the amount of the monthly lease payment. There are several tax issues that must be understood before entering into a lease agreement. A certified

public accountant or tax attorney should be consulted to clarify individual provisions of lease agreements (Box 19-2).

Tax Considerations of Buying vs Leasing

For tax purposes, an equipment lease must be managed differently than a bank loan used for the purchase of equipment. When money is borrowed from a bank, both principal and interest must be repaid. Only the interest, however, may be deducted. When an equipment lease is entered into, each monthly repayment is tax deductible. Therefore, 100% of the lease amount may be deducted.

Some consideration must be given to whether the lease deduction is advantageous for a given practice. It is often not particularly advantageous for a beginning practice, but for an established practice a lease arrangement might offer some tax benefits. Again, professional advice should be solicited before entering into an agreement.

Making the Appropriate Choices

There are practice-building and promotional aspects to having excellent instruments. Patients will judge the

---

Box 19-2 Common Provisions of Equipment Lease Agreements

Identification of the parties

If the lease is to be taken out by a professional association or corporation, limited liability company, S corporation or partnership, the lease agreement should be signed accordingly.

Description of the lease property

The practitioner will select the equipment that is to be purchased, and the leasing company will provide the funds to purchase it. The lease agreement needs to specify the equipment with specificity so that there is no mistake or question about the items subject to the lease.

Term of the lease

The lease period may vary from 1 to 7 years; some companies may permit even longer periods.

Option to purchase

At the conclusion of the lease period, the practitioner will have the right to purchase the equipment. The price can be set at the outset of the arrangement or may be expressed as a percentage that cannot be exceeded. If the practitioner does not wish to purchase the equipment, it is returned to the leasing company at the end of the lease term.

Cost of the lease

The interest, though higher than that charged by a bank, will be stable throughout the lease term. (However, if interest rates should go up significantly during the lease term, the interest rate charged by the leasing company may actually fall below the rate charged by a bank.) A monthly payment is established for the term of the lease, which does not change from month to month. (Some leasing companies offer a graduated payment schedule, whereby the lease payments are lower in the first years and gradually escalate over the later years of the lease term.)

Responsibility for repairs

The leasing company does not provide repairs; the practitioner will have to find an equipment dealer to perform repairs, and the practitioner will have to pay for them. However, the equipment manufacturer will provide maintenance and repairs during the warranty period.

Insurance

The practitioner will probably be required to purchase insurance sufficient to indemnify the leasing company in the event the equipment is lost by fire or other casualty.

Right of exchange

The practitioner may wish to exchange certain equipment before the lease term is concluded to obtain a newer model or a different piece of equipment altogether. The lease may recognize the right to perform exchanges (with proper adjustments in the cost of the lease).

Failure to make timely payment

The lease will provide certain remedies to the leasing company should the practitioner fail to make the lease payments as provided in the agreement. Among the remedies typically available to the leasing company are the acceleration of payments, increased charges for late payments, and seizure and sale of the equipment. The penalties for late payment should be clearly understood by the practitioner.

---

quality of the examination based on an impression of how up-to-date the instruments appear to be. Even if instruments are not new, they should look new. Automated and computerized instruments provide accuracy of measurement, state-of-the-art technology, public relations benefits, and savings of time because their use is delegated to support personnel. Informing patients about the special diagnostic instruments used in the practice is an excellent means of providing internal marketing, which can result in more word-of-mouth referrals. For that reason, new instrumentation is a great topic for newsletters, recall reminders, and office brochures.

The determination of the appropriate instruments and equipment for a given practice is one of the most important tasks a practitioner faces. As has been described, it is particularly important for beginning practitioners to be selective and to purchase only essential equipment to start a practice, adding on as necessary as the patient base and income grow.

Boxes 19-3 through 19-6 provide a summary of the equipment to be considered for a practice, organized by the room in which each instrument is typically used. A large range of costs and features usually are found for each instrument and, of course, some items are necessities, whereas others are luxuries.

Box 19-3 Equipment Check List

Data Collection Room
Basic
- Keratometer
- Telebinocular
- Color vision plates
- Stereopsis test
- Sphygmomanometer and stethoscope
- Lensometer
- Patient chair and examiner stool

Advanced (substitute or add to basic)
- Auto-refractor
- Non-contact tonometer
- Auto-keratometer/corneal topographer
- Auto-lensometer
- Auto-perimeter
- Retinal camera
- Rotating instrument table

Box 19-5 Equipment Check List

Laboratory
Optical
- Automatic diamond lens edger
- Hand edger
- Lensometer
- Layout marker and blocker
- Rimless grooving machine
- Edge polishing machine
- Lens tinting machine
- Chemical hardener
- Heat tempering oven
- Frame warmer
- Various dispensing tools

Contact Lens
- Contact lens modification unit and tools
- Radiuscope
- Shadowscope or dissecting microscope

Box 19-4 Equipment Check list

Examination Room
Basic
Refraction
- Examination chair
- Instrument stand
- Keratometer
- Chart projector and screen or chart display terminal
- Trial lens set and frame
- Retinoscope
- Examiner's stool
Ocular Disease Management
- Slit lamp biomicroscope
- Hand-held 60, 78, or 90 D lenses
- Goldmann tonometer
- Binocular indirect ophthalmoscope
- Direct ophthalmoscope
- Various hand-held devices for emergency and primary care
Additional
- Corneal topography analyzer
- Electrodiagnostic instrumentation
- Pachometer
- Slit lamp 35-mm camera
- Slit lamp video system
- Low-vision diagnostic aids
- Binocular vision testing and/or training equipment

Box 19-6 Equipment Check List

Business Office
- Telephone system
- Calculator
- Photocopier
- Answering machine
- File cabinets
- Postage meter
- Dictation equipment
- Computer system and printer
- Fax machine
- Light signal system (interoffice communication)

Acknowledgement

The authors of this chapter in the first edition of *Business Aspects of Optometry* were Neil B. Gailmard and John G. Classé.

Bibliography

Aldridge C: How to choose the right payment option: is it better to buy, lease or finance your new instrument? *Optom Management* 29(1):22-4, 1994.

Allergan, Inc: *Pathways in optometry.* Irvine, Calif, 1992, Author.

Arkin J: Time to replace your old equipment? Using these calculations, you may find it's costing you more than buying new. *Eyecare Bus* 3(12):61-2, 1988.

Baldwin BL, Christainsen B, Melton T: *Rx for success.* Midwest City, Okla, 1983, Vision Publications.

Barnett D: Are your instruments in tune with your practice? *Rev Optom* 129(8):19, 1992.

Bayusik L: The fine-tuning of an instruments market. *Eyecare Bus* 4(3):41,44-45,48, 1989.

Classé JG: *Legal aspects of optometry.* Boston, 1989, Butterworth.

Cleinman AH: Remove risk from technology investments. *Optom Management* 29(2):21, 1994.

Coady C: To lease or not to lease. *Eyecare Bus* 10(10):53, 1995.

Coleman DL: Your new ophthalmic equipment (first decide which is better for you. Then make sure you know the rules.). *Optom Economics* 2(4):30-3, 1992.

Donoghue SK: The paperless practice: the future is now. *Eyecare Tech* 3(2):13-6,26, 1993.

Gailmard NB: The Consultant's Corner: Are your investments secret information? *Rev Optom* 129(6):25, 1992.

Gailmard NB: When your practice screams for an extra exam room. *Rev Optom* 130(3):115-6, 1993.

Goldsborough R, Gailmard NB: Pick your exam room. *Rev Optom* 124(9):48-56, 1987.

Gorin SB: Equipment purchases: to lease or buy? *Optom Economics* 3(7):47-8, 1993.

Harris L: Build a testing room for the '90s. *Optom Management* 29(3):55-6, 1994.

Hayes J: How much to spend on new instruments. *Optom Management* 28(4):15, 1993.

Kirkner R: Instruments for the sake of patient care (editorial). *Rev Optom* 129(8):19, 1992.

Kreda SH: Enter the office of the future. *Optom Management* 30(4):31-2, 1995.

Legerton JA: Sound purchasing decisions (analyzing the what, when, why and how of purchasing ophthalmic equipment). *Optom Economics* 2(10):34-8, 1992.

Perry P: Look before you lease. *Eyecare Bus* 8(4):90-1, 1993.

Ramsay WK: Miniaturizing equipment: small and portable instruments for optometrists today. *Optom Today* 3(3):37,39, 1995.

Schwartz CA: Capitalizing on high-tech equipment. *Optom Economics* 3(5):28-31, 1993.

www.optometric.com. Online version of *Optometric Management* magazine, which offers product information and purchasing advice.

www.revoptom.com. Online version of *Review of Optometry* magazine, which offers product information and purchasing advice.

Chapter 20

Use of Computers

Stuart M. Rothman

The computer is no better than its program.
Elting Elmore Morison *Men, Machines and Modern Times*

The use of computers and computer systems has become commonplace in optometric practice, just as it has permeated health care and small business in general. The range of uses for these systems can be as limited as word processing on a single personal computer to as extensive as the paperless office on a multi-user system, with ophthalmic instruments data and practice management data fully integrated. This chapter describes the various roles and functions of personal computers in contemporary optometric practice. Specific patient management, business management, inventory management, and time management applications are discussed.

Use of the Personal Computer

The personal computer has revolutionized optometric office management in the same way it has revolutionized all small businesses. Computers save time by performing many of the functions that used to be performed by hand, and they also have expanded the capabilities of the optometric office to manage data.

Patient information, such as name, address, telephone number, birth date, and recall date, has been expanded by computerization to include diagnoses, insurance information, spectacle prescription, contact lens information, e-mail addresses, and various other marketing categories. A noncomputerized office has to create and maintain a separate file for each patient; when information is needed, it has to be retrieved by hand. The computerized office can store, obtain, and analyze information with the stroke of a few keys, which greatly expands the practice's ability to retrieve and sort the information collected.

Computers enhance communication between practitioner and patients, prospective patients, and potential referral sources. The merger of word processing with stored data allows a computerized office to send personalized letters to all these sources, permitting the office to market itself in ways that a noncomputerized office either cannot offer or can offer only with the expenditure of significant time and expense. The widespread use of e-mail allows communication with patients in ways that never existed before. E-mail allows for the rapid dissemination of information to patients and for patients to communicate with the office 24 hours a day, 7 days a week. The use of Web sites by optometric practices allows practitioners to enhance communication with patients and prospective patients before they come into the office and also allows practitioners to give patients in the office a way of obtaining more information about various services or products that the practice provides.

Financial management has been enhanced in the computerized office, from simple tracking of accounts receivable to accurate up-to-date summaries of the financial health of the practice and projections of future practice growth with changes in fees, addition of equipment, or use of ancillary personnel. Budgeting expenses and tracking the office expenses to the budget are easier to set up and monitor by computer, which allows the optometrist to self-monitor daily, weekly, monthly, or quarterly without having to wait for an accountant's report.

Computerized inventory management includes the tracking of ophthalmic materials such as frames and contact lenses, which allows for more efficient purchasing of these items by the practice. With the advent of frequent replacement and disposable contact lens wear programs, inventory management has become increasingly more important. The use of laser scanners and bar codes on these items by the optical industry makes inventory control even easier.

Computers also can be used for the management of patients. Equipment such as automated refractors, corneal topography units, automated lensometers, and visual field analyzers can be linked to personal computers to store pertinent data and to assist in the interpretation of this data, creating a "paperless" office environment. The use of computers in areas such as contact lens design, low vision care, and visual therapy has allowed optometrists to provide better, more efficient care to patients. Optometrists who are online have access to discussion groups and thus can acquire information on patient management, developments in clinical care, and ophthalmic products. Digital images of anterior segment disorders, retinal pathology, and corneal topography maps can be saved, stored, compared, and e-mailed for consultation with laboratories and specialists in the next town or across the country.

Specific Office Management Applications

Applications in the optometric office include patient information, insurance use, financial information, inventory control, services information, ophthalmic materials tracking, appointments, referrals, payroll information, appointment scheduling, marketing, and communications.

Patient Information

Computerization allows all the pieces of information about individual patients to be stored in one place. Information about patients can be categorized, sorted, and identified based on any one of the pieces of information that have been collected. For example, computer storage makes it possible for practitioners to learn the demographics of a practice. A practitioner considering a move to another location might want to analyze the patient population by zip code or address so that the most geographically desirable location for the move can be identified. Another application is marketing. Practitioners can perform internal marketing through the use of newsletters or other literature sent to a computer-generated lists of patients. Combining the use of demographic and marketing information allows the practitioner to know which newspapers might be best to place information in to

reach the largest number of patients in the practice. Or, the practitioner can use this information to market externally (see Chapter 32).

Typical patient information stored on a computer might include name, address, date of birth, telephone number, e-mail address, insurance information, referral source, the individual responsible for payment of fees, examination date, recall date, reason for recall, diagnoses, contact lens type, contact lens service agreement information, spectacle lens information, frame information, and account information (Figure 20-1).

Any of this information can be accessed, retrieved, sorted, and reviewed through the computer. For example, the office might want to inform all patients with high myopic refractive errors about a new type of lens material. Without a computer, retrieval of this information would require considerable staff time because individual patient files would have to be reviewed. With a personal computer, a list of the appropriate patients can easily be compiled, and mailing labels letters or e-mails can be sent to each patient, with minimal staff time and effort.

Insurance Information

In addition to allowing insurance information to be listed with other patient data, a computer will permit office personnel to more efficiently process and keep track of insurance payments. Many software programs print standard patient insurance forms, and most transfer information electronically (e.g., for Medicare patients). These procedures can hasten the reimbursement process and thus improve the office's cash flow. Many insurers insist on electronic claim submission via the Internet as a condition of participation in their managed care plans.

As more and more optometric patients obtain insurance coverage from third-party insurance plans, it will become necessary to monitor when payments are due from individual payers and to track third-party payment schedules. Many insurers now allow electronic filers to tap into their computer network to determine the status of claims being processed. Computerization also allows for easier and more efficient communication with third-party payers by permitting the use of standardized letters and forms.

Financial Information

Computerized billing and tracking of accounts receivable enables a practice to more efficiently bill and col-

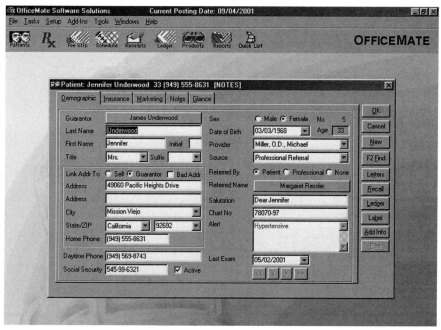

Figure 20-1 Patient information screen with information to be collected on each patient. This information can later be selectively retrieved. Patient data also can be sorted by various pieces of information. (Courtesy OfficeMate, Irvine, Calif.)

lect money owed. Charges for services rendered are entered in the office's practice management software with a breakdown of monies due from the patient and payments due from insurance companies. A receipt is printed for the patient at the time of the visit, and an insurance claim form is generated for the insurance company. Any balance due is applied to the patient and insurance company ledger for billing and tracking on a monthly basis. Many software programs allow the office to set payment schedules for patients. The computer will calculate interest charges and add them to a preprinted receipt that the patient is to return to the practice when money is due (Figure 20-2).

Tracking of accounts payable is made easier through computerized programs that act like a checkbook to record and categorize payments, write checks, and monitor accounts. Payment can be made electronically, saving the practitioner the time and expense of printing and mailing checks. These same programs also enable the office to obtain profit and loss statements as needed rather than having to wait for quarterly accounting reports. Budgets can be set up for the year, and expenses can be compared to the budget to allow the practitioner to more easily monitor cash flow and ensure available funds for taxes, retirement accounts, and purchases of new equipment.

The financial productivity of an office can be determined by the day, week, or year; as needed, income can be tracked for tax purposes. The financial contributions of the practitioners and staff also can be determined, an essential capacity in offices where practitioner income is divided on the basis of productivity or where bonuses are paid to staff based on performance or office productivity.

Inventory Control

Many practitioners maintain large inventories of contact lenses, on consignment, in the office so that patients can receive same-day service on replacement lenses or can be provided with lenses immediately after fitting. Management of inventory can be cumbersome without computerized inventory control. The computerization of inventory also makes it possible for the receptionist or contact lens technician to immediately tell a patient who is seeking a replacement lens whether the lens is in stock. The growing popularity of frequent replacement and disposable contact lenses places a much greater burden on inventory control. An efficiently run inventory control system can mean a substantial income savings for the practitioner.

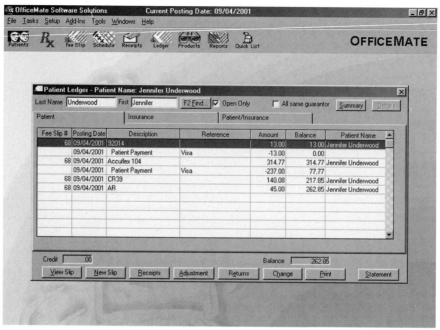

Figure 20-2 Patient receipt generated at the time of visit. (Courtesy OfficeMate, Irvine, Calif.)

Inventories of contact lens supplies and solutions also can be more effectively managed by computer. Many offices stock contact lens solutions for patients, and these solutions must be monitored for turnover rates and expiration dates. Determining when and how frequently solutions and other supplies must be repurchased can allow the office to take advantage of cost savings by buying supplies when they are discounted.

Most practices invest a substantial amount of money in a frame inventory. Computerized management of frames can provide information such as when the frame was purchased, how long it has been offered for sale, how frequently similar frames are sold, and whether similar frames are still in inventory. Reports can be generated by frame type, manufacturer, and cost. These reports can be used to make purchasing decisions for the practice (Figure 20-3).

Services Information

As patients are seen in the office, the type of services provided will be keyed into the computer. Computerization allows the office to track the services provided to any patient on any given day (Figure 20-4). This information is used to print a bill or insurance form for the patient at the time of the office visit. It also allows the office to keep track of the number of services provided and the income received by the prac-

tice from a particular service. The information also can be used to identify secondary services or specialized procedures and their use. Financial data can be used to allocate space and money for new equipment based on the amount of income generated by each procedure or service. For example, an optometrist who is considering the purchase of a corneal topographer but is not certain that it would be cost-effective would need to analyze the number of contact lens services provided in an average month and determine the increase in revenue from the number of patients who would require this test to clearly project the financial feasibility of the purchase.

Ophthalmic Materials Tracking

Patient orders for contact lenses and spectacles must be monitored for delivery time. Because patients expect prompt dispensing of ophthalmic materials, a failure on the part of the practice to provide timely service can result in loss of orders. Many ophthalmic laboratories now accept electronic transfer of information, which can eliminate the time-consuming method of messenger or postal delivery. Computerization of this aspect of optometric practice also can aid in the more efficient payment of laboratory bills by enabling credits and invoices to be followed-up more easily (Figure 20-5). Most vendors now have their own Web sites and allow

Company	Number	Frame Name	Color	Eye Size
Design	2685	Zenith 1 2207	6032	49
	2505	Zenith 2209	3031	49
	2510	Titanium 1 911	5011	43
	2511	P 835	5022	40
	2512	846	6021	48
	2513	6002	9031	47
	2538	5010	3822	46
	2625	6102	3522	51
	2347	P2201	903243	43
	2633	5014	4022	49
	2634	5017	6032	49
	2635	5012	5622	48
	2636	5018	4032	49
	2660	Pro vogue 6001	6031	45
	2661	Fourth dimension 5009	5522	50
	2626	6101	6022	49
	2331	7012	3531	44
	2328	P 625	DK MT BRN	38
	1940	P 1996	46/64	46
	1958	1992	46/46	52
	2130	P622 with clip	81	49
	1841	P2053	62	51
	2154	P1993	46/46	50
	2658	Zenith 2 2217	5031	50
	2515	6005	9531	49
	2235	P 2024	509032	48
	2236	P 2025	559022	53
	2508	Provogue 2 6009	4031	49
	2509	P833	9032	44
	2329	P320	660	50
	2330	P825	660	42
	2132	P903	5023	43

Figure 20-3 Report of frame inventory, listed by manufacturer.

ordering of materials 24 hours a day, 7 days a week on their Web site. Web sites also have been set up by various buying groups to allow purchasing of all contact lenses, frames, and office materials online.

Referral Information

The life blood of professional optometric practice is patient referral. Whether from existing patients, other health care practitioners, or community contacts, referrals keep pumping new blood into a practice. Being able to properly recognize and thank each referral source will make it more likely that these sources will continue to send new patients. Most practice management software programs facilitate the sending of thank you notices to a referral source. Many also will monitor the number of patients each referral source has contributed as well as the income generated by each referral source. For referrals from other health care providers, reports can be generated to allow the referring practitioner to keep up-to-date on a patient's progress. Managed care plans require prompt communication between the optometrist and the primary care physician gatekeeper. This communication is essential if the optometrist is to continue to receive referrals.

Payroll Information

As the number of employees in an optometric office increases, so does the time needed to handle payroll and tax reporting information. Computerization allows the office to calculate tax withholding, determine net salaries, and even print payroll checks. This information can be summarized and sorted by employees so that payroll taxes can be calculated quarterly as required. Information about employee salaries and tax withholding also can be printed on a year-end statement for use when completing tax returns.

Appointment Scheduling

A key element in practice management software systems designed for optometric offices is the appointment scheduler. In multipractitioner or multilocation

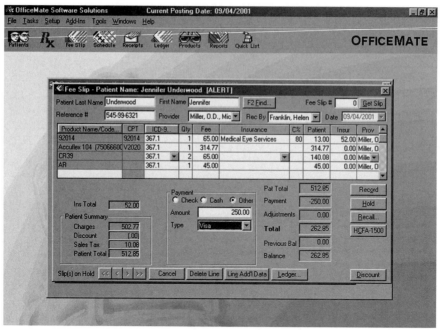

Figure 20-4 Services information for patients. (Courtesy OfficeMate, Irvine, Calif.)

offices, these systems can aid in more efficient use of time and can help to prevent improper scheduling. The use of ancillary staff in pretesting or assistants in contact lens training and vision therapy also can be more efficiently scheduled by computer. The computer can allocate the proper amount of time for a procedure, assign patients to a given practitioner, locate available appointment dates and times, and allow the viewing of all of the patients' appointments at a glance. Many offices will pre-appoint patients months and even years

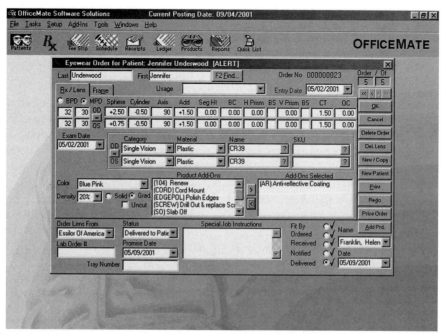

Figure 20-5 Tracking of ophthalmic materials orders. (Courtesy OfficeMate, Irvine, Calif.)

in advance in a perpetual appointment recall system. Computerization of this system allows the office to efficiently keep track of the appointments made, confirm them in advance, and refill the time slots if patients do not respond to or cancel scheduled appointments. Some companies have set up sites on the Internet where patients can book appointments, allowing patients the ability to schedule appointments even after office hours.

Marketing

A computer will make it easier to carry out all levels of a marketing plan. The first step is to identify a need or problem, such as the failure of many contact lens patients to renew their service agreements. The next step is to implement a marketing concept. For contact lens patients, a letter can be generated by the computer, reminding these patients that regular contact lens care is needed to maintain ocular health. An invitation to renew the service agreement can be included, offering an incentive if renewal is obtained by a specific date. The key element of any marketing plan is an ability to monitor the success of the marketing effort; then the return on investment can be determined. The computer is used to track patients to whom the letter was sent and the number of patients who responded positively.

Communication

Computers can be put to use in aiding communication with patients in various ways. Many practices now have their own Web site as a means of external and internal marketing. Various optical suppliers, managed care companies, and buying groups will help set up sites for practices doing business with them. Web sites allow the practitioner to get information to the public about a practice and the services provided. Patients looking for optometrists who provide specific services can now search on the Internet for practices in a geographic area. A patient who has been seen in the office can be asked to view the practice's Web site to obtain more information about specific services recommended.

Computerized patient history software, computerized report writing software, and computerized patient explanation software allow more efficient case presentation in the office. Patient history software allows patients to use touch-screen technology to describe ophthalmic and medical histories and to highlight reasons for visits, the desire for further information, and areas in which they have questions for the optometrist.

This information is sometimes required by managed care plans and allows for more efficient use of staff and optometrist time. It also allows the staff to tailor treatment recommendations based on patient needs. Patient explanation software (Figures 20-6 and 20-7) aids the optometrist and staff in describing various vision and eye health problems graphically so that the patient is more likely to understand and comply with treatment recommendations. Report-writing software allows the optometrist to quickly design reports either to patients or referring practitioners describing the patient's symptoms, findings, and recommendations.

How to Get Started Computerizing an Office

Computerizing an existing office is never an easy task. The actual procedures used can depend on the software system chosen. Certain software companies will load patient information into the system so that the office is "up and running." This process will cost more initially but can save money in the long run because staff time will not be required to enter information into the computer system. The office also will be fully functional on the computer for standard monthly procedures such as recall appointments and billing of accounts receivable. New patients will be added to the system as they come into the office.

Other software systems allow the office staff to enter data regarding patients with outstanding balances so that billing can be computerized from date of installation. Information on patients to be recalled is entered into the system monthly, requiring additional staff time before recall notices can be mailed. Full data on these patients are entered as they return to the office. For new patients, data are entered at the initial visit.

Some offices prefer to enter patient information as the patients return for care or when they are seen for the first time. This approach can require the least amount of additional staff time, but it has the disadvantage of delaying the computerization process because the staff has to go through both a computerized list and a noncomputerized list when sending out recalls, bills, or other patient correspondence. If the average patient visits the office once every 2 years, it will be at least that long before the office will be fully computerized.

Despite the initial disruptions to office procedure, computerization can benefit an office of any size. Smaller offices that seem to function quite efficiently without computers can still benefit from the additional

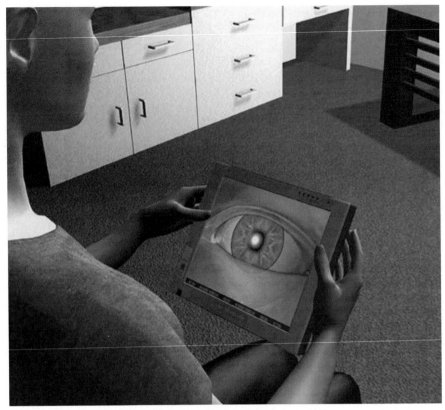

Figure 20-6 Use of patient explanation software. (Courtesy eyeMaginations, Towson, Md.)

capabilities that computerization offers. Costs of hardware and software products have regularly decreased, even while computer technology continues to expand. There is no "perfect time" to make the decision to computerize. Software will be improved periodically, and hardware can always be upgraded. Waiting until computer technology is "perfected" only means delaying the tremendous advantages of computerization.

For new offices, computers should be included as initial equipment in much the same way as a phoropter and ophthalmoscope are. The use of the computer in marketing, report writing, and patient communication will aid in the development of the new practice. The cost of computerization will be spread out during the lifetime of a practice loan in the same way as other optometric equipment.

Selecting Computer Software

For the computer novice, the use and applications of office computers can be discussed with fellow practitioners, experts in the field, and office staff of colleagues. Vendors from various companies can be found at large continuing-education seminars. Salespeople should be able to demonstrate the capabilities of software. Information can be obtained about the support the company offers, what is included in the price of the software, and how often upgrades are provided. Many companies offer demonstration videotapes of their software; these allow a practitioner who does not own a computer to get a feel for the capabilities of the software.

For the non-novice who has access to a computer, demonstration disks will give a more realistic demonstration of the ease of operation of the software. These demonstration disks typically allow the entry of data on a small number of patients or can be used for a specified period.

For the experienced computer user, testing a product in the office can be of value. Many experienced users decide to purchase a nonoptometric, commercially available database program. Such programs usually are less expensive than optometric software but require considerable time to program. The experienced user can use the software to customize a program that suits the particular needs of the office.

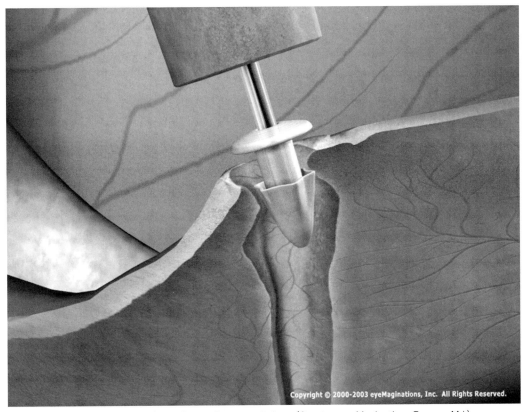

Figure 20-7 Example of patient explanation software for punctal plugs. (Courtesy eyeMaginations, Towson, Md.)

Prioritizing Use

Once the possible applications of software are understood, it should be determined how the computer will be used in the office. The initial investigation of a software package should reveal its strengths and weaknesses. In addition, knowing the functions that the computer must handle, along with the priority of functions, should assist the practitioner in making the software choice. For example, a program that is strong on inventory control will offer little benefit for an optometrist in a nondispensing practice. Most independent optometrists will find that a software program strong in patient information storage, billing, patient communication, and inventory control will meet all their needs. Separate modules or separate software products can be obtained for patient communication, accounting, and Web design.

Planning where the computer (or computers) will be located is essential in allowing for the full utilization of the computer program. It also will help determine the functions that will take priority on the computer. For example, personnel in an office with a sole computer that is located on the receptionist's desk will find it dif-

ficult to use the computer for inventory assessment and control by staff in the dispensary. Identifying the priorities for computer use will assist in the effort to establish hardware requirements and help to determine the number and location of computer workstations. Internal wiring must be planned for to allow for the networking of computer stations. The need for an independent server and the placement of the server are decisions that must be made in conjunction with the computer consultant. Any hardware and software should allow for expansion if the needs of the office change.

Knowing the Software Company

The software system should be "user friendly." Since the office staff will be the primary users of the system, the software should be designed with simple on-screen menus and explanations. This capability eliminates the need for extensive retraining every time a new staff person is hired. It also eliminates the new staff member's need to refer to a manual when using the computer for a waiting patient.

Support for the software can be provided in various ways. Some companies use a 900 telephone number, for which advice is billed at a per-minute rate. Other companies offer a yearly support fee, paid in advance, that allows the user to call for assistance. Many companies insist that the user purchase a telephone modem, which allows support personnel to view the problem on their own computer screens and make any corrections or adjustments.

Upgrades of hardware and software systems must be considered as a regular expense of doing business. As technology improves, these updates ensure that software is kept current. A company that issues regular updates stands behind its products and is investing in research for new products.

Hardware Requirements

The hardware requirements described here are for currently available optometric software. Hardware usually can be purchased from the software vendor or, separately, from a local hardware vendor.

Most optometric software runs on Windows-based operating systems. The software will specify the processing chip needed, the suggested speed of operation, the operating system, hard disk capacity, random access memory, and external disk requirements. Most software vendors recommend a tape backup system. Peripheral hardware such as internal fax modems and CD-ROM are now standard on most computers. Networking requirements include software and hardware connections to allow multiple-user stations. Remote software allows access to the computer system by the practitioner from home or a satellite office. Printer types include dot matrix, ink jet, or laser. The type of printer can be determined by the software system chosen and the type of correspondence used. Many offices use a dot matrix printer for multipart (NCR) forms and a laser or ink jet printer for all other office correspondence. Ink jet printers allow office personnel to print forms in various colors and are generally the least expensive and most common printers used today.

Hardware options include larger monitor, flat screen monitors (which take up less desk space), and laptop or notebook computers versus desktop models.

The computer workstation should be designed to provide maximum comfort and efficiency. Chairs should have proper back support and adjustable seats. Monitors should be placed slightly below eye level and should have antiglare screens. Keyboards should have wrist rests and should be adjustable so that the operator can reduce strain on upper back and neck muscles. Dot matrix printers, which are noisier than other printers, should be placed away from areas where conversations are held with patients or where telephones are located.

The time spent on the computer by staff members should be regulated if possible. If one person has specific responsibility for data entry, work periods should be of limited duration and periodic breaks provided. The workstation also should be properly designed.

Clinical Applications for Computers

Computers are beginning to have applications beyond those that provide standard office management. As technology improves, the potential for increased clinical use will expand. Some of the current software options include the following:

Report writing. This application allows the office to compile a full range of patient, referral source, and other practitioner reports by entering information from the patient examination.

Dispensing. Software availability includes a computerized display of lifestyle dispensing options; the ability to show patients their appearance with various frame shapes, sizes, and colors; and frame availability by manufacturer and distributors. New products take the computerized image of a patient's face and design an optically correct pair of spectacles with the proper eye-face-spectacle relationship. This can be done in the office or via the Internet.

Differential diagnoses and therapy. Software programs exist to analyze and store data for various diagnostic tests. These data can be used for determining the course or effectiveness of therapy. Today, most visual field instruments come with statistical software packages that analyze visual field defects, determine the probabilities of such defects, and compare multiple fields on the same patient. Software also exists to transfer and compare findings on various automated devices. Computerized nerve fiber layer and optic nerve analysis is now commonplace so that minute changes, not visible to even the most experienced retinologist, can be detected. This capacity can allow for more rapid diagnoses and treatment of conditions such as glaucoma. Databases also exist to help practitioners determine the differential diagnosis of pathologic conditions. Modems and communications software hold the promise of being able to transmit patient data, findings, or images to another location for immediate consultation.

Pharmacology. Current software allows a practitioner to enter the name of ocular or systemic medication taken by a patient and to obtain a list of ocular and systemic side effects. The information can be entered from a case history and printed for the practitioner before the patient is examined. This information also can be printed and given to the patient to take home as a reminder.

Vision therapy. Computer programs offer practitioners the ability to treat various binocular, oculomotor, and visual perceptual deficits. These programs are often highly motivating for younger patients because of their resemblance to computer games. Vision therapy programs replace older instrumentation that is no longer made and allow for easier quantification of patient progress during therapy. For practices that offer in-office training, the computer therapy programs allow increased flexibility by not requiring the constant supervision of the optometrist or therapist.

Contact lenses. Computers can aid in the design of rigid contact lens and specialty lens parameters. Corneal topography can be analyzed using photokeratography. This technique promises to allow more precise measurement of the cornea–contact lens relationship and of corneal changes that occur over time. Corneal topography software allows practitioners to determine how a particular contact lens might fit a patient's eye and can refine the lens design and fitting process, allowing for less trial and error.

Low vision. Computers can be used as low vision devices for the partially sighted and as aural word processing devices by the blind population. Various manufacturers produce computers that can be used with standard software to magnify the computer image to any level for the partially sighted; contrast and illumination also can be controlled. Talking computers are available to interface with standard software and enable blind patients to perform word processing and database management.

Personal digital assistants (PDAs). These hand-held devices can be used in conjunction with standard computer software to allow the optometrist to have examination room access to information such as differential diagnoses, pharmacologic side effects of systemic drugs, and potential side effects of ophthalmic medications.

Conclusion

Computer applications have produced dramatic advances, for both business and personal use. In the optometric office of the future, the computer will be one of the most important pieces of equipment used because it has the potential to manage both the business and professional care aspects of the practice. Because of this versatility of use, optometrists must understand and be prepared to apply computer technology to the wide array of business and patient care needs faced in private practice.

Acknowledgement

The authors of this chapter in the first edition of *Business Aspects of Optometry* were Stuart Rothman and Michael Usdan.

Bibliography

American Optometric Association: *Professional enhancement program. Monograph MN 16: optimize your professional opportunities through business equipment and computers.* St. Louis, 1986, Author.

Anonymous: Directory of automated instruments and lab equipment. *Eye Care Tech (Suppl)* 5(3):7-34, 1995.

Baggarly BA: Who's on line? *Optom Economics* 1(1):48-51, 1991.

Bailey GM: The paperless office: are we there yet? *J Am Optom Assoc* 70(10):667-71, 1999.

Baldwin BL, Christensen B, Melton JW: *Rx for success.* Midwest City, Okla, 1983, Vision Publications.

Beck D: The paperless office in the palm of your hand. *Rev Optom* 134(2):39-40, 1997.

Beirne M: Online appointments. *Rev Optom (Suppl)* 137(6):18A, 2000.

Castleberry K: Just how paperless can we get? *Optom Management* 32(1):42-5, 1997.

Davidson D: How to select hardware for your paperless practice. *Rev Optom (Suppl)* 135(9):14A, 1998.

Ensman RG: How do you rate on computer care? *Optom Economics* 4(4):28-9, 1994.

Freeman DN: Recall on line. *Optom Economics* 1(6):32-7, 1991.

Hamada K: The promise of paperless practice. *Optom Economics* 4(5):22-4, 1994.

Kirk V: How I went paperless. *Rev Optom (Suppl)* 135(9):10A-12A, 1998.

Kreda S: On the road to becoming paperless. *Optom Management* 35(5):57-8,60-1, 2000.

Lee J: Seven steps toward a paperless office. *Rev Optom* 137(3):47-8,50,52, 2000.

Liverpool LA: Ten questions about going paperless—answered! *Rev Optom (Suppl)* 135(9):7A-9A, 1998.

Maino J: How to network yourself. *Optom Management* 26(7):58, 1991.

Maino J: Why you should buy a clone. *Optom Management* 26(11):55, 1991.

Maino J: Optometric software: how 5 programs rate. *Optom Management* 27(7):41-4, 1992.

Maino J: A smarter way to shop for office software. *Optom Management* 27(3):51-2, 1992.

Maino JH, Maino DM, Davidson D: *Computer applications in optometry*. Stoneham, Mass, 1989, Butterworth.

Mathe N: Software guidance counseling. *Optom Management* 26(1):39-40, 1991.

Mathe N: Computers: the key to success in the 1990's *Optom Economics* 2(12):10-4, 1992.

Mathe N: Considerations when choosing a paperless office system. *Rev Optom (Suppl)* 135(9):14A, 1998.

Mayo WA: Optometric software looks ahead. *Optom Economics* 4(7):8-13, 1994.

Mortimer MD: Computerize without busting the budget. *Optom Economics* 1(1):42-5, 1991.

Nisbet RE: Buying a personal computer, part 1. *Vision Enhancement* 5(2):72-6, 2000.

Nisbet RE: Buying a personal computer, part 2. *Vision Enhancement* 5(3):147-53, 2000.

Ossip GL: Getting wired. *Optom Management* 32(3):49,51, 53-4, 1997.

Overberg TJ: A guided tour through the paperless office. *Rev Optom (Suppl)* 135(9):4A-6A, 1998.

Puzio FD: Are you ready for computerized medical records? *Optom Management* 33(5):44-6,48, 1998.

Sachs L: The right computer. *Optom Economics* 1(12):24-7, 1991.

Salsberg S: Computerized management systems in the clinical optometric setting: selecting appropriate software. *Practical Optom* 8(6):235-9, 1997.

Salsberg S: A software system for the paperless office. *Practical Optom* 11(4):152-8, 2000.

Schwaderer KN: Increasing your patient flow with computerization. *Optom Management* 33(7):30-4, 1998.

Sowby R: *Barstow: computerized for the 90's— take two*. Santa Ana, Calif, 1987, Optometric Extension Program Foundation.

Sterling R: Computerizing your office. *Optom Management* 33(3):50-2,54,56, 1998.

www.keyworlds.com/o/optometry-software. Online list of software for optometry practices.

www.optometric.com. Online version of *Optometric Management* magazine, which features computer products for optometric practices.

www.revoptom.com. Online version of *Review of Optometry* magazine, which features computer products for optometric practices.

Chapter 21

Selecting an Office Staff

Peter G. Shaw-McMinn, Daisy Rampolla, and Maria Robles

People who produce good results feel good about themselves.
Kenneth Blanchard *One Minute Manager*

In successful human resource management, all basic functions of management must be considered. These functions are planning, organizing, directing, and controlling. Many classic business texts add a fifth consideration–staffing–to this list. These five basic functions are considered in this discussion of human resource management for an optometric practice.

The objective that is addressed in this chapter is the selecting of efficient, enthusiastic staff. There is no office in which the instruments used, procedures performed, or materials dispensed contribute to the success of the practice and goodwill of patients more than the staff. When in place and functioning properly, the staff of an optometric office adds services to patients, assists with marketing efforts inside and outside the office, increases efficiency and productivity of the practice, and elevates the personal aspects of eye care.

When the five functions of management are described, there is inevitably some overlapping and considerable interdependence. All these functions must be addressed, however, to achieve the goal of implementing a management plan that will result in developing and maintaining an efficient, enthusiastic staff. In considering the goal of developing and maintaining such a staff, it might be asked, "Are efficiency and enthusiasm related?" The answer is clearly "yes." By producing good results (being efficient), people acquire a feeling of achievement (enthusiasm). This enthusiasm permeates the person, the practice, and the care being rendered to patients.

All employees need to know and feel the following six things if they are to be enthusiastic:
- Know they are needed
- Know what is expected of them and how to meet those expectations (proper training)
- Know there is a possibility for growth
- Know they are compensated fairly
- Know they are appreciated (recognition)
- Believe they are involved in the delivery of care and the growth of the practice (ownership)

These six things should be kept in mind as a management plan is developed.

Planning

To acquire an office staff, planning is a necessary first step. The planning process is used to determine the need for and qualifications of new staff members.

Need for Staff

Before hiring an employee, it is essential to determine the needs of the practice that the employee will fulfill. What responsibilities will this staff person have? In traditional personnel terms, what will be the workload of this employee? In this planning phase, it is necessary to determine how and why specific work functions are performed and to quantify their significance in terms of time and value to the practice. For an optometrist starting a practice with one employee, the primary responsibilities will probably be those of a receptionist. Even at this early stage of practice, however, a list of responsibilities should be developed. One optometric text on practice management lists 27 responsibilities for this job classification. The determination and listing of these responsibilities become part of the organizational aspect of the management plan.

When a new position is to be added to the staff, input should be obtained from current staff members (beyond the familiar cry of "we need more help"). Asking the staff to assess the responsibilities currently being performed by individual members–through the use of daily logs or time management sheets–permits quantification of the allocation of time and duties and helps to identify needs. This process also provides a role for employees in the planning process and serves as an occasion for employees to do a self-evaluation of their contribution to the delivery of care.

When a new position is created, the use of an appropriate title often helps the person fit into the staff. For example, if a second optometric technician were hired, with primary responsibilities in styling and dispensing, the appropriate title might be ophthalmic technician. For the first technician, if he or she has demonstrated leadership qualities, the title might be changed to senior technician.

In planning for the addition of a staff member, the economics of delivering care must be considered. As stated in the introduction to this chapter, there is no aspect of a practice that is more important to its success than the staff. It also can be the most expensive aspect of a practice if not planned wisely. From an economic standpoint, both original and additional staff members should increase the productivity of the practice. Increased productivity can be achieved by the delegation of responsibilities to staff members so that the practitioner's time is better used for the delivery of income-producing professional services. (This assumes that there is potential for the practitioner's time to be used more productively.)

Optometry students and new graduates often think they must work with a full range of paraoptometric personnel, but during the developmental phase of a practice the use of a large staff is not economically sound.

Findings obtained by American Optometric Association (AOA) Economic Surveys reveal that staff costs should average about 15% of the total gross income of a practice, with a range of 12% to 18%. Another guideline for staff costs also is based on practice income; it holds that a practice should have one full-time staff person for every $150,000 of gross income. A model for staff productivity has been proposed, using dollar productivity per hour per employee. Of course, actual figures will vary considerably with the type of practice and the optometric product being delivered. A practice performing a significant amount of in-office visual training that uses technicians would be labor-intensive and would have a higher percentage of gross income devoted to staff than would a primary care practice.

Qualifications of Applicants

During the planning phase, the qualifications of applicants should be carefully considered. These qualifications need to be commensurate with the specific staff responsibilities to be assumed. Although screening for these qualifications is clearly a part of staffing, the better the planning, the better the chance of finding someone who has these qualifications in the applicant pool. Each position will require a different prioritization of general abilities, in addition to specific knowledge or skills. General abilities needed might include dexterity, memory, verbal and nonverbal communication skills, ability to handle people, and telephone voice. Telephone voice would probably be the top priority if the position were for a receptionist with appointing responsibilities. If preparing reports were part of this same job, specific skills in typing or using a word processor would be critical. Minimum hiring standards should be part of planning. In busy offices that need a person to assume specific duties with minimum training, experience might be essential. A person with the right education and training usually will be an efficient and enthusiastic employee much sooner than someone trained on the job. The meeting of these standards will depend on the applicant pool, wage level, and competition for people with similar skills from other industries. People who are working as optometric technicians and who have formal academic training only account for 18% of the individuals filling these positions.

In a survey commissioned by Bayer Corporation, in cooperation with the National Science Foundation, the newest employees in America's workforce and their managers were asked to define the special skills needed to manage continuing change in the workplace. Both managers and employees agreed that the key skills were being able to solve unforeseen problems on the job (as opposed to referring unforeseen problems to others), adapting to changes in the work environment (as opposed to coping with a stable work environment), and doing their best work as a team (as opposed to doing their best work independent of others).

Organization

Organization is the management function of relating people, tasks (or activities), and resources to each other so that the practice can accomplish its objectives. Plans are carried out through the organizing process. Table 21-1 is an example of one organization model for optometric personnel.

In most optometric offices, staff persons will be needed to perform the functions of receptionist, ophthalmic technician, frame stylist, word processor, and office manager (see Table 21-1, top). There are optometric practices in which all of these functions are performed by one or two staff members and also by the optometrist. In larger group optometric practices, one or more staff members may be designated to one particular function, and there might be added areas of responsibility. For instance, ophthalmic assistants or optometric technicians could perform pretesting procedures, another staff member might perform all the insurance billings, and so forth. The organizational chart needs to describe the specific areas of responsibility for each position. For example, in Table 21-1 the "primary patient needs" of the receptionist is to answer the phone, make and confirm appointments, prepare patient files, and manage related duties.

Personality traits also should be considered. In Table 21-1, the "qualities" that are required to perform the "primary patient needs" are listed. For example, for a receptionist to perform "primary patient needs," he or she would need "qualities" associated with performing those tasks—such as being friendly, pleasant, polite, consistent, and patient with people.

Another consideration is the secondary skills required for a position. In Table 21-1 "secondary patient needs" and "management skills" required by the receptionist, ophthalmic technician, and office manager are described. Under "qualities," some of the personality traits required to perform those specific tasks are listed.

Whether it is a first or a subsequent employee that is being selected, a careful assessment should be made of the prospective employee's strengths and personality traits to determine the person's suitability for the position. It has often been said, "One can teach skills, but it is difficult to change a personality." Inappropriate matching of personality traits and staff positions will lead to stress, conflicts, high turnover rate, and a detrimental influence on the overall growth of the practice. Patients will be quick to notice changes and conflicts within the practice, and, although they will return to the office for optometric care, their enthusiasm to refer other patients to the practice will diminish.

When choosing the positions to fill in an office, careful consideration should be give to the titles used. For example, a receptionist is one of the most crucial employees in any optometric office; it is estimated that a receptionist will communicate with the patient four times more often than the doctor will. However, "receptionist" is often considered the position with the least status, and the job is commonly assigned small tasks that do not add significant value to the practice. The purpose or mission of a receptionist should be to provide a caring and competent atmosphere for patients, and too many responsibilities can detract from this primary duty. In fact, a busy receptionist may be so hurried trying to process patients that this purpose is forgotten. Although a receptionist can process about $30,000 per month, attempts to see more patients will result in increased accounts receivable, but also insurance claims processing delays, and poor recall of patients. So the purpose of the job and the title must be considered together.

Rather than receptionist, a more appropriate title might be patient manager, appointment secretary, front-desk coordinator, or patient relations coordinator. The title selected should be the one that best fits the responsibilities of the position and that adds value to the practice. These responsibilities may include those of hostess, time manager, accountant, finance manager, follow-up evaluator, and marketing manager. It is estimated that a good front-desk person normally earns up to seven times that person's salary in increased production if trained properly.

Through the years, three basic types of staff organizations have developed in the practice of optometry. They are referred to as type I, type II, and type III.

Type I Staff Organization

Type I is referred to as the "family" staff organization. It is composed of a solo practitioner and one full-time staff person, who performs most of the staff functions. The optometrist also helps in the dispensing and adjusting of glasses. In addition, there can be a part-time staff person, and the spouse of the optometrist is usually part of the office staff. The full-time staff person has been in the practice for many years and is an excellent employee but is not necessarily a "team player." The outstanding characteristic of this practice for the staff member is the closeness, friendship, and loyalties between the employer and the employee. If there are personal problems or tragedies, the support systems function just like those of a family. The staff wages and benefits might be less than that in other offices. The overall office efficiency and organization are not the strengths of this type of practice. The gross income of this type of practice does not change significantly over the years. In the type I practice there is a strong

Table 21-1 Organizational Model for Optometric Personnel

	RECEPTIONIST	OPHTHALMIC TECHNICIAN	FRAME STYLIST	TYPIST	OFFICE MANAGER
Primary Patient Needs	Answer phone Make/confirm appointments Prepare patient files Greet patients Record charges Deposit money and contact lenses Bill patients	Order prescription contact lenses Verify prescription contact lenses Deliver prescription contact lenses	Select frames	Type	
Qualities	Friendly Pleasant Polite Consistent Patient Courteous	Able to verbally instruct Mechanically inclined Patient Skilled in time management	Fashion and color sensible Patient Perceptive Detail oriented Sensitive	Organized Efficient	
Secondary Patient Needs	Bill insurance Record insurance payment Recall patient File charts Restock office supplies	Repair and adjust prescriptions Train patients in contact lens wear			
Qualities	Organized Efficient	Methodical			
Management Skills	Manage and control accounts receivables	Log and monitor prescriptions Restock contact lenses Restock contact lens solutions			Supervise Purchase frames Pay taxes and bills Reconcile bank accounts Resolve aging accounts receivable Maintain bookkeeping and accounting
Qualities	Decisive Direct Relentless "Respectable vs. likable"	Resourceful Creative Organized Judicious			Organized Respected Supportive of sharing goals Administrant Managemental Stable, consistent

← CROSS-TRAINING →

resistance to changes in staff organization and to the incorporation of changes in examination procedures. Because of the inflexibility of the type I practice, there is little acquisition and use of modern instrumentation or equipment.

Type II Staff Organization

The *type II* practice is referred to as the "saturated" practice. There usually is a solo practitioner and an associate optometrist, who works several days at the practice. The staff organization, staff salaries, and benefits are at higher levels than those of the type I practice. There are often three full-time and permanent staff members (or the part-time equivalent of three full-time staff members), and staff functions are divided among the three staff members, each having a primary area of responsibility. The staff members are excellent "team players," with one staff person extremely strong and perceived as the "leader."

The outstanding characteristics of the type II office is the efficiency of the office and the harmony. The office continues to grow and develop, and the instrumentation and equipment are usually updated. However, in general, the support systems, friendship, and closeness do not compare with that in the type I practice.

Type III Staff Organization

The *type III* practice, referred to as "the group," represents only a minority of optometric practices. There are at least three or more partners. The staff organization, salaries, and benefits are at the highest level of optometric practices. However, because of the large volume of patients and the use of many staff members, there is limited time in which to cultivate the friendship, loyalties, and closeness found in the type I (and, to a lesser degree, in type II) practice.

Matrix Organization

Another method of organization is the matrix system, used by Williams Marketing, Inc. Matrix organization is a way to build a team approach to patient care. All staff members have specific, designated responsibilities, and every person's name and particular responsibility is defined so that everyone in the organization, including new personnel, knows exactly where to go with specific questions. Responsibility for tasks is assigned according to the most logical individual, which means that the chief executive (doctor) can delegate tasks effectively, without fear of them getting "lost in the shuffle." This allows the doctor to focus more on patient care. Matrix management requires communication rather than authority. Staff members must support and help one another rather than work separately. This creates a cohesive team approach because everyone contributes.

Functions are divided into three management centers (front desk, clinic, dispensary), which are run by managers (Figure 21-1). Although management centers are separated within the matrix, the matrix interlocks staff members outside particular management centers by designating directors for five business functions (marketing, sales, patient care, finance, and quality control) and applying these functions to all three management centers. Isolation of employees is consequently eliminated. Because each individual in the management centers is assigned responsibilities, someone is immediately accountable for all functions. Because everyone contributes, there is cohesion and a shared sense of value.

In small practices the same person may serve as the manager of certain management centers and the director of certain functions. For example, the dispensary manager also may be the designated director of marketing and quality control. The chief executive (doctor) also may be the clinic manager and patient care director. The key to a matrix system is to ensure

	Marketing	Sales	Patient Care	Finance	Quality Control
Front Desk					
Clinic					
Dispensary					

Chief Executive

Figure 21-1　Matrix organization. (Courtesy Williams Marketing, Lincoln, Neb. Reprinted with permission.)

that the responsibility for duties falling under each management center and business function is specifically assigned.

Developing an Office Manual for Employees

After a thorough evaluation of the staff needs has been performed and the appropriate organization has been determined, it is mandatory that an office policy manual be written. If the office does not have a manual, the time should be taken to develop one. Even if a solo practice is started "cold," it should have a manual. The employment policy manual should include several basic topics (Box 21-1).

The AOA (and individual authors) have published guidebooks that go through each step of manual development. These sources should be consulted before attempting to draft a manual for a specific office.

Box 21-1 Topics to be Included in an Office Manual

Philosophy of care and of the office
Employee classification
Full-time, part-time, probationary
Equal opportunity statement
Policy of nondiscrimination
Duties and responsibilities of employees: staff functions
Employee conduct
  May include such issues as personal conduct, dress code, personal calls, personal visitors, punctuality, smoking, eating, drinking, chewing gum, grooming and attire
Working hours
Vacations, holidays, and leaves of absence
  May include such issues as paid vacations, holidays, sick leave or absence, emergency leave, leaves without pay
Payroll and employee benefits
Safety
Confidentiality
  May include provision that "violation of patient confidentiality" will be grounds for immediate dismissal
Performance and salary review
Patient complaints
Termination
  Voluntary, mutual, and involuntary
Jury duty
Bereavement leave

Designation of the Personnel Administrator

One of the significant advantages of a group practice is that one of the partners can be responsible for the management of the staff. Often this position merits special compensation because of the time commitment, stress, and pressure. In some practices, this administrator might give a performance review and evaluation for each staff member every 6 months, or at least once a year. During this review the administrator discusses the job description with the employee and measures performance against expectation, develops with the employee a plan for improvement, and provides feedback on employee strengths and weaknesses.

The personnel administrator also listens to staff complaints about the practitioners and the office. These complaints are then transmitted to the practitioners, who meet weekly to discuss issues as they occur. There also should be a staff meeting at least once a month. If it is at noon, a catered lunch could be served since the staff members are giving up their lunch time for an office meeting. The chair of each meeting is rotated among the staff. The administrator also determines staff vacation time for the calendar year and monitors sick and bereavement leaves and similar periods of absence.

Other models of an office hierarchy might have an office manager or personnel administrator who is not an optometrist. These administrators operate in a manner that is very similar to the process previously described, reporting frequently to the optometrist responsible for this part of the practice.

Many offices use front office coordinators or senior technicians as administrators to establish some vertical management. Whenever there is more than one employee, it is necessary to establish who is responsible to whom. Job classifications identify individual responsibilities, but there must be someone in the practice to see that these responsibilities are fulfilled on a day-to-day basis. The structure of any vertical management should be included in the practice manual or employee handbook.

Job Analysis

Once an organizational structure has been chosen, a job analysis must be performed to determine the specific responsibilities and tasks to be assigned to each staff member. Job analysis in some settings is no longer considered optional, rather being required in light of recent legal rulings that protect employee rights. These rulings indicate that a job analysis should provide the following:

- A thorough, clear, well-written, specific job description
- An indication of how often specific task behaviors should be evaluated
- An accurate evaluation of the job specifications, as provided by the U.S. Employment Service and U.S. Office of Personnel Management.

Legal considerations also affect the selection process when hiring new staff members.

Legal Considerations of the Selection of Staff Members

Employer-employee relationships, even in small optometric practices, are affected by a variety of both federal and state laws. Although some laws limit their application to employers having a minimum of 15 to 20 employees, others are more broadly applicable. The legislation therefore is applicable to most optometric practices. Because of their complexity, it is important to have competent legal counsel in dealing with these laws.

The Fair Labor Standards Act (FLSA) establishes minimum wage, overtime pay, recordkeeping, and child labor standards affecting more than 80 million full- and part-time workers in the private sector and in federal, state, and local governments.

The Wage and Hour Division (Wage-Hour) administers and enforces FLSA with respect to private employment; state and local government employment; and federal employees of the Library of Congress, U.S. Postal Service, Postal Rate Commission, and the Tennessee Valley Authority. For example, the Office of Personnel Management is responsible for enforcement with regard to all other federal employees.

Special rules apply to state and local government employment involving fire protection and law enforcement activities, volunteer services, and compensatory time off in lieu of cash overtime pay.

As of 2002, covered nonexempt workers have been entitled to a minimum wage of not less than $5.15 an hour. Overtime pay at a rate of not less than one and one-half times the regular rate of pay is required for each hour worked over 40 hours per week. Wages required by FLSA are due on the regular payday for the pay period covered. Deductions made from wages for items such as cash or merchandise shortages, employer-required uniforms, and tools of the trade are not legal to the extent that they reduce the wages of employees below the minimum rate

required by FLSA or reduce the amount of overtime pay due under FLSA.

Even though FLSA does set basic minimum wage and overtime pay standards and regulates the employment of minors, there are a number of employment practices that FLSA does not regulate. For example, FLSA does not require the following:

- Vacation, holiday, severance, or sick pay
- Meal or rest periods
- Premium pay for weekend or holiday work
- Pay raises or fringe benefits
- A discharge notice, reason for discharge, or immediate payment of final wages to terminated employees

Also, FLSA does not limit the number of hours in a day or days in a week an employee can be required or scheduled to work, if the employee is at least 16 years old. These matters are for agreement between the employer and the employees, or their authorized representatives. Under certain conditions, employers can pay a training wage of at least 85% of the minimum wage for up to 90 days to employees younger than 20. In addition to these issues, there are other conditions and exemptions in FLSA that should be considered.

The FLSA child labor provisions are designed to protect the educational opportunities of minors and prohibit their employment under conditions or in jobs that are detrimental to their health or well-being. These provisions include restrictions on hours of work for minors younger than 16.

The FLSA requires employers to keep records on wages, hours, and other items, as specified in Department of Labor recordkeeping regulations. Most of the information is of the kind generally maintained by employers in ordinary business practice and in compliance with other laws and regulations. The records do not have to be kept in any particular form, and time clocks need not be used.

The Civil Rights Act of 1964 and related amendments and executive orders prohibit discrimination on the basis of race, color, religion, sex, national origin, marital status, physical disabilities, military discharge, and arrest record. This legislation applies—and many state laws apply—to all employment practices, including hiring, firing, promotion, compensation, and other conditions of employment. A separate act, the Age Discrimination in Employment Act of 1967, and related amendments require employers to treat applicants and employees equally, regardless of age. Sexual harassment in the workplace also has become a highly sensitive issue in recent years, requiring employers to maintain a proper work environment.

Selection Process

One of the most frustrating aspects of private practice is personnel turnover. The finding, keeping, and training of personnel are part of an ongoing project and problem for most offices. Outstanding employees might leave to move out of state, get married, to have a child, or take other employment. Whatever the reason, the replacement of an employee should be regarded as an opportunity. A new face can bring a fresh attitude and ideas. Too often, practitioners keep employees who are chronically late, sloppy in their work, and snippy with patients, out of fear that they will not be able to find an adequate replacement. There are five basic steps that should be adhered to in the selection process: finding sources of competent applicants, screening applicants, setting up interviews, asking relevant questions during interviews, and checking applicant references.

Step 1. Sources For Applicants

There are several resources that can be used to search for employees, including employment agencies, technicians' schools, friends, patients, newspaper advertisements, optical companies, retail sales representatives, current patients, local churches, college placement services, Web sites, and employee-leasing agencies (which will frequently pre-screen candidates in response to specific needs).

Employment Agencies. Employees obtained from an agency come with a price. It is customary to pay the agency a fee of 1% for every $1000 of the employee's first-year salary. (This offsets the agency's costs for the advertising and screening of applicants.) If the practice is a small office, an agency may offer a discount. There usually is a 30-day trial period during which money is refunded if the employer or the employee is dissatisfied. If there is a problem within the first 90 days, the employment agency usually will guarantee to provide a replacement.

Optometric Technicians' Schools. Technicians who graduate from these schools have good background knowledge and some clinical training but are limited in number. A recent AOA survey reported that only 18% of employed optometric technicians had received formal training.

Friends. This source of employees has to be managed wisely. Hiring friends to work in an office can be a delicate situation. It can be difficult to introduce a business attitude into a relationship that has been built on an equal basis.

Patients. Satisfied patients make wonderful, enthusiastic staffers. They talk from personal experience about an office's good service and can be a great asset in promoting the office. Before a patient is hired, however, it should be determined that the patient possesses the required skills or is trainable.

Newspaper Classified Advertisements. There are several ways in which a newspaper advertisement can be used to attract applicants. One technique is to list a post office box number and request that applicants submit résumés; another is to list a private telephone number for applicants to contact for information on submitting their résumés. This technique can decrease the number of applicants because many employees applying for general office work or optical work do not have résumés. An alternative technique would be to ask for a letter of application rather than a résumé. The key to attracting applicants is writing an advertisement that makes the position or office sound exciting. People read into advertisements what they want, and generally what they want is excitement, fun, and a challenge.

Optical Companies. Super-opticals and chain locations usually are open 6 to 7 days a week, 12 hours a day. Many talented and experienced employees are not interested in working such an extensive work week. These individuals might even be willing to accept a decrease in salary for the more convenient hours of a private practice.

Sales Representatives in Optical Industry. Ophthalmic sales representatives are in a different office every day. They hear firsthand from employees if they are unhappy or are interested in moving for one reason or another. They can be very helpful in spreading the news that the practice is in the market for a new assistant.

Cosmetic or Jewelry Sales Representatives. Retail sales people in clothing, cosmetics, and jewelry have the personality and sales ability that adapts easily to the optical area. Many times, when hiring an experienced frame stylist, one also hires the stylist's old habits, such as prejudging a patient's spending ability.

Someone who knows how to provide a fresh attitude can bring a fresh approach as well.

Employee-Leasing Agencies. These companies interview, hire, and pay employees, saving the hassle that comes with frequent personnel turnover, the cost of benefits, and inconvenience of paying employment taxes. A fee must be paid to the agency, however, for the services and personnel obtained from the agency.

Web Sites. The Internet has changed the way information is obtained and exchanged. Many professional associations, optical companies, and employee agencies list employment opportunities on their Web sites.

Step 2. Screening Applicants

Screening applicants over the telephone is a crucial step in the hiring process. The interviewer should have a legal-size pad of paper by the phone, to note the applicant's name and the interviewer's first impressions. The sound and tone of the applicant's voice are important impressions. Is the voice harsh, the rate of speech too quick, or the tone of conversation false?

The "telephone personality" of the applicant also should be assessed. Close attention should be paid to the ease of conversation, the use of grammar, and any accent or dialect that is difficult to understand. During the telephone screening process, it is essential to stay in control of the conversation. The applicant's name and phone number should be obtained for future reference. (If the caller is not willing to provide this information, the conversation should be politely concluded.)

The caller usually will ask for a job description and the salary being offered. To stay in control, the interviewer should immediately ask the caller, "What are you doing presently?" This question will provide information about the caller's employment situation, such as whether the caller is unemployed and for how long that has been the situation. If the caller is working, the interviewer can find out where the caller is employed, what the caller's skills are, and the salary range expected.

Step 3. First Interview

The first interview should be handled by a senior employee. The office administrator should have applicants fill out an employment application. After all applications have been collected, the administrator can narrow the applicant field so that the practitioner only has to interview the best two or three prospects. Filling out an employment application provides not only pertinent facts about the applicants but also allows the applicant's handwriting and spelling skills to be analyzed.

One of the goals of a first interview is to size up the personal appearance of the interviewee. The cleanliness and neatness of the applicant's clothes and hair should be noted. A professional image is desired, and the person should be evaluated on that basis. The demeanor of the person also should be considered. The handshake can provide an indication of the person's personality, as can eye contact and the person's posture. Although the professional image of a person is composed of many factors, from a legal and an ethical standpoint the person's race, religion, sex, and age should not be considered. If the candidate volunteers any of this information, that is OK, but the topic should not be discussed at length.

To determine the questions that can be asked of a job applicant, the state employment department, the local Chamber of Commerce, professional organizations (such as the AOA), or the Equal Employment Opportunity Commission (EEOC) can be consulted. (The EEOC has a Web site at *www.eeoc.gov* that contains helpful information.) The same general questions should be asked of each applicant, and applicants should be managed similarly during the interview. Documentation should be as thorough as time permits. If an applicant is rejected, the decision should be based on objective standards only and documented accordingly. Personal comments about applicants should be avoided.

The interviewer should have prepared questions to ask. At the conclusion of questioning, the interviewer should ask whether the interviewee has any questions.

Step 4. Questioning the Applicant

There are a number of questions that are regularly asked during job interviews (Box 21-2). Often, the most important question to ask a prospective employee is, "What do you like to do best?" This question is asked to establish whether the interviewee's expectations and needs match the job description.

No matter what position a person is hired for, an employee will always gravitate toward the skills he or she enjoys most. A person can be hired as a receptionist, with duties of appointment making, collections, and recall, but if the person enjoys performing computer work, he or she will find ways to work at the computer, avoiding important job responsibilities.

Box 21-2   Fifteen of the Most Frequently Asked Interview Questions

- Tell me about yourself.
- Why are you interested in working for this company?
- Why do you want to leave your job?
- Why have you chosen this particular field?
- Why should we hire you?
- What are your long-range goals?
- What is your greatest strength?
- What is your greatest weakness?
- What is your current salary?
- What is important to you in a job?
- What do you do in your spare time?
- Which feature of the job interests you least?
- How do others describe you?
- What are your plans for continued study?
- Tell me about your schooling.

Suggested Reference Checklist

1. Applicant's name _____
   Date of reference check _____
2. Reference contacted _____
3. Employment dates _____ to _____
4. Salary history _____
5. Type of responsibilities _____
6. Attendance/punctuality _____
7. Special skills _____
8. Reason for leaving _____
9. Notice given _____
10. Severance pay given _____
11. Unemployment compensation _____
12. Is the applicant qualified for rehire? _____
13. Other comments _____
    _____
    _____

Figure 21-2 Example reference checklist for job applicants. (Courtesy American Optometric Association, St. Louis. Reprinted with permission.)

Thus it is best to determine beforehand whether the prospective employee's interests and the responsibilities of the position are well matched. Some doctors use psychological testing to learn more about applicants. There are commercially available tests that can be purchased for job applicants used to assess intelligence, aptitude, personality, interpersonal skills, and interests. For example, Schoer Medical Marketing Solutions sells tests to determine applicants' strengths, weaknesses, and attitudes. This company also offers a human resource guide that includes a new employee interview form, interview outline, technician interview form, applicant reference form, employment agreement form, employee review form, and an exit interview form.

Step 5. Checking References by Phone

After reviewing the applications and the results of the interviews and selecting the two best candidates, the references of these candidates should be evaluated over the telephone. If the applicant works (or worked) for a large employer, someone in authority should be questioned to verify the applicant's work history and establish that the person is right for the job (Figure 21-2).

There are a number of questions that can be asked. The first question, however, should be, "Is the employee punctual?" This question provides an indication of the responsibility and dependability of the person. The last question should be, "Would you rehire this employee?" This question allows for a "no"

response, while protecting the employer from possible legal entanglements.

Hiring Enthusiastic Top Performers

If staff members are enthusiastic, it is a way of saying, "I care." According to Scott T. Gross, author of *Positively Outrageous Service* (New York, Mastermedia, Inc.), there are four key characteristics to look for: "can do," "will do," "feel good," and "fit." "Can do" refers to a person with the knowledge and ability needed to complete the required task. Employees obviously should have the ability to achieve, but lack of ability is rarely the cause of job failure. The problem more often is that "can do" is overemphasized, at the expense of other important traits such as "will do," "feel good," and "fit."

If an employee can do the job but for some reason will not do it, all the training and experience in the world are of no value. Typically, it is inferred that the person is unmotivated. But that may not be completely accurate: the person just may not be motivated to do that particular job. Thus it is best to choose employees who can motivate themselves, want to achieve at a high level, and will do so without being prompted. Staff members who are energetic and willing to do the "something extra" that goes beyond expectations exhibit the "will do" trait that is found in top-performing employees.

The third trait to look for when building a staff is "feel good." If conversation with the applicant results in a strong, positive intuitive message, that same message will likely be communicated to patients. People who can make a favorable impression in a short period are usually welcome additions to an office staff.

Almost three of four individuals hired are chosen largely on the issue of "fit." Businesses are not essentially different from professional sports teams. It makes good sense that every new member of the team should be evaluated in terms of the potential to add to performance. Sony Corporation uses a series of five interviews to screen job applicants. The company looks for high achievers who earned an A or B grade average in school and who have a record of service in school or civic organizations. What is most interesting about the interview process is that Sony is less concerned with the content of the answers than with the conversational style and manner of the applicant. A new employee can be trained in the technical aspects of the business a lot easier than the employee can be trained to "feel good" and "fit." Some optometric offices have all employees interact with a prospective employee before the position is offered. Every employee must feel comfortable with the new prospect before he or she is added to the team.

Offering Employment

Once it has been decided that an applicant appears to suit the practice's needs, no time should be wasted in offering the position. Good employees are hard to find and can have other job offers to consider. During the interview, some of the benefits of working for the practice might have been discussed. During the job offer, it is necessary to negotiate the actual terms of the agreement, and—in so doing—to reach an agreement that fits the needs of both the practice and the new employee. The areas of concern in achieving this goal are preparing for the negotiation, items open to negotiation, a written agreement stating expectations, and what was agreed to by the parties.

Preparing for the Negotiation

Many job offers today are made over the telephone. The applicant is called, the job is offered, and a starting salary is specified. This approach can be adequate if no further negotiation of the employment terms is required. In most situations, however, there are many points open to negotiation, and this can necessitate a face-to-face meeting.

As in any negotiation situation, it is best to negotiate from a position of power, and that is most readily

achieved if the applicant comes to the office for the employment offer. In some situations, sitting behind a large desk might be preferred—to demonstrate a position of control. At other times, it can be better to be seated without anything between the two parties or to be seated next to one another. One of the considerations for choosing the setting is the employer's personal management style.

The terms of negotiation are based on how badly the practice wants or needs the potential employee. Employers should keep in mind that employees can be responsible for as much as two thirds of the gross income of a practice and that they can make or break a practice. Thus, it might be necessary to make numerous concessions for the right applicant. On the other hand, there are reasonable limits to any negotiation. The employer should determine and write down, before the negotiation, these bargaining limits. In so doing, specific limits should be decided for each of the following negotiable points:
- Responsibilities
- Hours
- Days
- Salary
- Education benefits
- Medical insurance
- Sick pay
- Vacation pay
- Personal time off
- Purchase of optical supplies
- Purchase of the practitioner's services
- Paid holidays
- Retirement plan
- Bonuses

Usually salary is the key item of interest to the new employee, particularly if the employee is young. If the employee has a family, medical insurance coverage might be more important. An older, single employee might be interested in retirement benefits. Employees older than 65 could be concerned with keeping their income lower because of Social Security benefits; they might prefer other forms of compensation, such as fringe benefits or personal time off. The employer should attempt to find out what compensation the prospective employee has decided is most important. Salary data for many occupations are now posted conveniently on the Internet. Salary survey sites deliver data organized by job title, industry, level of experience, company size, city, and even zip code. The information is based on hundreds of compensation surveys performed by industry and trade groups nationwide. These data could have the power to change salary negotiations in optometry forever, particularly when the salaries of receptionists, optometric assistants, optometric technicians, dispensing opticians, laboratory opticians, office managers, and optometrists become widely listed. Current Internet resources include *www.salary.com*; *www.careerjournal.com*; and *www.jobstar.org*. Other helpful Web sites include government sites provided by the U.S. Bureau of Labor Statistics, the California Employment Development Department, and the U.S. Census Bureau.

When making the employment offer, it is often advantageous to have a written document that can be used to record the negotiations.

Responsibilities

A responsibilities survey can be used to discuss the expectations of both sides (Figure 21-3). This survey is intended to allow the prospective employee to evaluate—on a 1 to 5 scale (1 being the most desirable and 5 the least)—potential or prospective work assignments. Use of such a survey can give the employer additional insight into the type of person who is being hired. Later on, if conflicts arise over work responsibilities, the survey can be used to document proof of what was discussed.

There will be a wide range of responses from the survey. Some potential employees will mark nothing less than a "2"; they might want to give the impression that they are willing to work in all areas. Other applicants might mark several areas with a "5." This response can indicate that the potential employee is inflexible and might not wish to change, or, perhaps he or she had some poor prior experiences; on the other hand, the response can indicate that the potential employee is straightforward and willing to communicate honestly.

Areas of Responsibility

Place 1 next to what you definitely wish to do and have done before.
Place 2 next to what you would like to try but have never done before.
Place 3 next to what you would do if asked.
Place 4 next to what you don't think you'd like to do but never tried.
Place 5 next to what you definitely don't want to do at this time.

Areas of responsibility:

__ Answering the telephone
__ Making appointments
__ Greeting patients
__ Distributing office information
__ Performing hostess duties
__ Seating patients in pretesting room
__ Answering patient inquiries into services
__ Obtaining patient case histories
__ Administering preliminary testing
__ Informing about office services and doctor's qualifications
__ Showing videotapes
__ Seating patients in exam room
__ Instructing about contact lens handling
__ Selecting frames
__ Discussing options on lenses and additional pairs
__ Writing up orders
__ Checking orders
__ Dispensing

__ Instructing about proper maintenance and adaptation for contact lenses
__ Explaining fee breakdown
__ Designing payment schedules
__ Writing up receipts and day sheet entries
__ Maintaining accounts receivable
__ Handling bank deposits
__ Maintaining inventory
__ Restocking supplies
__ Maintaining instruments
__ Maintaining facilities
__ Typing
__ Ordering office supplies
__ Assembling patient information packets
__ Maintaining public relations
__ Performing lab technician duties
__ Performing visual therapist duties
__ Performing low vision therapist duties

Figure 21-3 Example employee responsibilities survey.

The survey must be carefully reviewed by the employer. Does the completed survey of responsibilities fit the practice's needs? Do the likes and dislikes complement other employees? If not, can the practice settle for less than perfect? At what cost? The completed survey can affect the salary amount to be offered the prospective employee.

Probation Period

Since benefits do not begin until the probation period has passed, some potential employees might wish to have a shorter probation period. An offer of a lower initial salary in return for a shorter probation period might be acceptable to the potential employee.

Hours

The potential employee might prefer not to work past 5 PM. If that is the case, a lower salary could be acceptable. On the other hand, if the practice requires late hours, the potential employee might feel that additional compensation is deserved. Is the practice willing to pay more? How much? How will this affect other benefits?

Days

The days of employment require a negotiation strategy similar to the one used for hours. Is the applicant willing to work on Saturdays? How will the potential employee's attitude affect the salary offer?

Salary

Salary is the one item that will most likely be discussed when the potential employee first applied for the job. At that time a specific figure, or perhaps a salary range, would have been described. The employer must consider whether negotiations on other matters have altered the assessment of salary. Can a higher salary be traded for fewer fringe benefits? For example, the employer might be willing to pay a higher salary if the prospective employee agrees to work particular hours or on particular days or is willing to accept a limited number of personal leave or vacation days. The presentation of the offer is important. The employer should make the potential employee feel that the practice is willing to bend to suit the employee's needs. The employer also should stress the positive. The negotiation must stay, however, within the reasonable limits set.

The employer must constantly ask himself or herself, "How far am I willing to go to hire this person?" It should be remembered that, if too much is paid, others in the office might be resentful and that there is an important need to keep everything in equilibrium.

One way of offsetting a prospective employee's disappointment at the salary offered is to provide a bonus program. Such a program will give the confident employee a boost. The bonus system allows the employee to be paid more after the employee has demonstrated improvement in skills and thereby improvement in worth to the practice. A bonus system is often tied to the probation period. For example, an employee hired to work in the dispensary might be given the following offer: "I can pay you $8 per hour for the first month while we are training you how to do frame selection and adjustments. When you have demonstrated your proficiency at this skill, we will raise your salary to $9 per hour and begin training you in pre-testing and lab work. Once you've mastered the pre-testing skills, your salary will be $9.50 an hour, and then $10 an hour at the time you can complete the lab work independently."

The employee might be willing to settle for dispensing at $8 an hour and have no interest in laboratory work or pre-testing. At other times, the new employee will spend extra time and effort learning the added skills to obtain a higher salary. In either case, the pay will be what was expected for the responsibilities performed.

Employee development probably should not be open to negotiation. No matter who is hired, some time needs to be spent in integrating new employees into the office. An initial training period, continuing education, office meetings, and office retreats offer opportunities to increase the efficiency of the employee.

After all the negotiable points have been agreed on, they should be written down, and the new employee should be given a copy of the agreement. If everything has been presented properly, the practice now has someone who knows what responsibilities are expected, knows what can be expected as payment in return, and is eager to become a part of the team.

An employee file must be initiated, which at this stage should include job application, curriculum vitae, interview notes, and any pertinent documents or agreements.

Determining Compensation

To develop and maintain an efficient, enthusiastic staff the practice must offer salaries equal to or slightly more than the current pay scale in the area for persons with similar skills and responsibilities. The pay scale in the area can be determined by checking with other optometrists, health care providers, and businesses nearby. Positions with more responsibility or those that require special training will require a higher pay scale.

Salaries should be evaluated at least once each year. If an employee is exceeding the responsibilities assigned and is an asset to practice growth, that initiative should be rewarded. Most optometrists pay on an hourly basis rather than providing a weekly salary. There will be occasions when staff members have to remain after normal hours to fulfill responsibilities to patients. Staff members should be compensated for this time, and an hourly rate is more equitable than providing equivalent time off or adjusting the weekly or monthly pay of a salaried person. Many offices schedule full-time employees fewer than 40 hours a week to allow for this fluctuation in daily hours, thereby avoiding the payment of time and a half for overtime.

Fringe benefits usually are based on the practice location and size. Some offices pay bonuses, health insurance premiums, contributions to pension plans, and similar benefits. Other employers might not find it necessary to offer these types of benefits to keep satisfactory employees. An employer can offer many forms of benefits, although federal laws do not require them to be provided. If an employer decides to offer benefits, the same benefits must be offered to other employees that fall into the same employment category.

Fringe benefits are often as important to employees as salary. Important benefits include various pension plans; medical, dental, and optical insurance; vacation, sick, and holiday pay; educational and travel allowances; maternal leave; uniforms; paid parking; child care; and various periodic incentive bonuses. These benefits should be planned and budgeted for and included in the employee handbook.

Introducing New Staff to Patients

Staff turnover can create a negative impression in almost any practice. Patients may wonder why a staff member they've come to know and like has left voluntarily for another job. When turnover occurs repeatedly, patients may believe that the practice is not a pleasant place to work or does not provide adequate wages for employees. When there is turnover, it is important to present the changes positively to patients. Rather than allow patients to encounter the new staff member by chance, a careful introduction should be

orchestrated so that a favorable impression is conveyed. One way of doing this is to have the staff member write a letter of introduction to patients. The new employee should stress his or her enthusiasm and qualifications and explain how being part of the practice will benefit patients. Or, the practitioner can provide the information, stressing the items that are most positive to the practice.

Another excellent approach is to write an article in the practice newsletter. The focus of the article would be how much of an asset the new person will be to the practice and the new and interesting things he or she will be doing. The new staff member also can be featured in the reception area, on a bulletin board, or a movie-style display that patients can read. (A headline can be placed above the employee's 8×10 inch black-and-white photograph that reads, "Now Playing in Our Office . . . .") A newspaper ad also can be used to announce the addition of the new staff member.

The employee should be coached for the introduction to patients. Before the new employee meets even a single patient, he or she should memorize a list of facts about the practitioner and the practice. For example, at the very least, the new staff member should know the following:

- Each doctor's name, pronounced and spelled correctly
- How long each doctor has been in the practice and where he or she received professional training (also, one good thing about each doctor)
- Awards, honors, memberships, licenses, or special positions held by each doctor
- The practice's address and phone number (and Web site address and e-mail address, if applicable)
- A lay explanation of what optometry is and a short statement of practice philosophy
- Directions to the office, including parking and public transportation information
- The hours the office is open
- Names and titles of all employees and an explanation of each person's role
- The correct way to answer the phone
- Answers to patients' most frequently asked questions—about the services that are offered, fees, appointment availability, and so forth.

Other staff members can assist in the learning process by providing answers to these questions. If necessary, flashcards can be prepared to make learning easier for the new employee. Finally, the day will come when the new employee is introduced to his or her first patient. This is a moment that should not be allowed to go unnoticed. A photograph should be taken and an enlargement should be presented to the new employee with a degree of ceremony at the next staff meeting. Just like the "first dollar bill earned" that some businesses frame and hang, the photograph will celebrate the beginning of employment, and—over the years—hopefully serve to remind the employee of how much he or she has grown professionally as a staff member.

Conclusion

Mistakes are made by everyone in hiring. Many optometrists would list employee management as the single largest headache faced by the private independent practitioner. Determining reasonable terms, negotiating terms with the employee, and putting the terms in writing will facilitate the integration of the new employee into the team. Time and attention to such a process can save many hours in the future, prevent disagreement, and result in a smooth running office.

Acknowledgement

The authors of this chapter in the first edition of *Business Aspects of Optometry* were Donald H. Lakin, Ronald S. Rounds, Peter Shaw-McMinn, and Craig Hisaka.

Bibliography

Allergan, Inc: *Pathways in practice.* Irvine, Calif, 1995, Author.

American Optometric Association: *Practice enhancement program, MN5, optimize your professional opportunities through effective office staff policies and procedures.* St. Louis, 1984, Author.

American Optometric Association: *Practice enhancement program II, professional enhancement module, managing your practice plan, precourse workbook.* St. Louis, 1986, Author.

American Optometric Association: *Practice enhancement program II, professional enhancement module, your marketing plan module two, precourse workbook.* St. Louis, 1986, Author.

American Optometric Association: *Practice enhancement program, MN 1, optimize your professional opportunities through personal and professional goal setting.* St. Louis, 1986, Author.

Baldwin BL, Christensen B, Melton T: *Rx for success.* Midwest City, Okla, 1982, Vision Publications.

Blanchard K, Johnson S: *The one minute manager.* New York, 1993, Berkeley Publishing Group.

Blanchard K, Lorber R: *Putting the one minute manager to work.* New York, 1991, Berkeley Publishing Group.

Equal Employment Opportunity Commission: *Age discrimination in Employment Act regulations,* 29 CFR §1625.5.

Equal Employment Opportunity Commission: *Guidelines on discrimination because of national origin,* 29 CFR §1601.6(a)(2).

Equal Employment Opportunity Commission: *Guidelines on discrimination because of religion,* 29 CFR §1605.3.

Equal Employment Opportunity Commission: *Guidelines on employee selection procedures,* 29 CFR §1607.4c(2).

Gross TS: *Positively outrageous service.* New York, 1991, Mastermedia Limited.

Maslow AH: *Motivation and personality.* New York, 1987, Harper & Row.

McGregor D: *The human side of enterprise.* New York, 1985, McGraw-Hill.

Miller PJ: How to navigate the rigmarole of hiring. *Rev Optom* 137(2):33-5, 2000.

Moss GL: Use job analysis to hire the right employee. *Optom* 71(11):739-40, 2000.

Peters TJ, Waterman RH Jr: *In search of excellence.* New York, 1988, Harper & Row.

Sachs L: Introducing new staff to your patients. *Optom Economics* 4(10):15-7, 1994.

Stein H: Seven steps for interviewing and hiring employees. *Optom Management* 24(5):112–13, 1989.

Tecker IJ, Tecker GH: "Big boom theory." *Assoc Management* 43(1):46-7, 1991.

Winslow C: Elevate your receptionist to patient manager. *Rev Optom* 127(9):48-57, 1990.

www.obl.gov/elaws/flsa.htm. Fair Labor Standards Act advisor, which provides an online explanation of the law's requirements.

www.optometric.com. Online version of *Optometric Management* magazine, which provides advice about personnel management.

www.revoptom.com. Online version of *Review of Optometry* magazine, which provides advice about personnel management.

Chapter 22

Selecting and Using an Optical Laboratory

Craig Bowen

It has long been an axiom of mine that the little things are infinitely the most important.
Sir Arthur Conan Doyle *The Adventures of Sherlock Holmes*

Although most optometrists have accounts with many laboratories and frame companies, in the majority of practices, one source is used for more than half of the laboratory work. There are several factors that lead to the selection of a primary laboratory, including communication with sales representatives and laboratory managers; sources of frames; availability, service, and quality in obtaining frames; turn-around time; insurance provider status; inventory control of frames; quality lens control; laboratory service; pricing of materials; laboratory policies and the facility to expedite laboratory work and materials. These topics constitute the subject matter of this chapter.

Meeting with Optical Sales Representatives

Whether starting or buying a practice, it is necessary to establish a board of advisors: attorney, accountant, banker, financial advisor, and similar individuals with technical expertise. Another important advisor will be a trusted representative of the ophthalmic industry. To a considerable degree, financial success in practice will depend on that tangible aspect of the optometry product, the glasses dispensed. Approximately one third of the revenues generated in an optometric practice are used directly for the payment of ophthalmic materials.

Experienced laboratory representatives are familiar with the ophthalmic marketplace and can be used for advice on subjects as diverse as the tentative location of a practice, the demographics of eye care providers in an area, how to design and furnish a dispensing area, and how to budget for an initial frame inventory. It is a representative's business to know the current trends in the eyewear field and what has been successfully received by the public.

Once a relationship with a representative has been established, the representative becomes a source for the practice's eyewear. He or she will bring to the office products that the practitioner has seen advertised in journals or new products. These representatives also become the individuals who must be contacted regarding quality of work, laboratory services, and cost of materials. As a practice grows, representatives can provide an important service by educating staff members on the advantages of specific lenses and frames to patients. Many laboratories and suppliers will offer in-office, after-hours seminars to teach staff members how to present specific ophthalmic products to patients.

Sources of Spectacle Frames

Until the late 1960s, most spectacle frames were sold through wholesale distributors or optical laboratories. These companies were referred to as "full-service laboratories" and usually supplied frames from an in-house frame inventory while providing lenses and lens services from their surfacing and finishing laboratory. In addition, these companies usually sold full lines of ophthalmic equipment. During this era it was possible to deal with one optical laboratory. If all the frames in a practitioner's dispensary were from the same company that provided the lenses, orders for completed glasses could be phoned or mailed to the laboratory. Logistically, there is still a sizable advantage to working this way, and laboratories that maintain inventories of frames should be considered whenever they can satisfy the need for good service and price. Throughout the years, however, imported frames have become a bigger part of the ophthalmic market, and direct sales of frames by manufacturers have become very common. Many of these products are high-fashion frames or are provided to fill specific market niches. Imported frames have greatly expanded the frame market and also have changed the way frames are distributed.

Companies selling imported frames have their own sales representatives, and these individuals call on private practitioners for orders just as they call on national chains. These companies bill practitioners directly and often offer discounts on quantity orders or provide contracts to use a specific number of frames per month, quarter, or year. Most optometrists work with a number of these direct sales manufacturers so that a wide variety of eyewear can be offered to patients; the number of representatives usually is limited to three to four individuals. Such an arrangement increases the opportunity for greater volume discounts and decreases the time spent reviewing products.

Because of the financial advantages of ordering ophthalmic materials and contact lenses in large quantities, private practitioners have formed "buying groups." Originally these groups consisted of optometrists, opticians, or both who pooled their buying ability to negotiate with suppliers for the purchase of materials at discounted prices that approximated those being offered to national chains or very large practices. These buying groups have been quite successful, and some have expanded to regional size; a few have even been able to distribute their services nationally. Some are associated with optometric management consulting firms or national franchisers of ophthalmic materials. A few of the larger, more progressive "full-service" optical companies and laboratories are now negotiating with direct frame distributors to have the frames shown and sold by company representatives and billed at the lowest possible price to optometrists who order the frames through their laboratory. As single frames are needed for patients' orders, they are sent and billed to the laboratory, and the discounted cost, with a minimal handling charge, is passed on to the optometrist. The advantages of this process to optometrists are that the service is faster, there are fewer accounts to deal with, and frame materials can still be obtained at the lowest possible cost.

Frame Quality, Service, and Price

Quality, service, and price are three principal concerns when purchasing frames for a dispensary. Since frames vary considerably with regard to material, style, and features, quality is related to the suitability of the product for the specific type of patient for whom it is intended to serve. For example, a child's frame used for a Medicaid patient would need to be more durable than a fashionable, rimless mounting because eyewear for Medicaid patients must typically last several years before it can be replaced. Since most frames are ordered to fill a patient's immediate needs, service in getting frames promptly when ordered is critical to patient satisfaction. If frames can be sent directly from the frame board to the laboratory, production time is decreased; likewise, service to the patient is increased. Patients do not understand back orders, whether for initial orders, parts, or replacement frames. Most frame manufacturers provide a warranty for frames, with the minimum period being 1 year. The manufacturer's policy should be understood before putting a new frame in the dispensary. Availability of frames must be satisfactory both for the initial dispensing and for any follow-up services related to the frames.

There is a difference in the way that frames are priced by manufacturers. It is necessary to monitor what is paid for frames on a total and a per-unit basis to maximize value to patients, maintain fees for materials at a competitive level, and still have the dispensary make a financial contribution to practice overhead and income.

Inventory Control of Frames

Demographics of the practice population will dictate the makeup of the frame inventory. To obtain demographic data, both the current or projected patient base and the market area must be analyzed. Statistics on age, sex, and income provide a guide for the frame styles and price ranges that should be stocked. Optometrists (or their ophthalmic assistants) commonly make the mistake of purchasing products they like instead of what demographics tell them. Laboratory or frame representatives can help practitioners better understand the preferences and practices of a given patient population or practice area. This information and the anticipated volume of frame sales should serve as guides to inventory control.

It is necessary to have a plan for inventory control. The plan might be to achieve the goal of an inventory that turns over four times a year, an accepted industry goal for a reasonable return on the investment made in this part of a practice. Therefore, if the practice dispenses or plans to dispense 1200 frames a year, ideally the inventory should be held at 300 frames. This number might be too low, however, to allow presentation of a satisfactory variety of styles to patients. It can be necessary to accept a three- or even two-times turnover rate until the patient load increases to reach this four-times turnover goal. Depending on where the practice is located, the competition from other ophthalmic providers, and the demographics of the practice, 400 to 700 frames might be necessary. Considering all of these factors, the inventory plan should establish the total number of frames that is appropriate for the practice.

Having established the inventory number, frames must further be divided by sex and age. If the total number of frames is to be 500 and 60% of the patients in the practice are female, 40% are male, and 15% require child-sized frames, frames should be stocked as follows: approximately 250 women's frames, 175 men's frames, and 75 children's frames. Approximately 60% of the frames should be in the "stable" category—frames that are basic to the market, have long-range stability, and consistent turnover. "Fads"—frames that are momentarily popular—should be monitored closely. These frames are often shown and recommended by frame representatives. They usually are demanded by some patients, but for an abbreviated period. Fad frames can prove not to be popular in a particular practice, and therefore it is wise to inquire about return policies before purchasing them. The dispensary should offer some frames for sports and avocational use. These frames help to meet the various ophthalmic needs of the patient population, which is the primary goal of having a dispensary in the office.

The selecting and purchasing of frames is often delegated to the person responsible for the fitting and dispensing of ophthalmic materials. Selecting and purchasing frames can be best performed when a plan is in place and the person assuming the responsibility understands the plan, the goals of the dispensary, and the need for inventory control.

Most offices need an inventory log book or computer file to record the name or number of the frame, vendor, style, colors, sizes, price, and date received of all frames in stock. A log can be maintained on a rotary file and kept on or near the styling table. It allows the dispenser to have frame information at hand and also to determine which frame styles and types are being used most frequently. Computer files also may be used to maintain a frame stock inventory, but there must be a commitment by all staff members handling frames to keep the information up-to-date. The use of bar codes on frames also is used in some practices. This system works best when frames are being directly dispensed from existing coded stock.

In the past, because the variety of frames, styles, and colors was often limited and the investment in frame "samples" was much less, many optometrists ordered all frames from the laboratory rather than using frames from inventory. Since changes in the "samples" were much less frequent, as these frames became shopworn they were disposed of, with the loss being considered just a cost of doing business. In today's market, which requires a large number and variety of frames in most offices, if the frame selected by the patient is the proper size and color, it is usually removed from the display and dispensed to the patient. Dispensing from stock not only eliminates the cost of worn-out samples but also allows for replacement with newer frames, thereby providing a better service to patients. In addition, there is never a delay in obtaining a frame in stock. When dispensing from stock, frames should be available to replace those being sold. This reserve of frames can be as little as 10% of the frame stock, if the plan is to alternate the frames being shown. Some offices will obtain more depth in stock, particularly in the "stable" category, to replace frames removed for sale. There can be a cost advantage to buying some of these "stable" frames in quantity. If there is an in-office laboratory, a larger frame stock also can be required (see Chapter 23).

To obtain an ongoing control of inventory, it is necessary to compare what has been purchased to what has been sold. This process requires periodic review of the records of frame orders and sales. A computer makes the task easier, but it will still be necessary to take the time to make the comparison and take corrective steps as needed. A yearly count of the frame inventory certainly tells whether the buying plan has been followed, but the inventory can be out of control if not checked more frequently. Plans to stock inventory are based on dispensing patterns, which can and should be reviewed at least annually. The primary goal for the dispensing function of a practice is to meet the ophthalmic needs and wants of patients. The frames bought for this purpose are a critical part of providing total eye care and eyewear for patients.

The following "purchasing tips" should be kept in mind when buying frames:
- Practitioners should work only with vendors who will work with them.

- Practitioners should buy what sells rather than what they like.
- Purchasers should stick to a buying plan rather than buy the plan of a sales representative.
- Although a buying plan should be consistent, it should be periodically reviewed to determine whether results (e.g., returns, cancelled orders) might require a revision.
- If revisions are required, an alternative plan should be devised, followed, and monitored.

Supplying ophthalmic frames and lenses to patients is an important part of the optometric service. The use of quality materials and efficient laboratory service will help satisfy patients' expectations. Careful pricing of materials will keep the practice competitive.

Quality Control

Standards for prescription dress eyewear have been promulgated by the American National Standards Institute (ANSI); impact resistance standards for dress lenses have been adopted by the U.S. Food and Drug Administration. Accepted lens tolerances can be found in ANSI Z 80.1–1999, the current version of the dress eyewear standards (Tables 22-1 through 22-4).

To ensure the quality of lenses being dispensed, in-office lens (and frame) inspection and verification must be performed. The most important considerations are lens power and centering. Attention also should be given to surface lens defects and the edge finish. Lenses at the tolerance limit should be rejected if they could cause a problem for the patient. Lenses beyond the tolerance limit should be routinely rejected. Procedures for the return of rejected lenses should be discussed with the laboratory, which should be willing to correct defects promptly. With the state-of-the-art, high-tech equipment most laboratories use to lay out and edge lenses, quality should

not be a problem. If it is, another laboratory should be considered.

Laboratory Service

Patients expect a reasonable delivery time on their eyewear. The time required for an individual order will depend on the efficiency of the laboratory fabricating the eyewear and the method of delivery to the office. Assuming the laboratory has a good lens blank inventory, all orders should be ready to deliver within 48 hours. Lenses requiring special treatment or a coating that cannot be provided by the laboratory are the exception.

Surveys of laboratories reveal that the most common methods of delivery are United Parcel Service, the U.S. mail, overnight express, and the laboratory's own delivery service. The best method for any one practice will depend on where the practice is located. Delivery of orders should be discussed with the laboratory representative, and the method providing the quickest and most consistent delivery time should be used. Alternative methods for "rush jobs" also should be explored. Considerable cost can be attached to the delivery of orders, and this cost will be passed on to the patient either directly or indirectly. This factor should be considered and discussed when meeting with a laboratory representative.

Availability of frames is an important measure of service to patients. The inability of a laboratory to provide frames on a timely basis can be measured by the number of "back orders" or the length of time needed to complete orders. Frame lines that cannot be obtained in a timely manner and laboratories that cannot deliver frames should be discontinued. Patients should not be shown the frames of suppliers who do not have a stock of frames adequate to service the account.

Table 22-1 ANSI Z 80.1-1999 Tolerances for Single-Vision and Multifocal Lenses*

MERIDIAN OF HIGHEST ABSOLUTE POWER	TOLERANCE ON EACH MERIDIAN (A)	TOLERANCE ON NOMINAL VALUE OF THE CYLINDER (B)		
		0.00 UP TO 2.00 D	>2.00 TO 4.50 D	>4.50 D
0.00 up to 6.50	±0.13 D	±0.13 D	±0.15 D	±4%
>6.50	±2%	±0.13 D	±0.15 D	±4%

Modified from American National Standards Institute: Prescription Ophthalmic Lenses—Recommendations, ANSI Z80.1-1999. *Available from the American National Standards Institute, 11 West 42nd Street, New York, NY 10036. Reprinted with permission.*
The distance refractive power imbalance between a pair of lenses in each meridian shall not exceed ⅔ of the sum of the tolerances for each lens for that meridian.

Table 22-2 ANSI Z 80.1-1999
Tolerances on the Direction
of Cylinder Axis

NOMINAL VALUE OF THE CYLINDER POWER	UP TO 0.37 D	>0.37 UP TO 0.75 D	>0.75 UP TO 1.50 D	>1.50 D
Tolerance of the axis	±7°	±5°	±3°	±2°

Modified from American National Standards Institute: Prescription Ophthalmic Lenses—Recommendations, ANSI Z80.1-1999. *Available from the American National Standards Institute, 11 West 42nd Street, New York, NY 10036. Reprinted with permission.*

Table 22-4 ANSI Z 80.1-1999
Tolerances on Prism
Reference Point Location
and Prismatic Power

VERTICAL PRISMATIC POWER (PRISM DIOPTERS)	TOLERANCE (PRISM DIOPTERS)
0.00 up to 3.375	±0.33
> or Over 3.375	1 mm difference

Modified from American National Standards Institute: Prescription Ophthalmic Lenses—Recommendations, ANSI Z80.1-1999. *Available from the American National Standards Institute, 11 West 42nd Street, New York, NY 10036. Reprinted with permission.*

Comparing Prices for Frames

Quality of materials and service from laboratories should be the most important factors in obtaining eyewear for patients. However, price also is a consideration. There is competition between quality laboratories, and there is often a difference in how they price their materials.

Basic lens charges among laboratories are easy to compare because laboratories publish price lists. Add-on costs for certain lens powers, special base curves, oversize blanks, specific lens centering, prism, tints, coatings, and similar considerations are harder to compare. When these additional charges are added to the order by the laboratory, they must be passed on to the patient. Thus, the practitioner must know how much these charges are and when they apply because they must be built into the fee schedule used for patients. If two or more laboratories provide services, the practitioner should compare the invoices for similar prescriptions and determine the most reasonable fee for the services.

It is standard practice for laboratories to award discounts to practitioners who pay their laboratory bills promptly. Many laboratories also offer different prices based on the volume of orders. These business practices encourage optometrists to use a single source for all laboratory work. These advantages always should be discussed and explored with laboratory sales representatives.

Use of discounting techniques can make a big difference in the pricing of ophthalmic materials and in the contribution of the sales of materials to practice income and profit. Ideally, an internal accounting system (e.g., computer program) should be able to identify profit and cost centers in the practice. Comparing the cost for materials in the practice to average costs for the profession is one method of evaluating fees for materials and laboratory bills. Surveys of laboratory costs usually report their findings by comparing the cost of materials to the practice gross income. Over the years, surveys of optometrists have shown that laboratory bills constitute 28% to 30% of gross income. If the cost of materials exceeds $35,000 for every $100,000 of gross income the practice produces, the material costs are too high or the fees for materials are too low (see Chapter 30 for a further discussion).

Understanding Laboratory Practices

Many laboratories have policy statements regarding the management of practitioner accounts. These policies should be reviewed with the laboratory representative. Some manufacturers will guarantee patient satisfaction—often in the form of warranties—to encourage

Table 22-3 ANSI Z 80.1-1999
Tolerance on Addition
Power for Multifocal and
Progressive Addition
Lenses

NOMINAL VALUE OF ADDITION POWER	UP TO 4.00	>4.00
Nominal value of the tolerance on the addition power	±0.12 D	±0.18 D

Modified from American National Standards Institute: Prescription Ophthalmic Lenses—Recommendations, ANSI Z80.1-1999. *Available from the American National Standards Institute, 11 West 42nd Street, New York, NY 10036. Reprinted with permission.*

the prescribing or dispensing of new products to patients. The laboratory is given the responsibility of ensuring that these policies are properly administered. Does the policy mean the laboratory will remake an order in another lens material at no charge? Will a credit be given to the account if the new lens material is more expensive? Will a voucher or certificate be issued by the manufacturer? Practitioners should understand laboratory policies before using any products being presented.

Laboratory policies vary on remake orders and doctor errors. Any remakes that are necessary because the ophthalmic materials do not satisfy ANSI tolerances should be performed on a no-charge basis. Some laboratories will charge 50% or less on the remake if an order is transmitted incorrectly by the practitioner. The same policy often is offered if it is necessary to modify an order after the spectacles have been dispensed to the patient because of doctor error. These policies should be clarified when a practitioner first establishes a working relationship with a laboratory. They can make a difference in satisfaction with the laboratory and also in the cost of doing business.

Placing Laboratory Orders

Transmission of orders in an expedient, accurate, and complete manner is a joint responsibility of the practitioner and the laboratory. Before the advent of toll-free telephone numbers and facsimile transmission and in the days of dependable mail service, laboratory orders were mailed at the end of the day. The use of mail was more likely if the optometrist was in a different city or state than the laboratory. Many laboratories still encourage the use of mail since written orders can be processed as they are received, when personnel are available. Mail delivery also reduces the expense of needing staff to take phone orders. The advantage of telephone orders is that they enable the laboratory to maintain personal contact with the optometrist or office staff while ensuring that all information to fabricate the eyewear will be received. In addition, laboratories with a computer inventory of frames can alert the caller to any possible delays in the order or can request that the frame be sent if it is not in stock.

Currently, the preferred method for communicating laboratory orders is by facsimile transmission and Internet access. Although the use of facsimile transmission saves staff time at both the office and the laboratory, it also requires that orders be complete and legible. Ordering by the Internet avoids legibility issues, and the transmission is virtually immediate.

There are times when UPS, U.S. mail, or an express service might be required for an order–for instance, when using a laboratory that does not supply frames or when using a large number of frames from other vendors. In these instances, the most expedient way to get the order completed is to send the frame, from stock, to the laboratory. Ordering the frame from another vendor and having it sent directly to the laboratory also might be necessary. If the frame received is the incorrect color or size, the error cannot be recognized by the fabricating laboratory. A practitioner must inspect and verify orders before the eyewear is dispensed to patients, however, and the in-office inspection by the staff should detect the error before the eyewear is dispensed to the patient.

Conclusion

The dispensing of eyewear has been the basis of optometry's unified service to the public. Although there are many challenges in carrying out this important professional function, the selection and use of efficient laboratories and ophthalmic suppliers will contribute greatly to making this a satisfying part of practice.

Acknowledgement

The author of this chapter in the first edition of *Business Aspects of Optometry* was Donald H. Lakin.

Bibliography

Allergan, Inc: *Pathways in optometry*. Irvine, Calif, 1990, Author.

American Optometric Association: *Caring for the eyes of America–a profile of the optometric profession*. St. Louis, 1992, Author.

Anonymous: Eight ways to improve your spectacle dispensing. *Rev Optom* 138(10):18-9, 1994.

Anonymous: Ophthalmic suppliers and sources directory: optical laboratory supplies. *Rev Optom* 31(3):115-9, 1994.

Aron F, Bennett I: The 1990s, a decade for ophthalmic lenses: results of AOA surveys of laboratories and practitioners. *Optom Economics* 2(10):17-21, 1992.

Bargman B, Yoho A: Get more out of your optical lab. *Optom Management* 28(5):33-6, 1993.

Bennett I: Pricing ophthalmic frames. *Optom Management* 23(11):101-3, 1988.

Bennett I: *Management for the eyecare practitioner*. Stoneham, Mass, 1993, Butterworth.

Bierstock SR: Inventory control for the optical dispensary. *Ocular Surg News* 12(6):23, 1994.

Brassfield A: We tamed the frame game. *Optom Management* 29(9):83-6, 1994.

Brogan R: After the implementation: increased patient returns and a higher level of quality dispensings. *Optician* 205(5399):19-20, 1993.

Bruneni JL: Dispensing new frame materials. *Optom Economics* 3(9):10-5, 1993.

Carlson AS: The importance of good dispensing in the modern optometric practice. *S Afr Optom* 52(3):15, 1993.

Edlow R, Aron F: Labs, frames, buying groups: results of three AOA practice characteristics surveys. *Optom Economics* 1(3):33-5, 1991.

Fanelli J: How to stock your primary care practice. *Rev Optom* 126(2):73-6, 1989.

Gailmard NB: Consultant's corner: make your patients start seeing double. Imaging system helps patients decide on frames. *Rev Optom* 131(9):27, 1994.

Gottlieb H: Finding lost profits in ophthalmology: medical eyewear dispensing requires service-oriented mindsets. *Ocular Surg News* 12(10):18, 1994.

Gregg CP: The optical laboratory: state of the art today. *Eyecare Tech* (Suppl) 3(1):42-4, 1993.

Kirkner R: Frames market outlook: time to pay the piper— get ready for higher prices and standardized bar coding. *Rev Optom* 129(9):59-65, 1992.

Lee J: How to avoid the "7 deadly sins" of dispensing. *Optom Management* 29(6):44-6, 1994.

Maul JR: Getting control of your frames. *Optom Economics* 1(5):22-3, 1991.

Outcault RF, Johnson PM: Setting up to sell: is your dispensary merchandising keeping pace with the demands of today's patients? *Optom Economics* 4(9):27-8, 1994.

Schwartz CA: Minimize inventory and maximize return: put stock where it's needed, when it's needed. *Rev Optom* 129(9):51-4, 1992.

www.optometric.com. Online version of *Optometric Management* magazine, which offers information about ophthalmic materials.

www.revoptom.com. Online version of *Review of Optometry* magazine, which offers information about ophthalmic materials.

Chapter 23

In-House Laboratories

Craig Bowen

Don't be penny wise and pound foolish.
Benjamin Franklin *Poor Richard's Almanac*

At the time Benjamin Franklin wrote the often-quoted words stated above, the predecessors of modern optometrists were laboring in optical shops. In these shops, run by opticians, the need for vision testing became apparent, and during the 19th Century the "refracting" optician emerged. When, at the end of the 19th Century, these individuals sought legal recognition as an independent profession, they separated themselves from "dispensing" opticians. Through the years, a guiding principle of clinical optometry has been that the practitioner who performs the examination is the best individual to determine the suitability of the eyewear prescribed. For this reason, the fabrication of eyewear has been a consistent part of optometric practice. Even though optometry has continued to evolve into a primary eye care profession, the fabrication and dispensing of ophthalmic materials have remained important parts of an optometrist's service to the public.

Surveys of practice patterns conducted during the 1980s and 1990s indicated that optometrists were increasing fabrication and dispensing services so that they could provide the quickly produced, cost-efficient, high-quality eyewear demanded by today's consumers. An essential part of the effort to provide these services is to establish an in-office finishing laboratory. The 2001 American Optometric Association Scope of Practice Survey revealed the following:

- About 50% of practitioners edge their own lenses
- Almost 60% tint lenses themselves
- Nearly 50% provide coatings (e.g., ultraviolet, scratch-resistant)

It seems likely that these numbers will only increase in succeeding years.

There are several considerations regarding patient care, equipment needs and costs, staffing, lens inventory maintenance, space requirements, and liability issues that influence the use of in-house laboratories. Perhaps the most important consideration, however, is the improved service that can be offered to patients. Optometrists who would require several days to deliver eyewear to patients can reduce the period to 1 to 2 days, or even a matter of hours if necessary. The "one-hour" service promoted by large chains and optical corporations is not demanded by most patients. In fact, patients often are skeptical of immediate service and worry that the quality will be inferior to eyewear that requires more time to fabricate. Optometrists in private practice can assure patients of quality service, and they also can control the timing of orders. If there is a need for a particular order to be completed rapidly, it can be given precedence. Patients are particularly grateful for timely service during emergencies. This capacity can assist greatly in the effort to maintain a patient's loyalty to the practitioner.

There also is marketing potential in having an in-house laboratory. Even without promotion, most patients perceive an in-office laboratory as being an asset. Patients assume that the practitioner has become more up-to-date and that a more efficient service will be provided. Optometrists who have in-house laboratories might find that the quality of ophthalmic materials is more consistent than when materials are obtained from outside laboratories. Certainly, the level of responsibility for eyewear increases when there is an in-house laboratory. The same strict tolerances for lens powers, lens centering, and finishing work must be provided by the in-house laboratory as would be expected if the work were done independently. That means there will be a "spoilage rate" as part of the cost of doing business. In well-run laboratories, this rate should be no more than 2% to 4%. To maintain a low rate, there must be a commitment by the individuals performing the laboratory work to the delivery of high-quality materials. If work is produced that does not meet accepted tolerances, however, it must be rejected and remade (see Chapter 22). In fact, this work is more rapidly performed and better controlled if it is performed in-house; reinspection and dispensing can more likely be provided within the time frame expected by the patient than if an outside laboratory has to remake, reinspect, and redeliver the order.

Cost also is a factor in deciding to install an in-office laboratory. The escalating fabrication cost for eyewear obtained from outside laboratories is cited by many optometrists as a key reason for establishing an in-house laboratory. When using outside laboratories for all fabrication work, the cost of ophthalmic materials averages 28% to 30% of gross income. This expenditure is obviously sizable, but is the effort to reduce laboratory costs "penny wise and pound foolish"? The costs of maintenance for machinery and of ophthalmic materials can cut—or even eliminate—profits, especially in practices with low lens volumes. The number of lenses that will be finished in-house is an important factor in determining whether a laboratory will be worth the financial commitment. Careful recordkeeping will be necessary to determine whether profit is being realized. Sound financial management demands that the optometrist determine the costs of operating a laboratory and make an effort to control those costs. There will be capital outlay for equipment, expenses related to maintenance, costs related to the purchase of materials, additional expenditures for utilities (e.g., electricity, water), and wages to be paid for labor.

Even after taking into account all the aforementioned factors, many optometrists have found the operation of an in-house laboratory to be highly successful, although profitability is directly tied to the number of lenses finished per week. For example, in practices that finish 40 to 60 pairs of lenses per week, optometrists report savings of $6 to $8 per pair on stock single vision lenses and $10 to $12 per pair on bifocals. These savings also can make the optometrist more competitive in terms of the prices for ophthalmic materials.

Labor costs will affect economic projections considerably. In practices with a low volume of orders, it might be appropriate to use the "unfilled" time of office staff for the finishing work or to have the optometrist perform it rather than to hire another employee. Optometrists just beginning a practice will most likely not have the patient volume to justify setting up an in-house laboratory. As the practice becomes established, however, the viability of a laboratory becomes more certain. In fact, there are cases in which optometrists in young practices have found that working in their own laboratories contributed to availability, service, and cost containment more than working for other practitioners outside the office one or two days a week.

In a multipractitioner office, an in-house laboratory can be quite successful. The per-unit cost can be competitive, not only with the costs of outside laboratories but also with those of buying cooperatives composed of groups of optometrists. A full-time employee—often an optician—will probably be necessary because of the volume of orders. Overhead costs should be computed so that the "break even" volume can be determined. For example, it can be calculated that 300 pairs of lenses must be finished per month to break even. All orders greater than that figure represent profit. The effect of a financially successful in-house laboratory will be to lower the cost of ophthalmic materials to less than the 28% to 30% of gross income that is typical for most practices; in fact, material costs can drop considerably less than 30% when volume is high. Optometrists successfully using in-house laboratories routinely report savings of up to 25% to 35% of laboratory costs. The availability of these laboratory services, when combined with a quality product, will inevitably contribute to practice growth.

The usual interest is in finishing laboratories, but with the newer available equipment that allows a practitioner to control the entire service, the surfacing function of lens fabrication has been added to some in-office laboratories. The use of surfacing equipment requires a higher volume to break even or generate a profit for the practice.

Equipment Need and Costs

There is considerable variance in the cost of equipment needed to set up a finishing laboratory (Figure 23-1). Costs will depend on the functions to be performed—edging, tinting, coating, or all three—and whether new or used equipment is purchased (Figure 23-2). A practitioner must consider whether it is wise to spend the money required to purchase modern high-tech equipment. At optical shows for optometrists, at least one out of eight exhibitors will display new optical laboratory equipment. Patternless edgers can be purchased with computer memory and different types of finish; such an item can be the centerpiece of a laboratory. Much of this equipment does not require the skills of a

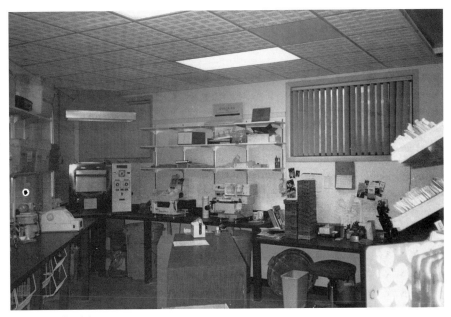

Figure 23-1 View of an in-office laboratory.

trained laboratory optician to operate and can be a good investment. Surveys of optometrists with in-house laboratories indicate that the cost of finishing laboratory–equipment ranges between $7000 and $20,000. A list of basic equipment needed to start a finishing laboratory and a brief description of the function of each piece of equipment can be found in Box 23-1.

With more than 80% of the ophthalmic lenses sold today being made of plastic (including polycarbonate), many practitioners choose not to fabricate glass lens orders and thus do not invest in chemical treating units. Box 23-1 does not include a heat treatment or chemical hardening unit. If a practitioner decides to include glass lenses, a chemical treating unit should be

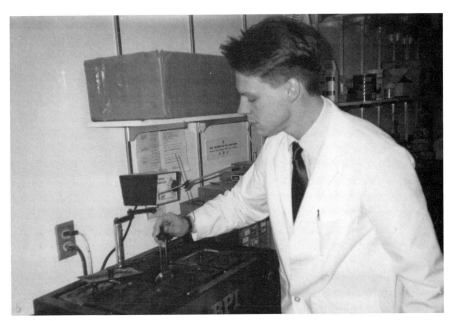

Figure 23-2 Lens-tinting device.

Box 23-1 Basic Equipment For an In-House Finishing Laboratory

Edger: Cuts the unfinished lens to the shape of the frame. An extra set of diamond wheels is suggested, for use when the regular wheels must be sharpened. Many edgers are available that dry edge CR-39 and polycarbonate lenses with all types of finishes—groove, facet, bevel—in about 40 seconds.

Lens groover: Used for nylon suspension frames.

Layout marker: Marks the optical center of the lens.

Layout blockers: Holds the lens in place during layout marking.

Blocker: Holds the lens in place during edging or grooving.

Frame warmer: Available with many different types of heat conductors; some also have coolers.

Lensmeter: Internal-reading models and projection-type models are available.

Lensclock: Measures the base curves of the lens.

Dying tank/tinting unit: For tinting lenses.

Coating machine (open): For special lens coatings.

Drop ball testing apparatus: To verify impact resistance.

---

considered. A realistic projection of the number of glass lenses that will be fabricated should be undertaken before investing in this equipment.

The cost of a surfacing laboratory also is dependent on the range of equipment purchased. Most optometrists put this cost at between $40,000 and $80,000. A surfacing generator, two-cylinder machines, computer, and layout blocker make up the largest part of this investment. When put into operation, the surfacing laboratory will realize savings of up to 70%, as compared with outside laboratory costs for bifocal, progressive, polarized, and high-index lenses. To break even, approximately 25 to 30 pairs of lenses must be surfaced each day. There are a number of injection mold systems for plastic lenses on the market. The same thing also can be said of wafer systems. The optometrist considering these two methods should explore the equipment currently on the market, and before making a purchase, visit the offices of optometrists who already are using the equipment.

As of 2000, approximately 9% of optometrists performed lens surfacing themselves (Figure 23-3). About 75% of these practitioners did the work in the office; the other 25% sent the work to a separate facility.

Nearly half of all optometrists offered lens coating services. Of these practitioners, a little more than half did the work in-office, and the remainder sent the work to a separate facility that they own.

No matter what equipment is purchased, if something goes wrong with it, a service representative should be available right away. The ability to troubleshoot and operate equipment is usually acquired with experience. Optometrists who are novices at working with laboratory equipment should probably purchase it new. Often, when new equipment is delivered, it is set up by the seller, who also will provide instruction to the practitioner and the staff.

Laboratory Staff

The first step in human resource management is to have a plan. In Chapters 21 and 25 the economic aspects of quantifying the personnel needs of a practice are discussed. If an in-house laboratory is to be a service and profit center for the practice, economic planning is critical. A full-time employee might not be necessary for this service. The employee's status is usually dependent on the size of the laboratory. When beginning a laboratory, if a technician or optician currently employed by the practice has the necessary technical background or is interested in running a laboratory, this individual can be assigned part-time laboratory duties. This person should possess good organizational skills and be able to run the laboratory as an assembly line, keeping several jobs in progress at one time. This person also should be orderly and efficient and take as much pride in the work produced as the practitioner. The time devoted to laboratory functions should be charged to optical supplies to run the laboratory as a separate profit center. The time charged to optical supplies should be equal to the time actually spent on laboratory work. It is best to have the laboratory person be responsible for ordering uncut lenses and maintaining stock lenses (Figure 23-4).

In some practices, workers from other offices or optical laboratories can be chosen to "moonlight" when the laboratory is first started. If the optometrist does not have the time or background to train a staff member, an experienced optician can serve as a teacher for a staff member who wants to learn laboratory work. Equipment manufacturers and distributors usually offer optometrists an in-office training program for the staff. Training can include instruction on how to use the equipment and pertinent nomenclature. Knowledge of parts facilitates repair—especially when that repair must be performed via telephone—because the

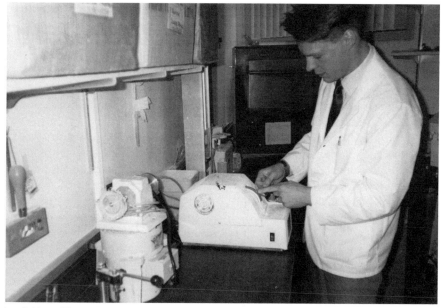

Figure 23-3 Hand-polishing of lens edges.

technician can precisely describe the part or function that requires repair.

If there is enough work to keep an employee busy full time and the practitioner is fortunate enough to hire a trained laboratory optician, it might be necessary to orient this person to the private practice environment. Most successful optical laboratories are very production oriented. Although skilled and efficient, a laboratory optician might have a factory attitude toward work. It is hoped that a practice will be service oriented; desired work patterns and practice goals should be discussed at the time of hiring.

Finding trained laboratory technicians can be a problem, especially in smaller communities. Some larger cities will have optical laboratory technician programs that are taught in trade schools. These

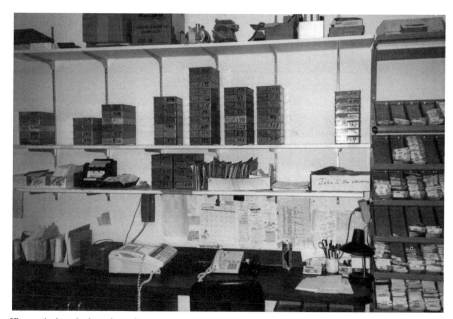

Figure 23-4 In-office ordering desk and stock area.

schools are good sources for employees. Often, individuals working in large laboratories want to move into a clinical environment. An in-house laboratory will provide an opportunity to make this move, and an offer for the individual to participate in dispensing can prove to be an additional inducement. A "help wanted" advertisement or an advertisement offering to train a qualified applicant will often bring additional individuals into the applicant pool. The ophthalmic industry is a relatively small community, and a conversation with local optometrists, frame sales representatives, or employees of the practice can result in the recommendation of qualified individuals.

Lens Inventory

To intelligently develop a plan for lens inventory, it is necessary to know what materials will be prescribed and the relative frequency with which they will be used. Many in-house laboratories limit inventory to plastic and polycarbonate lenses because glass lenses must be hardened to impart impact resistance to the lenses. Lenses purchased for stock can be bought in quantity at a lower price than on a per-lens basis. Usually an optical supply house will offer the best price on quantities of 75 pairs or more. When the initial order is made, and continuous re-ordering for stock is anticipated, the practitioner can usually negotiate with the seller to obtain the same per-unit price on reorders for stock or for lenses out of the stock range. As stock is taken from inventory, lens envelopes should be used to place reorders, which can be daily, or at least weekly, based on volume. Practitioners in metropolitan areas may consider ordering all lens blanks from a local laboratory. Delivery of stock can be assured on the same day it is ordered in many cases. This has the advantage of saving the cost of inventory management and the expense of the tax burden on property in some states.

Most in-office laboratories start with two pairs of lenses for each parameter stocked. In plastic, stock should be maintained up to plus or minus 3 diopters for spherical lenses and up to 2 diopters for cylindrical lenses. If scratch-resistant coatings are frequently used in the practice, coated blanks should be considered because they are the least expensive method to offer coated lenses. Pricing should be investigated for various size lens blanks. Because the minimum thickness of minus lenses is in the center, using larger blanks than needed will not affect the quality of the work. With plus lenses, larger blanks will affect quality because smaller lenses are needed for smaller eye sizes. Depending on the number of lenses that will be needed and the variables chosen, the cost of a plastic lens inventory can vary somewhat from practitioner to practitioner.

If polycarbonate and high-index plastic lenses are not used frequently, they should be ordered on a per-case basis. Because of safety considerations, many practitioners routinely prescribe polycarbonate lenses for all children, monocular patients, active adults, and patients who need them for athletic use. If polycarbonate materials are frequently prescribed, they should be stocked in the same manner as other plastic lenses. Polycarbonate and other high-index materials used for high prescriptions are usually ordered on a per-case basis since they are often beyond stock range and need to be surfaced. Because of the higher unit cost of polycarbonate lenses, a polycarbonate lens stock will require a slightly higher investment.

If a practitioner decides to fabricate glass lenses, stock should include spherical lenses up to plus and minus 2 diopters and up to 2 diopters of cylinder for each power. All compound multifocals are surfaced lenses. Stock multifocal spherical lenses usually are available in plus powers only. Most in-house laboratories do not stock these lenses. Practitioners must know the ranges stocked by optical supply houses and use them when patients require this type of lens. Stock multifocal spherical lenses usually are less expensive than are surfaced bifocal blanks. When buying uncut surfaced lens blanks in multifocals or single-vision lenses beyond stock ranges, laboratory representatives should be asked for their volume uncut price list. Many full-service laboratories have a small differential in price between uncut blanks and complete prescriptions to maintain the same profit margin on both. Laboratories with greater surfacing capabilities and an awareness of the market niche of in-house fabricating practices are considerably more competitive in pricing uncut lens blanks.

These considerations should be explored and the practice volume should be realistically evaluated before investing in a lens surfacing operation. If another practice has invested in a surfacing or lens molding system and has a surfacing capacity beyond its needs, this situation also could be a good source to explore.

Space Requirements

The location of the laboratory and its space requirements will vary considerably, depending on volume and how fabrication is perceived as part of the optometric product. Ideally, the laboratory should occupy a separate room, at least 10 × 10 feet, with adequate ventilation (for chemicals). The laboratory will require several countertop electrical outlets, and these outlets should be on two or three different circuit breakers to prevent the blowing of fuses. Since a finishing laboratory tends to be noisy, it should be located as far from the examination rooms as possible.

For a busy practice with a full-time employee performing both glass and plastic lens finishing and a second employee performing the ordering, there should be at least 400 square feet of space. If lens surfacing is included, 1000 square feet will be needed. In computing the cost of materials sold, the expense of this space (and maintaining it) must be considered.

When planning an office that includes a laboratory, these location and space requirements should be discussed with the designer. Some practitioners might plan the location of the laboratory adjacent to the frame room, with a window that allows patients to look into the laboratory; this emphasizes the image of a "complete" eye care facility. In such cases, the laboratory can even be located in the front of the office and enclosed with a soundproof glass window so that, on entering the facility, patients can see that eyewear fabrication is part of the service. Other practitioners might want the laboratory placed out of sight in the back of the facility to maintain a more "professional" image. This function of optometric practice often polarizes practitioners who want optometry to be accepted as a primary eye care profession while continuing to meet the needs of patients for quality eyewear. Only a realistic assessment of the marketplace will lead to the appropriate decision for any one practice.

Liability Issues

The advantages of having an in-house laboratory are affected by the added legal responsibility of fabricating lenses that are sold directly to patients. From a liability standpoint, the most important consideration is impact resistance.

Federal regulations regarding impact resistance—which have been incorporated into American National Standards Institute standard Z80.1–1999–state that all dress lenses shall be capable of withstanding a drop ball test. The standard provides, however, that plastic, laminated, and raised edge multifocal lenses can be tested in statistically significant samples by the manufacturer. Therefore, only glass lenses have to be tested individually for impact resistance by the fabricator of the eyewear.

If prescription safety eyewear is provided, a different set of requirements must be met. The requirements for safety lenses—which are described in ANSI standard Z87.1–1998–require a drop ball test; a minimum lens thickness (3 mm); and the use of a logo, which must be placed on the lens edge by the lens fabricator. Safety lenses must be placed in a safety frame (identified by the Z87 logo) to constitute "safety glasses."

All optometrists should have adequate professional liability insurance. Practitioners who dispense eyewear should have coverage for both negligence and product liability claims. Because assistants or opticians are commonly involved with the fabrication and dispensing of ophthalmic materials, the policy should cover claims arising out of their actions (see Chapter 11). Coverage also should provide for instances in which these employees are injured (e.g., from accidents occurring during the fabrication or dyeing of eyewear). Worker's compensation coverage may be available, depending on the size of the practice. All optometrists who fabricate materials in the office should be sure that liability insurance covers these eventualities. The best way to check insurance coverage is to review the policy with an insurance agent and to have the agent identify the specific language that provides coverage.

Liability claims involving the fabrication of eyewear are not common because optometrists are required to inspect eyewear to ensure that it meets legal standards for impact resistance. Optometrists who establish in-house laboratories should make certain that these obligations are met before eyewear is dispensed.

Acknowledgement

The author of this chapter in the first edition of *Business Aspects of Optometry* was Donald H. Lakin.

Bibliography

American Optometric Association: *Caring for the eyes of America—a profile of the optometric profession.* St. Louis, 2002, Author.

Anonymous: Practice management, retail and lab software. *Eyecare Tech* 3(2):17-9,22-5,34, 1993.

Aron F, Bennett I: The 1990s, a decade for ophthalmic lenses: results of AOA surveys of laboratories and practitioners. *Optom Economics* 2(10):17-21, 1992.

Barnett D: The building blocks of an in-office lens lab. *Rev Optom* 129(10):37-40, 1992.

Bostick D: Surfacing solo: making a lab work for you. *Optom Management* 25(4):59-62, 1990.

Bulmlein S: Introducing in-practice prescription laboratories. *Optician* 201(5300):18-21, 1991.

Hunter MA: Profile of Greames Optical: full comprehensive prescription laboratory. *Optom Today* (Britain) 33(19):22, 1993.

Kloos SA: Running your own in-office lab, ups and downs. *Optom Management* 24(5):57-60, 1989.

Legerton JA: In-office laboratories: control or chaos? *Optom Economics* 3(10):24-8, 1993.

Maino JH: Moving the in-house lab into the 21st century. *Computers in Eyecare* 2(3):51-4, 1992.

Ossip G: Should you start a finishing lab? *Optom Management* 28(10):32-4, 1993.

Rusynko T: Don't lose your edge with an on-site lab—they're not for everyone. *Rev Optom* 130(9):45-8, 1993.

Underwood WB: Setting up your own in-office lab: what you should know. *Eyecare Tech* 4(1):63-4, 1994.

www.optometric.com. Online version of *Optometric Management* magazine, which offers information about ophthalmic materials.

www. revoptom.com. online version of *Review of Optometry* magazine, which offers information about ophthalmic materials.

Section Five

Practice Administration

Chapter 24

Organizing an Office

Craig Hisaka, John G. Classé, and C. Thomas Crooks III

Good order is the foundation of all good things.
Edmund Burke *Reflections on the Revolution in France*

In the past, it was possible for practitioners to completely ignore the business operation of a practice and concentrate on serving patients, yet still earn a comfortable income. Today—with the soaring cost of operating an optometric practice, the decrease in third-party reimbursement rates, a competitive marketplace, the expanding scope of optometric care, and the influence of managed-care organizations on health care services—neglect of business issues will result in an inefficient practice. This lack of efficiency will require the practitioner to work longer hours to meet expenses and will cause an erosion of the quality of care.

There are two components of an optometric practice: a professional component and a business component. The *professional component* involves the practitioner's efforts at providing quality care to patients. The optometrist is trained to provide care; thus, a practitioner spends most of the day in this area. To provide quality care, the practitioner invests time and money to improve technical skills and purchases modern instrumentation to improve accuracy and efficiency of testing. The *business component* involves the administration of the practice. Even though the optometrist might not be trained in this area, it should be given as much time, effort, and energy as the professional component. The skills and personality needed to be an effective manager and administrator are different from the skills required to be an effective health care practitioner. Maximizing the efficiency of the business component of a practice will result in an environment in which the practitioner will be able to provide the best quality of care for patients. If a practice is not efficient, organized, and properly managed, the quality of care eventually will be compromised. In any community, the most successful practitioners are those who provide a high quality of care due to the acceptance and integration of successful business concepts into the practice.

The purpose of this chapter is to provide basic guidelines for organizing a private practice. Ideally, if a practitioner spends 40 hours seeing patients, the practitioner should spend the same amount of time—40 hours—in office administration. However, the reality is that most practice time will be allocated to patient care. Despite the burdens of these professional duties, there are some essential administrative tasks that must be performed. If the practice is new, there are a number of responsibilities that the practitioner faces in just preparing the practice to open for business.

Getting Started

When beginning a private practice, it is essential that the practitioner obtain a support network of advisors. Professional consultants can provide valuable advice, and good business strategies are as important to the stability of a practice as are satisfied patients. The practitioner should establish relationships with a banker, attorney, accountant, and insurance agent. These relationships are essential to the organization of a practice. A banker is needed because loans and business and personal checking accounts need to be obtained at a full-service bank. An attorney can be consulted for advice and assistance related to the type of business organization being formed (i.e., sole proprietorship, partnership, limited liability company, professional association or corporation, S corporation) and the legal steps required to begin the business (see Chapters 6 through 8). An accountant is needed to provide advice and assistance about the withholding and paying of taxes. An insurance agent should be consulted to obtain office contents, disability, office overhead, life, and premises liability insurance; malpractice coverage; or any other insurance coverage needed for the protection of health, home, and personal property (see Chapters 9 through 12).

One of the most valuable means of evaluating a potential advisor is simply asking other professionals about the advisor's reputation. If other health care providers have found the advisor's services to be helpful and reasonable, it is a good sign. A meeting should be scheduled to discuss how the advisor can be helpful and the cost of the advisor's assistance. At this meeting it is appropriate to inquire about the advisor's years of experience and how the advisor keeps up-to-date with current trends, legislation, and client needs.

A key task for the beginning practitioner is the formation of an office staff. To identify potential staff members, advertisements or other means of contacting qualified applicants should be used. The standard process of interviewing and evaluating of candidates should be followed (see Chapter 21).

Another important task is to contact representatives of optical laboratory and frame and contact lens manufacturers. A frame and contact lens inventory must be assembled, and accounts must be opened at the optical laboratories with which the practice will be doing business (see Chapter 22). In addition, inventories of supplies—such as ophthalmic drugs and solutions, stationery, business cards, appointment reminder cards, recall notices, magazine subscriptions, prescription pads, examination forms, and record folders—should be ordered. Fee schedules also need to be set (see Chapter 34).

The practitioner must enroll as a provider in third-party health care plans such as Medicare, Medicaid, Vision Service Plan, and medical insurance (e.g., Blue Cross/Blue Shield). Although Medicare and Medicaid are federal programs, enrollment is performed at the state level, through bureaucracies that administer these programs. If there are health maintenance organizations or other types of managed care panels in which the practitioner wishes to participate, enrollment must be solicited (see Chapters 36 and 37). It usually requires several weeks for the enrollment process to be completed, and ample time should be allocated.

If the practitioner is not already a member of the state optometric association, an application should be obtained and submitted.

Telephone service should be initiated (deadlines for inclusion in the annual directory need to be ascertained), and accounts with utility companies (electricity, gas, water) should be opened. Answering and paging services should be contacted, and janitorial services need to be obtained.

The visibility of the practice is important in attracting patients. Signs for the office, announcements of the opening in the newspaper, Yellow Pages listings, and other means of putting the public on notice should be secured.

These are but a few of the many tasks that await the new practitioner. A checklist should be devised so that omissions are kept to a minimum (Box 24-1).

Patient Management

Efficient patient management requires a coordinated effort from both practitioner and staff, combined with well-rehearsed patient flow, effective communication, scrupulous bookkeeping, and conscientious attention to detail. To provide orderly management, the practitioner must organize the facility, staff, and paperwork. Staff members must be instructed about how the system is to be run. Ongoing evaluation is an integral part of an efficient office; regular meetings between practitioner and staff to identify and eliminate deficiencies are necessary. Coordination of effort can be achieved with adequate planning and experience, but cohesion between practitioner and staff requires a different form of interaction: trust. The staff must trust the practitioner to establish a workable plan, and the practitioner must trust the staff to carry it out. The trust between practitioner and staff must be mutual; if it is not, it will be apparent to patients that such is the case. Patients seek a satisfying relationship with both practitioner and staff. This requires that they be treated with respect, be rendered competent service, and be given individual attention. When these objectives are achieved, trust is the result. Trust is the cornerstone of patient loyalty, and it is an inevitable ally of efficient management.

The four cornerstones of effective patient management are availability, efficient patient flow, communication, and troubleshooting.

Availability

Inefficient appointment schedules have long been a problem for optometrists. The availability of the practitioner is based on the policy decisions adopted by the practice:

- What days will the office be open?
- What will be the office hours?
- How much time will be allocated for each appointment?

Box 24-1 Timetable of Things to Do When Starting a Private Practice

1 Year Before Starting a Practice

Obtain demographic and health resource data on the chosen practice location from books, guides, and the local Chamber of Commerce.

Visit the community to discuss the need for optometric services (optometrists, dentists, physicians, pharmacists, bankers, teachers, school nurses, real estate agents).

Talk with representatives from ophthalmic laboratories about opening a practice in the community.

Make site visits to determine the practice location. If possible, make a final decision on the practice location.

Contact the state board of optometry about the requirements for licensure. Obtain a copy of the state optometry laws.

Check on membership in local, state, and national professional societies.

Determine the date that information must be submitted to be included in the white and Yellow Pages telephone directories. If possible, reserve an office telephone number.

Visit banks to meet bank officers. Obtain a loan application from the loan officer and determine the information and format needed to submit a proposal to obtain practice financing.

At the bank selected, open personal and business checking accounts.

Prepare a loan proposal to obtain the necessary capital for equipment and operation of the practice. Submit the application within the appropriate deadline.

9 Months Before Starting a Practice

Check the office site and determine whether leasehold improvements will be needed. Obtain necessary estimates for the improvements.

Check with the local city hall or zoning board to determine the requirements of zoning ordinances that apply to the site chosen.

Determine office layout and design.

Determine office and professional equipment that will be needed.

Select professional advisors (accountant, attorney, banker, insurance agent, real estate agent).

Obtain bids on the purchase of office and professional equipment. Compare leasing versus purchasing.

6 Months Before Starting a Practice

Obtain the services of an answering service (physician's exchange, beeper service, call forwarding).

Meet or talk with representatives of Medicare, Medicaid, and other third-party insurance carriers. Obtain provider numbers, prevailing fee schedule (Medicare), insurance claim forms, and copies of procedure codes (CPD-4) and diagnostic codes (ICD-9).

Obtain application for hospital privileges.

Order office record system.

Plan and order an accounts receivable or payable system.

Plan and order payroll accounting system.

Order sign for office.

Notify frame, contact lens, and pharmaceutical representatives of the practice.

Obtain county and city occupational licenses (from the county or city clerk or city hall).

3 Months Before Starting a Practice

Obtain professional liability insurance coverage.

Obtain office insurance (office overhead coverage, office liability, business interruption, employee fidelity bond, office contents). Umbrella coverage provides comprehensive catastrophic coverage for liability claims that are beyond the limits of regular insurance.

Determine whether worker's compensation is required by state law by consulting with the state worker's compensation board or industrial commission.

Obtain health and accident insurance coverage for yourself and employees.

Obtain disability insurance coverage.

Obtain life insurance coverage.

Obtain automobile insurance coverage.

Arrange for telephone service and installation. Determine the telephone equipment and system to be purchased.

Continued

Box 24-1 Timetable of Things to Do When Starting a Private Practice—continued

3 Months Before Starting a Practice—cont'd

Order office opening announcements. Discuss the placement of advertisements in local newspapers.

Meet with local physicians who are potential referral sources. Send follow-up letters.

If there is a local referral service through the optometric society, provide the information needed to be listed.

Check on membership in local civic and religious organizations and join as appropriate.

Arrange for movers, if necessary.

Write preliminary job descriptions for employees. Obtain a sample office procedures manual.

Begin the effort to locate employees for the office (advertising, interviewing).

Apply for a federal employer identification number from the Internal Revenue Service (form SS-4).

Apply for a state employer identification number through the state employment office or Department of Labor.

Obtain the *Small Business Tax Guide* (publication 334) and *Your Federal Income Tax Guide* (publication 17) from the Internal Revenue Service. Obtain the appropriate tax forms from the IRS and the state employment office or Department of Labor.

Obtain payroll withholding booklets for federal, state, and local taxes from the IRS.

Review tax withholding and reporting requirements with an accountant or tax attorney.

Choose and order an appointment scheduling book or system.

Arrange for appropriate office support services as needed (janitorial, snow removal, laundry service, lawn care).

Order clinical supplies and set up an inventory control system.

Order necessary business supplies (appointment cards, business cards, letterhead stationery and envelopes, patient recall notices, petty cash vouchers, deposit stamps for checks, prescription pads, purchase orders, preprinted telephone message pads).

If desired, meet with collections attorneys or agencies about the collection of unpaid accounts.

Determine fee schedule.

Select and order magazines for the reception area. Also select and order professional journals.

Purchase office equipment and furniture and arrange for their delivery to the office.

Arrange for laboratory services at optical laboratories.

Notify area pharmacies that you are starting a practice.

Select any patient information materials and have them printed or delivered.

Obtain a postage meter and a bulk mail permit, if necessary.

1 Month Before Starting a Practice

Start setting up the office.

If necessary, have the utilities turned on.

If not previously arranged, have signage displayed.

Hire and begin training office personnel, with emphasis on telephone techniques, appointments, collections procedures, office policies.

Begin making appointments.

Establish a petty cash fund.

Have announcements of the office opening published in the local news media.

Mail out announcements of the opening to local physicians, pharmacists, health groups, school nurses, and others as appropriate.

Hold an "open house."

Begin seeing patients.

Modified from Park DL: Optimum timetable for starting your practice. Uriah, Calif, 1990.

• How will the practitioner's absences be managed?
• How will emergencies or "walk-ins" be served?

These are decisions that must be made at the outset of a new practice. Modifications can be incorporated into the schedule as time permits.

Office Hours

Determining the days and hours available for patient examination depends on several factors: the cost of staff and office overhead, the needs of the patient population being served, the quality of life the practitioner wishes to enjoy, and similar considerations. When debating the scheduling of weekend or evening office hours, the practitioner should consider the long-term ramifications. Once these times are offered, it can be difficult to eliminate them. In competitive areas, where it is common to have two working spouses, it might be necessary to offer expanded hours of operation.

In many practices, the newest associates see patients in the evenings and on Saturdays. Since more than 70% of U.S. family households have both the husband and wife working outside the home during the daytime hours, evening and weekend appointments are highly desirable in many communities. In fact, seeing patients in the evenings and on weekends allows new associates to develop their skills sooner and become partners. More important, patients deeply appreciate the extended office hours, and being open during unconventional business hours shows that the practitioner cares about the patients' needs.

Patient Scheduling

The allocation of time for appointments will differ according to service. Contact lens fits, eye health assessments, glaucoma follow-ups, and low vision examinations all require different amounts of time. The practitioner must determine the time to be allocated for each service, and the receptionist who schedules appointments must be told how to provide the proper amount of time for each patient. Of particular importance is the use of pupillary dilation, which adds time to the examination and changes the flow of patients.

Patient scheduling is a reflection of the philosophy of care. In many practices, each patient is scheduled for 30 to 45 minutes or even an hour. The visual analysis not only consists of the traditional optometric procedures but also routine pupillary dilation and examination using the binocular indirect ophthalmoscope; assessment with a 60, 78, or 90 D fundus lens; Goldmann tonometry; blood pressure measurements; automated perimetry; and other tests. It is common to recall patients every one or two years for a routine visual analysis.

Checkup visits for contact lenses are typically scheduled for 15 to 30 minutes. A patient who is interested in being fitted for contact lenses is scheduled for a 1- to 1½-hour examination. Office visits are usually 15 minutes. There are two basic scheduling methods. The "stream" method of patient scheduling requires appointments to be equally spaced throughout the day in 1-hour or 1½-hour intervals. The "wave" method

entails scheduling patients in groups—for example, two patients are scheduled at 8 AM; one at 8:45 AM; and two at 9:30 AM. If one patient is late or if the optometrist needs more time with a patient, the wave will help average the time spent with each patient.

The use of pupillary dilation extends the amount of time needed for examination and disrupts the examination sequence. During the 15 to 30 minutes needed to achieve adequate dilation, the patient should be removed from the examination room so that it can be used for the evaluation of another patient. A special room can be set aside for patients who are waiting for dilation. They can be taken to the dispensary, they can be given a visual field test, or they can be returned to the waiting room. Management must be coordinated between practitioner and staff to ensure that efficient use is made of this time and that unnecessary delays are avoided.

It might be necessary to rehearse the movement of patients on a drawing of the office layout and to have "walk-throughs" to ensure that patient flow is properly controlled. Meetings between the practitioner and staff members also can be used to identify problems and arrive at solutions.

Absence of the Practitioner

Practitioner absence not only affects availability but also disrupts continuity of care. If a practitioner is not available because of vacation, illness, or continuing education, a patient in need of care must seek another eye care provider. Coverage by other practitioners during these periods must be planned, and patients calling for care must be appropriately notified or directed to substitute clinicians by the practitioner's staff.

Patients seeking emergency or urgent care do not often call for appointments. An efficient office must be able to offer services to "walk-in" patients who require timely diagnosis and treatment. To manage these patients, many offices leave appointment slots open just before lunch and in the late afternoon, to ensure that time is available for examination.

When a patient calls for an appointment, the preferred method of scheduling is to offer the patient two specific dates and times and to permit the patient to choose the one that is most convenient. If neither time is acceptable, a third, compromise choice can be offered. The patient's name, status (new or former patient), and telephone number should be noted in the appointment log or computer entry. Because changes in scheduling of appointments are inevitable, log information is written in pencil. Erasures can be used when necessary to change and refill appointment slots. Computerized appointment systems also should be flexible.

The patient should be reminded of the appointment before the scheduled time, and the receptionist should note in the log that this reminder has been given. A list of each day's appointments should be prepared for the practitioner and posted in the examination room or on the door to the room. A master list of patients can be maintained on computer, which also can keep track of "no shows," recalls, and referrals.

Patient Flow

Patient flow for a new practice can be divided into the following three phases: the initial buildup of a patient base, which generally requires 5 to 7 years; the plateau, a period of 2 or 3 decades during which the practitioner enjoys a fairly stable patient base and income; and the preretirement phase, a period of declining practitioner involvement and patient flow, which can last 5 to 10 years.

For each of these phases, the demands of patient flow are different. At all phases, however, efficient movement of patients through the office is necessary to reduce patient waiting time, eliminate unnecessary delays, and keep "chair time" to a reasonable level. Efficiency is especially desirable when a practitioner has only one examination room. Of particular importance is the scheduling of patients. This has to be carefully planned but can be disrupted by the cancellation of appointments, appearance of unexpected "walk-ins," late arrival of patients, or misallocation of time for examination.

As soon as a patient enters the office, management is necessary. Time spent waiting to be examined should be kept to a reasonable minimum. This time can be used for the filling of forms and providing pertinent information. If a technician is available to assist the practitioner, the patient can be moved to a room for preliminary testing. This room can be an examination room or another room used for the purpose of initial evaluation. Then the patient can be moved to the examination room so that the practitioner can perform the necessary testing. After the practitioner has finished, the patient usually must be taken to the dispensary and, after that, to the waiting room or administrative office where financial details can be settled.

Patient Communication

Nonverbal communication is of well-established importance: dress, conduct, and physical environment all assist in creating an impression—favorable or unfavorable—of the practitioner. Various written and verbal communications also are influential in the formation of a favorable impression of practitioner and practice. The most important forms of communication include the following:

- Reception of patients in the office
- Telephone conversations with patients
- Oral and written communications in the office
- Mailings to the patient

Each of these forms of communication requires a brief commentary (see also Chapter 26).

Reception of Patients

The reception room should be comfortable, clean, and capable of putting the patient at ease. Numerous decisions must be made to create an environment that achieves these goals. Is smoking permitted? Is there a play area for children? Is there adequate room for all patients? Are toilet facilities conveniently available, and are they handicapped accessible? Is there a wide range of current reading material? Similar questions also need to be asked with regard to the decor of the reception room and the conduct of the receptionist. Unless all these considerations are planned for (and evaluated periodically), an undesirable impression can be conveyed.

Telephone Conversations

The manner in which telephone queries are handled by a receptionist is of great significance; patients are commonly won or lost on the basis of these brief conversations. Practitioners must ensure that receptionists receive proper training in this vital area of patient communication. Many sources can be consulted to obtain this training, including telephone companies, practice management consultants, and various publications. Some basic considerations include the following:

- The telephone voice and personality of the receptionist should be an asset at all times.
- Telephone "busy signals" should be avoided with the use of the proper telephone technology.
- The receptionist should be capable of succinctly answering patient questions about examination fees and charges for materials.
- Telephones should be available in key areas of the office, such as the reception desk, the dispensary, and the practitioner's office.
- Receptionists should be able to triage patient complaints and schedule patients who require emergency or urgent care for same-day examinations.

Receptionists are often questioned by patients about matters of clinical care that are outside their area of expertise. Receptionists should understand how to manage these situations so that patients are not offended and erroneous information is not conveyed.

Paper Flow

The average office has the following three typical avenues of distribution and dissemination of paper: information given directly to patients; prescriptions and other records of care; and follow-up mailings such as bills, recall notices, and newsletters.

Patient information includes brochures, instructional booklets, fitting agreements for contact lenses, and similar documents. These items can be especially useful with contact lens patients, when medicines are prescribed, or if patient education is needed for a complex condition such as glaucoma.

Records should be carefully controlled, especially in light of confidentiality requirements established by the federal government (see Chapter 28). Although the practitioner is the owner of the record, the patient generally has a right to review the information in the record, and that right should be respected. Policies for the release of contact lens prescriptions should be adopted in all offices and should conform with the requirements of state law. When patients move or change practitioners and request the transfer of records, it is preferable to provide a summary rather than a verbatim copy. The practitioner should always retain the original record for the period required by law.

Follow-up mailings such as newsletters can be used to provide information on new services or instruments, cards thanking a source of referrals can be used as a practice builder, and computer-generated reminder notices can personalize the effort to provide recall. The ways in which follow-up mailings can be used to communicate more effectively with patients are limited only by the ingenuity of the practitioner.

Management does not end after a patient leaves the office. It might be necessary to schedule the patient to return for the dispensing of ophthalmic materials, to recall the patient for further examination, or to refer the patient to another health care provider. The appropriate steps must be taken to ensure that the patient understands when and where to go. Patient communication is an integral part of efficient management.

Troubleshooting

It is inevitable that, occasionally, difficulties will arise in the management of patients and that troubleshoot-

ing will be required. These problems are often of acute onset, trying to both the practitioner and the staff and difficult to resolve. If managed improperly, the effect can involve not just one patient, but several. Patient control is more easily achieved if procedures have been developed for management. Also, patient satisfaction is more likely.

Although there are numerous potential sources of conflict with patients, the most common situations involve fees, ophthalmic materials, and prescriptions. Some pointers for troubleshooting in these situations include the following:

With the complexities of third-party care, mistakes do occur. Make sure a knowledgeable staff member (or the practitioner) reviews the billing before telling the patient no mistake was made.

Complaints about fees should be answered honestly and openly; candor is never inappropriate in such a situation.

Be certain that spectacles are correct before debating with a patient.

Do not be reluctant to recheck refractions or other sources of patient dissatisfaction.

If ophthalmic materials are incorrect, make them right.

Try to resolve patient disputes in an amicable fashion. Arguments do not contribute to the benefit of the practice.

Establish a written office policy for the release of contact lens prescriptions.

To reduce conflicts over contact lens prescriptions, deemphasize charges for materials such as contact lenses and place more emphasis on fees for services.

Use prepaid service agreements for contact lens patients.

Offer patients a spectacle prescription (if needed) after the examination is concluded.

One of the keys to effective troubleshooting is to project confidence when dealing with the patient. Confidence is an attribute that is easily communicated to a patient, and it also is just as evident in its absence. To feel confident, technical expertise is required. Education does not end after graduation from school; it persists throughout the professional lifetime of the practitioner. Knowledge is often the difference between settling a problem and leaving the patient dissatisfied. Optometrists should work diligently to keep up with technical developments and to use them for the benefit of those they serve.

Another key to projecting confidence is to have an established method for management of the problem.

Such methodology is usually the result of experience or trial and error, but common sense often will go a long way in attempting to resolve patient disputes. Both practitioner and staff must discuss and develop ways of efficiently dealing with patient management problems. Efficiency is a learned skill that repays many times the time spent in its acquisition. It is of unquestionable assistance in developing effective patient control.

Personnel Management

Undisputedly, among the most challenging tasks faced by a practitioner are the hiring, training, supervision, and dismissal of personnel. These tasks are described in detail in Chapters 21 and 25. The organization of personnel and the description of their duties is best achieved through the use of an office procedures manual. This manual should outline the standard operating procedures that have been agreed on for the orderly, day-to-day management of the practice. The specific duties assigned to each employee, employee compensation, procedures for personnel evaluation and dismissal, and many other items are described in the manual. It is a necessary first step in the management of a practice's greatest resource, the people who work in it. Exemplar manuals can be obtained from various sources and can be used as the "template" for a manual specifically written for the practice.

Financial Management

In an efficiently run office, procedures are established to manage the finances of the practice. In general, the practitioner must set reasonable fees, ensure that they are properly billed and collected, monitor practice expenses and adjust them as necessary, exercise control over inventories of ophthalmic materials and supplies, and guard against loss from waste and theft.

Fees

After fees have been initially established, the practitioner must monitor costs and expenses to determine when fees should be increased. The decision to change fees must be adequately explained to staff members so that they can answer patient queries properly. Because fees are among the most common causes of conflict with patients, staff members must be able to explain clearly what charges are for and how they can be paid.

It is not unusual for the fee schedule to include "professional courtesy," which is a means of reducing or eliminating the fees charged to certain individuals—

usually other health care providers—who, in return, provide a similar courtesy to the optometrist. Immediate family members usually are included in the arrangement.

Fee schedules set by third-party health care programs such as Medicare and Medicaid and by vision and medical service plans are invariably different from those charged by the practitioner on a fee-for-service basis. Familiarity with these programs is essential to practice administration today because they are the source of about two thirds of patients for the average optometrist.

Taxes

As an employer, a practitioner has the responsibility to determine the proper withholding of taxes for employees. This obligates the practitioner to determine the appropriate amounts for federal, state, and local income taxes; Social Security and Medicare; and other deductions available to employees, such as retirement plans, medical savings accounts, or other benefits (see Chapter 40). These funds have to be properly collected, deposited, and then transferred on a timely basis to the appropriate federal or state agency.

If an employee is to assist in tax bookkeeping, the practitioner must be certain that this individual is knowledgeable and diligent because the practitioner is responsible for inadequate deductions or delays in payment. For this reason, it is essential that practitioners have a basic understanding of business taxation, so they can properly supervise the in-office tax process (see Chapter 39). Of course, self-employed optometrists also must pay taxes, which necessitates familiarity with principles of individual income taxation and another set of forms and deadlines (see Chapters 38 and 40).

Tax errors can be expensive and time-consuming to remedy. For private practitioners, having a readily available professional tax advisor is both prudent and necessary.

Billing and Collections

Office policies must be set for the awarding of credit and for the billing of accounts (see Chapter 35). Staff members responsible for the collection of payment must understand these policies and apply them fairly and uniformly. Because of the complexity of third-party reimbursement plans, in a busy office it will be necessary to have a staff member assigned to the billing and collection of these accounts. Changes in billing methods are frequent, and reimbursement problems can arise quickly if appropriate attention is not devoted to program details.

An office policy for the collection of unpaid accounts must be set by the practitioner. Accounts receivable should be monitored monthly to ensure that these procedures are effective and that a disproportionate number of accounts do not go uncollected.

Periodic Economic Evaluation

It is essential to list monthly expenses so that they can be properly monitored for any significant changes. Typical monthly expenses involve quite a number of items (Box 24-2).

Ideally, the expenses on the monthly expense sheet should be monitored each week. If an expense is unusually high, it will be necessary to review the records for the past 12 months and compare the amounts. For example, if health insurance costs for employees increase substantially from the previous year, the person in charge of the office's insurance plans should call insurance agents and try to get a more cost-effective health plan. Observing present trends can provide valuable information in planning for the future. For instance, by refinancing loans at lower rates, the practitioner can reduce monthly expenses. Variable expenses should be monitored to minimize the likelihood of being forced to make large increases in fees or to see more patients to offset an increase in expenses.

An economic analysis should be performed periodically to determine the progress of the practice toward reaching its financial goals (see Chapter 41). Fees must be periodically evaluated and adjusted to compensate for added costs and expenses.

Inventory Control

Because optometrists sell spectacles and contact lenses, inventories must be maintained for these ophthalmic materials. An inventory control system—utilizing a ledger or a computer—must be established (see Chapter 20).

Protection Against Embezzlement

A surprising number of optometry practices are plagued by employee theft. Few optometrists think about this possibility before it occurs and therefore do not have office procedures to prevent employee theft. Preventive policies should be effective but not offensive to employees.

The simplest and least intrusive method of protecting against loss by embezzlement is to obtain appropriate insurance coverage. If economic loss is incurred, the policy will provide reimbursement.

Box 24-2 Typical Monthly Expenses

- Rent
- Health and dental insurance
- Loans and interest for loans
- Life disability, and professional liability insurance
- Salaries
- Payroll taxes
- Answering services
- Janitorial services
- Retirement plans
- Utilities
- Telephone service
- Postage
- Office supplies
- Printing
- Computer supplies
- Legal and professional fees
- Lease payment
- Convention and seminar fees
- Promotional and advertising fees
- Donations
- Subscriptions to magazines and professional materials
- Dues for professional organizations
- Business and property tax
- Automobile expenses
- Unemployment insurance
- Miscellaneous expenses

Conclusion

When an optometry school graduate enters private practice, there inevitably will be a "learning curve" as the graduate acquires needed experience with office administration and patient management. The young practitioner might have to spend just as much time attending to the business tasks of a practice as the time spent actually seeing patients. Being involved with office administration might seem to be an undesirable task for many practitioners; however, for those who become owners of practices, knowledgeable administrative techniques and prudent business strategies are necessary for a practice to operate smoothly and efficiently. Such practices enjoy a high level of morale—on the part of the practitioner as well as the staff. Just as important, these practices are perceived as "patient friendly" by patients and are inevitably popular and successful.

Bibliography

Allergan, Inc: *Pathways in optometry.* Irvine, Calif, 1995, Author.

Andrews FJ: Choosing your "experts" wisely. *Optom Management* 24(7):64-8, 1988.

Baldwin BL, Christensen B, Melton T: *Rx for success.* Midwest City, Okla, 1982, Vision Publications.

Bennett I: Dealing with patient complaints, remakes. *Optom Management* 24(2):94, 1988.

Bennett I: Keeping your office expenses in line. *Optom Management* 24(5):29-39, 1988.

Bennett I: *Management for the eyecare practitioner.* Boston, 1993, Butterworth-Heinemann.

Christensen B: Personalities: can you mix and match? *Optom Management* 25(12):29-33, 1989.

Coleman DL: Protect yourself from employment lawsuits. *Optom Economics* 1(11):47-8, 1991.

Coleman DL: Your new ophthalmic equipment (first decide which is better for you. Then make sure you know the rules). *Optom Economics* 2(4):30-3, 1992.

Day J: Turning the heat on employee pilfering. *Optom Management* 25(9):84-91, 1989.

Fischer BA: Fine tuning the message. *Optom Economics* 2(1):12-21, 1992.

Gailmard NB: Guide to diagnostic instruments and equipment. *Rev Optom* 130(3):111-28, 1993.

Goldberg F: Foolproof records that stand up in court. *Optom Management* 25(11):59-70, 1990.

Goldsborough R: Five ways to ease the strain of opening cold. *Rev Optom* 124(5):97-103, 1987.

Handler G: Remember the person behind the eyes. *Optom Management* 25(2):88-92, 1989.

Hayes J: How much to spend on new instruments. *Optom Management* 28(4):15, 1993.

Internal Revenue Service publication 15, *Employer's tax guide (circular E).*

Internal Revenue Service publication 334, *Tax guide for small business.*

Internal Revenue Service publication 583, *Starting a business and keeping records.*

Internal Revenue Service publication 1518, *Tax calendar for small business.*

Legerton JA: Sound purchasing decisions (analyzing the what, when, why and how of purchasing ophthalmic equipment). *Optom Economics* 2(10):34-8, 1992.

Melton JW, Phillips JH, Plank KE: Answers for success. *Optom Economics* 2(4):34-6, 1992.

Miller PJ: How to prevent employee theft. *Optom Management* 24(9):62-6, 1988.

Morrison RJ: Quality, caring, and marketing. *Optom Economics* 1(6):28-31, 1991.

Palmer DM: Telephone techniques. *Optom Economics* 1(3):18-21, 1991.

American Optometric Association: Practice Enhancement Program: *Optimize your professional opportunities through patient communication in your practice. Professional enhancement monograph, MN 17.* St. Louis, 1986, Author.

American Optometric Association: Practice Enhancement Program: *Optimize your professional opportunities through patient communication in your community. Professional enhancement monograph, MN 18.* St. Louis, 1986, Author.

American Optometric Association: Practice Enhancement Program II: *Professional enhancement module, managing your practice plan, precourse workbook.* St. Louis, 1986, Author.

Schulman E: What patients need to know. *Optom Economics* 1(9):12-5, 1991.

Sherburne SO: Handling the problem patient. *Optom Economics* 1(11):25-7, 1991.

Stein H: Communication skills: do you rate a ten? *Optom Management* 26(1):65, 1991.

Stein H: Communication skills, part 2: opportunities for success. *Optom Management* 26(2):59, 1991.

www.optometric.com. Online version of *Optometric Management* magazine, which offers articles about practice administration.

www.revoptom.com. Online version of *Review of Optometry* magazine, which offers articles about office administration.

Chapter 25

Managing an Office Staff

Peter G. Shaw-McMinn, Daisy Rampolla, Maria Robles, and Craig Hisaka

Nothing great was ever achieved without enthusiasm.
Ralph Waldo Emerson *Circles*

Successful human resource management requires that attention be given to the basic functions of management: planning, organizing, and directing and controlling personnel. This chapter describes the direction and control of office staff. Directing staff members begins with training.

Training of Staff

Training of staff is an ongoing process. Technology improves, economic conditions change, and commitments need to be redefined. An efficient practice continues to evolve policies that are appropriate for the times and to reconfirm policies that work well. To remain efficient, time must be set aside for continued employee development. An American Optometric Association survey of practicing optometrists showed that the average amount of time devoted to training per month was 2.8 hours. The same survey revealed that the minimal amount of training these optometrists thought should be provided was 6.1 hours per month. This result indicates that optometrists believe staff members do not receive as much training as is desirable. The amount of time needed by the employees of a particular practice, however, will depend on the goals set for the practice and the abilities of both employer and employees to achieve those goals.

Goals and Objectives of Training

The American Optometric Association survey also showed that practitioners believed the objectives of training should be in the following areas:
- 71%, communication with patients
- 61%, technical skills
- 54%, ophthalmic dispensing
- 53%, general knowledge
- 43%, office policies

In a partnership or group practice, one way of identifying the areas to include in training is to survey the optometrists involved (and, if available, the office manager). Using a checklist can be helpful (Figure 25-1). If patient surveys or suggestions have been used, they should be checked for the areas that patients rated as less than excellent. These areas should be considered for training topics. Another source of topics can be gleaned from looking over the evaluations of each employee. Areas of weakness within the practice can be identified and prioritized, and objectives for training can be created to remedy problems. An example of such a training program is found in Box 25-1.

Training Techniques

There are several options available to the practitioner when choosing a way to train the staff in appropriate behavior. Opportune moments, performance reviews, lunch meetings, staff meetings, retreats, and continuing education seminars all provide opportunities for the training of employees. The choice of technique depends on the objectives and goals of the training.

Opportune Moments

During the course of working with an employee, positive or negative behavior can be observed. Practitioners should look for positive behavior and reinforce it whenever possible. The reinforcement and accompanying dialogue can be used to train the correct behavior.

VI   YOUR STAFF

Exercise 2.18

Staff assessment checklist

Although your primary responsibility is providing vision care for your patients, you are also an employer. Here is a checklist of staff activities. Go through it quickly, indicating your actual assessment of your staff members. Put an X in the third column if you'd like to see improvement in certain areas.

	Yes	No	Wish would improve
1. I like being in charge of my office.			
2. I like my staff members to wear uniforms.			
3. I like my staff members to make all my appointments.			
4. My receptionist has a pleasant telephone voice.			
5. My receptionist is courteous.			
6. My receptionist is patient.			
7. My receptionist knows when an emergency occurs and knows when to interrupt me.			
8. My staff members keep my files in order.			
9. My staff members keep my billings up-to-date.			
10. My staff members are well groomed and project a neat, clean appearance.			
11. My staff members know my office policies and follow them.			
12. My staff members are on time for work.			
13. My staff members respect and keep patient information confidential.			
14. My staff members get along well with patients.			
15. My staff members get along well with each other with a minimum of friction.			
16. My staff members get along well with me.			
17. My staff members know how to generate appointments for me.			
18. My staff members, on their own, know how to generate income in my office.			
19. My staff members are competent in all areas of my practice.			

Figure 25–1 Staff assessment checklist. (From American Optometric Association. *Practice enhancement program II, professional enhancement module, managing your practice plan, precourse workbook.* St. Louis, 1986, Author. Reprinted with permission.)

For example: A practitioner notices that the receptionist has appeared indifferent to telephone callers who ask for the price of contact lenses. However, in response to one of these calls, the receptionist gives an excellent explanation of the choices and services the office provides; this is followed by the scheduling of an appointment. The practitioner should reinforce this behavior by telling the receptionist that his or her management of the caller was exceptional. The reason for approval should be explained. In this case, the receptionist initially avoided the issue of cost by describing the advantages of using the office, educated the patient about the complexities involved in fitting contact lenses, and explained the range of fees in such a way that the patient was confident enough to set an appointment. This moment results in making the employee feel good, reinforces positive behavior, and improves patient satisfaction.

At other times it can be difficult to catch the employee doing the right thing. When the practitioner is feeling patient and the employee is in the right mood, a poor performance should be discussed in a nonthreatening way. The practitioner should do this privately and as soon as possible after the poor performance.

For example: A practitioner hears the receptionist answer a patient's inquiry about the price of contact lenses by saying, "Contacts are $400 a pair. Interested? Goodbye." This moment can be used by the practitioner to review office procedures and policies about

answering such questions. It is hoped that in the near future, the receptionist will be overheard answering such inquiries more appropriately.

Opportune moments can provide informal settings for learning. A study by the U.S. Department of Labor shows that 70% of workplace learning is informal. Chatting on the job, discussions during lunch, and exchanges at breaks offer good environments for stress-free learning. Some offices place pads and pencils in employee break rooms and encourage unofficial gathering of staff.

Lunch Meetings

Some offices have a difficult time finding a few hours to set aside for training. Since most people eat lunch at some time, lunch meetings can be held to satisfy a limited objective. There are many distractions that can occur during a lunch meeting, however, and the stress of a lunch meeting can cause fatigue in the afternoon and affect employee performance or morale. For these reasons, it is best to choose lighthearted, less important activities and objectives during a lunch meeting. An example of an appropriate topic would be a brief presentation on what it means to be "patient centered." This could be followed by a brainstorming session and the identification of staff behaviors that indicate services are patient centered (see Box 25-1).

Staff Meetings

Regular staff meetings can provide the time necessary to mold a cohesive team that is consistent in providing services. Enough time must be set aside for planned objectives. Whatever time is allocated, there must be a plan with objectives and outcomes in mind. The meeting should not be left open without defined goals because the effort to reach objectives can pay large dividends in the long run.

Examples of activities for staff meetings include the following:
• Role-playing sessions
• Question and answer sessions
• Surveys
• Pretesting procedures
• Discussion workshops
• Problem-solving panels
• Demonstrations
• Lectures

The activities chosen can depend on the management style in use. Too often, when using a lecture format, it is assumed that everything said will "sink in." Although lectures can be effective on some occasions, there are times when the information will not result in any behavior changes. Generally, employees will learn best by getting involved and participating in an activity.

There are two adages to keep in mind when training staff members. One is, "No one ever fell asleep while talking." The other is, "The best way to learn is to teach." These sayings reinforce an important point—the most successful sessions can be those in which the optometrist says the least.

The usual staff session begins with a review of the previous meeting and a summary of the success of previous changes (Box 25-2). Then a staff member is asked to provide a brief presentation. The member might be chosen because he or she understands the topic best or because of an ability to demonstrate it most skillfully. The practitioner assists or provides resources to the staff member so that an adequate presentation can be given.

Before the presentation, a pretest can be given to staff members to determine their level of knowledge and to focus their thoughts. The order of questions can be designed to lead the group through levels of increasing awareness. Questions are designed to incite discussion and not necessarily to elicit right or wrong answers.

The practitioner then serves as the facilitator to lead the group through each question. The employees save their pretests and are allowed to jot additional notes as they go along. It is stressed that the pretest is to be used by the individual staff member and will not be seen by anyone else. If done properly, the practitioner will have very little to say other than to focus staff involvement on the questions and the ultimate goal and objectives of the meeting.

Awareness is of little value without action. Goal sheets for the meeting are prepared by the practitioner. Typical goals include behavioral changes and measurements (Figure 25-2). These changes are then discussed at the beginning of the next meeting.

Retreats

When great change is desired—and more time might be needed to discuss objectives than the time afforded in a staff meeting—it can be of value to close the office for a day and hold meetings away from the office. This type of intervention is especially effective when dealing with sensitive issues or defensive staff. Part of the day can be designed as a reward to lighten the concerns of attendees. Retreats can vary from an all-expenses-paid trip to a vacation spot to a day at a local meeting facility. A sample retreat agenda is provided in Box 25-3. An

---

> **Box 25-2 A Typical Agenda for a Staff Meeting**
>
> I. Report of results from interventions recommended at last meeting (each individual staff member)
> II. What is meant by patient-centered care (senior staff member)
> III. Pretest activity
> IV. Discussion of pretest questions (practitioner, facilitator)
> V. Recommendations for change
> VI. Assignment of responsibilities
> VII. Topics for next meeting

---

information packet, typically including articles and background information on the chosen topic, is distributed to staff members a week or so before the retreat.

One of the advantages of setting aside an entire day is that the progress toward the objectives can be measured, and, if problems arise, tempers flare, or someone becomes upset, time can be taken to relax or refocus the group. A nice advantage of having free time is that there is the opportunity to take each employee aside and discuss issues privately in a nonthreatening environment. Staff members also can take the opportunity to informally discuss pertinent issues with each other. As a facilitator, the practitioner's main responsibility is to keep everyone focused on the issues and to steer them toward desired outcomes.

Training can be time consuming and sometimes frustrating, but the rewards can be tremendous when a program is properly carried out. Studies show that patient load can be increased by 35% for each properly trained optometric technician. Unfortunately, studies also show that nearly half of all employees hired for a given job turn out to have been poor choices. The average length of employment is only 3.6 years. In corporate practices, employee turnover is 25% to 50% a year.

For these reasons, taking the time to develop the staff into a cohesive, happy team that reflects a competent, cohesive, happy practice will be worth the time and effort invested.

Dismissing Employees

If a practitioner is making a reasonable effort to train and control staff members, the employee who is not able to become an efficient and enthusiastic member of the team will know there are problems and will probably resign. Everything should be documented in

SAMPLE GOAL SHEET

Today's Date _____

Specific goal:

    – Specific benefits of reaching goal:

Target date:

Where am I today with regard to the goal?

Obstacles to achievement:

Checkpoint dates:

    – Intermediate Goal #1

    – Intermediate Goal #2

    – Intermediate Goal #3

    – Intermediate Goal #4

Plans for surmounting obstacles:

Specific actions to take to form new habits:

Date Goal Was Met: _____

Figure 25-2 Sample goal sheet.

Box 25-3 A Sample Retreat Agenda

Valentine's Day Retreat
9:00 Meet at office. Overview of day's activities.
9:15 Pretest: "What the Experts Say About Providing Services to Patients."
9:30 Champagne breakfast at Mimi's Cafe.
10:00 Brainstorm activity, "The First 5-10 Minutes of the Patient Visit."
10:30 Brainstorm activity: "Follow-Up Your Patients."
11:00 Tour of Dr. Stanley's office.
12:00 Role-playing activity: "How to Say Goodbye to the Patient."
1:00 Lunch at Knotts Berry Farm followed by free time at the amusement park.
4:00 Prioritizing; setting goals and objectives.
5:00 Agenda for next meeting. Adjournment.

each employee's file, including the curriculum vitae, résumé, or letter of application sent before employment; the interview notes; results of training programs; progress with training; evaluations; reprimands; warnings; and attendance record.

When it is necessary to dismiss an employee, these items should be reviewed with the individual in a nonconfrontational manner. The good things that the employee has done should be pointed out, so that he or she can see that the evaluation is a balanced one and can understand the achievements and the problems that have been encountered during the course of employment.

Most practices have a probation or trial period for new employees. This is usually 60 to 90 days. Performance should be carefully monitored during this period. If training is not progressing at an agreed-on schedule, this would be the best time to terminate the employment. Many optometrists are hopeless optimists and assume that, despite a difficult start, things will get better, but often they do not.

Some practices request 2 weeks' notice from an employee when the employee wants to or has to leave employment. It is fair for the employer to offer the same notice. If an employee cannot reasonably contribute to the practice after being informed of termination, the 2 weeks can be used as paid time for the employee to find other employment. This is optional and is not required under the Fair Labor Standards Act.

There are causes for immediate dismissal, and these causes should be included in the employee handbook for each practice. Examples are provided in Box 25-4.

When an employee is dismissed, that employee might be eligible for unemployment compensation. Each state has specific eligibility requirements that must be met by a dismissed employee to receive unemployment compensation. If an employee does receive this compensation, the former employer will be required to pay an additional amount of money into the state compensation fund; the amount is based on the number of former employees drawing this compensation.

Exit Interviews

Every practice experiences some turnover of personnel. An exit interview allows the employer to learn how to improve the workplace for other employees. Typical questions that are asked include the following:
- Did the job meet your expectations?
- Why are you leaving?
- What did you like and dislike about our office?
- What specific suggestions for improvement could you make?

These questions should be used as a starting point for more in-depth discussions. The feedback received can prove to be extremely valuable.

Controlling Staff Members

The controlling aspect of management involves setting standards, measuring performance, and taking corrective actions. To successfully carry out this function with staff members, they must first feel that they are a part of the practice.

Mission Statement

The office manual should include a mission statement for the practice. Employees must feel that they are a part of the practice, and including them in the mission statement, as well as in the long-term objective of the practice, fulfills this need. This mission statement should be read by all employees (Box 25-5).

Employee Evaluations

Evaluations of all employees should be performed at least once a year. During training periods, evaluations can be provided weekly. These evaluations should be written and made a permanent part of the employee's file. An example employee performance review is provided in Figure 25-3. This format permits the evaluator to address the employee's quality of performance, quantity of responsibilities, and knowledge of the job. In preparing for the evaluation, it is a good idea to keep notes about employee performance, using specific dates. The notes should include employee successes, problems, and any questions about employee performance. Before the evaluation the record should be reviewed, and examples should be used during the dis-

---

Box 25-4 Example of Causes for Dismissal

The following can be cause for immediate dismissal. Any employee dismissed for cause will not be entitled to a minimum notice nor termination vacation pay. This list is not to be construed as inclusive:
- Inefficiency or inability to perform assigned duties
- Excessive absenteeism or tardiness
- Poor personal hygiene
- Dishonesty
- Breach of confidentiality or professional ethics
- Refusal to perform assigned duties
- Theft
- Embezzlement or mishandling of funds

Box 25-5 Example Mission Statement

- To provide our patients with quality eye/vision care, therapy, ophthalmic materials, and contact lenses in a professional, efficient, and friendly setting.
- To operate as a profitable, secure, and growing optometry practice; to provide maximum care at a fair cost.
- To be dedicated to providing growth opportunities, a caring environment, and an improved life for all staff members.

EMPLOYEE PERFORMANCE REVIEW

Name: _____

Today's date: _____

Date hired: _____

Period covered: _____ to _____

Position: _____

Evaluated by: (signature) _____

Please rate the employees in each of the areas below, using the following scale. Your evaluation should reflect on impartial judgment that is based on the entire period covered—not upon isolated incidents.

Outstanding: Employee exhibits consistent, superior ability, far in excess of job requirements.
Very good: Employee exhibits ability above that expected for the position.
Satisfactory: Employee meets the position requirements.
Fair: Employee exhibits ability below job requirements. Some improvement needed.
Unsatisfactory: Employee exhibits ability far below requirements. Much improvement needed.

1. QUALITY:
  a. Produces error-free work
  b. Handles assignments with thoroughness

2. QUANTITY:
  a. Produces an acceptable volume of work
  b. Completes tasks promptly

3. JOB KNOWLEDGE:
  a. Knows job duties
  b. Knows office policies and procedures

4. DEPENDABILITY:
  a. Arrives on time
  b. Has good attendance record
  c. Completes a consistent quantity of work with
    acceptable quality

5. ATTITUDE:
  a. Cooperates with associates
  b. Maintains pleasant demeanor
  c. Conforms to office policies and procedures

6. INITIATIVE:
  a. Needs minimal supervision
  b. Completes more work than expected

7. APPEARANCE:
  a. Dresses according to office standards

8. PERSONAL FACTORS:
  a. Concentrates on work rather than personal factors

9. OVERALL PERFORMANCE:
  a. Employee's strong points
  b. Areas that need strengthening

Figure 25-3 Employee performance review.

cussion. Many human resource experts recognize that annual performance reviews can be threatening to employees, and some believe ongoing performance discussions throughout the year are more productive. However, all experts agree it is necessary to provide regular feedback to employees.

Setting Individual Goals

The use of performance evaluations is the first step in helping employees identify individual goals that will carry out the practice's mission.

The secret to employee development is good communication. Nowhere is this more evident than during a periodic review of the employee's performance. The perceptions of the evaluator can be quite different than those of the employee. How the performance review is conducted can be critical to morale and to the future productivity of the employee.

A good way to begin the first evaluation of an employee is to have the employee complete a self-evaluation survey. Figure 25-3 is one example of a format that could be used. This self-evaluation will provide the evaluator with insights into the employee's perceptions of performance. If these perceptions differ from those of the evaluator in many areas, it might be best to choose only a few areas on which to concentrate. The evaluator should not forget, however, that 90% of all employees rank themselves in the top 10% in regard to performance.

The evaluator's survey should be reviewed with the employee, including performance scores and the reasons for these scores. Pertinent comments should be written for future review. Together with the employee, the evaluator should compose goals, a plan to reach these goals, and the consequences that will result if the goals are not reached. After the review, the employee must sign the evaluation and the plan. This information should be used to increase or decrease employee bonuses. If the desired behavior requires little effort to correct, the time spent for the evaluation and goal setting can serve as a training period for the employee.

Monitoring Implementation of Changes

Sometimes, despite all the preparation, planning, and training, the behaviors sought do not occur. This situation is particularly likely in an office where employees have been following unchanging routines for a long period. In this type of office, a daily worksheet can serve as a helpful reminder to encourage employees to change the routine according to recommendations.

On the daily worksheet, the employee must note when the new procedure is used. Employees should be assured that this extra time will be required only until the new changes become part of their routine. The practitioner might wish to monitor the employees' efforts to incorporate changes into the office routine by using personal observations.

Directing Staff Members

The manner chosen to communicate with employees is referred to as *leadership style*. Many business authors use the term management style instead because communications will, unquestionably, affect the entire manage-

ment process. Generally, there are two extreme types of management style, with most managers' style falling somewhere in between. The most authoritarian style is the military approach, in which the manager tells the employee what to do and the employee follows the instructions without question. The opposite style is one in which the manager orchestrates situations so that the employee realizes what to do and does it because the employee believes it is in the best interest of the office. Each style has its advantages and disadvantages.

Douglas McGregor calls these management styles theory X and theory Y in his book *The Human Side of Enterprise* (New York, McGraw-Hill). The two theories are briefly described in Box 25-6.

Management style X means that the manager must control everything that goes on in the office and every decision that must be made by employees. The manager must constantly monitor the employees' performances. A specific procedures and policy manual is necessary to direct the staff to handle every situation the way the manager wants it handled.

This management style seems easier because no effort is made to convince staff members to understand or support changes. Their duty and job are simply to carry out orders, not question why. On the other hand, this management style requires more time. The employees must be constantly monitored or they might not provide services correctly because they were not told how to handle a particular situation. The employees will hesitate to act and might, in fact, be ineffective without the manager present. A large policy and procedures manual will be needed; large manuals are difficult to memorize and time consuming to create.

Management style X can be summarized by the statement, "Management is getting people to do things your way." Management style Y is completely different. Staff members participate in the decision making and are allowed to decide how to best handle situations. Office policy and procedures are decided by a group effort, with most input obtained from those providing the services. The manager offers resources and training to help the employees reach their goals for the office.

Initially, this management style seems slow and laborious because meetings must be held, levels of awareness must be raised, and alternatives discussed. Staff members must first realize that change is necessary, research the options, and finally agree on the policy to be implemented. Once the policy has been decided, implementation is usually much quicker and easier because staff members "own" the changes. They understand the need for change and can adapt the philosophy behind the change to every situation. The

Box 25-6 Management Styles

Theory X

Assumptions about the average person

Works as little as possible

Lacks ambition, dislikes responsibility, prefers to be led

Inherently self-centered; indifferent to organizational needs

By nature resistant to change

Gullible, not very bright

Assumptions about management personnel

Responsible for organizing staff, equipment, and supplies in the interest of economic ends

Direct staff efforts, motivate them, and control their behavior to fit the needs of the organization

Must persuade, reward, punish, and control staff activities; otherwise staff members would be passive or resistant to organizational needs

Theory Y

Assumptions about the average person

At least potentially mature

Trustworthy

Able to handle responsibility

Motivated by organizational goals

Will use self-control and self-direction

Assumptions about management personnel

Responsible for organizing staff, equipment, and supplies in the interest of economic ends

Believe it is their responsibility to provide opportunities to develop abilities

Provide guidance

Encourage growth

Remove obstacles

Arrange the work environment so that employees can achieve their own goals while meeting the goals of the practice

Modified from McGregor D The human side of enterprise. New York, 1960, McGraw-Hill.

employees are able to work independently and are not afraid to offer novel options for consideration. The staff members treat the business as their own because, in a large sense, it is. This management style can be summarized by the statement, "Management is the ability to let other people have your way."

Which style is best for a given practitioner? One employer might prefer to choose the style that comes most naturally. Another employer might choose the style to which employees respond best. Still another manager might change management styles from one to the other because change is generally more productive than rote routines.

There are arguments that can be made in favor of each rationale.

Selecting a Natural Management Style. Choosing a style that comes naturally requires the least amount of effort on the manager's part. One means of determining management style is illustrated in Figure 25-4. This exercise provides insight into individual management tendencies.

Selecting a Style to Which Employees Respond. Through experimentation, a manager finds the management style that each employee seems to respond to best. Time and effort can be reduced by predicting the management style that will be most effective in obtaining the best productivity from an employee. To make these predictions, it is helpful to look at the value systems of different groups of people. Managers should not be surprised to observe that an employee's value system is very different from the manager's own value system.

Changing Management Styles. There might be times when a change in management style is needed. Different types of employees, different types of practice environments, or even staleness in a practice can necessitate a change. When altering management styles, however, the changes should be readily apparent to all employees. Otherwise, confusion and dissatisfaction can result.

Motivating Employees

The information used to predict the response of employees to a management style also can be used to motivate them. There are a number of common factors that motivate individuals in general. By applying Maslow's hierarchy (Figure 25-5) to the profession of optometry, optometrists can learn what will be most effective in motivating employees.

Physiological Needs

All people have bodily needs such as food, water, rest, exercise, shelter, and protection from the elements. The motivation of staff members is obviously beyond this basic level.

Security and Safety

People require protection against threats, dangers, and deprivation. Many people fear losing their job, benefits

Management Style Questionnaire

The purpose of this exercise is to give you a general idea of your management style. For each statement listed check whether you mostly or completely agree with it or whether you mostly or completely disagree with it.

Respond to all the statements.

Scoring directions follow the questionnaire.

Statement	Mostly or completely agree	Mostly or completely disagree
1. Since patient contact is critical, I try to provide all direct patient services myself.		
2. When I've tried to delegate patient services to an assistant, I've found patients got poorer service.		
3. To assure the right decision is made, I make all the decisions myself.		
4. I expect employees I've hired to learn to do things my way.		
5. I hardly ever hear any complaints from my employees.		
6. The important thing is that employees understand what I want of them.		
7. I assign tasks to whoever is capable of handling them.		
8. There are few employee problems that cannot be solved by better pay.		
9. Employees who insist on making all of their own decisions should open their own business.		
10. It's just not possible for everyone to make a living doing what they enjoy.		
11. The average employee is basically self-centered and indifferent to the goals of my practice.		
12. I allow employees to post humorous sayings about how this office is run, and there are many.		
13. My best technique in dealing with an employee grievance is to assert my leadership in determining what I need to do to correct the situation.		
14. If I let my employees make their own decisions, I will lose control of my practice.		

Figure 25-4 Management style questionnaire. (From American Optometric Association. *Practice enhancement program II, professional enhancement module, managing your practice plan, precourse workbook.* St. Louis, 1986, Author. Reprinted with permission.)

Continued

Statement	Mostly or completely agree	Mostly or completely disagree
15. As manager, I am responsible for everything my employees do.		
16. The function of the manager is to set out and enforce clear rules; the function of the employee is to follow them.		
17. Allowing employees to attend optometric conferences and workshops cuts into their working time and may give them ideas to look for work elsewhere or about ideas for equipment or procedures that I can't afford to implement. It will only make them restless.		
18. If individuals are allowed to make their own decisions, they will not be for the good of the office, but for their own benefit.		
19. I enjoy optometry, and I'm unwilling to devote less than my full time to patient care.		
20. I'm in optometry to make a good living by providing quality optometric care. If I let my employees get too independent, I'll lose all my cost controls and jeopardize the profitability of my practice.		

Scoring directions

Now add up the number of your "Mostly or Completely Agree" answers.

If you checked 15 to 20 "agree" answers, you run a very "tight ship." Your style is highly directive, what is called a Theory X management style.

If you checked 7 through 14, your management style includes a number of practices that are consistent with a more participative management style.

If you checked 1 through 6 "agree" responses, your management style is highly participative, and you delegate not so many tasks as you do responsibilities in achieving shared goals. Your management style might be characterized as a Theory Y management style.

Figure 25-4, Cont'd

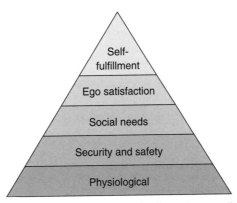

Figure 25-5 Maslow's hierarchy of needs. (Reprinted from AH Maslow: *Motivation and personality.* New York, 1970, Harper & Row.)

such as medical insurance, or an adequate income after retirement. To provide motivation, employers should offer regular performance reviews, with emphasis on feedback that stresses the positive aspects of job security. Updates should be provided on the status of employee benefits and their economic value. Bonus or profit-sharing plans also can be offered, contingent on level of performance. Retirement plans also can be provided. The employer should be reassuring when discussing job security and business stability.

Social Needs

People have interpersonal needs, such as belonging, association, acceptance, and giving and receiving friendship and love. Participation in certain activities on behalf of the practice can reinforce these feelings and provide motivation. Attendance at continuing education courses; staff participation in the determination of office policies and procedures; use of staff ideas to improve office functions; membership in various professional organizations and societies; and the periodic use of group functions, such as office retreats and informal staff birthday celebrations, can all achieve this goal.

Ego Satisfaction

People need self-esteem, which comes from self-confidence, independence, and achievement. People also enjoy a sense of reputation, which confers status, recognition, respect, and appreciation. The satisfaction of these needs can greatly improve motivation.

These needs are satisfied by promotions, assignments that provide added responsibilities, participation in the training of new staff members, or evaluations or opportunities in which positive feedback is supplied about performance. Patients should be encouraged to include staff members when offering thanks for services. Employees should be allowed to write or sign memos to other staff members; display an outstanding employee's name in work areas; mention accomplishments in front of patients and peers; and market the employee to patients through the use of biographical sketches, comments on signs, displays of awards and certificates, business cards, and name tags with an office title.

Recognition can be demonstrated by giving flowers, candy, lunches, theater tickets, or other rewards to employees. Saying "thank you" to employees, particularly in public, is effective. So is a letter to the employee, noting a job well done.

Self-Fulfillment

Motivation involves realizing one's own potential, continued self-development, and creativity in its broadest sense. This final area of need is said to come from within. Self-fulfilling employees are motivated through introspection, a recognition of what is important to them. They are able to focus on satisfying their personal needs and require no outside motivation. A manager must provide the resources and the opportunity for employees to reach their fullest potential by using the office as a vehicle to attain self-fulfillment.

Motivating employees must take into account their needs and wishes. The manager must be able to recognize "true" rewards, which differ from individual to individual. When providing a reward, the manager must ask, "Is this reward really what the employee considers special?"

A motivation plan can accompany a training program. Each opportunity to improve staff performance also can be used to motivate employees. Retreats, staff meetings, lunch meetings, performance reviews, and opportune moments all can be used to reinforce positive behavior and encourage more of the same. Perhaps the most powerful opportunity of all is the opportune moment when an employee is caught doing something the right way. This moment should be seized because such acknowledgment builds enthusiasm like nothing else.

Managers have at their disposal many strategies with which to motivate employees. Effective managers will use as many of these strategies as they can. They will note which strategies work best with individual employees. They will use these strategies to mold the staff into a team that works together to reach the goals of the practice. Management style strategies should be planned and implemented with the same attention that would be given to the planning and conduct of a vision examination. Managers should never forget to set aside sufficient time for administrative duties and responsibilities. If management is properly performed, this time will be enjoyably spent working with an efficient and enthusiastic office staff.

Acknowledgement

The authors of this chapter in the first edition of *Business Aspects of Optometry* were Donald H. Lakin, Ronald S. Rounds, Peter Shaw-McMinn, and Craig Hisaka.

Bibliography

American Optometric Association: *Practice enhancement program II, MN 5, optimize your professional opportunities through effective office staff policies and procedures.* St. Louis, 1984, Author.

American Optometric Association: *Practice enhancement program II, professional enhancement module, managing your practice plan, precourse workbook.* St. Louis, 1986, Author.

American Optometric Association: *Practice enhancement program II, professional enhancement module, your marketing plan module two, precourse workbook.* St. Louis, 1986, Author.

American Optometric Association: *Practice enhancement program, MN 1, optimize your professional opportunities through personal and professional goal setting.* St. Louis, 1986, Author.

Baldwin BL, Christensen B, Melton T: *Rx for success.* Midwest City, Okla, 1982, Vision Publications.

Blanchard K, Johnson S: *The one minute manager.* New York, 1993, Berkeley Publishing Group.

Blanchard K, Lorber R: *Putting the one minute manager to work.* New York, 1991, Berkeley Publishing Group.

Hayes J: Keep staff members "in the loop." *Optom Management* 29(5):24-8, 1994.

Maslow AH: *Motivation and personality.* New York, 1987, Harper & Row.

McGregor D: *The human side of enterprise.* New York, 1985, McGraw-Hill.

Peters TJ, Waterman RH Jr: *In search of excellence.* New York, 1988, Harper & Row.

Tecker IJ, Tecker GH: "Big boom theory." *Assoc Management* 43(1):46-7, 1991.

www.optometric.com. Online version of *Optometric Management* magazine, which provides advice about personnel management.

www.revoptom.com. Online version of *Review of Optometry* magazine, which provides advice about personnel management.

Chapter 26

Patient Communications

Stuart M. Rothman, Harry Kaplan, and Craig Hisaka

What we got here is a failure to communicate.
Frank R. Pierson *Cool Hand Luke*

Successful health care practitioners find that the way they communicate with patients can be just as important as their clinical proficiency. Modern practitioners often spend as much time explaining procedures, tests, treatment options, and recommendations as actually examining the patient. This chapter reviews the basic tenets of effective communication, while providing a basis for patient communication in an optometric office setting.

A Standard Model of Care

The classic disease model of health care can be analyzed in the following six stages:
- The period when the patient is at no risk
- The period when the patient is at risk due to change in age or environment
- The period after an agent strikes, during which the patient is in danger of acquiring the disease
- The period when signs are present
- The period when symptoms appear and the patient complains
- The period when disability results

In the past, health care focused on the last three stages of disease. Patients sought care only when they were in pain and extremely uncomfortable. Because a community's health care practitioners were educated and highly trained, they were respected and often revered. Communication between practitioner and patient was comparable to that between parent and child—the practitioner told the patient what to do; the patient listened and complied. The practitioner's advice was never openly questioned by the patient, who always assumed a passive role. This paternal model of health care persisted for many decades.

Today, the dynamics of health care and of the doctor-patient relationship have changed. Contemporary practitioners are likely to be treating patients of equal education and economic level. Patients are more informed about health and the factors that relate to health. They also understand that health care needs to move beyond a pure disease model of care. Successful patient communication depends on the willingness of practitioner and staff to accept the patient as an equal and to consider the patient a participant in the treatment regimen. Practitioners also must appreciate that a patient who understands diagnoses and treatment options will be a more compliant patient, with the attendant long-term benefits to health that this understanding brings.

A successful practitioner knows the expectations brought to the doctor-patient relationship. The practitioner should enter the relationship expecting to provide the highest level of care. When providing care, the practitioner expects the patient to comply with recommendations and to establish and maintain an open line of dialogue regarding needs, wants, and results. The patient's expectations include being treated with respect, kindness, and compassion in a highly ethical and professional manner. In any relationship, there can be different expectations by both practitioner and patient with each individual encounter. The practitioner who is able to fully understand the expectations of the patient at each encounter will be the one who establishes a long-term relationship with the patient.

The Need to Communicate Effectively

In today's competitive health care environment, patient communication is a key element in the successful delivery of care. The importance of patient communication can be attributed to the following factors:

Patients are more aware of health care issues and are more knowledgeable about the treatment options available to them. This has been dramatically advanced by the media and the proliferation of Internet use.

There is more competition for health care revenues, and this has led to increases in the advertising of health-related products and treatments.

Increased specialization in health care has forced patients to triage themselves so that they can see the specialist who best meets their needs.

Second opinions for major treatment options are expected by practitioners, patients, and insurance companies.

The risk of liability claims has increased the need for informed consent, requiring patients to understand the risks and benefits of treatment options.

The increasing automation of tests and procedures has allowed for greater use of technicians and assistants. In the efficient delivery of health care, the practitioner acts as an interpreter of information and has more time to discuss findings, diagnoses, and treatment options.

Setting the Stage for Effective Communications

For effective patient communication to occur, the practitioner must identify the message or image to be conveyed to patients by the office. This message or image should be communicated to every patient or potential patient at every encounter with the practitioner or staff. It also should be conveyed in every other type of communication that comes out of the office.

The most important messenger that any practitioner will have is the office staff. The staff will be the first personal contact that a potential patient has with the office. Staff members also will be the first contact the patient has when arriving at the office. Effective patient communications require that the right staff members be hired and that they be trained to communicate properly. Even if an office has a staff manager, it is ultimately the practitioner who must select, train, and monitor staff members.

Telephone Communications

Most patients have their first personal contact with an office through the telephone. This first encounter must convey warmth, caring, competence, and efficiency. The staff member responsible for answering the telephone must direct full attention to the person calling and must avoid diversions that convey a negative message. Many practice consultants advise putting a smiling face or humorous saying near the telephone to remind the staff member to convey a positive image to the patient. It is a good idea to have carefully scripted responses to common questions that might be asked in routine telephone conversations. This is most important in making an appointment for a patient. Not only is it important for the staff person to get the patient's name and phone number, but the type of appointment needed, the type of insurance, and the referral source also might be required. Patients must be informed of the information that must be brought with them to the appointment. Some practitioners prepare audiotapes of experienced staff members responding to questions so that they can be used during training of new staff members. Telephone communications require that a protocol be observed when responding to callers. Some common requirements are listed in Box 26-1. As optometrists increasingly engage in the treatment of eye disease, it is essential that the person answering the phone be trained to properly triage callers. Staff members must be told

---

Box 26-1　Telephone Etiquette

Do's

- Answer the telephone with a smile.
- Treat the patient the way you would want yourself or your family to be treated.
- Talk slightly slower than normal conversation and enunciate clearly.
- Offer to call a patient back rather than put the patient on hold for longer than one minute.
- Stay as close as possible to the office telephone script.
- Try to reinforce a caring, concerned attitude.
- Remember that the office is there to serve the patient, not the other way around.

Don't

- Be abrupt with the patient.
- Rush the patient.
- Continue to put the patient on hold more than once or keep the patient on hold for longer than 30 seconds without checking with the patient.
- Give professional advice.
- Assume that the patient understands everything about what the office does or the services it provides.

what constitutes an emergency or what is urgent, so that prompt and appropriate care is provided.

Communication Through Marketing

Marketing comprises the whole range of efforts that go into building and maintaining a professional practice. To be most effective, the message that is communicated must be consistent, fill a need in the community, and be communicated in such a way that patients and prospective patients understand the potential benefits of having this need fulfilled. Specific marketing strategies will be based on the needs of a particular community, but there must be consistency in the message conveyed to the patient. Various themes can be observed in the advertising used by large corporations. These themes range from quality of care to specific product promotions with emphasis on price. Once a marketing niche is established, it becomes difficult to change the image that has been created. Therefore, the initial message needs to be appropriate for the practice.

Prospective patients will find out about an office either through word of mouth; an insurance plan listing; external marketing using Yellow Pages listings, newspapers, television or radio; or via a Web site on the Internet. Before making the decision to call an office for an appointment, these patients have made a decision that the office can provide the care they need in a setting that they are comfortable with. It is essential that these external marketing sources reflect the image that is to be conveyed to the public. They allow the office to present a capsulized image of itself. There also must be follow-through in supporting this image in the office and throughout the patient's experience in the office.

Communication in the Office

The following factors contribute to effective communication with patients while they are in the office: the appearance of the office and of practitioner and staff, efforts to alleviate patient apprehension, use of printed materials, and verbal communication.

Office Appearance

Patients expect to be cared for in an office that is clean, neat, uncluttered, and up-to-date. The reception room should be large enough to accommodate several patients without being crowded. The furniture does not need to be of "living room" quality but should not be sterile and impersonal. Refreshments, such as coffee and soft drinks, convey a caring attitude. Patients should be offered a choice of materials to view while they are waiting to be seen. Brochures, pamphlets, books, magazines, and videotapes can be used to entertain and inform patients while they wait.

One of the biggest complaints by patients is the time that must be spent waiting to be seen by practitioners. Patients are expected to arrive at or before their appointment times. They, in turn, expect practitioners to begin the examination within a reasonable period after the scheduled appointment time. No amount of plush furniture, entertainment, or refreshments will negate a one-hour wait. On days when the office is running well behind schedule, a call to the patient at home or work should be standard procedure.

Patient treatment rooms should convey a feeling of security to the patient. Equipment does not need to be brand new but it should be in excellent working order and have a modern appearance. Even though the patient might not know the difference between a phoropter that is 20 years old and one that is new, an examination chair that is worn will be readily apparent.

Patient expectations usually are highest in the dispensary. If the patient has been to or seen a "super-optical" showroom, an inevitable comparison will be made. The patient might not expect to see the same number of frames displayed but will expect to see frames arranged in an attractive and tasteful manner. The appearance of the dispensary can be crucial in the patient's decision to purchase eyewear. The image and feeling that the dispensary conveys to the patient will affect the patient's impression of the quality and value of the eyewear being displayed.

Practitioners should set aside a portion of each year's budget for the purchase of new equipment or for the improvement of the office. Existing patients will notice changes that have occurred in the office and will talk about these changes to friends and relatives. This enthusiastic promotion of the practice can help pay for the changes many times over.

Personal Appearance

As competent and as caring as a practitioner might be, the patient will form an impression at the first encounter that can be quite difficult to change if it is negative. This first impression depends as much on the practitioner's appearance as it does on what the practitioner says or does. The office staff also can convey a negative first impression. There are many schools of thought about what constitutes appropriate attire for practitioner and staff. Authority can be conveyed by more formal attire, such as a white clinic jacket or uniforms, but this image can be offset by too much formality. Comfort is important, but practitioner and staff should be dressed in attire that patients are comfortable with as well. Proper attire can vary from one part of the country to another, and even within a relatively small area. What is appropriate for a large city might not be appropriate for a rural community just a few miles away. Appearance also can vary depending on the type of patient seen in the office (e.g., children as compared with adults). Practitioners must take note of all these factors and determine the type of image that is appropriate for the practice and patient population.

Alleviating Patient Apprehension

Many patients come to the office of a health care provider with a sense of apprehension. This feeling is not limited to new patients—it can be held by existing patients as well. New patients are entrusting their health and well-being to an individual they only know by the recommendation of a friend, relative, other practitioner, or preferred provider insurance listing. Aside from the uncertainties these patients might have about this new practitioner, there are the obvious concerns about vision or health that caused them to seek care in the first place. Existing patients share this apprehension, whether they are seeking care for a problem or for

a routine examination with no symptoms. Very few people can "be themselves" under these circumstances. Understanding this apprehension can help practitioner and staff make patients feel more at ease, allowing the practitioner to obtain greater insight into the person being treated and generally permitting better treatment to be provided. The patient's openness also will lead to greater willingness on the part of the practitioner to communicate treatment options and will lead to greater understanding of treatment options by the patient.

Calling the patient by name and discussing the patient's hobbies, family, work, and avocational interests help the practitioner and staff relate on a more personal level while also alleviating the patient's apprehension about the office visit. The patient should feel that he or she is being given the undivided attention of the doctor and the staff throughout the encounter.

Use of Printed Materials

Many offices offer printed materials that describe the practice (e.g., a "welcome to the office" brochure), the services that the office provides, new ophthalmic materials available in the dispensary, or the treatment options for various ocular conditions. Representative brochures are found in Figure 26-1. Printed materials

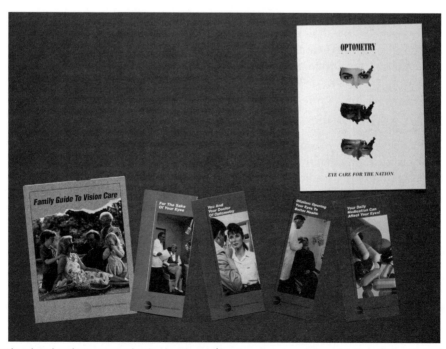

Figure 26-1 Sample printed patient communication brochures. (Courtesy American Optometric Association, St. Louis. Reprinted with permission.)

are useful because they provide information even after the patient has left the office. More important, they reinforce, in writing, the information presented verbally during the examination. These brochures can be designed by the practitioner and printed at a modest cost, or they can be purchased from various suppliers such as private companies, contact lens and frame companies, optical laboratories, and professional organizations such as the American Optometric Association.

Videotapes also can be used to disseminate information to patients and, in fact, are enjoying increasing popularity. Tapes can be used for instruction in the office or lent to patients for viewing at home. Subjects include contact lenses, vision training, and treatment options for various conditions. Depending on the subject matter, they can be obtained from private companies or professional organizations (Figure 26-2).

Report-writing computer software allows the practitioner to custom design a report to a patient about symptoms, diagnoses, and recommendations. This can be given to the patient as the patient leaves the office or sent to the patient a few days after the visit. In either case it helps to reinforce what was discussed during the examination and allows the patient to synthesize the information in a more comfortable, less stress-producing environment.

Software also is available (Figures 26-3 and 26-4) that can graphically explain certain symptoms and treatment recommendations. It is said that a picture is worth a thousand words, and these three-dimensional moving computer-generated images extend the capabilities of a two-dimensional static picture.

Verbal Communication

There is no substitute for the face-to-face contact that practitioner and staff have with the patient in the office.

The case history is one of the most important parts of the examination because it establishes the personal and clinical relationship between practitioner and patient. A good clinician will listen as the patient describes the chief complaint and, as necessary, will help the patient articulate the problem being described. The information conveyed will guide the clinician's examination while ensuring that the clinician addresses the patient's concerns. Preprinted patient history questionnaires allow the practitioner to focus on the major concerns of the patient but should not be used as a substitute for a face-to-face patient history. Similarly, computer touch-screen history programs also allow the practitioner to know in advance what the patient is concerned about and can more concisely direct the history.

Describing the purpose of testing as it is performed will make the patient feel more informed and enable

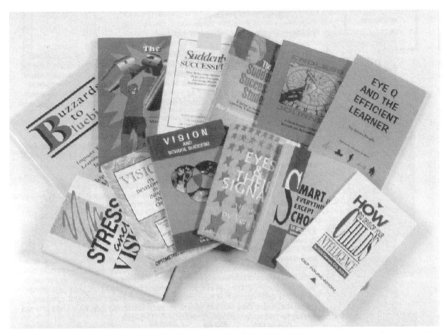

Figure 26-2 Sample educational resources used to educate patients. (Courtesy Optometric Extension Program, Santa Ana, Calif. Reprinted with permission.), Santa Ara, Calif.

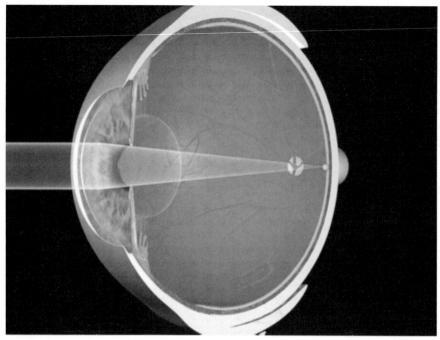

Figure 26-3 Example of computer-generated information for patients; this sample illustrates emmetropia. (Courtesy Eyemaginations, Towson, Md.)

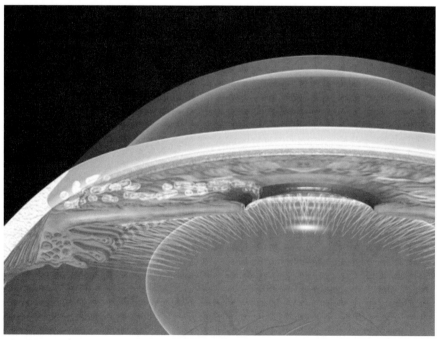

Figure 26-4 Example of computer-generated information for patients; this sample illustrates open-angle glaucoma. (Courtesy Eyemaginations, Towson, Md.)

the patient to become more of a participant in care. It also will educate the patient about the services that are being provided. For tests that are performed by ancillary staff, a scripted description of the purpose and procedure of the test should be used.

The case disposition must address the needs of the patient. A clinician's ability is directly related to his or her capacity to describe how the patient's problem relates to the testing performed and how the treatment prescribed can alleviate the problem. This means talking to the patient in terminology the patient can understand. Effective communication also can involve using demonstration aids so that the patient can better visualize what is being described. Examples of some of these demonstration aids are provided in Figure 26-5. The case disposition might require the practitioner to present the patient with various treatment options and describe the pros and cons of each option. Effective communication means listening as well as talking. The patient should be guided toward the best solution so that the patient participates in the decision-making process and understands the outcome.

There might be instances when the practitioner has to act like a practitioner of the past and inform the patient of the actions that must be taken. These situations usually involve direct risk to patient health and well-being, such as sight-threatening diabetic retinopathy. Even in these instances, it is important that the practitioner be able to effectively communicate dangers and risks to the patient to ensure patient compliance.

The issue of informed consent also must be considered in cases that pose a risk of injury. The patient has a right to know the risks, hazards, and likely outcomes of a recommended procedure or treatment and to be informed of the alternatives to that particular test or treatment. Informed consent also requires disclosure when suspicious findings or abnormalities are detected.

The latter obligation is the toughest test of the optometrist's communication skills. For example, a patient with elevated intraocular pressure must be informed of the potential significance of this finding and advised of the specialized testing that must be performed to rule out the possibility of glaucoma. The practitioner must convey the need for testing and the need for long-term follow-up even if the results are negative, so that the patient understands and agrees to periodic assessment for disease.

Communication with Patients After They Leave the Office

Effective patient communication occurs not only when patients are in the office but also after they have left. Patients who encounter a problem, such as with ophthalmic materials, often will not call the office to describe the problem; instead, they simply will not return for further care. They might also tell relatives and friends about their problem. The successful office can prevent such situations from occurring. Problems can be

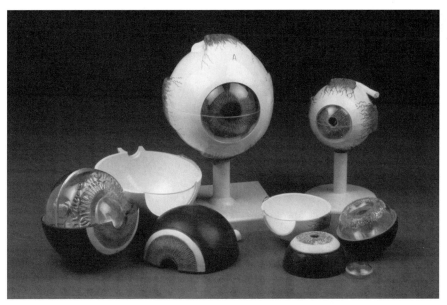

Figure 26-5 Models for explanation of vision problems. (Courtesy American Optometric Association, St. Louis. Reprinted with permission.)

identified by calling patients after services or materials are provided to ensure that they are satisfied. Many offices will conduct periodic patient surveys to obtain feedback about office policies and patient management.

The success of an office in handling patient problems is determined by the attitude of the practitioner and staff. The office should regard patient complaints as an opportunity to regain trust and confidence and should convey a positive attitude. The office that handles these problems defensively will further antagonize the patient.

Satisfaction will be determined by the patient's perception that treatment exceeded expectations. Dissatisfaction occurs when patients perceive that they have not gotten what they expected. Satisfaction can be increased by elevating the patient's perception of treatment or by decreasing the patient's expectations. After the fact—when patients have already been provided with treatment—it is difficult to lower their expectations. Therefore, decreasing patient expectations is not a practical alternative. The most successful strategy is to elevate the perception of treatment. This should be the goal of the office.

Communicating with Special Patient Populations

There are three populations that require special communication techniques: the elderly, persons with disabilities, and children.

The Elderly

The office that communicates well with elderly patients and makes them feel comfortable will invariably do a better job of serving this growing segment of the U.S. population. The elderly population is the group most likely to experience diminished visual performance, and it is important that they be made to understand the age-related visual changes that can occur. More than any other age group, they will be apprehensive about eye health because of the increased prevalence of glaucoma, age-related maculopathy, and cataracts among their friends and contemporaries. They also can be undertreated for systemic conditions that have ocular manifestations, such as diabetes and hypertension. Their understanding of these conditions might come from what they have learned from friends, relatives, or the media. The key to successful management of these patients is to set realistic expectations. Age-related vision changes are common. The case disposition should describe these changes in terms the patient will

understand. Demonstrations, pictures, and videotapes will help elderly patients understand their condition and the visual limitations that can occur. A staff person should assist elderly patients when they are asked to use computer-assisted history or testing software.

The practitioner should be aware of any hearing or mobility problems that a patient has before bringing the patient into the examination room. The practitioner and staff should be especially conscious of talking directly to the patient, not to a caretaker or relative accompanying the patient. Eye contact and clear enunciation are especially important. Elderly patients should not be addressed by first name, especially by practitioners and staff who are younger than the patient is.

Elderly patients do not like to feel rushed during an examination. They might have concerns that they will not share with the clinician until they feel comfortable doing so. The practitioner who is a skilled communicator will be able to guide the patient to the important areas of the case history without making the patient feel rushed. Unrushed communication should continue throughout the examination to make the patient feel at ease and reassured. Elderly patients with visual problems might not give clear, consistent subjective responses. These responses should be verified for consistency and should be confirmed by objective findings when possible. Clinicians should never forget that subjective responses become less reliable if patients feel that they are being rushed.

The office staff can be tremendously helpful in making an elderly patient feel welcome and in conveying a caring attitude. Offering the patient a cup of coffee or tea on a cold winter's day, calling a taxi for the patient when the examination is concluded, referring to the patient by name, inquiring about the patient's children and grandchildren, and reinforcing the practitioner's recommendations can go a long way toward creating enthusiasm in elderly patients.

Patients with Disabilities

Many of the communications procedures used for elderly patients also are applicable to patients with disabilities. However, several additional procedures need to be offered. Disabled patients will want to know that the practitioner and staff feel comfortable dealing with them. The office staff needs to convey this attitude to patients when the appointment is made, before the patient ever enters the office. The office policy regarding patients with disabilities should be determined in advance. Nothing destroys confidence more than a receptionist who puts the patient on hold while checking to see whether the practitioner will see the patient. Practitioners should adopt a policy that is in keeping with legal requirements. Federal, state, and local laws regulate access to health care offices and providers, and office policies should be consistent with these laws.

The office staff also should be aware of how to handle the office visit by a disabled patient. Care involves not only direct communication to the patient but also indirect communication—how to seat the patient during pretesting or how to manage the special visual requirements and restrictions that influence eyewear selection and dispensing.

Many patients with disabilities will come to the office with a friend, relative, or caretaker but are able to understand and make decisions and should be treated accordingly during testing and case disposition. The practitioner and staff should talk directly to the patient, not to the person accompanying the patient. Patients with disabilities should be treated like any other patient in terms of respect and equality.

Children

Many practitioners find that the pediatric population is their most difficult patient group. Children do not respond and act like adults when visiting a health care provider. It should not be forgotten that a child does not make the decision to be examined. This decision has been made for them, and it takes a special ability to get them to cooperate and participate in care. Children have a keen sense of knowing whether a practitioner or staff member feels comfortable with them. They do not like to be ignored or talked down to. They want to feel that the practitioner and staff are concerned and interested in them and their lives. They want to be comforted during testing and reassured that they are safe and secure with the care provided by the practitioner and office staff.

The office environment should be inviting to children. A corner area of the reception room can be made into a children's play area with a child-size table and chairs, puzzles, books, and games. All of these items should meet applicable safety standards for children. Some offices use videotapes to entertain children when they are waiting, though they should be offered only if they can be made unobtrusive to any adult patients who also might be waiting.

Parents might not want to discuss their concerns with the child in the room, requiring that the case history be taken with the parent before the child is brought into the room for examination. Many practitioners do not wear white clinic jackets when examin-

ing children, preferring a more informal appearance. The office should be equipped with instrumentation that is specifically designed for children's visual abilities. Objective pretesting can be used to obtain initial information and limit fatigue. Given the limited attention span of children, testing should be performed quickly, with the most important tests, as determined by case history, performed first. Nonthreatening aids like hand puppets and cartoons can be used to maintain visual attention during testing. The practitioner might find it useful to discuss the case disposition with the parent before or after speaking directly to the child.

Using positive reinforcement, behavior modification, and a reward system can help make the practitioner's job easier during testing by making the child more cooperative. It also can leave the child with a positive impression of the experience. Using colorful stickers, toys, or treats can go a long way toward putting a smile on the face of the child as he or she leaves the office.

Conclusion

In today's competitive health care marketplace, the office that communicates a caring, compassionate, and competent impression to patients is able to succeed and flourish. More than any other skill, effective communication will attract patients, create a favorable image of the practitioner and staff, and motivate patients to return for future care. With effective communication, satisfied patients will become enthusiastic patients. This should be the ultimate goal of any patient encounter.

Bibliography

American Optometric Association: Practice enhancement program. *Optimize your professional opportunities through patient communication in your practice. Professional enhancement monograph, MN 17.* St. Louis, 1986, Author.

American Optometric Association: Practice enhancement program. *Optimize your professional opportunities through patient communication in your community. Professional enhancement monograph, MN 18.* St. Louis, 1986, Author.

Anan B: Understanding the older patient population. *Optom Management* 25(11):35-41, 1989.

Bailey RN: The doctor-patient relationship: communication, informed consent and the optometric patient. *J Am Optom Assoc* 65(6):418-22, 1994.

Baker WJ: Listening will improve your hearing. *Optom Management* 23(7):57-61, 1987.

Baldwin BL, Christensen B, Melton JW: *Rx for success.* Midwest City, Okla, 1983, Vision Publications.

Barber A: Communication: speaking and listening skills. *Behavioral Aspects Vision Care* 41(1):24-9, 2000.

Bennett I: Dealing with patient complaints, remakes. *Optom Management* 24(2):94, 1988.

Bremer A: Caring for older adults. *Optom Economics* 1(10):14-6, 1991.

Brooks DJ: Kid stuff. *Optom Economics* 1(9):42-5, 1991.

Brownlow C: *Communication and compliance.* Rancho Cordova, Calif, 1998, Vision Service Plan.

Christensen B: Personalities: can you mix and match? *Optom Management* 25(12):29-33, 1989.

Classé JG: *Legal aspects of optometry.* Boston, Mass, 1989, Butterworth.

Ettinger E: *Professional communications in eye care.* Boston, Mass, 1994, Butterworth.

Fischer BA: Fine tuning the message. *Optom Economics* 2(1):12-21, 1992.

Gailmard NB: Managing the grief patient. *Optom Economics* 1(8):18-21, 1991.

Handler G: Remember the person behind the eyes. *Optom Management* 25(2):88-92, 1989.

Harvey B: Clinical communication skills: general principles of interpersonal communication. *Optician* 215(5640):22-7, 1998.

Harvey B: Clinical communication skills: patient personality traits. *Optician* 215(5653):23-6, 1998.

Jameson M, Muhr C: Telephone triage in a primary care practice. *Optom Economics* 5(1):46-50, 1995.

Lee G: Serving hearing impaired patients. *Optom Economics* 4(11):8-12, 1994.

Legerton J: Our two most powerful tools. *Optom Economics* 4(6):20-2, 1994.

Levoy B: Proper etiquette with disabled people. *Optom Economics* 2(5):41-2, 1992.

Lill DJ, Cotham JC, Thomas JC: Listen up. *Optom Economics* 1(4):24-8, 1991.

Manso VA: Communication skills for the optical dispensary. *Eyequest* 4(3):66-72, 1994.

Marino D: Managing the hearing impaired. *Optom Management* 24(10):67-71, 1988.

Melton JW, Phillips JH, Plank KE: Answers for success. *Optom Economics* 2(4):34-6, 1992.

Miles LL: Staff to patient communication. *Optom Economics* 3(3):22-3, 1993.

Miller PJ, Miller RW: How to manage patients with emotional problems. *Optom Management* 25(9):97-100, 1989.

Morrison RJ: Quality, caring, and marketing. *Optom Economics* 1(6):28-31, 1991.

Palmer DM: Telephone techniques. *Optom Economics* 1(3):18-21, 1991.

Persico J: What does your reception area say about you? *Optom Management* 27(7):33-8, 1992.

Robinson C: Communication in practice. *Optometry Today UK* 39(2):38-9, 1999.

Schulman E: What patients need to know. *Optom Economics* 1(9):12-5, 1991.

Scipione PA: Capturing and keeping the senior patient. *Optom Management* 25(11):24-8, 1989.

Sherburne SO: Handling the problem patient. *Optom Economics* 1(11):25-7, 1991.

Stein H: Communication skills: do you rate a ten? *Optom Management* 26(1):65, 1991.

Stein H: Communication skills, part 2: opportunities for success. *Optom Management* 26(2):59, 1991.

Stein H: Dress for success, yes! *Optom Management* 26(3):51, 1991.

Stein H: Turn complaints into compliments. *Optom Management* 26(5):61, 1991.

Torgenson N: Creating an energized office. *J Optom Vis Development* 29(4):224-6, 1998.

Watts R: Putting communications technology to work. *Eyecare Technology* 6(6):39-40, 1996.

Werner DL: Ethics and the presbyopic patient. *Optom Economics* 4(3):15-8, 1994.

Wilson J: Communication skills. *British J Optom* 7(1):31-2, 1999.

Wright R: The best foot forward. *Optom Economics* 1(1):46-7, 1991.

Zaba J: Catering to the children in your practice. *Optom Management* 25(1):80-2, 1989.

www.keyworlds.com/o/optometry-software. Online list of software for optometry practices.

www.optometric.com. Online version of *Optometric Management* magazine, which offers articles about effective communication.

www.revoptom.com. Online version of *Review of Optometry* magazine, which offers articles about effective communication.

Chapter 27

Interprofessional Relations

Sam Quintero and Jack Bridwell

A little sincerity is a dangerous thing, and a great deal of it is absolutely fatal.
Oscar Wilde *The Critic as Artist*

Interprofessional relations are a necessity for all health professions in their commitment to the well-being of patients. As a primary eye care profession, optometry has increasingly enjoyed the benefits of receiving referrals and consultations from other health care professionals, while steadily providing referrals and consultations to them. This interprofessional activity is vital to the development and maintenance of a healthy practice and to the establishment of a good working relationship with many kinds of health care providers. The value of interprofessional relations is obvious at the individual practitioner level. Referrals and consultations from one type of health practitioner to another are a daily occurrence in communities everywhere.

Practitioners should attempt to identify all optometric and nonoptometric referral sources in the community. Interprofessional referral and consultation techniques also should be explored because they will result in better patient care and management. Better-organized health care delivery is likely to result from interdisciplinary interactions and cooperation. Patients are likely to receive more efficient diagnosis, treatment, and management of health problems. It is likely that, in the long run, such collaborative efforts will benefit the consumer as well as the health professionals. Characteristics of resourceful referral and consultation partnerships include developing professional relationships, marketing to target professionals, professional communication and reporting, professional courtesies, and remembrances for referring and consulting sources. These characteristics are the subject of this chapter.

Developing Professional Referrals and Consultations

It is a healthy practice that has the confidence of other professionals who refer patients or seek consultations. These professionals can be other optometrists, other eye care professionals, practitioners in other fields of health care, and professionals whose work is not in health care. To develop such a referral and consultation base requires a willingness on the part of these professionals to entrust their patients to the optometrist.

It is important to understand the difference between a referral and a consultation. This distinction is medicolegal in nature and important for purposes of liability. In a *referral*, the eye care professional is required to use "due care" in the selection of a practitioner to whom the patient is being referred. Due care is construed to mean the practitioner chosen is competent to perform the necessary services that are deemed necessary. In this instance, the eye care professional will not be liable for the actions of the practitioner to whom the patient was referred, provided the referring eye care professional has no responsibility for the care of the patient while the patient is under the care (treatment/management) of the other practitioner. On the other hand, a *consultation* is considered to be a joint undertaking between two or more professionals. In a consultation the patient receives diagnosis or treatment by one provider that is offered in conjunction with the care being rendered by another provider. In this instance, if there is negligence by either party, then both parties could be held responsible or liable for any harm the patient may have experienced while under the care of the consulting practitioner.

Why Should a Practitioner Refer or Consult?

In general, referrals are made from one health care professional to another if the service needed is beyond the scope of licensure or training of the practitioner seeking the interprofessional relationship. Legally and ethically, referral is required when specialized testing or treatment is needed that cannot be provided by the referring practitioner. In comparison, a consultation is voluntary and is sought to use the expertise of more than one health care professional in the management or treatment of a patient's condition.

Certain procedures can be so time consuming that it is not cost-effective for a practitioner to perform them, necessitating that the patient be sent to a colleague or specialty clinic, even though the referring practitioner is legally allowed to provide the procedure.

If a practitioner does not possess the specialized equipment or instrumentation needed to make a diagnosis or provide treatment, the practitioner must refer the patient so that the appropriate care can be rendered.

A practitioner's interprofessional relations should exemplify confident and competent interactions. It is essential that the communication between practitioners regarding the patient include what is known about the patient's condition, the status of the condition at the time of referral, and what is needed in the way of additional care.

Why Don't Practitioners Refer?

Practitioners may choose not to refer for several reasons. Many times a practitioner enjoys performing a particular procedure to gain further experience or wants to do the procedure because of the challenge the procedure presents. In a beginning practice that is not yet established, a new practitioner might be motivated to perform a wide range of procedures for economic reasons. Sometimes there is fear that failure to perform certain procedures can result in loss of professional prestige and recognition. Actually, when a patient is referred to a highly qualified individual, the benefit is usually significant and results in an even higher professional regard for the referring practitioner.

There is always the concern that not only the patient but also the patient's family might never return after a referral. In fact, more often than not after a successful referral, the entire family becomes loyal to the referring practitioner. Conscientious practitioners who seek to provide the highest level of care will always gain the respect of patients and their families.

It is important to remember the referring practitioner expects excellent professional care, good communication, and eventual return of the patient.

How to Encourage Referral Sources

Optometrists should consider several factors when attempting to develop referral sources. First, skill must be attained in a specific area of practice. A high level of skill is often achieved by limiting practice to a specific specialty, such as contact lenses, low vision, or binocular vision. In such a practice, the optometrist can expect more referrals from primary eye care practitioners. If it is not practical, because of economic considerations, to limit the practice to a specialty area, then patients referred for consultation should be returned to the referring practitioner. Under no circumstances should the consultant provide primary eye care for these patients. A report should be sent to the referring practitioner after testing or treatment has been completed. This report should describe how the patient's problem has been determined and, in clear, concise terms, the results of the treatment or disposition of care.

A new practitioner should be willing to accept difficult cases—difficult cases that are extremely time consuming often will be the first ones that another practitioner refers. These cases might not have a cost-effective result, but success with difficult cases ultimately will provide referrals of patients whose treatment will be more cost-effective.

To gain the respect and confidence of referral sources, a new optometrist must gain prestige by obtaining success in a chosen area of practice. An effort should be made to become a diplomate of the American Academy of Optometry in an area of expertise. The Academy provides a rather rigorous examination, both written and practical, that must be passed to obtain recognition. Efforts also should be made to publish in professional journals. These publications can be presented to potential referral sources when appropriate. A recognized expert will be asked to lecture at continuing education programs. The greater the number of lectures, the greater the exposure and the more opportunity for receiving referrals from other practitioners.

Establishing interprofessional relationships for referral and consultation requires maintaining a confident attitude and expecting positive results.

If specializing, the practitioner should have state-of-the-art, highly specialized instrumentation. If such instrumentation is not available to the average practitioner, it provides a rational reason to refer to the "specialist." The specialist always must be available for telephone consultation with referring doctors at any time. Sometimes the specialist can be required to offer advice regarding patients not yet referred.

To succeed with difficult cases, the optometrist must expect to spend as much time as required to fully satisfy the objective of the referral.

Finally, it is essential to send patients back to the referring practitioner. If patients are not returned, further referrals are unlikely.

Marketing to Targeted Professionals

The many types of health care professionals located in the general area should be identified. Many such professionals are listed in Box 27-1.

Meeting with Local Health Care Professionals

A detailed list of all health care professionals in the area should be developed. A new practitioner should personally visit each of these health care professionals. Optometrists need to meet face-to-face with other professionals, if at all possible, in the optometrist's office so that the professionals can see the optometrist's practice. A tour of the office and face-to-face discussions are most important and must be conducted with the individuals who actually make the referrals. It is critical to demonstrate that the optometrist possesses the proper basic and clinical science training and equipment and is readily available to participate in care. During the visit, the practitioner should ask whether the professional may be used as a referral source for specific problems. It is important to exchange ideas about prescribing and treatment philosophies and to discuss how patients are to be managed. Practitioners should talk specifically about the information to be provided and management protocols. Discussions should include the types of patients to be referred, particularly if specialty services are provided. A week or two later the practitioner should mail a copy of an office brochure with a brief cover letter to the professional.

From time to time, articles relating vision to systemic disease can be found in professional journals, medical-pharmaceutical updates, and timely news items. A copy of such an article can be sent to the

---

Box 27-1 Health Care Professionals

1. **Family practice/general practitioners** are truly primary care providers.
2. **Pediatricians** also may be primary care providers.
3. **Dermatologists,** although secondary providers, often see patients who present for primary care and who may require the services of an optometrist when the dermatologist has completed treatment.
4. **Allergists** can be an excellent source of referral because many allergies are eye-related and may create vision problems.
5. **Internists** are similar to family practitioners because many symptoms of problems in internal medicine, such as headaches, are eye- and vision-related.
6. **Cardiopulmonary specialists** see optometric patients who will need co-management if they are taking certain medications.
7. **Plastic surgeons** frequently require the services of an optometrist for their patients after eye surgery, and specifically, blepharoplasty. Many contact lens problems need treatment after surgery.
8. **Podiatrists** see and treat many elderly patients who also require continuing eye care. They work well with optometrists.
9. **Chiropractors** see patients who complain of headaches that might necessitate ophthalmic management.
10. **Industrial physicians** frequently see patients with injuries, such as foreign body injuries, that benefit from optometric care.
11. **Nurses** are extremely good referral sources because patients who complain of eye strain, headache, and red eyes often seek their advice first. They are respected and trusted by other health care professionals. They are influenced and motivated by quality care. The positions that nurses might fill include:
    - Corporate staff nurses
    - Clinic nurses
    - Hospital nurses
    - School nurses
    - Visiting and licensed vocational nurses

appropriate professional; included should be a brief note indicating that the professional might find the article of interest.

Working with Ophthalmologists

A mutual referral relationship with a local ophthalmologist must include a one-on-one discussion of vision care philosophies, including protocols to be used for the co-management of specific vision and eye health conditions. To initiate referral relationships, the practitioner should research the ophthalmologists within a wide radius of the practice. Most important are those physicians who do not offer services similar to those of the practitioner (including those who have optometrists on staff). Surrounding colleagues should be asked to whom they refer.

Each practitioner must fully understand and respect the other to establish a successful relationship. For a beginning optometrist, it is helpful to discuss specific referral procedures, such as when to refer, how to make an appointment, what to provide in a referral letter, and when the ophthalmologist will provide written follow-up after the consultation. When co-management is necessary, protocols for care should be established and reduced to writing. Table 27-1 provides an example of a co-management protocol.

For an optometrist to establish a long-term relationship with an ophthalmologist, each practitioner must understand and agree on the other's philosophy of care. For the patient's benefit, there should be no duplication of testing except when absolutely necessary. Information should be freely shared and care coordinated to eliminate duplicative or unnecessary follow-up.

A similar rapport must be established with a retinal specialist for the management of patients with diabetes, vitreous disorders, and retinal diseases. Inter-referral relationships with neuro-ophthalmologists, oculoplastic specialists, and other ophthalmologists will be less frequent, but the same frank discussions and agreements are needed to ensure strong professional relationships.

Working with Co-management Centers

Eye care referral and surgical centers have been established nationwide. These centers capitalize on the value of inter-referral relationships. For years, referral was primarily from optometrists to ophthalmologists. Referral and surgical centers have been able to bring ophthalmologists and optometrists together in an association that produces the most efficient health care delivery system for eye care. Each professional practices at the highest level of competency. The initial evaluation and follow-up are provided by the optometrist and surgery is performed by the ophthalmologist. Patients referred for care often receive medical and surgical treatment that is beyond the scope of practice for the referring optometrist.

Table 27-1 Sample Co-management Protocol*

CATARACT		
POST-OP VISIT	**PROCEDURES**	**EXPECTEDS**
1 day surgeon		Follow-up report
1 week surgeon	BVA, IOP, SLE, refraction	Follow-up report
4 week OD	Refraction	Follow-up report
6 week OD	BVA, IOP, SLE dilated fundus examination	Follow-up report
9-12 months OD	Evaluate capsule	Follow-up report
	Retinal examination	
	IOP check	
Medication tapering protocol—suggested		
1 week	Tobradex qid	
3 weeks	Pred Forte tid tapered by 1 drop/day	
	each week for 3 weeks as inflammation subsides	

Courtesy Dr. Randall Reichle, Eye Associates of Houston, Houston, TX.
*Contact the co-management center immediately when patient response is outside normal limits.
BVA, best visual acuity; IOP, intraocular pressure, SLE, slit lamp examination.

Because information must be freely transferred between the referring practitioner and the co-management center—often on a timely basis—facsimile transmission is necessary. The use of fax machines permits medical information to be instantly shared by practitioners, allowing diagnostic and treatment decisions to be made on the basis of current data. Use of facsimile transmission has become state-of-the-art in eye care and should be considered a necessity when working with co-management centers.

Obtaining Referrals from Optometrists

Because of the expanded scope of optometric practice and the advanced education (such as residency training) available in many areas of optometry, more and more optometrists are now specializing in limited areas of eye care. If an individual practitioner does not provide specialized services, professional ethics and legal standards of care can demand that patients who require specialized services be referred to the appropriate optometric or other health care specialist.

Optometrist-to-optometrist referrals can become problematic if the practitioner referred to performs the slightest service ordinarily performed by the referring doctor. It also is essential to ensure the patient is returned to the referring doctor and that the relationship is a reciprocating one. Therefore, the practitioner referred to must make an appointment for the patient to return to the referring doctor.

Examples of specialized practice include pediatrics, low vision, diagnosis of disease, contact lenses, and sports vision.

Pediatric Care. The pediatric specialist will have a practice that is geared toward the young patient, including children's waiting room furniture, pediatric acuity and visual skills assessment charts, up-to-date electronic training equipment, and an unusually large selection of children's eyewear in the dispensary.

The pediatric optometrist offers developmental vision services and treatment for conditions such as strabismus, amblyopia, visually related learning disabilities, and vision perception problems. Today's pediatric optometric specialist also might be well versed in the fitting of infant or newborn eyeglasses. Contact lenses also can be fitted when necessary due to prematurity, surgery, or other related conditions. Pediatric optometrists work closely with teachers, counselors, and family members to ensure that there is continual feedback on any progress achieved in the treatment of the child's condition.

Low Vision. Although there are some "stand alone" low vision clinics, most low vision specialists are located in a facility that provides other vision and eye care services. These optometrists are located in facilities because it is difficult for a low vision practice to be financially self-sustaining. The low vision specialist provides a lengthy examination and uses unique equipment in the evaluation of the visually impaired patient. This equipment usually includes specialized low vision acuity and visual field tests, as well as a large variety of sizes and powers of magnifiers, handheld and spectacle-mounted microscopes and telescopes, lights, and electronic low vision aids such as closed circuit televisions. As the U.S. population ages, referrals for low vision care are sure to grow. The low vision specialist works closely with other optometrists, ophthalmologists, and state agencies that fund low vision care.

Diagnosis of Disease. In the past, when a medical workup or report was needed by an optometrist, the patient was referred to an internist or specific medical specialist. In many instances, patients did not return after referral—physicians often sent referred patients to an ophthalmologist for follow-up care and rarely returned them to the optometrist. The optometrist rarely received reports about referred patients or even an acknowledgment of the referral.

The eye care referral center concept was born in the 1980s. Services offered through these referral centers include electrodiagnostic testing, fluorescein angiography, threshold visual field testing, medical care for ocular diseases, treatment of ocular emergencies, and most types of eye surgery. Contact lenses, refractive care, spectacles, low vision aids, and visual training usually are excluded from the care given at these centers.

Since the implementation of these centers, optometrists have been able to participate in the decision-making process for patient care. Most of these centers use an optometrist for the clinic director and a physician for the medical director. Because patients are returned to the referring practitioners, these organizations have ensured that optometrists will play a role in the continuing management and follow-up of patients. The feedback received from the referral centers also improves optometrists' education regarding the latest in disease diagnosis and treatment.

Optometric referral centers traditionally offer postgraduate continuing education courses for local and referring practitioners. For local optometrists, these centers usually provide medical care for patients during periods when the optometrists are out of their offices for sickness, vacation, or emergencies.

Contact Lens Specialists. Most contact lens specialists limit their practices to the fitting and care of contact lens patients. Many work primarily with the "hard to fit" patient. These specialists have the expertise to fit patients with dry eye syndrome, astigmatism, and presbyopia. They have the knowledge and ability to fit unusually shaped and traumatized corneas. Because they are usually on the "cutting edge" of contact lens development, these practitioners often participate in clinical trials of new contact lens materials and solutions.

Sports Vision Specialists. Some optometrists offer sports vision as a subspecialty. Sports vision optometrists provide expertise at all levels of competition, from professional leagues to children's sports. These practitioners detect vision problems affecting athletic performance, prescribe special eyewear for sports and leisure activities, provide training to enhance athletic performance, prescribe protective eyewear to prevent eye injuries, and manage eye injuries suffered during athletic competition. Like the highly competitive athletes they serve, vision care in this field is state of the art and requires the use of highly specialized equipment and techniques.

Professional Communications

Optometry's role in health care has expanded significantly, requiring optometrists to describe patient findings and recommend management to other practitioners in the health care field. Optometrists are called on by other health care disciplines to perform specific tests and procedures for patients. Optometrists might offer more services than at any time in the profession's history, but they must rely on others in the health care field to work cooperatively for the benefit of patients. This approach is relatively new to many practitioners who have been in practice for 10 or more years. Emphasis is on personal communications among practitioners—such as letters of referral, consultation and summary reports, and thank you letters or summary reports for patient referrals.

Letters of Referral

When referring patients to another practitioner or health care facility, certain procedures and protocols should be followed. To ensure that the patient receives the care desired, the appointment for the referral should be made while the patient is in the office. The office to which the patient is referred should be informed of the needs of the patient so that a timely appointment can be scheduled and the appropriate tests performed. A referral letter should be written and sent so that it arrives before the date of the future appointment (Figure 27-1). Timely arrival can require sending the letter by facsimile transmission if a same-day referral is arranged.

A referral letter should describe any or all of the following:
- Patient's name, age, sex
- Date of examination
- Chief complaint and symptoms
- History of past and current eye care
- Pertinent health history, including medications being taken
- Significant tests performed and findings obtained
- Diagnosis and treatment
- Reason for referral
- Date of referral appointment

Copies of any pertinent test results (e.g., visual fields) should be attached.

Consultation and Summary Reports

Consultations for Medicare-eligible patients operate under special rules that have been in effect since 1992. Many of these rules have been adopted in some format by major medical insurance companies. Patients might need consultation for one or more of the following reasons:
- Further testing before a definitive diagnosis is made
- Second opinions to confirm diagnosis or treatment
- Suggestions regarding ways to approach the treatment of a specific condition

When a patient is referred for a consultation, the referring practitioner should note the reason for the consultation and request a timely telephone call or written summary report from the practitioner to whom the patient has been referred.

Thank You for Referrals and Summary of Findings

When a patient is referred to an optometrist for treatment, diagnosis, or advice, a summary letter describing test results or recommendations for care should be sent by the optometrist to the referring practitioner or facility as soon as possible. In many instances, a telephone call on the day of the visit can be provided. Words of thanks should be part of the beginning and ending of the call or letter. The summary of testing and results or recommendations should be brief, if possible, and a copy should be retained for the optometrist's file.

Dr. M. Dee
1122 Friendly Street
Friendly, TX

Re: Mrs. I.M. Patient

Dear Dr. Dee:

I am referring Mrs. I.M. Patient, a 41-year-old white female seen in our office on April 5th, to you for treatment of diabetic retinopathy.

Mrs. Patient has been treated for diabetes for the past 11 years. She frequently fails to take her oral medication, however, and seldom checks her blood glucose level. She reports not having seen her family physician for 18 months.

Examination findings are as follows:

Best visual acuity	OD 20/30^{-3} OS 20/20^{-2}
Pupils	OD 4 mm R/D3/C3 No APD OS 4 mm R/D3/C3
Versions	Unrestricted
External assessment	Unremarkable
Intraocular pressures	OD 17 mmHg OS 16 mmHg
Fundus examination	Numerous dot and blot hemorrhages extending over four retinal fields in each eye. Hard exudates in and surrounding the macula in each eye, with retinal thickening. There is a hemorrhage in the macula of the right eye. Fundus photography was performed for documentation.
Amsler Grid	Positive OD

Impression: Preproliferative diabetic retinopathy, with clinically significant macular edema.

Mrs. Patient is being referred to you for fluorescein angiography and possible laser treatment. Please let me know if I can be of any further assistance in the care of this pleasant lady.

Sincerely,

Dr. Primary Care

Figure 27-1 Sample referral letter to an ophthalmologist.

A letter should communicate the necessary information in an easy-to-read format. The practitioner should read and check each letter for spelling and accuracy of information before signing it. A sample letter is provided in Figure 27-2.

Professional Courtesies and Exchange of Services

There are many ways of handling professional courtesy. Each practitioner should be guided by local and customary practices among health care practitioners in the community.

A common policy is to exchange services only and to exclude costs related to laboratory charges. Under such a policy, an optometrist and the optometrist's family can receive medical and dental care services without cost but must pay for the actual cost of materials such as gold fillings, bridgework, major medical tests, and medical appliances. Physicians, dentists, and other health care professionals (and their families) who are examined by the optometrist would enjoy the same courtesy, paying only for ophthalmic materials and not for services.

Just as frequently, many professionals exchange all the costs of care and treatment that are not reimbursable by third-party insurance carriers.

Dr. John C. Wright
1234 Aqueous Way
See Port, VA 35434

Re: Patient Tom Jones

Dear Dr. Wright:

Thank you for referring Mr. Jones for low vision care. When he was seen on Jan. 4th he related his entire visual and physical case history. Your letter explaining his diabetic retinopathy was most helpful. His chief complaint was his recent inability to read fine print.

His vision was evaluated using a complete series of magnifiers and microscopic low visual aids. His best vision result was achieved while using a 4x aspheric hand-held magnifier. He was pleased with his vision (J-1) while using this aid.

Our technician provided complete instructions regarding the use of this aid, and it was dispensed to him today. Mr. Jones was advised to return to your office for your continued care. I appreciate the opportunity to participate with you in his care.

Sincerely yours,

Dr. Low Vision

Figure 27-2 Sample thank you letter for a referral.

Successful optometrists will have the opportunity to examine most of the community's health care providers, as well as many nurses and ancillary medical personnel. It is always a rewarding policy to provide 10% to 20% professional courtesy to as many of the ancillary personnel as possible because they appreciate the gesture and they frequently make referrals.

When professional courtesy is offered, the same level of care should be offered as would be provided to a fee-for-service patient.

Developing and Cultivating Professional Relationships Through Common Interests

Generally, people who work or play together develop a common bond of trust and respect. Referrals are inevitable when a personal relationship occurs.

Communities usually offer many opportunities for professionals who share common interests to meet. Professionals possess leadership skills and usually share common interests in education, local government, and community service organizations. They share a civic responsibility to promote growth and excellence in the community. The opportunity to serve in charitable and service organizations is particularly meaningful. Although the primary goal of participation should be "service above self," as the Rotary Club's motto states, participation will nurture friendship as well as a professional association with others who share a civic-

minded attitude. Most professionals will pursue sports, social, or self-improvement activities. Among professionals who share similar interests, friendship is common. Such individuals are often mutually supporting and provide referrals to one another. Friendship becomes the basis for the sharing of care among patients.

Remembrances for Referring Practitioners on Special Occasions

The traditional Christmas or Thanksgiving gift to special referral sources can range from the inexpensive to the elaborate, depending on the extent of the relationship. The most important consideration is a "thank you" for the trust and confidence reposed in the optometrist. A thoughtful letter of appreciation can be as meaningful as, or, in some cases, even more meaningful than, the gift. Whatever is given, it is best to be original—the novel gift can be very effective and is more easily remembered. It also is essential to keep track of each year's gift to avoid duplication year after year.

A unique way to thank special referral sources can be used any time of the year—theater tickets or tickets to popular sporting events. Invitations for dinner or cultural events are always appreciated. Social occasions in which spouses or family members participate can further bond the relationship and cultivate strong professional ties.

Non–Health Care Professionals

In general, by developing a superb reputation for expertise and by developing the credentials of a true specialist, optometrists can become important referral sources for non–health care professionals. Accountants, attorneys, architects, and engineers understand the effort that is required to obtain an advanced degree. They can become excellent patients if they understand and appreciate the quality of optometric education and service. In turn, they should be afforded the respect and consideration that is merited by the years of education and training necessary in their fields of expertise.

Acknowledgement

The authors of this chapter in the first edition of *Business Aspects of Optometry* were Jack Bridwell, Michael Usdan, and Paul Farkas.

Bibliography

Anonymous: Meeting report: making effective referral decisions. *Optician* 194(12):14, 1987.

Baldwin B, Christensen B, Melton J: *Rx for success*. Midwest City, Okla, 1983, Vision Publications.

Balliett G: *Practice management*. New York, 1978, McGraw-Hill.

Bennett I: Building a practice the write way. *Optom Management* 19(6):63, 1983.

Bennett I: Bettering O.D.-M.D. referral relationships. *Optom Management* 24(12):43-5, 1988.

Bennett I: *Management for the eyecare practitioner*. Stoneham, Mass, 1993, Butterworth.

Biaggio MK, Bittner E: Psychology and optometry: interaction and collaboration. *Am Psychol* 45(12):1313-15, 1990.

Brahe NB: *15 Days to a great new practice*. Appleton, Wis, 1971, Project D Publications.

Brumberg JB: *Efficient ethical private practice*. Dania, Fla, 1981, Independent Ophthalmic Publishing.

Byers S, Cornett S: Nurses help lead interprofessional team. *Ohio Nurses Rev* 65(1):8, 1990.

Classé JG: *Legal aspects of optometry*. Boston, 1989, Butterworth.

Cohen A: Issues and problems relating to reporting relations in a medical center and comprehensive health care environment. *Optom Vis Sci* 73(5):321-2, 1996.

Cohn S: The referral revolution. *Optom Management* 21(11):26-30,32,34,39,42, 1985.

Elmstrom G: *Advanced management for optometrists*. Chicago, 1974, Professional Press.

Farkas P: Build a better contact lens practice. *Optom Management* 17(7):53, 1981.

Farkas P: Developing a contact lens practice. *Contact Lens J* 20(8):15-7, 1993.

Farkas P, Kassalow TW, Farkas B: Eight tips to build your contact lens practice. *Optom Management* 21(1):68-73, 1985.

Farkas P, Kassalow TW, Farkas B: "Extending" your extended wear practice. *Optom Management* 21(6):47-55, 1985.

Fortner C: Building cooperation with physicians: an interview with Charles Fortner. *Am Pharm* 30(2):24-6, 1990.

Gregg J: *The business of optometric practice*. New York, 1980, Advisory Enterprises.

Hillier CG, Rosenow EL: Optometric vision therapy rehabilitation in hospitals. *J Optom Vis Dev* 30(Summer):83-5, 1999.

Horder J: Working with general practitioners. *Br J Psychiatry* 153(10):513-20, 1988.

Hubler R: Confident, competent referrals. *Optom Economics* 2(9):15, 1992.

Jackson WE: Family physicians: their referral potential. *Optom Management* 25(7):79-84, 1989.

Kerfoot K: "Managing" professionals: the ultimate contradiction for nurse managers. *Nurse Economics* 6(6):321-2, 1988.

Mariano C: The case for inter-disciplinary collaboration. *Nurse Outlook* 37(6):285-8, 1989.

Mitchell G: Working with school nurses: improving children's vision and building relationships. *J Am Optom Assoc* 70(11):738-40, 1999.

Moss GL, Shaw-McMinn PG: *Eyecare business marketing and strategy*. Boston, Butterworth-Heinemann, 2001.

Munson BJ: Doctor to doctor. *Optom Economics* 1(10):35, 1991.

Richter S, Ettinger E: Study of physicians overlooking eye care, New York. *AOA News* 31(11):1-4, 1992.

Roberts BL: Communication between optometrists and physicians in referrals. *J Am Optom Assoc* 42(1):64-8, 1971.

Sachs L: Professional courtesy. *Optom Economics* 1(11):39-41, 1991.

Shaver DV Jr: Opticianry, optometry, and ophthalmology: an overview. *Med Care* 12(9):754-65, 1974.

Thurburn L, Annunziato T: *Modern optometry—1990; a practice management guide*. Houston, Texas, 1990, Practice Management Associates.

Walls LL: Issues for optometrists relating to interprofessional relations in a hospital and medical center. *Optom Vis Sci* 73(5):307-8, 1996.

Winslow C: Put some muscle in your referral relationships. *Rev Optom* 130(4):34-6, 1993.

Chapter 28

Recordkeeping Basics

John G. Classé

He listens well who takes notes.
Dante Alighieri *The Divine Comedy*

Recordkeeping is a necessary obligation in the practice of optometry. The primary reason for maintaining records is to facilitate management of a patient's case and to provide a current, comprehensive account of the care and treatment undertaken by the practitioner. It also is necessary to substantiate reimbursement under third-party vision and medical reimbursement plans, especially Medicare. Appropriate documentation is a necessary aspect of risk management and for the defense of malpractice claims (see Chapter 11). All optometrists should carefully organize, maintain, and preserve their patient records and should be aware of the legal ramifications of recordkeeping.

Paper or Electronic Recordkeeping?

A basic question facing any practitioner is how to maintain records: on paper, electronically, or a combination of the two methods? The answer often depends on the size and degree of computerization of the practice. Practitioners may not have the time and resources necessary to compile solely electronic records or convert paper records to electronic versions that can be called up, analyzed, and shared through computer programs (see Chapter 20). For this reason, the great majority of practices have paper records, although some patient information is recorded and transferred electronically (such as information for reimbursement under third-party programs). Regardless of the manner in which patient information is maintained, there are important management issues that every practitioner must address, including ownership and control of records, their form and content, the release of information, use of records as evidence, and retention of records.

Ownership and Control

The ownership of patient records in a solo practice vests with the individual practitioner who maintains them. Consequently, an associate who is employed by an optometrist has no claim to ownership of the records of patients seen by him or her in the practice, such records being the property of the employer. The ownership of patient records in a partnership or limited liability company will depend on the provisions of the partnership or limited liability company agreement. Ordinarily, these agreements will specify some form of co-ownership between the partners. A corporation will customarily own the records of the patients seen by employee practitioners. If an optometrist is the employee of a hospital, customarily all records are the property of the hospital and the practitioner has no right to claim them. Optometrists who have sold their practices or retired or whose patients have resorted to successor doctors are ethically obligated to transfer patient records or copies of them to the current optometrist when the patient so requests. The same is true for the estates of deceased optometrists.

The owner of patient records has the right of physical possession and control. As a general rule, such owners should not permit removal of the record from their control, except by court order. Therefore, neither the patient nor the patient's authorized representative (i.e., attorney) has a right to possession of the record, but the practitioner's right of physical control does not mean that the patient and variously interested third parties have no legal right of access to the record and the information it contains. Through numerous laws and court decisions patients have been given the right to view and copy their records or to appoint authorized representatives to examine them (discussed infra).

Form and Content of Records

The form, organization, and content of an optometrist's patient records are best determined by professional standards and not by specific legal requirements. Professional standards of practice for optometrists require that entries in the patient record contain a certain minimum of information, which is intended to provide proper substantiation of the care rendered to the patient. In maintaining records it is essential to document when and why the patient was seen, what was diagnosed, and what was done in terms of treatment. The problem-oriented record is an excellent way to organize this information.

The *problem-oriented record system* is solution-oriented and enables the practitioner to manage patients in a logical and efficient manner by helping to define problems, plan for their resolution, and properly monitor their progress. When used appropriately, the problem-oriented record system also provides the documentation that is essential for medicolegal purposes while necessitating minimal time for recording and interpretation.

There are four steps to the problem-oriented system of recordkeeping: formulating an adequate data base, compiling a problem list, formulating a plan to solve the identified problems, and using progress notes for follow-up.

Data Base

The data base begins with the collection of information sufficient to allow the practitioner to perform an adequate examination. The amount of information necessary to constitute an adequate data base will vary from patient to patient and from case to case but should include the chief complaint and all information essential to the proper evaluation of this complaint (patient profile, history, and examination findings).

The patient profile should include data such as age, race, sex, marital status, occupation, avocation, and special needs.

The history should include the chief complaint, history of present illness, ocular history, past medical history (including review of systems), family health history, and affect (alertness). Examination findings should include all pertinent tests and observations necessary to satisfy the standard of care (Figure 28-1).

Various forms may be used to record this information, and there are many sources from which personalized forms may be obtained to inscribe patient data efficiently and thoroughly.

Problem List

The use of a problem list enables the practitioner to review past and current problems at a glance, thereby assuring thoroughness and continuity of care. The list is based on positive examination findings and is an ongoing account of the problems that require management. The list is added to as old problems are resolved or as new problems develop and forms the basis for the diagnostic or therapeutic efforts undertaken by the practitioner (see Figure 28-1).

Plans

A plan must be developed for each problem, whether the problem is to be managed by the practitioner, co-managed in consultation with another health care provider, or referred to another practitioner for specialized care. The plan may consist of further diagnostic testing, the use of a specific treatment, or educational efforts directed at the patient. In formulating plans for specific problems, the practitioner should consider each of these components and note them in the patient record (see Figure 28-1).

The importance of patient education should not be overlooked. In some cases the practitioner will have a clinical and legal obligation to communicate with the patient concerning examination findings, to inform the patient of meaningful symptoms, or to warn of the risks associated with the use of certain ophthalmic products. Better understanding may be achieved in many cases through the use of printed forms, which also can serve to remind the patient of the importance of timely care.

Progress Notes

A practitioner may use progress notes to monitor any efforts to solve a particular problem, and when used the notes should be numbered and titled to correspond to the complete problem list for the patient (Figure 28-2). Progress notes also can be used for the evaluation of a specific chief complaint or for episodic care. In both instances the progress notes should follow a specific format, which requires

Text continued on p. 276

UAB School of Optometry
Primary Care Optometry Service

PATIENT: I. Need Care #123456
DOB: 5-15-43   AGE: 59
DATE: 6-27-02   DOCTOR: John G. O'Dee   INTERN: Stu Dense

PATIENT HX:

CC _decreased visual acuity OD at distance – near acuity "good" with readers_

HPI _decreased acuity x 6 months – seems to be getting worse_

PMH/ POH:

HTN (+/−)
CVA (+/−)
Other (+/−)
CAT (+/−)
Eye Sx (+/−)
Other (+/−)

DM (+/−)
Heart Dz (+/−)
LPE _6 weeks ago – all "OK"_
GLC (+/−)
Eye Injury (+/−) _trauma OS x 20 yrs_
LEE _4 years, Dr I. Care_

THY (+/−)
Pul Dz (+/−) _surgery to remove fluid from lung_
Dr _Paul Monary_
BV (+/−)
CL Wear _none_
Dr

FMH/FOH:

HTN (+/−)
CVA (+/−)
CAT (+/−)
Other Eye Dx (+/−)

DM (+/−)
Heart Dz (+/−)
GLC (+/−)

THY (+/−)
Other (+/−)
Blindness (+/−)

MEDS _none_

ALLERGIES _denies any allergies_

P/S: Voc _teacher_   Avoc _golf_   Tob (+/−)   ETOH (+/−) _2/day_ Other

ROS: GEN (+/−)   SKIN (+/−)   H/N (+/−)   ENT (+/−)   RESP (+/−)   CV (+/−)   GI (+/−)

UG (+/−)   MS (+/−)   NEURO (+/−)   HEM (+/−)   ENDO (+/−)   PSYCH (+/−) _oriented to time and place_

REFRACTION:

Current Rx: _near use only_   Date Rx obtained _4 years old_

	Sph	Cyl	Axis	Add	Seg type	Prism
OD	+2.25					
OS	+2.25					

VA SC DIST OD _20/40⁻²_ OS _20/50⁺¹_ OU _20/30⁻²_ NEAR OD _.40/1M_ OS _.40/1M_ OU _.40/1M_
CC DIST OD _____ OS _____ OU _____ NEAR OD _____ OS _____ OU _____

R OD _+1.00 −0.25 x 085_ VA _20/40⁺²_ **K** OD ___/___ @___ clr/distort
OS _+1.25 DS_ VA _20/30⁻²_ OS ___/___ @___ clr/distort

M₁ OD _+0.50 −0.25 x 048_ VA _20/40⁺²_ **M₂** OD _____ VA _____
OS _+0.75 −0.50 x 030_ VA _20/20_ OS _____ VA _____

ADD OD _+2.50_ VA _.37M_   METHOD _TF_   RANGE OD _25-53 cm_
OS _+2.50_ VA _.37M_   OS _25-53 cm_

TRIAL FRAME _preferred +2.50 over +2.25_

Confrontations _full OS, constricted OD_ Versions _full and smooth_   Pupils _PERRL 4+, neg APD_
Cover Test DIST _ø_   NEAR _4ᐃ XP_   THRU _sc_   BP _142/75 RAS_ @ _11_ (AM) PM
OTHER TESTS:

Figure 28-1 Sample examination form illustrating documentation of data base, problem list, and plan. (Courtesy UAB school of Optometry, Birmingham, Ala. Reprinted with permission.)   Continued

PATIENT: I. Need Care   **DOB:** 5-15-43
DOCTOR: John G. O'Dee   **DATE:** 6-27-02

OCULAR HEALTH:

T (G)P/Tpen OD __24__ OS __23__ @ __10:45__ (AM) PM
Ist Fluress apprehension moderate

SLIT LAMP EXAM:

DILATE _1gt T 1%, 1gt PE 2.5%_ @ __10:50__ (AM) PM
Dilation warning given __SD__ (initial)
FUNDUS EXAM: (BIO) DO MIO Lens: 60 78 90 (SF)

OS rosette cataract

LIDS/LASHES __no ptosis, lashes clear OU__

CONJ __pingueula N+T OU__

CORNEA __arcus 360° OU__

IRIS __intact OU__

AC __deep and open OU__

ANGLE __1:½ T 1:¼ N OU__

LENS __NS 2⁺ OD, 1⁺ OS   traumatic cataract OS__

ONH __margins distinct, NRR eroded vertically OD__

C/D __OD ·6/·8   OS ·5/·6__

MACULA __FLR(+) avascular OU__

VESSELS __A/V ²/₃ tortuous OS>OD__

POST. POLE __no hemorrhages or exudation OU__

VITREOUS __attached OU__

PERIPHERY __lattice inferiorly OU__

lattice degeneration
w/o holes

ASSESSMENT:	PLAN:
① Glaucoma suspect	① RTC x 1 day for threshold visual fields and gonioscopy
② Nuclear sclerosis OD>OS	② Monitor x 1 year
③ Traumatic cataract	③ Monitor x 1 year – look for angle recession during gonioscopy
④ CHA OU and presbyopia	④ Prescribe M, with +2.50 add – patient educated on lens design options for golf

FINAL RX:

	SPH	CYL	AXIS	ADD	PRISM
OD	+0.50	−0.25	048	+2.50	
OS	+0.75	−0.50	050	+2.50	

RTC: (1d) 1wk 1mo 3mo 6mo 1yr 2yr

FOR __visual field testing, gonioscopy__

INTERN __Stu Dence__

I have seen the patient personally and performed key parts of the examination.
ATTENDING __gJ O'Dee__   O.D.

Figure 28-1, Cont'd

PROGRESS NOTE

PATIENT: I. Need Care

DATE: 6-28-02   DOCTOR: John G. O'Dee

S   RTC x 1 day for completion of evaluation for POAG. Gonioscopy and
    threshold visual fields to be performed today.

O   dist | sc / 20/40⁻² | near | sc / .40/1M | PERRL 2/2- neg APD
    20/50⁺¹   .40/1M   EOMs F&S
    20/30⁻²   .40/1M

    Tapp <23/24 sualtg @ 11³⁰ am   Gonioscopy OD   OS
         1 gt Fluress

    Fields 30-2 performed with reliable results for
    both eyes. Nasal and arcuate field loss
    consistent with POAG noted OD, and a
    nasal step OS indicative of early POAG.

A   POAG OD>OS
    Angles are narrow but open.

P   Begin Travatan OU q pm 1gt. Return in 1 month for IOP check and
    repeat visual fields.

I have seen the patient personally and performed key parts of the examination.

_____
Faculty/Resident Signature

Figure 28-2 Sample progress note.

a four-step evaluation, often referred to by the mnemonic *SOAP*:

- *S*ubjective complaint or updated case history
- *O*bjective findings or observations
- *A*ssessment of findings or progress of case
- *P*lan for the problems listed in the assessment

The SOAP format is widely used by the medical profession and readily accepted in legal proceedings.

Documentation for Medicare Patients

Special obligations exist for Medicare patients. Medical insurance plans such as Medicare have formalized the manner in which medical diagnoses and procedures must be documented and reported. Medical diagnoses may be found in the federal government's *International Classification of Diseases (ICD)* handbook, which is used by the Health Care Financing Administration (HCFA, renamed Centers for Medicare and Medicaid) for the Medicare program. Five-digit codes are used to represent the medical diagnoses listed in the handbook; these codes are reported by providers for purposes of reimbursement. For example, the code 365.01 means "glaucoma suspect."

Procedural codes are listed in *Current Procedural Terminology (CPT)*, which is published by the American Medical Association. CPT has been adopted for use in the Medicare program. These five-digit codes represent the services provided to patients and are reported for purposes of reimbursement. For example, the code 92083 corresponds to "threshold visual fields."

For a provider to appropriately code and bill a Medicare patient, the diagnosis (ICD) code must relate to the procedure (CPT) code. For example, the case of a patient who presents for treatment of a corneal abrasion and whose examination is given a procedural code for a comprehensive examination would be miscoded if the examination in fact consisted of a history, acuities, and slit lamp evaluation.

The key consideration is the reason for the patient's visit; reimbursement "depends on the purpose of the examination rather than on the ultimate diagnosis of the patient's condition." For example, a presbyopic patient who presents for examination with a complaint that the bifocal does not seem to be strong enough but is found to also have open-angle glaucoma does not have a medical diagnosis for purposes of reimbursement because the medical finding does not correspond to the complaint. Even though open-angle glaucoma is listed as a diagnosis, it cannot be used for reimbursement of this examination. Subsequent examinations will qualify for medical insurance reimbursement,

however, because the patient will be returning for treatment of a medical condition.

Diagnostic codes are fairly straightforward, since all that is required is that they be looked up in the CPT handbook. Procedural codes are more complex because there are two types of procedural codes currently in use—92000 codes and 99000 codes (see Chapter 37). These codes are monitored for accuracy through audits, and providers are expected to understand and adhere to them when submitting claims for reimbursement. If the level of reimbursement exceeds the actual level of service, the provider can be held responsible for the excess amounts paid and be required to forfeit not only the overbilled amounts but also penalties, based on the amounts overpaid.

Release of Patient Information

One of the most important issues in the management of patient records is the release of information. There are significant differences in the obligation faced by practitioners, based on whether the information is being released to the patient or to a third party.

Release of Information to Patients

The right of patients to inspect and copy information in medical records has been established by both statutes and court decisions. Federal and state freedom-of-information acts require the release of copies of patient records on demand by the patient. State optometry practice acts provide for disciplinary actions to be instituted against practitioners based on allegations of unprofessional conduct if they refuse to comply with requests for information or copies of records. Optometry board rules or regulations also have been enacted that require optometrists to release patient information when presented with a valid request. Again, failure to comply subjects the optometrist to the possibility of disciplinary action.

In addition to these provisions, courts have been active in defining the rights of patients to medical information. Although decisions have recognized that health care practitioners have a right to withhold information from patients, the circumstances under which this right may be exercised are generally limited to life-threatening conditions and psychological dysfunction. In these cases the courts have weighed the patient's right to obtain the information and the practitioner's right to keep what is believed to be harmful revelations from the patient. Situations under which an optometrist could invoke such a defense would be extraordinary.

Thus patients are generally entitled to obtain their health care information from optometrists.

The release of prescription information to patients is subject to special federal and state laws.

Spectacle Prescriptions. All practitioners are required to comply with the prescription requirements of the Federal Trade Commission's (FTC) "Eyeglasses Rule," which is applicable in every jurisdiction. The basic provisions of the rule are as follows:

- The doctor must offer a copy of the spectacle prescription to the patient at the conclusion of the examination.
- If the doctor determines that there is no reason to prescribe spectacles, no prescription needs to be tendered to the patient.
- If the patient is wearing spectacles, and no change in the prescription is required, the prescription still must be offered to the patient even though there will be no change in the spectacles.
- The prescription must contain information sufficient for spectacles to be obtained, and it must be signed by the doctor; if state laws or board regulations require specific information to be provided, the doctor must include the additional information in the prescription.
- A doctor can charge a fee for writing a prescription if all patients are charged a fee for this service (and not just patients who choose to obtain their spectacles elsewhere).
- An expiration date can be placed on the prescription as long as it is reasonable (the expiration date may be regulated by statute or board rule in the jurisdiction–1 year is a commonly accepted period).
- A fee can be charged for verifying spectacles obtained from another ophthalmic provider.
- No disclaimers can be placed on the prescription.

Violations of the rule are punishable by a fine of up to $10,000 per offense.

Contact Lens Prescriptions. The FTC "Eyeglasses Rule" does not apply to contact lens prescriptions. The obligation to provide contact lens information to patients is determined by state laws or board rules or regulations. The majority of jurisdictions require the release of contact lens information, but usually only if an examination for contact lenses has been performed and the patient has worn the lenses for a specified period to ensure that acuity, physiological response, and comfort are adequate. In some jurisdictions specific information must be included in a contact lens prescription. Because of these differences, individual state laws or board rules or regulations must be consulted to determine whether prescriptions must be released to patients and to ascertain the information that must be provided.

Whenever contact lens prescriptions are provided, it is in the best interests of both patient and practitioner to include as much information as possible and in all cases to include at least the minimum amount of information specified by state law (see Chapter 31).

Release of Information to Third Parties

The release of information to third parties has been the subject of considerable regulation by the government, particularly since the development of electronic records and reimbursement systems based on the transmission of information through computers. In general, it has long been held that patient information should not be provided to a third party without the patient's consent and that this consent is best documented through a signed release. (Similarly, when an optometrist requests patient information from a doctor or institution, the optometrist should be certain to have a signed, current release from the patient directing the doctor or institution to send the record or summary to the optometrist.) In addition, whenever patient information is to be divulged to a third party, only as much information as is necessary to comply with the request should be provided. The full patient record must be released only on rare occasions (such as when there is a statutory obligation to do so or the practitioner has received a legal order to do so due to litigation). In most instances, a letter containing a summary is sufficient, and the practitioner should transmit only the information actually requested, retaining a copy of the summary for inclusion in the original record.

Because of third-party insurance programs and electronic transmission of information, concerns have arisen about the confidentiality of patient information and how it can best be safeguarded. These concerns have led to the passage of a landmark federal law, known as the Health Insurance Portability and Accountability Act (HIPAA).

Confidentiality and the Health Insurance Portability and Accountability Act

HIPAA was passed in 1996 to make health insurance "portable" so workers would not lose their insurance when they changed jobs. The law also included provisions intended to increase the use of electronic transactions and established privacy protection for health care information. If legislation providing regulations for HIPAA was not passed within 3 years, however, it was left to the U.S. Department of Health and Human Services (DHHS) to do so. Congress failed to pass the legislation. Accordingly, DHHS has promulgated three types of regulations: setting standards for electronic transactions; setting certain security standards; and setting standards designed to ensure the privacy of health care information. Practitioners were expected to comply with the last standard—the "privacy rules"—by 2003.

The HIPAA "privacy rules" are extensive, but contain the following three basic requirements:

- HIPAA creates restrictions on the use or disclosure of "individually identifiable health care information"
- Rights are established with respect to a person's own "individually identifiable health care information"
- Health care providers are required to take certain administrative actions that are intended to protect the privacy of "individually identifiable health care information"

Optometrists are deemed "health care providers" under HIPAA. Any information created or received by an optometrist from a patient that identifies the patient is defined as "individually identifiable health care information" and thus subject to HIPAA.

The first HIPAA requirement involves restrictions on the use of health care information: optometrists "cannot use or disclose protected health information, except as permitted or required by the rules." There are 10 disclosure exceptions, the most important being the following:

- With the patient's consent (HIPAA requires that the consent be in writing and describes what must be in it)
- Without consent for treatment, payment, or certain health care operations (e.g., emergencies, if there are barriers to communication)
- With a specific authorization (if disclosure is sought for reasons other than treatment, payment, or general health care operations)
- With a written contract for "business associates" (such as nonemployee claims processing, quality assurance, billing)

When using or providing protected health care information, reasonable efforts must be made to limit information to the minimum necessary to accomplish the use or disclosure.

The second HIPAA requirement establishes the following privacy rights:

- Every practitioner must have a "privacy notice" for patients, the contents of which are established by HIPAA
- Patients are given the right to inspect and obtain copies of their medical and billing records
- Patients have the right to ask the practitioner to amend records
- Patients can request an account of all disclosures of personal health information by a provider within the preceding 6 years (except those for treatment, payment, or health care operations)

The third HIPAA requirement establishes several administrative requirements to ensure compliance with the privacy rules, including the following:

- A "privacy officer" must be appointed by the provider
- Employees must undergo training so they understand HIPAA
- Safeguards must be put in place to ensure that the privacy of personal health information is protected
- A complaint process for patients must be established
- Sanctions must be imposed on employees who do not comply with HIPAA provisions
- Patients cannot be required to waive HIPAA rights as a condition for treatment nor can they be punished for exercising these rights
- Policies and procedures must be documented in writing

Sample agreements have been published by the American Optometric Association to serve as exemplars for HIPAA documentation, including *notice of privacy practices*, which describes how patient information may be used and disclosed and how patients can get access to it (Figure 28-3), and *patient authorization*, which allows for the release of identifying health information (Figure 28-4). Practitioners must have similar agreements and use them appropriately to avoid HIPAA violations.

HIPAA represents the first effort to impose national standards for the protection of health information. DHSS enforces the HIPAA requirements, and penalties range from a $100 fine per violation to fines as much as $250,000 and up to 10 years in prison for malicious use of records.

Records as Evidence in Litigation

The patient records of optometrists are generally open to legal scrutiny in virtually all jurisdictions, a fact that adds extra importance to a practitioner's recordkeeping burden. Whenever optometric patients are parties to litigation, the likelihood is great that the optometrist's

Text continued on p. 283

Effective date of notice: _____

NOTICE OF PRIVACY PRACTICES

_____, O.D.
[mailing address]
[phone number]
[fax number]
[E Mail]
[office contact person]

THIS NOTICE DESCRIBES HOW MEDICAL INFORMATION ABOUT YOU MAY BE USED AND DISCLOSED AND HOW YOU CAN GET ACCESS TO THIS INFORMATION. PLEASE REVIEW IT CAREFULLY.

We respect our legal obligation to keep health information that identifies you private. We are obligated by law to give you notice of our privacy practices. This Notice describes how we protect your health information and what rights you have regarding it.

TREATMENT, PAYMENT, AND HEALTH CARE OPERATIONS

The most common reason why we use or disclose your health information is for treatment, payment or health care operations. Examples of how we use or disclose information for treatment purposes are: setting up an appointment for you; testing or examining your eyes; prescribing glasses, contact lenses, or eye medications and faxing them to be filled; showing you low vision aids; referring you to another doctor or clinic for eye care or low vision aids or services; or getting copies of your health information from another professional that you may have seen before us. Examples of how we use or disclose your health information for payment purposes are: asking you about your health or vision care plans, or other sources of payment; preparing and sending bills or claims; and collecting unpaid amounts (either ourselves or through a collection agency or attorney). "Health care operations" mean those administrative and managerial functions that we have to do in order to run our office. Examples of how we use or disclose your health information for health care operations are: financial or billing audits; internal quality assurance; personnel decisions; participation in managed care plans; defense of legal matters; business planning; and outside storage of our records.

We routinely use your health information inside our office for these purposes without any special permission. If we need to disclose your health information outside of our office for these reasons, [we will] [we usually will not] ask you for special written permission.

[We will ask for special written permission in the following situations: _____ .]

USES AND DISCLOSURES FOR OTHER REASONS WITHOUT PERMISSION

In some limited situations, the law allows or requires us to use or disclose your health information without your permission. Not all of these situations will apply to us; some may never come up at our office at all. Such uses or disclosures are:

- when a state or federal law mandates that certain health information be reported for a specific purpose;

- for public health purposes, such as contagious disease reporting, investigation or surveillance; and notices to and from the federal Food and Drug Administration regarding drugs or medical devices;

- disclosures to governmental authorities about victims of suspected abuse, neglect or domestic violence;

- uses and disclosures for health oversight activities, such as for the licensing of doctors; for audits by Medicare or Medicaid; or for investigation of possible violations of health care laws;

- disclosures for judicial and administrative proceedings, such as in response to subpoenas or orders of courts or administrative agencies;

- disclosures for law enforcement purposes, such as to provide information about someone who is or is suspected to be a victim of a crime; to provide information about a crime at our office; or to report a crime that happened somewhere else;

Figure 28-3 Sample notice of privacy practices, required by HIPAA, describing how patient information may be used and disclosed and how patients can get access to it. (Courtesy American Optometric Association, St. Louis. Reprinted with permission.)

Continued

- disclosure to a medical examiner to identify a dead person or to determine the cause of death; or to funeral directors to aid in burial; or to organizations that handle organ or tissue donations;

- uses or disclosures for health related research;

- uses and disclosures to prevent a serious threat to health or safety;

- uses or disclosures for specialized government functions, such as for the protection of the president or high ranking government officials; for lawful national intelligence activities; for military purposes; or for the evaluation and health of members of the foreign service;

- disclosures of de-identified information;

- disclosures relating to worker's compensation programs;

- disclosures of a "limited data set" for research, public health, or health care operations;

- incidental disclosures that are an unavoidable by-product of permitted uses or disclosures;

- disclosures to "business associates" who perform health care operations for us and who commit to respect the privacy of your health information;

- [specify other uses and disclosures affected by state law].

Unless you object, we will also share relevant information about your care with your family or friends who are helping you with your eye care.

APPOINTMENT REMINDERS

We may call or write to remind you of scheduled appointments, or that it is time to make a routine appointment. We may also call or write to notify you of other treatments or services available at our office that might help you.

OTHER USES AND DISCLOSURES

We will not make any other uses or disclosures of your health information unless you sign a written "authorization form." The content of an "authorization form" is determined by federal law. Sometimes, we may initiate the authorization process if the use or disclosure is our idea. Sometimes, you may initiate the process if it's your idea for us to send your information to someone else. Typically, in this situation you will give us a properly completed authorization form, or you can use one of ours.

If we initiate the process and ask you to sign an authorization form, you do not have to sign it. If you do not sign the authorization, we cannot make the use or disclosure. If you do sign one, you may revoke it at any time unless we have already acted in reliance upon it. Revocations must be in writing. Send them to the office contact person named at the beginning of this Notice.

YOUR RIGHTS REGARDING YOUR HEALTH INFORMATION

The law gives you many rights regarding your health information. You can:

- ask us to restrict our uses and disclosures for purposes of treatment (except emergency treatment), payment or health care operations. We do not have to agree to do this, but if we agree, we must honor the restrictions that you want. To ask for a restriction, send a written request to the office contact person at the address, fax or E Mail shown at the beginning of this Notice.

- ask us to communicate with you in a confidential way, such as by phoning you at work rather than at home, by mailing health information to a different address, or by using E mail to your personal E Mail address. We will accommodate these requests if they are reasonable, and if you pay us for any extra cost. If you want to ask for confidential communications, send a written request to the office contact person at the address, fax or E mail shown at the beginning of this Notice.

- ask to see or to get photocopies of your health information. By law, there are a few limited situations in which we can refuse to permit access or copying. For the most part, however, you will be able to review or have a copy of your health information within 30 days of asking us (or sixty days if the information is stored off-site). You may have to pay for photocopies in advance. If we deny your request, we will send you a written explanation, and instructions about how to get an impartial review of our denial if one is legally available. By law, we can have one 30 day extension of the time for us to give you access or

Figure 28-3, Cont'd

photocopies if we send you a written notice of the extension. If you want to review or get photocopies of your health information, send a written request to the office contact person at the address, fax or E mail shown at the beginning of this Notice.

- ask us to amend your health information if you think that it is incorrect or incomplete. If we agree, we will amend the information within 60 days from when you ask us. We will send the corrected information to persons who we know got the wrong information, and others that you specify. If we do not agree, you can write a statement of your position, and we will include it with your health information along with any rebuttal statement that we may write. Once your statement of position and/or our rebuttal is included in your health information, we will send it along whenever we make a permitted disclosure of your health information. By law, we can have one 30 day extension of time to consider a request for amendment if we notify you in writing of the extension. If you want to ask us to amend your health information, send a written request, including your reasons for the amendment, to the office contact person at the address, fax or E mail shown at the beginning of this Notice.

- get a list of the disclosures that we have made of your health information within the past six years (or a shorter period if you want). By law, the list will not include: disclosures for purposes of treatment, payment or health care operations; disclosures with your authorization; incidental disclosures; disclosures required by law; and some other limited disclosures. You are entitled to one such list per year without charge. If you want more frequent lists, you will have to pay for them in advance. We will usually respond to your request within 60 days of receiving it, but by law we can have one 30 day extension of time if we notify you of the extension in writing. If you want a list, send a written request to the office contact person at the address, fax or E mail shown at the beginning of this Notice.

- get additional paper copies of this Notice of Privacy Practices upon request. It does not matter whether you got one electronically or in paper form already. If you want additional paper copies, send a written request to the office contact person at the address, fax or E mail shown at the beginning of this Notice.

OUR NOTICE OF PRIVACY PRACTICES

By law, we must abide by the terms of this Notice of Privacy Practices until we choose to change it. We reserve the right to change this notice at any time as allowed by law. If we change this Notice, the new privacy practices will apply to your health information that we already have as well as to such information that we may generate in the future. If we change our Notice of Privacy Practices, we will post the new notice in our office, have copies available in our office, and post it on our Web site.

COMPLAINTS

If you think that we have not properly respected the privacy of your health information, you are free to complain to us or the U.S. Department of Health and Human Services, Office for Civil Rights. We will not retaliate against you if you make a complaint. If you want to complain to us, send a written complaint to the office contact person at the address, fax or E mail shown at the beginning of this Notice. If you prefer, you can discuss your complaint in person or by phone.

FOR MORE INFORMATION

If you want more information about our privacy practices, call or visit the office contact person at the address or phone number shown at the beginning of this Notice.

---tear here---

ACKNOWLEDGEMENT OF RECEIPT

I acknowledge that I received a copy of [*name of O.D.'s*] Notice of Privacy Practices.

Patient name _____

Signature _____ Date _____

Figure 28-3, Cont'd

_____, O.D.
[*address*]
[*phone number*]
[*fax number*]
[*E Mail*]
[*office contact person*]

AUTHORIZATION FOR RELEASE OF IDENTIFYING HEALTH INFORMATION

Patient name_____

Patient number _____

Patient address _____

Patient phone number _____

I authorize the professional office of my optometrist named above to release health information identifying me [including if applicable, information about HIV infection or AIDS, information about substance abuse treatment, and information about mental health services] under the following terms and conditions:

1. Detailed description of the information to be released:

2. To whom may the information be released (name(s) or class(es) of recipients):

3. The purpose(s) for the release (if the authorization is initiated by the individual, it is permissible to state "at the request of the individual" as the purpose, if desired by the individual):

4. Expiration date or event relating to the individual or purpose for the release:

It is completely your decision whether or not to sign this authorization form. We cannot refuse to treat you if you choose not to sign this authorization.

If you sign this authorization, you can revoke it later. The only exception to your right to revoke is if we have already acted in reliance upon the authorization. If you want to revoke your authorization, send us a written or electronic note telling us that your authorization is revoked. Send this note to the office contact person listed at the top of this form.

When your health information is disclosed as provided in this authorization, the recipient often has no legal duty to protect its confidentiality. In many cases, the recipient may re-disclose the information as he/she wishes. Sometimes, state or federal law changes this possibility.

[For marketing authorizations, include, as applicable: We will receive direct or indirect remuneration from a third party for disclosing your identifiable health information in accordance with this authorization.]

I HAVE READ AND UNDERSTAND THIS FORM. I AM SIGNING IT VOLUNTARILY. I AUTHORIZE THE DISCLOSURE OF MY HEALTH INFORMATION AS DESCRIBED IN THIS FORM.

Dated _____ Patient signature _____

If you are signing as a personal representative of the patient, describe your relationship to the patient and the source of your authority to sign this form:

Relationship to Patient _____ Print Name _____

Source of Authority _____

Figure 28-4 Sample authorization to release identifying health information, required for compliance with HIPAA. (Courtesy American Optometric Association, St. Louis. Reprinted with permission.)

records, if needed for the purposes of litigation, will be obtainable.

Attorneys will seek by means of pretrial discovery to obtain information from the records of patients who are parties to litigation or from documents that they believe will aid the preparation and trial of the lawsuit. Depositions and orders to produce will be the usual means of obtaining this information. If the attorney seeks to have such information entered into evidence at court, the attorney will serve the optometrist with a *subpoena duces tecum*, which orders the optometrist to appear with the record in a court or other duly constituted tribunal that has jurisdiction over the pending litigation. In most instances the optometrist will not be a party to the lawsuit, merely the person in possession of records that may or may not be relevant to the case. Therefore, the fight over what is pertinent or admissible will be between the opposing attorneys, and the optometrist will rely on the rulings of the court as to whether to provide the information. If the optometrist is a party to the case, then the dispute is of more immediate interest, and the optometrist should obey the instructions of the optometrist's attorney in handling and discussing patient records. It should be mentioned that there also is no privilege of confidentiality under federal law, and so the Internal Revenue Service can obtain access to optometric records for tax purposes.

Of course, the most worrisome type of litigation is a malpractice case in which the optometrist is the defendant. More likely than not, in such a lawsuit the patient record will either be the cornerstone of the optometrist's defense or the optometrist's Achilles' heel. Well-documented records may be of critical importance in proving that no negligence occurred or in refuting the patient's allegations of improper diagnosis or treatment. Even though proper completion of all records on each patient is obviously time consuming and probably an active nuisance, an optometrist who is sued by a patient (usually a considerable time after treatment has been terminated) will be in a much more favorable position if the optometrist's records indicate clearly that proper treatment was given. On the other hand, records that disclose negligent treatment will materially benefit a patient's case. Records that have been altered for any reason, even the most innocent, should always include notations of the date and reason for the change. If a negligence suit is filed subsequent to alteration of a record, and that alteration is apparent, it will undoubtedly be construed as a dishonest attempt to avoid liability.

Because patient records are entered into evidence with great frequency, extraneous comments should be assiduously avoided. In particular, comments that denigrate the patient or members of the patient's family should be omitted since they convey the impression that the doctor is not interested in the patient's welfare.

Retention of Records

An important consideration in the maintenance of records is how long they must be retained. Although optometrists do not collect the kind of information that is likely to be used in litigation, there is always a chance that an optometrist could be an important witness or party to a legal claim filed long after the patient has been dismissed. Ideally, no patient records should be thrown away, and there are ways to preserve records (especially if electronic copies are kept) without incurring great expense or requiring copious amounts of space. But, if records are to be eventually discarded, the optometrist should be sure that they have been retained for the period of time required to satisfy the following:

- State laws or optometry board rules or regulations
- HIPAA requirements
- The statute of limitations for tort or contract actions
- The statute of limitations for actions brought by Medicare or other third-party insurance programs

These periods vary from jurisdiction to jurisdiction and range from 1 to 15 years. A prudent practitioner should consult with legal counsel before discarding patient records to ensure that pertinent time periods have been satisfied. If records are stored, they should be kept in a facility where they will not be damaged or destroyed.

Conclusion

A beginning practitioner must make some important decisions about records and documentation in conjunction with the computer hardware and software selected for the office. Office protocols for the release of information must be established and must conform to the demands of HIPAA and pertinent state laws or board rules or regulations. In addition, appropriate measures must be taken to store and maintain records during the period necessary to comply with legal requirements.

Bibliography

American Optometric Association: *Scope of practice: patient care and management manual.* St. Louis, 1986, Author.

Avery M: *Medical records in ambulatory care.* Rockville, Md, 1984, Aspen Systems Corp.

Classé JG: *Legal aspects of optometry.* Boston, 1989, Butterworth.

Classé JG: *Standards of care for primary eyecare.* Columbus, Ohio, 1998, Anadem Publishing.

HIPAA regulations can be obtained online at *www.hhs.gov/hipaa.*

Holder A: *Medical malpractice law.* New York, 1976, Wiley & Sons.

Morris RC, Moritz AR: *Doctor and patient and the law,* ed 5. St. Louis, 1971, Mosby.

The "Eyeglasses" trade regulation rule can be found at 16 C.F.R. §456 (1978).

Weed L: *Medical records, medical education, and patient care.* Cleveland, Ohio, 1970, Press of Case Western Reserve.

Weed L: *Implementing the problem-oriented medical record.* Seattle, 1976, Medical Computer Services.

www.keyworlds.com/o/optometry-software. Online list of software for optometry practices.

Chapter 29

Recall Systems

Craig Hisaka

It ain't over 'til it's over.
Yogi Berra *Comment on 1973 baseball pennant race*

The scope of care in optometry has changed significantly during the past few decades. With this change in scope of practice and approach to services, there has been a concomitant change in the purpose and design of recall systems. In the past, the underlying motivation of a recall system was perceived as a strategy to "build a practice." The notion of "goodwill" was associated with recall systems because of the ability of these systems to sustain a practice. There have been several traditional reasons proffered for the use of such systems. A recall system provides an opportunity for the practitioner to get better acquainted with patients through regular interaction. Patients who enjoy a friendly relationship with a practitioner will (it is hoped) be more inclined to adhere to recommendations made by that practitioner. In recall sessions, the optometrist can regularly offer recommendations for preventing eye problems and detect problems unknown to the patients. Recall encourages patients to return for examinations—an important consideration because, frequently, patients will not take the initiative to return, even when they are satisfied with the care and treatment received.

Today, recall systems also are vital because they provide the practitioner with a mechanism to identify and monitor patients who are at risk for or suffer from pathological conditions. Recall serves as a way for the optometrist to keep patients informed of ocular health status and to properly evaluate and treat (when necessary) existing eye conditions. In fact, the concept of recall has been incorporated into the standard of care. Because of modern technology and instrumentation, the expanded scope of optometry, and the responsibilities of a primary care provider, the purpose of recall essentially has been redefined.

An inadequate recall system, which results in untimely examination of patients, can result in permanent harm and injury and lead to litigation. Therefore, a successful recall system must be a feature of any practitioner's office. In this chapter, various types of recall systems are described, beginning with the most fundamental consideration—implementation of a system that is compatible with the practitioner's philosophy of care.

Philosophy of Care

The philosophy of the practice often dictates the approach to and the organization of the recall system. The aggressiveness of the system chosen must be acceptable to the practitioner or practice and should not reflect adversely on the professionalism of either.

Methods of Recall

After examination, the practitioner must determine when the patient needs to return for further care. Depending on the patient's status, the appointment could be the next day, week, month, or year. The patient must be given a reminder of the appointment date. The patient needs to be given sufficient notice in advance of the appointment so that it can be changed if necessary, but it should not be so far in advance that the patient will forget. The time frame also needs to be such that, if the patient cancels the appointment, there is adequate time to schedule another patient in the vacated time slot.

There are three basic methods of providing recall to patients: mail, telephone, or a combination of both. (Mail and telephone systems actually tend to use both methods, but for the purposes of this discussion mail and telephone systems are classified as being primarily one of these methods.)

Mail Recall System. The mailing system is traditional and is used by most optometrists and dentists (Figure 29-1). It is probably the easiest system for an office to adopt. Since this approach is nonaggressive, the perception by patients should be favorable. In such a system a card is mailed notifying the patient that it is time for an examination to be scheduled or reminding the patient that a follow-up appointment has been scheduled. The patient is asked to call the office to make or confirm the appointment.

Because this recall system is passive, the patient response is lower than that with the other two methods. Also, the costs of printing and mailing makes this system expensive, and it can be time consuming for the staff. The system can be made more personal by using attractive cards or envelopes with picture stamps instead of metered postage, personalized messages generated by computer, and addresses written by hand instead of printed labels.

Telephone Recall System. The telephone recall system allows personal contact with patients. Because it is personalized, it creates a positive perception. However, patients who cannot say "no" when called may fail to appear at the scheduled time, and therefore the "no-show" rate still can be substantial. This method allows a practitioner to obtain information about why patients have not returned and, if applicable, the reasons why they sought care elsewhere. This valuable information can assist the practitioner in improving the practice.

In implementing a telephone recall system, a staff member is assigned specifically to call patients. If the calls are to remind patients of scheduled appointments, patients to be seen in the morning are called the afternoon before the appointment and patients to be seen in the afternoon are called the morning of the appointment. If the purpose of the call is to schedule patients for new appointments, calls usually are made in the late afternoon or early evening. If a patient cannot be reached by telephone, a letter or postcard is sent—letters make a better impression and other information can be provided in the letter. If the patient does not respond to the first recall attempt, a 2-year recall process is started. Approximately 1½ years after the last examination, the patient is telephoned and a letter or postcard is sent stating "second reminder." Approximately 2 years after the examination, another recall letter is mailed and a follow-up telephone call is made. After approximately 28 months, a fourth recall attempt is made via telephone, postcard, or letter. Then, at about 34 months the last telephone call is

UAB OPTOMETRY **Primary Care Vision Service**

A friendly reminder.......
at your last visit, we reserved
this time for your next visit

Day _____   Date _____

Time _____

**Please call us at 934-3089 to
confirm that this date and time is convenient !**

Figure 29-1 Sample postcard for mail recall. (Courtesy School of Optometry, University of Alabama at Birmingham. Reproduced with permission.)

made, and correspondence stating "final reminder" is sent. If the patient does not respond, the patient's record should be placed in the nonactive file.

Combination Mail and Telephone Systems. As is evident from the preceding discussion, most recall systems use a combination of mail and telephone to contact patients. Usually mail is the means attempted for first contact with the patient, and the telephone is used to confirm that the card or letter was received and that the appointment will be kept or scheduled.

For annual or 2-year recall appointments, a card is sent reminding the patient that it is time to call to schedule an appointment. If the patient does not respond within a certain period (usually 1 month), the patient is contacted by telephone to ensure that the card was received and to determine whether an appointment can be scheduled. If an appointment is made, the patient is contacted by telephone the afternoon or morning before the appointment as a reminder. Combination mail and telephone systems usually provide a higher percentage of appointments made and kept than do systems that are strictly by mail or telephone.

Use of a Preappointment System

With this recall system, an appointment is always scheduled before the patient has left the office, even for examinations 1 to 2 years in the future. A specific date and time are selected and entered into the appointment book or computer. 2 to 4 weeks before the scheduled date, the patient is called and reminded of the appointment, which can be rescheduled if necessary. If preferred, a card can be sent to the patient approximately 1 month before the scheduled appointment. It contains the date and time of the appointment and asks the patient to call the office to confirm that the patient will be able to come as scheduled. If the patient does not respond to the card by 1 to 2 weeks before the appointment, a telephone call must be made to confirm the appointment or to schedule a new date and time.

The advantages of preappointing are that the appointment book stays full, avoiding seasonal slow periods, and it is less costly than other methods of recall since it does not necessarily involve printing and mailing expenses. The disadvantages of this method are that it requires careful coordination of effort to ensure that preappointed patients are properly confirmed or rescheduled and that patients can misinterpret the purpose of preappointing if the system is not properly explained. Patients may perceive this method as aggressive and more attuned to filling appointment slots than providing needed care. If done appropriately, however, the "no-show" rate is the lowest for all the recall systems.

Setting a Reasonable Recall Schedule

Recommended guidelines for the examination of children and adults, drawn from the consensus of opinion in the profession, have been established by the American Optometric Association. These clinical practice guidelines generally require different recall periods for asymptomatic individuals who are not at risk than for individuals who are at risk for ocular disease (Table 29-1).

Table 29-1 AOA Clinical Practice Guidelines for Examination of Children and Adults

	EXAMINATION INTERVAL	
PATIENT AGE	**ASYMPTOMATIC/RISK-FREE**	**AT RISK**
Children		
Birth–24 months	By 6 months of age or as recommended	By 6 months
2–5 years	At 3 years of age	At 3 years of age or as recommended
6–17 years	Before first grade and every 2 years thereafter	Annually or as recommended
Adults		
18–40 years	Every 2–3 years	Every 1–2 years or as recommended
41–60 years	Every 2 years	Every 1–2 years or as recommended
61 years and older	Annually	Annually or as recommended

From *American Optometric Association:* Clinical practice guidelines for comprehensive adult eye and vision examination and for pediatric eye and vision examination. *St. Louis, 1995-96, Author.*

Use of Computers to Facilitate Recall

Using a computer can be as useful, if not imperative, for recall systems as it is for other areas of office management. Every practice should have some type of computer system. Since specific information pertaining to patients can be easily identified by using a data base, it is simple for staff members to produce a list of patients due for recall. Also, staff members can measure the effectiveness of the patient recall system by using the computer to create information that can be easily read and interpreted (see Chapter 20).

One of the advantages of computer recall is that mailings can be personalized. Specific messages can be addressed to individual patients, creating a personal touch that assists in the effort to get patients to respond. Computerized recall also works well with preappointment systems, but such a system does require operation by a knowledgeable staff member.

When Patients Ignore Recall Attempts

Patients have a variety of reasons for not responding to recall notices. Common reasons for patients' failure to make recall appointments include shortage of financial resources, satisfaction with vision, perception that the optometrist's fees are not competitive, or dissatisfaction with the optometrist's practice.

The most effective way to determine why a patient has not returned for an appointment is by calling the patient. A telephone call under such circumstances requires the office staff to be tactful. When making such a call, the staff member first inquires about the patient's well-being in general and then explains that a review of the person's file indicates that the patient has not been in the office for a significant period and that this has caused some concern. Next, the staff member suggests that the patient come in for an examination. If the patient's response is not positive, the staff member attempts to learn whether the patient would like another reminder at a later time. If the patient does not want further communication, the call is ended.

When a patient decides to remain inactive, an exit survey should be sent. A letter stating that the optometrist is looking for ways to improve the delivery of health care and asking that the patient complete the survey anonymously should accompany the survey. The survey—concisely written and containing a limited number of multiple choice or true-false questions—should elicit responses about the optometrist's fees, location and physical facility, convenience and availability of appointments, professional demeanor, staff, parking and public transportation, services, and selection of eyewear and contact lenses. A self-addressed, stamped envelope should be enclosed with the survey for the patient's convenience.

If a patient is being recalled to provide follow-up for an eye problem and the patient fails to keep the appointment, the practitioner should have a staff member call the patient to determine why the appointment was not kept and to schedule the patient for a new date and time. If a patient with a problem fails to appear despite repeated efforts to schedule the patient for follow-up, the practitioner should send the patient a letter (by certified mail with return receipt requested if documentation of receipt is necessary). The letter should advise the patient of the necessity for further examination, describe the possible complications that might result if an examination is not performed, and urge the patient to call to schedule an appointment. A copy of the letter should be retained in the patient's file.

Conclusion

Patients tend to make appointments when they recognize a vision problem or have some uncertainty about their vision or eyes. Many patients would not return for regularly scheduled examinations without receiving a recall notice. Therefore, a recall system is important, but its effectiveness depends on the practitioner's and staff's understanding of the system and on the ability of the office to adhere to its procedures. To be successfully implemented, a recall system must not only be appropriately structured but also provide a true benefit to patients. This value to the patient is the most important element of any recall system.

Acknowledgement

The authors of this chapter in the first edition of *Business Aspects of Optometry* were Craig Hisaka and John Rumpakis.

Bibliography

Bergman L: Winning way with direct mail. *Optom Economics* 1(5):8, 1991.
Crooks CT III: The ultimate recall system. *Optom Economics* 1(12):34-7, 1991.
Freeman D: Taking the headache out of recall. *Optom Management* 25(7):87-92, 1989.
Freeman D: Recall on line. *Optom Economics* 1(6):32-7, 1991.

Hubler R: Beyond the postcard. *Optom Economics* 1(12):12-6, 1991.

Sachs L: Back to the fold: are you making every effort to bring inactive patients home to your practice. *Optom Economics* 1(5):39-42, 1991.

www.optometric.com. Online version of *Optometric Management* magazine, which provides articles on recall methods.

www.revoptom.com. Online version of *Review of Optometry* magazine, which provides articles on recall methods.

Chapter 30

Ophthalmic Dispensing

Diane Robbins-Luce and Greg Luce

The engine which drives enterprise is not thrift, but profit.
John Maynard Keynes *A Treatise on Money*

During the past several decades, optometry students have not held optical dispensing in high regard. Increasingly, there are more appealing and more challenging areas of specialization within the scope of optometry. It must be remembered, however, that even during these times of primary care, the majority of patients who seek the services of an optometrist do so for the purpose of refractive correction with eyeglasses. Patients do not understand the lack of interest in the mechanics of eyeglasses—any reduced status that dispensing might hold is in the minds of practitioners. To patients, eyeglasses are an important, sometimes vital, aid to vision.

It has long been understood that no matter how expert a practitioner's clinical services might be, the finished pair of glasses that are on the patient's face will be the long-lasting proof of excellent optometric care. Eyeglasses, if they are of high quality, can serve to build an excellent reputation and can become a major referral stimulus for the optometrist. Conversely, glasses that perform poorly and cause problems can be the source of many negative comments by the patient.

If these factors are not enough to encourage the student of practice management to excel in optical dispensing, it should be realized that in most practices the sale of optical materials contributes more to the typical practice's gross income than all areas combined—about 55 cents on the dollar. A practice that does not provide dispensing services usually can double its gross income if dispensing is added.

Assuming that optical dispensing and laboratory services are delegated to technicians and assistants, it is almost always financially attractive to provide dispensing. Patients generally prefer the full-service concept of eye care, as evidenced by the fact that most independent practitioners have a very low percentage of patients who have their spectacle prescriptions filled by another dispenser. A major benefit of receiving both clinical services and optical materials from one office is that the patient only needs to turn to that office in the event of problems.

The actual duties of the selection and dispensing of eyewear are generally delegated to an optometric technician, frame stylist, or optician. This approach is a sensible one, allowing the optometrist to function at the highest level of skill and to concentrate on the diagnosis and management of eye conditions, while serving as a supervisor with regard to optical dispensing. Many educational programs exist today for the training of technicians to completely manage and operate an optical dispensary, but the majority of individuals who perform this function are trained on the job.

Image of the Dispensary

Various styles of optometric practice include dispensaries that convey different images. The form of the dispensary can range from the traditional, specialized service available only to the patients of the private practice to the highly retail and commercialized optical superstore. Patients will differentiate between a retail and professional image largely on their initial impression when entering the office. If the frame showroom area is the first room entered from the outside, the image is largely retail. This design is often found in optometrists' offices in which the optical dispensary serves as the reception room or there is no reception room. If the outside entrance opens into a traditional reception area, the impression is one of professional eye care.

A good approach to the separation of the retail and professional aspects of a practice is to have two separate entrances—one of them leading to an optical dispensary and the other one leading to the practitioner's office waiting room (Figure 30-1). This concept does provide some advantages in that it retains the professional image of a health care practitioner while still attracting patients who would like to purchase eyeglasses separately. This arrangement could incorporate the use of a separate business name for the optical dispensary. The name selected could be used in exterior signage and would allow the practitioner to feel more comfortable with the advertising of optical services in the local media. Care should be given to such external marketing, however, to ensure that the public is being sent the desired message concerning which aspect of care is emphasized as primary and which is deemed to be secondary.

There are obvious advantages and disadvantages to having a separate optical dispensary. In one regard, it should not be allowed to be so separate that there is no connection, visible to the public, between the optometrist and the dispensary. When that connection is broken, so is the loyalty that retains patients and causes them to purchase optical materials from the practice. It can be desirable to have the dispensary still function under the organization of the practice—this

will allow for one set of accounting records to be maintained and also allow the patient to simply write one check for clinical services and eyeglasses.

Having a separate optical dispensary also requires a larger staff. It is important for each entrance to have a receptionist or technician always available to greet patients when they enter. This is not only good etiquette and a custom that is expected by patients in a service-oriented business but also is necessary in the optical dispensary to prevent the problem of shoplifting.

As defined for the purposes of this discussion, optical dispensing includes the following functions:
- Lens design (and selection of options)
- Frame selection and measurements
- Ordering and verifying of eyeglasses
- Dispensing and adjusting of eyeglasses
- Maintaining and repairing of eyeglasses

The appearance of the optical dispensary is extremely important to the successful operation of the business (Figure 30-2). When a patient enters the optical dispensary, that individual becomes a consumer. Consumers make many subconscious judgments that affect their purchasing habits. The decor and appearance will influence the consumer's decision to purchase a product and even how much the consumer will pay. The optometrist's dispensary has a distinct advantage over other optical dispensaries because the optometrist

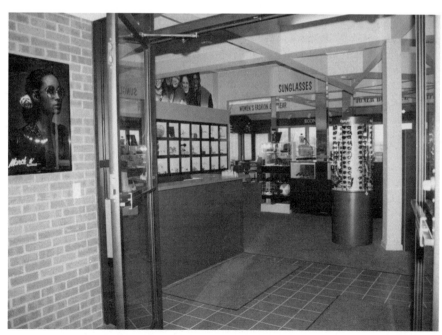

Figure 30-1 Separate optical entrance. (Courtesy Gailmard Eye Center, Munster, Ind.)

already has provided professional and clinical services to the patient and has gained the patient's trust. It is not sufficient to rely solely on this professional relationship, however, because the optical dispensary should appeal to the patient on its own. The optical dispensary must be continuously updated and periodically redecorated with additions such as wallpaper, carpeting, new paint, and new furniture. Patients will judge the entire operation of a practice by what they understand, and they understand retail merchandise displays. Even though it is a considerable expense, the optical dispensary must be kept modern and tasteful.

See Chapter 18 for further discussion of the design of the optical dispensary.

Frame Display Options

It is important to display the inventory of frames in a way that highlights them in an impressive manner. There are many options available through professional optical design companies; these companies will fabricate custom frame bars or sell ready-made ones. Frames often are displayed in categories or sections such as men's, women's, and children's groupings. Additional areas can be added, such as sports eyewear and nonprescription sunglasses (Figure 30-3). A decision should be made as to whether patients are allowed to browse and try frames on or whether they will be seated and frames will be shown one at a time by a technician.

A good merchandising idea is to display more upscale and expensive frames in a different environment. It has been observed that displaying a few very expensive frames will help sales of medium- to high-priced frames because it desensitizes the consumer who might have "sticker shock." Antique furniture can provide an interesting backdrop for a more spread out merchandising effect of individual frames on pedestals. Manufacturers and frame suppliers will provide excellent ideas for merchandising and showcasing their products. A display kit that promotes one style of a frame in several colors is appealing in any location in the dispensary. Observing the window displays and accessory displays in fine department stores is an excellent way to learn professional display techniques.

Frames can be displayed on glass shelves that allow them to sit singly and with temples open. This frame display method tends to make a smaller inventory look larger because it is spread out. The use of frame bars generally places a larger frame inventory into a smaller space.

Dispensing tables should be readily available as a workplace for frames, clinical records, and accessories (Figure 30-4). These dispensing tables also can serve as a counter so that optical measurements can be taken accurately and prescription eyeglass orders can be written. These tables also can be the area where fees are explained and presented to the patient. The dispensing tables, which are used for frame selection, also can

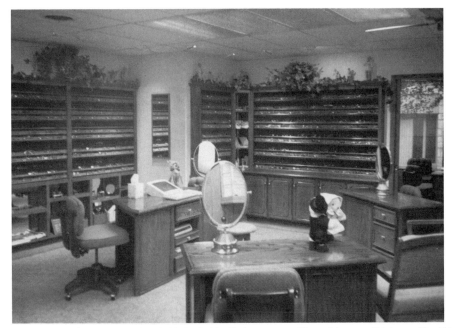

Figure 30-2 Optical dispensary. (Courtesy Drs. Bob Baldwin, Bobby Christensen, and Russell Laverty, Oklahoma City, Okla.)

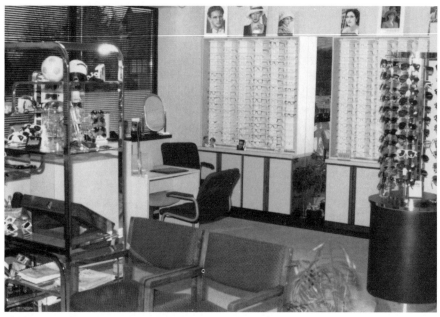

Figure 30-3 Optical dispensary. (Courtesy Dr. David Hansen, Des Moines, Iowa.)

double as tables to be used for delivering finished eyeglasses and providing eyewear adjustments. It should be remembered, however, that the use of these tables might be in great demand, and this can make it inconvenient for patients who wish to select a frame if all tables are being used for deliveries and adjustments.

One alternative, if space permits, is to have separate dispensing counters, booths, or small private rooms to deliver and adjust eyewear (Figure 30-5). This specialized delivery and dispensing section also emphasizes the service aspect of dispensing glasses. The basic dispensing tools and frame warmer can be positioned in a nearby location, preferably with a sink also available. This design allows the patients to see some of the basic adjustments being performed on their eyeglasses and saves the technicians the many

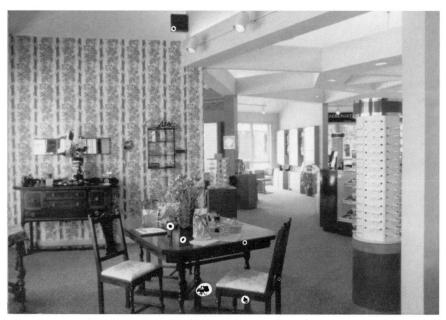

Figure 30-4 Optical boutique area. (Courtesy Gailmard Eye Center, Munster, Ind.)

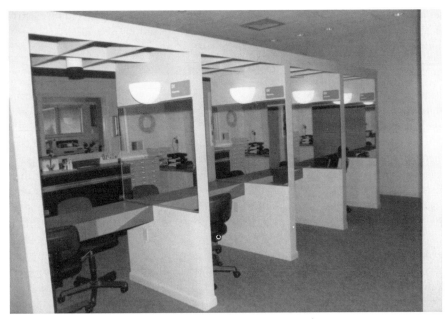

Figure 30-5 Eyeglass adjustment booths. (Courtesy Gailmard Eye Center, Munster, Ind.)

steps that must be made to walk back and forth from a separate laboratory.

Lighting is a very important consideration in a dispensary. As experts in visual science, optometrists should display excellent lighting techniques. It is generally noted that skin tones are much more attractive to a person under incandescent or natural lights. The use of track lights or other spotlights can add a pleasing appearance to patients trying on frames and viewing themselves in mirrors. General overall lighting with fluorescent lights is practical in commercial buildings. Indirect fluorescent lighting, where the light is bounced off ceilings or other surfaces, tends to make the light more pleasing. The use of daylight through skylights and windows adds a third type of lighting and can contribute to an attractive blend of all three. One additional consideration in lighting is the use of back-illuminated frame bars. This is an individual decision because, although the frame bars are quite eye appealing when frames are lit from behind, the actual color of a frame is much harder to see when displayed on these frame bars. The frame often must be removed from the frame bar and viewed in a separate light for the color to actually be appreciated.

Frame Inventory Management

Ordering and buying frames are described in Chapter 22. The first consideration is the number of frames that should be on display and carried in inventory. This frame number will vary widely, from a range of approximately 500 frames in a small office to more than 3000 frames in a typical super-optical environment. The size of the practice, the budget available, and the marketing strategy of the practitioner will dictate the number of frames to carry. The practitioner will need to consider the number of men, women, and young patients so that the appropriate percentage of frames will be carried for each category.

It is possible to display all frames, but some offices keep an additional stock so frames can be replaced. Keeping frame boards completely filled with minimum empty spaces makes them more attractive and appealing and also makes it easier to spot potential theft problems. An assistant can check the frame displays every morning and be certain that all empty spots are filled with frames, even if sunglasses or safety frames must be used. It can be an advantage to the large practice to try to use frames from the frame board as much as possible rather than ordering frames to be supplied by the laboratory. This practice has the major benefit of reducing back order problems, which often can occur without the knowledge of the optical staff and delay an order unexpectedly. Additionally, using frames directly off the frame board creates a constant turnover of inventory, which means frames will always be new and not shopworn.

Obviously, the optometrist (or staff members) periodically must meet with frame manufacture sales representatives to buy new frames and replace those that have been sold. This meeting should be arranged by appointment and given due time and consideration since it represents the products that will be shown and dispensed. Frame representatives can provide a valuable service by conducting an inventory of their products and keeping records of what was sold since the last purchase. There generally will be more frame vendors who wish to do business with the optometrist than the optometrist can reasonably manage. It is generally necessary to restrict the number of vendors to those who provide the best products, service, discounts, and return policies.

It can be a good strategy to provide as much business as possible to a limited number of vendors so that the practice becomes an important account to these companies. This important account relationship can result in better buying programs and discounts from the vendor.

The optometrist or staff member who buys frames must stick to a budget and not buy under pressure. The professional sales person is very skilled at selling, and the optometrist must be able to say "no." It also is advisable to try to buy for the entire market of patients and avoid simply purchasing what the buyer personally likes. A wide range of frame prices should be available, and a good mix of frame sizes (large and small), materials (metal and plastic), and styles (conservative and high fashion) should be obtained. Attention must be given to older stock that has not sold; these frames should be returned within the company's return policy. Sales representatives sometimes are not anxious to facilitate returns, so the frame manager must be attentive to this task. Another consideration when buying frames is the use of buying groups, which can help obtain better discounts for an independent practitioner when the number of purchases is small.

Many computer software programs are available for eye care practices, and these programs can provide valuable assistance in inventory management. Computer programs are useful for frames but also can be applicable for uncut ophthalmic lenses and contact lenses. Various printed reports can be generated, and this information can make frame buying more intelligent and scientific. Of course, to obtain excellent data from the computer, considerable effort is required to input the necessary information when new frames are added and when display frames are sold. Each frame must have an inventory number or bar code placed on

it that is typed in or entered by electronic wand during each transaction (Box 30-1).

Lens Design

Lens design is an aspect of dispensing that is all too often forced into a secondary role even though it is really more important than the selection of the frame. Patients understand the process of frame selection very well because they try on the frames and look at them and touch them. The lens is not well understood, however, because of the complexities of different types of prescriptions, the placement of optical centers, the use of oversize blanks, the need for antireflection or ultraviolet coatings, and the various styles of multifocals that can be chosen. It is a good practice to begin the dispensing visit with a discussion of the lenses, before frames are considered, perhaps at an in-office "lens design center." This special area is devoted to samples and demonstration lenses in the form of uncut lens blanks and mockup eyeglasses. Box 30-2 provides some ideas on the kind of information that can be provided.

The process of designing lenses and selecting options simply begins by educating the patient. It is the dispenser's duty to inform each patient of the newest available technologies for ophthalmic lenses. Patients have a right to know what new products are available, and the dispenser should avoid prejudging what the patient will or will not want or can afford. The key to patient education is the use of demonstration items and literature. Nothing can explain different types of bifocals better then having actual eyeglasses made up with different types of bifocals. These items also are perfect when attempting to answer questions such as, "How thick will the edges be in a certain size

---

Box 30-1 Advantages of Computerized Frame Inventory Management

- Current inventory always available in wholesale or retail dollar amounts and in number of units.
- Inventory reports by frame type, manufacturer, supplier, or model.
- Inventory aging reports: listings of frames, quantity, and date acquired.
- Reports of frames that are on order or at the laboratory.
- History of sales per month by manufacturer or model.
- Reports are of assistance when buying and reordering frames, for accounting needs, and theft control.

Box 30-2 Lens Design Center Demonstration Items

Uncut Lens Blanks

- Grey and brown plastic tints from #1 to #5 for fashion and sunglass
- Other tint colors including rose #1 and #2 and gray/green sunglass
- Gradient tint samples
- Photochromatic plastic and glass and polarized samples
- Glass lens coatings for color and mirror
- High-index plastic vs. CR-39 in same prescription (e.g., −6.00 D)
- Polycarbonate and aspheric lenses

Mockup Spectacles

- Right lens rolled and polished, left lens normal, in wire frame
- Right lens A/R coat, left lens normal
- Progressive lenses with plano at distance and +1.50 adds
- Right lens executive bifocal, left lens FT-35
- Various bifocal and trifocal styles
- Various high-plus and minus powers in different eye size frames

frame?" or "How does this look with an antireflection coating?" or "How does a lens look when the edges are rolled and polished?" The manufacturer for a nominal fee can provide samples of eyeglasses or lens blanks.

Lifestyle Dispensing

The educational approach leads to the concept of lifestyle dispensing. This term refers to finding out more about a patient's needs in daily activities and providing additional pairs of eyeglasses or special lens options to help the patient with those needs. Obviously, this procedure requires more in-depth questioning with regard to patients' occupational and vocational interests. Examples of needs that can be satisfied with lifestyle dispensing include golfing, fishing, special safety glasses for the work environment, or special reading glasses for computer use. Some practices use a printed questionnaire to find out about lifestyle needs, whereas others simply use a friendly verbal interview.

A side benefit to good lens design is increased optical sales in the form of second pairs, sunglasses, and lens add-on options, but the primary outcome is eyewear that provides optimal visual performance for the

patient in his or her daily life. The practitioner's philosophy will determine how much salesmanship should be used during dispensing. One must be careful not to take this technique too far so that it becomes a high-pressure sales tactic that can adversely affect the doctor-patient relationship.

Technicians who serve as frame selection assistants or frame stylists should be trained to assist patients with proper frame sizes and shapes. Frame stylists must be trained to note the lens prescription first so that this information can be considered when determining the type of frame to use. Additionally, training in color, style, and the selection of proper shapes for facial features is appropriate. The use of video cameras has become useful in helping patients view themselves while wearing potential new eyeglass frames. This technique has some obvious benefits since some patients cannot see well when trying on sample frames that do not contain a lens prescription. Seeing oneself on video also permits angles of view that a mirror does not achieve. The use of a video camera can be somewhat time consuming but, in a high-service practice, does differentiate the practice from the competition.

Frame and Lens Pricing

The most popular method for setting fees for ophthalmic materials is to use a markup system. The amount of markup can vary from two to three times the wholesale cost. Informal surveys should be performed to determine the markup rate for various optical materials in a given area. The marketing philosophy and positioning of the practice will dictate if this practice should be on the high, middle, or low end of the price scale. Prices can be marked on small adhesive stickers that serve to show the patient the cost as the patient tries on the frames. A popular idea is to use a clear label and apply it to the demonstration lens that comes with the frame. Lens prices generally are listed on a printed fee schedule that can be kept near the dispensing tables. This list can show different prices for the different types of lenses—spheres, sphero-cylinders, single vision lenses, bifocals, and progressive addition lenses. Also, various lens options can be listed as add-on prices. A quality, wholesale laboratory's finished lens price list can be used as a guide for determining the patient cost for these options.

An alternative method for the pricing of frames and lenses has been the use of dispensing and prescription fees. These fees represent the profit that would be made on the service aspect of dispensing. When using these methods, optical materials generally are priced at wholesale cost, with a slight add-on margin to allow for operational costs. Dispensing fees and a low materials fee are often used by third-party companies in an effort to control costs. It has been noted that patients might not accept dispensing fees as easily as they accept a markup on ophthalmic materials.

As part of good dispensing service, the dispenser should be trained to review and explain all fees that are charged for optical materials and, if necessary, the other professional and clinical fees charged to the patient at the current visit.

Nonprescription Sunglasses

One area of dispensing that seems to be of growing interest is the provision of nonprescription sunglasses. Optometrists routinely educate patients about the importance of protection against ultraviolet radiation and the value of quality optics. This would naturally support the dispensing of nonprescription sunwear. Even though the majority of nonprescription sunwear purchases takes place in department and drug stores, there is a market for higher-quality sunglasses sold through eye care professionals. A requirement for success in sales of nonprescription sunglasses is a significant investment in inventory (Figure 30-6). The consumer wants selection and variety. Historically, optometrists have not been pleased with sales of nonprescription sunglasses, but this lack of success can be due to the practice of carrying a small inventory of sun-

glasses by ophthalmic frame companies that are not known by the public. Name brands have great appeal to the public. Promotion to the public might be necessary in the form of media advertising. A natural market for sunglasses is the contact lens population, who would have an interest in nonprescription sunwear.

Advertising

The advertising of dispensing services must be performed carefully so as not to adversely affect the image of a professional practice. The practitioner's "philosophy of practice" should be used to establish the goals of external marketing before any advertising campaign is started. The practitioner must consider the position of the practice first and then adopt a promotional campaign that will meet the goals of the practice image. Advertising is a major investment for a practice and speaks loudly to the public about its image. It is best to use advertising agencies for assistance, but this assistance does require a significant budget. Frame manufacturers can provide professional camera-ready advertisements and even cooperative funding for advertising when it is performed within their guidelines.

Eyewear Delivery

The delivery of finished prescription eyeglasses involves the services of adjustment and fitting. Office policies for the notification of patients and for the dis-

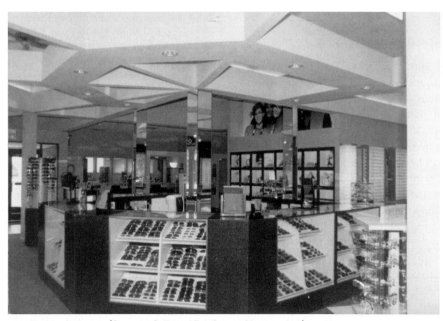

Figure 30-6 Sunwear display showcase. (Courtesy Gailmard Eye Center, Munster, Ind.)

pensing of eyewear should be adopted. Some practices offer dispensing of eyeglasses by appointment only, but this method can result in delays and inconvenience for the patient. If the practice has adequate staff members who can dispense eyeglasses, appointments will not be necessary for this rather brief service. Patients who simply walk in to pick up eyeglasses generally will understand a short wait of 5 or fewer minutes. Excellent eyeglass dispensing involves the following:

- Adjustment of the frame to the patient's face and head to ensure proper fit and comfort
- Instructions to the patient on the use and care of the new eyeglasses
- A review of the lens options that were ordered

The technician dispensing the eyeglasses should ask the patient whether the type of eyewear being provided has been used before. If it is new to the patient, instructions on adaptation symptoms as well as how to use the eyewear properly can be appropriate. A reading card should be handy, to allow the patient to test nearpoint vision and to learn to use different parts of multifocal lenses. An additional technique that should be included in dispensing is the routine review of special options that were incorporated into the eyeglasses. Patients forget the purpose of extra options such as antireflection coatings, photogrey tints, scratch-resistant coatings, and similar items, and the dispenser should use this opportunity for one last review of the options ordered and their purpose. This review also can spark referrals when the patient wears the new glasses and finds the options helpful. Patients should be instructed to return at any time if frame adjustments are needed.

A progressive practice must be aware of the importance of the time taken to fabricate eyeglasses. It is no longer common for 2 weeks to be required to fabricate a pair of glasses, and yet some special lens designs and special frame orders can necessitate a waiting period as long or longer. The important consideration when encountering such orders is to keep the patient informed. It is very important to call the patient if any delay is encountered in the fabrication of new eyeglasses, rather than waiting for the patient to call and ask why the eyeglasses are not ready.

Eyeglass Warranties

A more consumer-oriented approach has developed in dispensing, as various marketing strategies have been adopted by optical chain stores and private practices. Eyeglass warranties have become popular and gener-

ally extend for 1 year from the date of dispensing. Sometimes an additional charge is required for such a warranty, and sometimes the warranty is provided to all patients at no additional cost. Typically, the eyeglass warranty will provide for the repair or replacement of any broken part of the frame or lenses with a "no-fault" guarantee so that no matter how the glasses are broken, a repair or replacement is made.

Sometimes these warranties can have a "one-time only" stipulation, whereas other warranties can be unlimited throughout the year. The eyeglass warranty does remove any potential disagreement about whether the eyeglasses performed adequately, were defective, or were abused by the patient. A separate warranty usually accompanies scratch-resistant plastic lenses and typically provides for replacement at no charge if the lenses scratch within 1 year. These warranties are easy for a practitioner to provide, since both frames and scratch-resistant lenses usually are under warranty by the manufacturer.

Managing the Unhappy Patient

There will always be a small percentage of patients who are unhappy with their vision or have difficulty with adaptation to new eyeglasses. Additionally, problems will occur in which lenses fall out and screws and temples come loose. An office policy should be established for the management of unhappy patients. The best policy is the age-old "the customer is always right" approach. Policies should be developed to easily and fairly handle a refund in the event a patient requests one—although solving the problem is a better resolution. All efforts should be made to rectify any problems the patient has as quickly as possible. Generally, job remakes and corrections should be made at no charge to the patient if they occur within a reasonable amount of time. Assistants should allow patients to have access to the prescribing practitioner, usually with a free appointment, if complaints of a visual nature are received.

Additional optical policies can include the use of a payment plan. It is common to accept major credit cards, and this provides an easy way for practices to avoid offering credit to patients. It is common for the office to require a 50% deposit when eyeglasses are ordered, with the balance due at dispensing. Whatever policy is selected, it is vital that patients be informed in advance of what is expected of them. This philosophy can prevent awkward situations, such as instances in which patients arrive to pick up glasses but are not ready to pay. It is difficult to turn patients away or to take back glasses that have just been fitted.

Acknowledgement

The author of this chapter in the first edition of *Business Aspects of Optometry* was Neil B. Gailmard.

Bibliography

Allergan, Inc: *Pathways in optometry.* Irvine, Calif, 1992, Author.

Baldwin BL, Christensen B, Melton J: *Rx for success.* Midwest City, Okla, 1983, Vision Publications.

Barnett D: Is your dispensary a sight for sore eyes? *Rev Optom* 129(9):51-9, 1992.

Bennett H: Is your optical a hit or a dud? *Rev Optom* 137(9):39, 2000.

Bennett I: *Management for the eyecare practitioner.* Stoneham, Mass, 1993, Butterworth.

Brooks C, Borish I: *System for ophthalmic dispensing,* ed 2. Boston, Mass, 1996, Butterworth-Heinemann.

Drew R: *Professional ophthalmic dispensing.* Chicago, 1970, Professional Press.

Dunleavy B: Lens choices. The frame factor. Available at: *http://www.2020mag.com/Issues/1997/November/lens.htm.*

Dunleavy B: Lens choices. Through the looking glass. Available at: *http://www.2020mag.com/Issues/1998/Feb/lens.htm.*

Dunleavy B: The doctor is in. Available at: *http://www.2020mag.com/Issues/1998/oct/mp.htm.*

Gailmard NB: Make your optical dispensary separate—but not too separate. *Optom Management* 18(10):21-5, 1982.

Gailmard NB: How I improved our eyeglass delivery time. *Rev Optom* 124(5):33, 1987.

Gailmard NB: Meet the service challenge. *Rev Optom* 126(7):23, 1989.

Gailmard NB. Managing the grief patient. *Optom Economics* 1(8):18-21, 1991.

Gailmard NB: The Consultant's Corner: a premium lens at a lower premium. *Rev Optom* 130(3):33, 1993.

Guerrein R: Viewpoint: don't dispense with dispensing. *Optom Management* 29(2):11, 1994.

Kirkner R: Ophthalmic dispensing: getting ahead of the curve. *Rev Optom* 137(11):53, 2000.

Kirman B: Keep the right frame sizes on the board. *Optom Management* 29(3):46-50, 1994.

McMillan PH: Dispensary design trends. *Eyecare Bus* 9(10):20-4, 1995.

Schwartz C: Minimize inventory and maximize return. *Rev Optom* 129(9):51-9, 1992.

Weber J: *101 Dispensing tips and procedures.* Melville, NY, 1994, Marchon Eyewear.

Winslow C: You can improve your eyeglass service. *Rev Optom* 128(10):39-42, 1991.

Winslow C: Your stylist's biggest frame-buying blunders. *Rev Optom* 128(10):31-4, 1991.

www.optometric.com. Online version of *Optometric Management* magazine, which provides articles on ophthalmic dispensing.

www.revoptom.com. Online version of *Review of Optometry* magazine, which provides articles on ophthalmic dispensing.

Chapter 31

Building a Contact Lens Practice

Richard D. Hazlett, C. Denise Howard, and Janice M. Jurkus

If you build it, he will come.
William P. Kinsella *Shoeless Joe*

Contact lens–related patient care is an integral aspect of the modern practice of optometry. For many optometrists, the time spent on and income derived from contact lens services represent a significant component of practice activity and practice income. Illustrating the importance of contact lens services, economic surveys performed by the American Optometric Association have repeatedly found that virtually all practicing optometrists provide contact lens care.

Although practitioners have traditionally considered contact lens care to be a specialty area, thanks to current contact lens technology, contact lenses can be regarded as an option for the majority of patients needing vision correction. Since individuals fitted with contact lenses often experience superior vision, tend to be loyal to the practice where they were fitted, and offer significant economic benefits for the practice, it behooves optometrists to develop this aspect of practice.

A significant number of contact lens patients are obtained through referral. Methods used to encourage referrals from other health care providers are described in Chapter 27. However, practitioners also can build a contact lens practice through marketing efforts directed at existing patients and at the public at large. This chapter describes various means for creating such a contact lens practice.

Obtaining New Contact Lens Patients from Referrals

A referral base can be created by a practitioner who communicates effectively with patients, emphasizes personal attention, and attends to the unique aspects of presenting visual problems. Additionally, any special techniques or unusual lenses used in fitting the patient, if pointed out, often result in an inspired patient who will tell others about the practitioner's expertise as a contact lens clinician.

Contact lens patients especially like to feel that a practitioner is at the cutting edge of care and that the newest developments are being used. If a practitioner can obtain the newest instrumentation for the diagnosis and management of contact lens patients—and makes the patient aware that advanced instrumentation is being used—this, too, will encourage the patient to inform acquaintances of the advanced state of the practitioner's practice. This information also can result in new referrals.

Contact lens patients are more likely to refer other patients when they are enthusiastic contact lens wearers. How does a practitioner create enthusiasm? Enthusiasm is generated by reinforcing the patient's perception that he or she is receiving special care from the best practitioner. There are several ways to create this favorable impression.

Problem Solving

Patients will be enthusiastic if a practitioner has the reputation of being a problem solver. If a patient has troublesome contact lens problems that are solved, the practitioner benefits not only from an appreciative patient but also is likely to receive additional referrals because of this demonstration of clinical expertise.

This is especially true if the patient's problems have been overlooked or unresolved by other practitioners.

Supportive Staff

A well-trained supportive staff that shows individual concern for patient needs and enthusiasm for patient success will promote patient loyalty and referrals. Therefore, it behooves practitioners to make a significant investment in staff training, with an emphasis on showing staff how to become sensitive to individual patient needs.

In-Office Contact Lens Development from Former Patients

Many primary care patients are excellent candidates for contact lens wear. One way to encourage these individuals to consider contact lenses is by creating a newsletter (Figure 31-1). The newsletter should include the most up-to-date information about contact lenses and about how the office is implementing new developments. Printed contact lens promotional material should be available in the office and visible to patients waiting to be seen for primary eye care. This material can be printed—in the form of either reprints of articles or brochures supplied by lens manufacturers—or it can be in the form of verbal encouragement by the staff. It is essential in a contact lens practice that a significant number of staff members and practitioners wear contact lenses and believe in the product. There is nothing more credible than an enthusiastic staff member who is wearing contact lenses. Staff members should discuss their contact lens experiences in the most positive manner.

In-office referrals are often gained through enthusiastic patient interaction. Primary care patients should be able to meet lens wearers in the office and to hear firsthand about the advantages and benefits of lens wear. In addition, audiovisual aids should be available in the reception area. Answers to commonly asked contact lens questions can be conveniently provided by either a videotape or a laser disc. The video cassette recorder or laser disc player should be operated unobtrusively by a staff member.

Marketing

Several different marketing approaches can be taken to build a contact lens practice. The approach chosen should be appropriate for the practice and the type of contact lens patient the practitioner wishes to attract. As with all other aspects of marketing, a carefully thought out plan is a necessary first step.

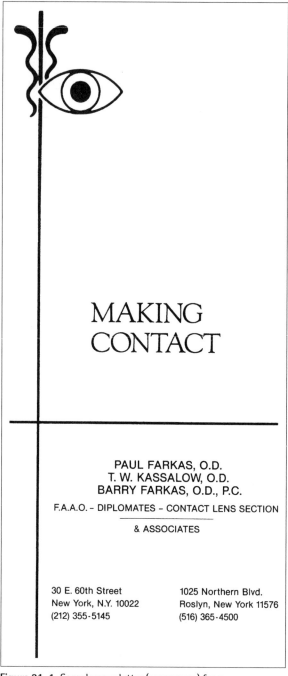

MAKING CONTACT

PAUL FARKAS, O.D.
T. W. KASSALOW, O.D.
BARRY FARKAS, O.D., P.C.
F.A.A.O. – DIPLOMATES – CONTACT LENS SECTION

& ASSOCIATES

30 E. 60th Street
New York, N.Y. 10022
(212) 355-5145

1025 Northern Blvd.
Roslyn, New York 11576
(516) 365-4500

Figure 31-1 Sample newsletter (cover page) for a practitioner providing contact lens care. (Courtesy Dr. Paul Farkas, Boca Raton, Fla.)

Developing a Marketing Plan

When developing a marketing plan, practitioners must first define goals and objectives. To set goals, the current situation must be analyzed. A well-crafted *positioning statement* will help the practitioner focus on desired objectives. This statement should elucidate the characteristics the practitioner wishes the practice to portray, such as quality of care, convenience, fashion, price, specialized services, or new technology. It will have an important bearing on all aspects of marketing, especially for a new practice, where it can influence the practice name, location, office decor, products supplied, and even the type of employees hired.

For a new practitioner with no marketing experience, a local advertising agency can help with these important facets of the marketing plan. If professional advice is to be solicited, it is recommended that the practitioner interview several agencies and select the one that best matches the practice's goals and resources. If this approach is not affordable, another possibility is to contact the head of the marketing department of a local college or university to determine whether there are any talented students who may be able to help with this aspect of the practice marketing effort.

Research

When considering how to attract potential contact lens patients, practitioners can obtain valuable marketing information from contact lens companies, which are familiar with the demographics and buying habits of the type of patients being sought. Once the type of patient the practice wishes to attract has been identified and the message to be conveyed to these patients has been established, the practitioner can consider different methods of attracting these patients and select those that best fit the practice's needs and budget.

Media Planning

There are many variables that will help determine the media to be used to build a contact lens practice. In large markets, it may be too costly to use radio, television, and newspapers, but there are creative ways to get public relations exposure to these media.

Public Relations

An ideal way to develop public relations is to become one of the local experts the news media will rely on when there are interesting developments in the contact lens field. A way to start is to contact local news departments with new information about advances in contact lens practice. This may result in

an interview or an appearance on the local news. The best approach is to prepare a news release about the innovation and include personal experience or information about the research. If the information is well prepared and well documented, it is likely to be well received and the practitioner most often will be credited.

When a practitioner opens an office, changes locations, speaks at a conference, receives an award, adds a new employee, or promotes staff members, a press release can be issued. Over time, these small efforts add up to exposure in the market. Also, talk show radio hosts are always looking for guests and are usually receptive to the idea of interviewing an expert on health-related topics.

A form of free marketing that has proved to be quite successful in developing a contact lens practice is authorship of articles appearing in well-known magazines or newspapers that are widely read by the practice's patient base (Figure 31-2). The best choices are fashion magazines or a reputable newspaper. In addition to personal practitioner interviews, an article published in a local newspaper about new contact lens developments can create interest in the practice. In fact, such an article will often be saved by a potential patient and will stimulate a future visit to the optometrist's office. With limited time and resources, this approach is favored as perhaps the most effective way of bringing new contact lens patients into a practice.

Employing a public relations professional also can be an effective means of marketing to the public, but a sophisticated public relations firm usually recommends a budget that is greater than the average individual practitioner can afford. Optometrists do benefit from professional public relations efforts that are paid for by contact lens companies or interested optometric organizations. However, use of a public relations firm puts the practitioner's best image forward in the media, and this benefit can be helpful.

Radio

If a marketing budget will allow for radio advertising, it can be an effective way to reach potential contact lens patients. Repeated exposure is the key to results. There are two basic ways to buy radio time. One is to purchase a series of radio spots that are repeated within a given time period, and the other is to buy sponsorship of a news show or traffic reporting spot for a specific time. Radio advertising can fail to be cost-effective if it does not reach the appropriate audience, which is why

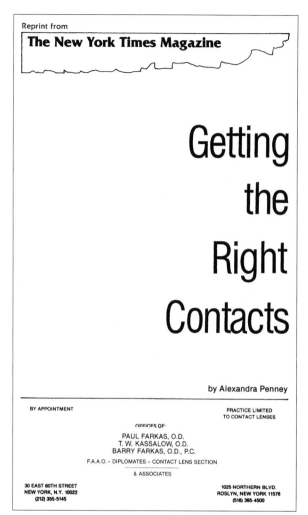

Figure 31-2 Example article published in the local media. (Courtesy Dr. Paul Farkas, Boca Raton, Fla.)

the time that radio spots are run is so important to the success of the effort.

Television

Television is a good medium for attracting contact lens patients, but unless a practice has multiple locations, it is unlikely that television advertising will be cost-effective, especially in large market areas. In smaller markets, television can sometimes be used with consistency by buying less expensive air times such as late night or early morning programming.

Print Media

In large markets, newspaper advertising can be very expensive, but there are ways to reduce cost. Most of a

practice's patients either work or live within a five-mile radius. Often, newspaper advertisements that will be distributed only in an area close to the practice location can be purchased. These limited distribution sections of newspapers are often called the "neighborhood section," and ads purchased in these sections can be cost-effective, even for single location practices. It also may be cost-effective to buy ads in smaller papers, such as a newspaper produced for a particular suburb or college campus. There are specialty publications in larger markets that are entertainment oriented and that may appeal to the same demographic mix as many contact lens practices. These advertisements may be cost-effective for some individual offices. Another option is to advertise in the events programs of local high schools or the program of the symphony or opera, depending on the type of contact lens patient desired.

Yellow Pages advertising has become an almost essential part of any contact lens marketing plan. The majority of patients use the Yellow Pages to make telephone contact with optometrists to find office locations (Figure 31-3). It is recommended that an advertising professional be used in the design of Yellow Pages ads. An ad size should be selected that will get attention but not be larger than judged necessary to achieve the desired results.

Direct Mail

Direct mail should be part of any marketing plan, including patient reminders for checkups and recalls. Post card mailings can be very reasonable in price and quite effective. Announcements should be mailed to surrounding residential areas when a new office is opened or a move is made. A direct mail house or an advertising agency can help with this effort. As a practice grows, a newsletter can be a valuable resource for attracting contact lens patients. Newsletters may be purchased from a number of sources or produced in-house. In either event, the newsletter should be easy to read and informative. It should highlight any new contact lens services or products being offered and provide educational information regarding successful contact lens wear as well as interesting facts about vision. Newsletters mailed to established patients, as well as to homes near to the office, have proved to be a cost-effective way of vitalizing a contact lens practice.

Internet Marketing

Many practitioners have created their own Web sites on the Internet as a part of their contact lens marketing

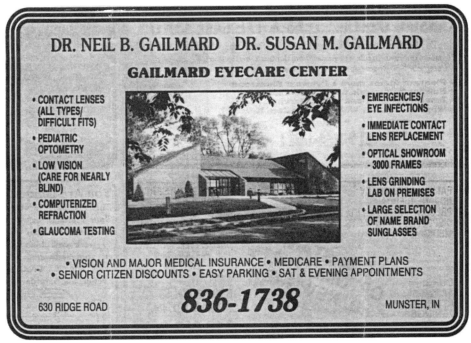

Figure 31-3 Sample Yellow Pages advertisement. (Courtesy Dr. Neil B. Gailmard, Munster, Ind.)

plan. This approach has limited value in attracting new patients to the practice, but it can be an effective tool for communicating with an established patient base. A growing number of contact lens practitioners have found it beneficial to offer a Web site that allows patients to order replacement contact lenses directly.

Marketing Results

It is sometimes difficult to judge marketing results because patients often do not volunteer information about how they found a practitioner. In fact, a large group practice that conducted an aggressive marketing campaign for new patients found that, when they asked new patients how they became aware of the office, 92% said they were referred by a friend. When asked whether they had heard of the office from any source other than from the friend that referred them, the answer from patients was almost universally yes. It should be remembered that all marketing efforts make an impression, and thus marketing must be consistent with the practice's goals so that it delivers the message and image desired. The overall growth of the contact lens practice should be the measure of the office's contact lens marketing success.

Contact Lens Assistants

Many aspects of contact lens care can be performed cost-effectively by a well-trained assistant. Consequen-

tly, many duties in contact lens practice are delegated to assistants, including ordering and verification of contact lenses, training of patients in techniques for insertion and removal of lenses, and education of patients in the use of proper lens care regimens. However, assistants must be properly trained, and their scope of responsibilities must be clearly defined.

Training Assistants

There are various ways for an assistant to obtain training. The best means is through formal course work. There are formal training courses for optometric technicians offered at community colleges and at selected colleges of optometry. Although these individuals learn basic skills in a teaching institution, most require on-the-job training to ensure that they conform to the standards of a specific practice. The majority of contact lens assistants are trained in an optometric office. It is easiest to train a contact lens assistant who is presently a contact lens wearer. These individuals are more sensitive to the problems and needs of a potential contact lens patient and have personal experience as a wearer to guide them.

Many times, because of relocation or other circumstance, an individual with an extensive contact lens background can be hired by a practice. Although these individuals understand the basics of contact lens care, it is generally necessary to give them additional on-the-job training to conform to the standards of practice. In fact, all contact lens technicians should be required to attend ophthalmic assistants' courses offered at state and regional educational meetings. Attendance at continuing education courses not only adds new knowledge but also helps keep the assistant motivated and enthusiastic.

Contact lens assistants should know their personal limits and should understand the degree of autonomy allowed to assistants under state law. Any questions of a professional nature concerning the limits of responsibility should be brought to the supervising optometrist for resolution. In many states, trained ophthalmic dispensers can practice contact lens fitting under the direct supervision of an optometrist. In addition, these individuals can act as supervisors to contact lens assistants with less training.

It is possible, by having well-structured office procedures, to allow employees who are contact lens assistants to make independent decisions. These independent decisions can be outlined in their scope of work and are described in the office handbook (see Chapter 21).

Scope of Work

To have a well-run contact lens practice, contact lens assistants should have clearly defined responsibilities that are described in writing. The scope of these responsibilities will vary from practice to practice, but basic skills that are generally required include the following:

Telephone skills are essential. A contact lens assistant should be able to answer many procedural contact lens questions by telephone. On occasions when patients do not return for follow-up care, these assistants should be trained to call patients and encourage them to return. The contact lens assistant should be made aware of the philosophy of the office regarding fees and should be able to intelligently discuss and answer any questions that a potential contact lens patient might have about fees.

The assistant should understand why a contact lens patient must return for a follow-up appointment and what procedures will be performed during that visit. The contact lens assistant should be trained to understand rigid gas-permeable and hydrogel lenses and also should understand the use of solutions, eye makeup and eye makeup remover, and face creams by contact lens wearers.

In most states the contact lens assistant can legally use an automatic refractor, objective or subjective refracting system, keratometer, or lensometer. This use of assistants changes the role of the optometrist from a data collector to a data analyzer and decision maker, decreasing the contact lens practitioner's costs while maintaining professional quality.

The assistant should understand that questions beyond the scope of his or her expertise must be brought to the attention of the supervising optometrist. By using assistants to their optimum capacity, optometrists can work at their highest level of professional capability in the most cost-effective manner.

Contact Lens Inventory

For practitioners who fit contact lenses, there is an inevitable need for trial lens sets and a contact lens inventory. A balance must be achieved between the size of the inventory and its cost-effectiveness.

The larger the inventory, the greater the number of options the practitioner can offer to patients. On the other hand, the larger the inventory, the greater the expense of maintaining it. The advantage of maintaining a large inventory—in addition to permitting the patient and the practitioner the maximum choice of product—is the ability to dispense lenses to the patient on the same day the lenses are fitted or needed. Because U.S. citizens live in a society that treasures immediate results, the sooner the patient can receive the lenses, the happier the patient will be. Moreover, there is a great advantage to be realized in terms of quality control. The larger the inventory, the greater the opportunity to replace a lens on the same day.

The disadvantage of a large inventory is that lenses not in use have already been paid for and can constitute a significant expense. The advent of disposable and planned replacement lenses has placed new demands on inventory. This issue should be managed with the "just-in-time" approach, which allows the manufacturer to maintain a large inventory and uses overnight mail and messenger service to replace depleted inventory. Another disadvantage of a large inventory is the problem of obsolescence. It is essential that any arrangements made with a manufacturer include the return of unopened vials for full credit. The final disadvantage of a large inventory is a lack of inventory control. With proper computerization, however, an effort at inventory control can be made.

Practitioners need fitting sets of lenses made by various manufacturers, including different polymers, which allow the broadest range of parameters in hydrogel products. In addition, the contact lens practitioner should select a favorite daily wear, extended wear, and disposable lens, which should be well inventoried. The practitioner should not inventory lenses that are dispensed under different brand names but have the same parameters and polymer.

The inventory should have one favorite daily wear, rigid gas-permeable lens that is inventoried on a consignment basis. The rest of the available rigid gas-permeable lenses should be small fitting sets. It is unnecessary to inventory every type of lens because required lenses can be received by overnight mail with the "just-in-time" replacement philosophy.

It is inadvisable to try to inventory toric and bifocal lenses since the number of parameters that are available makes stocking these materials extremely expensive. Patients wearing custom-designed toric lenses, which might take several weeks to produce, should be advised of this fact. In many instances, patients will then decide to keep an unopened backup pair in the event of an emergency.

Every effort should be made to negotiate with contact lens laboratories to persuade them to consign lenses at minimum cost rather than to require outright purchases. The type of arrangement that can be made with a specific laboratory depends on the practitioner's negotiating skills and the volume of contact lens patients.

There is no exact formula for maintaining a contact lens inventory to maximize practitioner efficiency and patient convenience while minimizing inventory expense.

Reorder Methods for Contact Lenses

There are many reordering systems, but the two basic methods are replacement ordering and computerized systems. An inventory sheet with minimum numbers of lenses will determine when inventory is low, based on a weekly count. More lenses of the most frequently used powers (i.e., −2.00 to −4.00 D) should be maintained in inventory. Using bar codes, a computerized inventory system permits the practitioner to keep current on lenses that need to be reordered.

In most areas, contact lens sales representatives will visit an office, count the number of inventory lenses that have been dispensed, and reorder them for the office. In this way, each time a lens is dispensed, another lens of the same parameters is placed back into inventory.

Replacements also can be made by having the practitioner or staff order a replacement lens each time a lens is dispensed. The lens is ordered from the laboratory as a "stock lens."

Bar coding and automatic ordering by computer also can be used. Computer systems are now being updated to allow for bar coding that will result in automatic reordering.

Contact Lens Fee Structure

The contact lens fee structure can be broken down into fees for services and fees for materials. The fee for services is determined by the value of the practitioner's time—this includes the practitioner's charge for services, in addition to the base chair cost (see Chapter 41). Consideration also should be given to the fees charged for contact lens services in the community. Materials charges are based on the cost of lenses. A fee is added to the cost of the lenses to compensate for mailing and handling expenses, which can be as much as two times the cost. The amount to be added will be influenced by the cost to patients of obtaining similar materials in the community.

Replacement lenses usually are provided at a predetermined cost based on the fee policies of the office. A frequent replacement lens program establishes the cost of office visits and lens replacement as a fixed dollar amount per year and guarantees the patient a certain number of lenses per year. A disposable lens program is like a frequent replacement system—the patient pays a fixed amount per year and receives a certain number of lenses and certain enumerated services. A structured program encourages patients to use the lenses dispensed each year and reduces the tendency of patients to hoard or stockpile supplies of lenses.

Refund Policy

Each office should establish a fair adjustment policy for patients who cannot be successfully fitted with lenses. The value of such a policy cannot be overemphasized because it allows an escape clause for both the practitioner and the patient if the fitting does not succeed.

The contact lens patient who cannot be successfully fitted can be a management problem for the practice. The practitioner can spend an enormous amount of time, effort, and money constantly replacing lenses in the hopes that the fit will succeed. It is often preferable to inform the patient that the fitting was not successful and offer a refund.

Refunds can be made by returning part of the fee for materials, but a more desirable approach is a refund composed of other types of ophthalmic materials (such as sunwear). When a refund is given, the patient should be asked to sign a written release indicating that a refund was received and that the practice is no longer obligated to continue contact lens services.

Contact Lens Fitting and Service Agreements

Documentation of contact lens fitting and follow-up is essential, and written agreements are a necessary part of contact lens practice. Both fitting agreements and service agreements should be used.

Fitting and Informed Consent Agreements

A written contact lens fitting agreement is a valuable component of contact lens practice management. The agreement should address issues of patient compliance with wearing schedules, contact lens care and handling, and needed follow-up care.

The agreement also should specify the exact fees that are being charged for the contact lens care, including the cost of the original lens supply and replacement lenses. It also should specify the cost of needed follow-up care and should include a discussion of a refund policy if the patient proves to be unsuccessful as a contact lens wearer.

For extended-wear contact lens patients, the agreement must contain language that informs the patients of the risks of overnight wear and of the alternative modalities that are available (see Chapter 11). A properly worded agreement, signed by the patient and the doctor (or doctor's representative)—a copy of which is given to the patient, with the original retained in the record—will provide written evidence that the patient was properly informed if there should be any legal dispute.

Service Agreements

The use of prepaid agreements for contact lens follow-up care is thought, by many practitioners, to be an extremely valuable management tool. These agreements allow patients to pay in advance for follow-up visits and to receive solutions and contact lenses at a reduced fee (Figure 31-4). The benefits generally include a fixed number of visits per year, while the fees include the cost of the service contract and the charges for lens replacements. In general, the presentation of the service contract should be made at the completion of the initial contact lens fitting procedure. It should be offered by the practitioner as part of the treatment plan and further described by the assistants before asking the patient to sign a contact lens fitting agreement.

Contact Lens Prescriptions

The Federal Trade Commission requires practitioners to provide patients with a prescription at the completion of an examination conducted for the purpose of prescribing spectacles (see Chapter 28). However, there is no federal requirement to provide a copy of a contact lens prescription; the release of contact lens prescriptions is controlled by state law. These requirements vary from state to state: some states leave it to the discretion of the practitioner to determine whether a patient is to be given a contact lens prescription, but the majority of states require prescriptions to be released, usually under certain circumstances and at specific times in the contact lens fitting process. In most states the obligation to release the prescription is not incurred until the patient has been successfully fitted with lenses, as demonstrated by postfitting follow-up visits. Individual state laws must be consulted to determine exact legal obligations.

When a contact lens prescription is provided, it should include all pertinent parameters of the lens, the specific lens material, whether lens wear is daily or overnight, and a reasonable expiration date.

Contact Lens Solutions

Most contact lens offices provide complimentary solutions for lens cleaning and disinfection at the time contact lenses are dispensed. After the patient uses the initial supply, many practitioners prefer to sell a 3- to 6-month supply of solutions to the patient, thus ensuring that the patient will continue to use the recommended solutions. At the very least, to encourage compliance, the solutions and their usage should be spelled out in a written contact lens fitting agreement.

Contact Lens Follow-up Care

Follow-up care is an inherent aspect of contact lens practice. After the final lens design has been determined, it is appropriate to see the patient for a 1-week and then a 1-month follow-up visit to ensure that the patient is enjoying optimum vision, comfort, and physiologic response. Three-month checkups are recommended for patients using lenses overnight. Six-month checkups are recommended for individuals who are daily wear contact lens patients.

By Appointment

Practice Limited
To Contact Lenses

PAUL FARKAS, O.D.
T.W. KASSALOW, O.D.
BARRY FARKAS, O.D., P.C.
F.A.A.O. - DIPLOMATES - CONTACT LENS SECTION

AND ASSOCIATES

30 East 60th Street
New York, NY 10022
(212) 355-5145

1025 Northern Blvd.
Roslyn, NY 11576
(516) 365-4500

CONTACT LENS SERVICE CONTRACT

This is to certify that _____ has contracted, for a fee of **$150.00**, to receive the following services through: **July 22, 2002.**

1. Two (2) office visits to maintain optimum performance of your present contact lenses.

2. Unlimited replacement of contact lenses (of like material) at the following rate:

   Daily Wear Hydrogel Lenses replaced at $70.00 per lens.

3. An office visit within 30 days of dispensing of a lens replacement will be included at no charge while the Service Contract is in effect.

4. Special visual evaluations outside of normal contact lens follow-up care are not included in this contract. The customary fee for these services will be reduced by 10%.

Sincerely,

Barry Farkas, O.D.

Dated:

Figure 31-4 Sample prepaid service agreement. (Courtesy Dr. Paul Farkas, Boca Raton, Fla.)

It has been shown that the most effective way of ensuring that patients return for appropriate follow-up care after a fitting is to schedule the follow-up before the patient has left the office (preappointments). This approach to scheduling will be most effective when the doctor not only specifies the date but also emphasizes the importance of the follow-up visit to the patient. Office staff members who schedule the follow-up appointments also should reiterate the reason for the next visit in terms that will emphasize the benefit to the patient.

To further secure success of the preappointment scheduling approach, the patient should be called by telephone 3 to 7 days before the appointment to confirm the date and time of the scheduled visit. Additionally, if the appointment is scheduled more than 3 months ahead, a written confirmation should be mailed 1 month before the scheduled appointment.

The recall approach that is most efficient for a particular practice is the approach that should be used; however, a consistently used follow-up evaluation system is essential for the patient's continued success with contact lenses and the maintenance of good ocular health.

If patients fail to keep scheduled follow-up appointments, an effort should be made to reschedule them. It has been shown that the most effective means of rescheduling patients is by telephone. This approach offers an opportunity to discuss the value of the next appointment with the patient personally and to resolve any issues that may have prevented the patient from returning to the office. If telephone recall attempts are unsuccessful, a written notice should be sent to the patient describing the importance of the recommended follow-up care and giving the patient an opportunity to make an appointment (Figure 31-5).

If after a reasonable time (6 months to a year), the patient has failed to keep recommended follow-up appointments, further efforts should be made to determine the reason for the patient's noncompliance. It may be determined that the patient simply chooses not to return, or that the patient has discontinued contact lens wear, or has sought care from another practitioner.

In any event, at this point the patient should be informed in writing of recommendations for further eye care and that the patient is being placed on the practice's inactive list.

Conclusion

This chapter summarizes how to develop a contact lens practice from within an existing patient base as well as how to efficiently administer a contact lens practice for optimum benefit to patients. The methods described are used in successful contact lens practices throughout the United States. Although not every approach is universally suitable, most of these suggestions should be helpful to any practitioner, whether the practitioner fits contact lenses on a full-time basis or as necessary as part of a primary care practice.

By Appointment   Practice Limited
                                                                  To Contact Lenses

PAUL FARKAS, O.D.
T.W. KASSALOW, O.D.
BARRY FARKAS, O.D., P.C.
F.A.A.O. - DIPLOMATES - CONTACT LENS SECTION

_____

AND ASSOCIATES

30 East 60th Street   1025 Northern Blvd.
New York, New York 10022   Roslyn, New York 11576
(212) 355-5145   (516) 365-4500
FAX: (212) 308-3262   FAX: (516) 365-6580

Dear:

Your record indicates that we have not had the opportunity of checking your vision and general ocular condition for quite some time.

Unlike eyeglasses, where only the visual acuity is the determining factor, contact lens wearers require semiannual checkups to determine whether any corneal changes have taken place. Occasionally adjustments, polishing, or cleaning techniques are necessary to insure continued lens comfort. Changes can occur even after several years of successful contact lens wear, which can lead to discomfort and lower wearing time. In addition, new products are occasionally introduced which can improve your overall contact lens comfort and visual performance.

Our prime concern is that you continue to achieve optimum performance from your contact lenses.

Sincerely,

Barry Farkas, O.D., F.A.A.O.

Figure 31-5 Sample reminder of a missed appointment. (Courtesy Dr. Paul Farkas, Boca Raton, Fla.)

Acknowledgement

The authors of this chapter in the first edition of *Business Aspects of Optometry* were Paul Farkas and Neil B. Gailmard.

Bibliography

Bennett E: The profitability of RGP lenses. *Contact Lens Spectrum* 10(1):16, 1995.

Bennett I: *Management for the eyecare practitioner.* Stoneham, Mass, 1993, Butterworth.

Bevington RC: Stay successful with disposable lenses. *Contact Lens Spectrum (Suppl)* 14(5):11s-3s, 1999.

Classé JG: Management of contact lens prescriptions. *Optom Clin* 4(1):93-102, 1994.

Cosgrove J: Successful contact lens practice. *Contact Lens Spectrum* 15(11):42,44,46, 2000.

Farkas P: How to find the perfect aide. *Optom Management* 10(9):18-21, 1974.

Farkas P: A rational refund policy. *Contact Lens J* 20(2):23, 1992.

Farkas P: Developing a contact lens practice. *Contact Lens J* 20(8):15-7, 1993.

Farkas P: Practicing optometry today: Setting high standards and living up to them. *Optom Today* 3(5):30-2,34, 1995.

Farkas P, McGlone V: Before planning for the future evaluate the present. *Contact Lens Spectrum* 10(7):46-7, 1995.

Gailmard NB: Contact lens strategies for a consumer-driven market. *Optom Management* 34(2):17s-9s, 1999.

Ghormley NR: Contact lenses are profitable. *Optom Economics* 2(8):30-1, 1992.

Kattouf RS: Competing on convenience and price. *Optom Management* 31(9):34,36,38, 1996.

Koetting RA: Marketing contact lenses in a competitive world. *Contact Lens Spectrum* 14(9):25-6,28-29, 1999.

Koffler BH: 8 reasons to add contact lenses to your practice. *Rev Ophthalmol (Suppl)* 7(1):6,8,10, 2000.

Lee J: Five ways to keep your contact lens practice competitive. *Rev Ophthalmol* 5(3):51,54-5, 1998.

Nelson A: Seven staff motivators for building your contact lens practice. *Rev Optom* 132(1):39, 1995.

Tuberty P: Making your bottom line come alive. *Optom Management* 33(2):36, 1998.

Wagner H, Janoff LE, Patrick A: Quality assurance in a cornea and contact lens service. *Optom Education* 25(1):15-20, 1999.

www.clspectrum.com. Online version of *Contact Lens Spectrum* magazine, which contains articles on contact lens practice.

www.optometric.com. Online version of *Optometric Management* magazine, which offers information on contact lens practice.

www.revoptom.com. Online version of *Review of Optometry* magazine, which offers information on contact lens practice.

Chapter 32
Marketing

Lawrence S. Thal and Craig Hisaka

You can tell the ideals of a nation by its advertisements.
Norman Douglas *South Wind*

Like a nation, the ideals of an optometric practice can probably be determined by its advertisements. However, advertising should not be confused with marketing. Comparing the definition of these two terms illustrates their differences. As applied to optometry, *marketing* can be defined as "the total of activities by which the provision of services and transfer of materials from optometrist to patient are effected." In comparison, *advertising* would be defined as "the art or practice of calling public attention to one's product, service, needs, or related matters—especially by paid announcements in newspapers and magazines or over radio, television, or other media."

As these definitions indicate, an advertisement is a message—printed in a newspaper or magazine, broadcast on radio or television, sent to individuals through the mail, or disseminated in some other fashion—that attempts to convince readers or listeners to favor a particular optometrist or buy a particular product. Surveys of optometrists have revealed that 27% of patients choose their optometrist or ophthalmologist on the recommendation of relatives or friends and, for an established practice, more than 65% of patient flow is derived from previous patients. In many practices, therefore, advertising could be used only to compete for the remaining 10% of patients. This might explain why many practitioners have concluded that advertisements, in the long run, do not really increase earnings. Recent studies have shown that television, radio, and newspaper advertising produce only 5.6% of new patients and Yellow Pages advertising, 4.6%.

It is because of marketing, not advertising, that the majority of patients continue to return to optometrists year after year for care. The goal of marketing is to acquire, satisfy, and retain patients. It is clear that

optometrists who understand the needs of their patients and seek to satisfy them tend to be more successful than optometrists who do not. Even though marketing has evolved into a potentially complex and diverse field, which includes a wide variety of special functions—such as advertising, public relations, market research, and so forth—the basic needs of most patients usually are not complex. Their needs are best satisfied by listening, providing education, and being able to convey a caring attitude. It is unfortunate that patients usually are not qualified to determine how much a practitioner knows. It is easy, however, for a patient to gain a sense of how much a practitioner cares.

External Marketing

The most commonly used external marketing technique is advertising.

Advertising

The aim of advertising is to influence consumer choice. A magazine, television program, or any other advertising medium is judged by an advertiser according to "exposure opportunity"—the number of people who might see the advertisement—and "message opportunity"—the way an advertisement communicates via a particular medium.

In considering "exposure," advertisers speak of "reach," which signifies the number of people who see or hear the advertisement at least once, and of "frequency," which is the average number of times each person is "reached." An advertisement's total impact is indicated by its number of "gross impressions"—reach times frequency. A further aspect of exposure is cost, which usually is stated as "cost per thousand gross impressions" (CPM). Another aspect is "target reach," which is the number of people within a specific audience who have seen the advertisement. Often, advertisers want to reach only one segment of an audience—for example, women, teenagers, presbyopic individuals, or new residents of a particular community. Exposure, reach, and frequency are factors that influence the selection of advertising media, including television, radio, newspapers, magazines, or direct mail.

Television provides high exposure and low CPM. It is not efficient for specific targets. Because it supplies sound, pictures, and movement, it offers the most complete message opportunity. Unlike printed media, however, its messages are ephemeral, disappearing after being broadcast. Television receives approximately 21% of total advertising expenditures in the United States.

Television is the most striking communications medium in the world today, and radio is listened to as never before. Exposure through broadcast media reaches an extensive audience. Television and radio stations often allot time for public service programming, including interviews and listener call-in shows. These formats are excellent opportunities for participation as an eye care expert.

Radio is good for targeting various geographic, age, or interest groups. Its CPM is very low. Like television, its messages are conveyed only when being broadcast. Because radio offers nothing but sound, it is the most limited medium. Radio receives approximately 7% of the total advertising expenditures in the United States.

Broadcast promotion is expensive and requires considerable expertise in writing, production, and media selection. To be effective, broadcast promotions must air for a sustained length of time. Intermittent announcements are costly and often ineffective. With the exception of practitioners who have practices in extremely competitive environments, most optometrists find the paid use of broadcast media to be expensive and unnecessary.

Newspapers have much lower exposure than television or radio but reach a higher percentage of the areas they cover. They are excellent for geographic targeting. Newspapers receive the highest proportion of total advertising expenditures (approximately 30%). Many optometrists have instituted media relations programs, which consist of sending short news releases to local newspapers on a regular, year-round basis. The news release usually offers helpful eye care advice or provides information on optometric public service activities. By sending out releases on a regular basis,

optometrists establish visibility and credibility among editors, increasing the probability that they will be written about in newspapers or consulted on eye-related articles.

Optometrists have received positive media exposure by supplying eye care columns for local newspapers. The American Optometric Association (AOA) offers a series of columns with accompanying artwork for this purpose.

Paid announcements in large newspapers and magazines usually are not necessary for most optometric practices. When used, announcements must be published for a substantial period to attract attention, gain acceptance, and foster recall. Many optometrists find that other, more targetable communications are more effective.

Magazines provide less exposure than does television, radio, or newspapers but are highly selective with respect to audience interests. Magazines reproduce more attractively than newspapers, but newspapers are printed more frequently. Magazines receive approximately 9% of total advertising expenditures in the United States.

Direct mail is not inexpensive, but it is the most selective of all media. The advertiser typically uses mailing lists containing only the names of people within the selected audience. Listings are chosen for particular features, such as age, geography, sex, income, or other characteristics. Direct mail can offer lengthy messages, but it has the disadvantage of being easily discarded by the recipient before being examined. Direct mail receives approximately 14% of total advertising expenditures in the United States.

A variety of printed materials can be used effectively to keep the optometrist's name visible to current patients and to raise his or her profile in the community. Some proven strategies include the use of brochures and pamphlets, literature published by the AOA, letters and mailings, news releases, practice newsletters, personal letters, and telephone listings.

Brochures and Pamphlets

Distributing educational brochures is an excellent way to increase patient and community awareness of professional services, to build an identity with civic and community organizations, and to educate and inform individual consumers. Sending brochures not only gets eye care information into patients' homes but at the same time reminds them that the practitioner is a concerned professional. Patients might pass the brochure on to neighbors or friends—all potential patients.

Regardless of where or when literature is distributed, it is important for it to contain the practitioner's identity. Literature should be tastefully printed with the optometrist's name, office address, and telephone number, making it easy for a recipient to obtain more information or make an appointment.

American Optometric Association Literature

An excellent source of educational literature is the AOA. Member optometrists can obtain professionally written and designed materials covering nearly every aspect of eye care.

Letters and Mailings

Another effective technique for keeping a continuous flow of information to patients is to create special mailings. Birthdays, holidays, and other special occasions offer opportunities for optometrists to personalize their relationship with patients.

News Releases

Many optometrists have found that sending news releases to local newspapers is an effective public relations strategy. A news release might focus on a new staff member or associate, a new service, a screening that the optometrist is sponsoring, or a human interest story about the optometrist or one of the optometrist's patients.

Practice Newsletter

Newsletters are versatile, economical, and well-received marketing tools. They help the optometrist keep in touch with patients between office visits and provide information about the office staff, patients, new products and services, and advances in eye care.

Personal Letters

Personal letters or announcements, sent to patients and referral sources, are good vehicles for announcing a new location, additional services, a new partner or associate, or a change in office hours. Direct mail adds importance to an announcement that otherwise might be hidden in a newsletter.

In general, printed media—newspapers, magazines, or direct mail—offer a significant advantage: they can be saved for future reference.

Telephone Listings

Another form of printed media is the telephone book. The Yellow Pages is the one form of advertising that all optometrists use. There are two types of Yellow Pages listings—trademark listings and display advertising. The trademark listing is a 1-inch by 1-column advertisement that can include a name line, a certain number of words, and the logo of a society, with a listing of local members beneath it. A display advertisement can be up to half a page in size and can refer readers to the trademark listing. Whether or not an optometrist chooses to use a display advertisement, a trademark listing for the local optometric society is often considered a necessity.

Even though advertising is a very effective method for reaching a large audience quickly, it is an extremely expensive option for most health care professionals. By effectively using less aggressive and less costly communication techniques, many optometrists find that a telephone directory listing is the only form of paid promotion they need to market their practice. If a practitioner decides to use some form of advertising, however, it will be necessary to devise a marketing plan.

Components of a Marketing Plan

Components of a marketing plan consist of a mission statement, goals, and strategies. A sample marketing plan is illustrated in Box 32-1.

Mission Statement

The mission statement describes the basic purpose of the practice and what the optometrist seeks to accomplish through it. The marketing goals break down the mission statement into the five or six major tasks that the practitioner must accomplish to achieve or come close to achieving the mission. Once the practitioner has set these goals, the ways in which they will be met can be established. These methods constitute the practitioner's marketing strategies which, once set, lead to a tactical plan to implement each strategy.

Marketing Goals

Before a practitioner decides on marketing goals, the current marketing situation must be analyzed. For example, the practitioner might want to work with young children and increase the number of patients seen so that more than 50% of the practice is devoted to pediatric care. If the school population is decreasing, however, and if there are several other optometrists in the community who specialize in pediatric care, this goal might not be realistic. Therefore, goals must reflect reality. That reality includes the opportunities and problems that affect the practice.

Box 32-1 Sample Marketing Plan for an Optometric Practice

Mission statement

To provide high-quality, reasonably priced primary eye care with special emphasis on services for children and to educate patients and the community about the importance of ongoing, routine eye care.

Goal #1

Attract 50 patients (younger than 12 years old) during the next 6 months by improving communications with parents of school-aged children.
  Strategy: Write articles for practice newsletter on eye conditions that affect children. Emphasize the practice's special expertise in diagnosing and treating these problems.
  Strategy: Write a news release for the local newspaper discussing children's eye problems and treatments.
  Strategy: Volunteer to speak at a meeting of a parent-teacher organization or other community group whose members are parents of school-aged children.
  Strategy: Organize a children's eye screening at a local shopping center or participate in community-wide health screening or "Save Your Vision Week" event.

Goal #2:

In the next 12 months, make children's frames account for 20% of dispensary business.
  Strategy: Increase by 20% the number of children's frames in the dispensary.
  Strategy: Create a children's corner in the dispensary with special decor and display area.
  Strategy: Write an article for practice newsletter on children's frames (e.g., special features, how to select children's frames). Create an attractive "fact sheet" using this same information and display it prominently in the office or use as a handout to parents of school-aged children.

Modified from Allergan, Inc: Pathways in optometry. *Irvine, Calif, 1994, Allergan.*

Suppose, for example, that a department store chain is going to offer eye care at a shopping mall near a practitioner's office. The optometrist might see this as a real threat–patients could be lost to the store. In response, the practitioner might set a goal to minimize the risk that the store represents to the practice. On the other hand, the optometrist might see department store eye care as an opportunity. It could be a chance for the practitioner to highlight and contrast the services being offered by his or her practice compared with those offered by the store. By having this store nearby, the practitioner can capitalize on the differences. Either way, the practitioner has identified the effect that this external factor has on the practice and can plan a response to it.

Marketing Strategies

Strategies are the way that a practitioner meets the goals that have been set. Strategies are based on target markets and the marketing mix.

Before selecting a strategy, two things must be decided about the current market. First, is the practitioner going to provide services to all segments of the market, or will the practitioner concentrate marketing efforts on one particular target segment? Second, should the practitioner choose to target one or more market segments, and which would they be? The major benefit of target marketing is that it allows the practitioner to concentrate marketing efforts and resources.

Another factor that affects the selection of strategies is the marketing mix. There are four basic considerations. An optometrist's "service" is eye care, "place" is the setting in which that care is delivered, "price" is the fee charged for services, and "promotion" refers to the way the practitioner communicates with current and potential patients. The practitioner analyzes each of the four areas and looks for ways to enhance them when formulating marketing strategies.

Only after a practitioner has analyzed the market and formulated goals is he or she ready to begin marketing activities. Participating in marketing activities without a clear set of goals is a scatter-shot approach, one that can keep the practitioner busy without producing significant results.

Advertising Effectiveness

A 1991 study of the amount spent on advertising by 3432 California optometrists in solo practice found several characteristics to be statistically significant. Practices that spent the most on advertising had the following results:

- More patients seen per week
- More total time spent fitting contact lenses
- Less time spent with individual patients receiving contact lenses
- Higher gross income
- More technicians employed
- Lower fees
- Less time spent per patient examination
- Less time spent on health portions of examinations
- Patients on a more frequent recall schedule

Practices that spent the least on advertising had the following results:

- More time spent per patient examination
- Higher net-to-gross income ratio
- Larger patient backlog

Because many studies of advertising effectiveness have been performed, with highly variable results reported, it is left to each practitioner to determine how to use advertising within a specific community. Since an advertisement conveys the ideals of a practice, a practitioner must be very careful not to damage an otherwise good public impression. Advertising actually can be destructive if it is aimed at a target audience but is considered inappropriate by that audience. Most Americans have seen advertising that they find to be offensive. Although it can be assumed that an advertisement in poor taste will alienate consumers from the product, the advertiser who uses it has apparently been convinced that this method of advertising is, in fact, effective.

An example of advertising with a poor effect is "price advertising." Lower prices are thought to be synonymous with lower quality. As some ophthalmic chains have found, the power of advertising—when based strictly on cost—does not well serve the advertiser in the long run. Although price advertising is known to be effective in building a short-term response, it also can destroy the consumer's perception of the advertiser's professional abilities, hindering the advertiser's capacity to develop a loyal customer base for the long term. As a result, the traditional means of attracting patients to chains—advertising low prices, convenience, and variety of products—has not met with long-term success.

Some of the commercial chains have, in fact, chosen to abandon the discount market—a small and low-profit segment of the industry—in favor of advertising campaigns aimed toward the value market, which is made up of patients who desire quality care. This market belongs largely to private optometrists, who in 2000 provided 39.8% of all eye examinations and

accounted for 35.6% of the total ophthalmic market. In 2000 optometrists performed 57.4% of all examinations, and ophthalmologists performed 42.6%.

State laws and board rules can include specific regulations about advertising. They should be consulted before an advertising program is initiated as part of a marketing effort.

Legal and Ethical Aspects of Advertising

Optometry boards have a long history of opposition to advertising. Despite the advent of precedent-setting decisions by the U.S. Supreme Court recognizing the right of professionals to advertise, boards may continue to initiate actions to prevent unfair or deceptive advertising of ophthalmic goods or services.

The ban on advertising by professionals began in the 1930s. In the 1950s the U.S. Supreme Court stated that it could "see no constitutional reason why a state may not treat all who deal with the human eye as members of a profession who should use no merchandising methods for obtaining customers." In the majority of states, the high court's opinion resulted in laws or board rulings that prohibited or restricted advertising by optometrists.

Deceptive tactics that led to these restrictive state statutes and regulations included "bait and switch" advertising. Cut-rate prices would be advertised by the business, but the low-priced items would be either "unavailable" or "unsuitable" for the potential purchaser, who would end up buying an expensive item instead. Another reprehensible tactic was "capping and steering," in which advertising was used to lure people seeking ophthalmic materials to an unscrupulous practitioner. After the practitioner had "capped" the individual by determining the spectacle prescription, the individual was "steered" to the business for the sale of expensive eyewear. Underlying these and other despicable practices was the power of advertising, which, although undeniably abused, achieved its single purpose—to attract business. Advertising is not profitable unless a volume business is sought, and it is this fundamental purpose of advertising that is at odds with the concept of professionalism and quality of care.

Since the 1970s the Supreme Court has recognized that certain commercial advertising by professionals should be afforded constitutional protection. However, states are still allowed to set reasonable restrictions to ensure that consumers receive truthful and nondeceptive advertising (Box 32-2). Exact provisions vary from state to state, and state laws and board

---

Box 32-2 Examples of State Restrictions on Advertising

- Optometrists must be able to substantiate all claims made in advertisements and any claims must be accurate. It is unlawful to disseminate any form of public communication containing a false, fraudulent, misleading, or deceptive statement.
- Guarantees, if stated, must be adhered to and spelled out.
- Reference to price in an advertisement should be exact. Terms such as "from $19.99," "as little as," or "as low as" should not be used since these are potentially misleading.
- Advertising professional superiority or advertising that an optometrist performs professional services in a superior manner is prohibited.
- It is illegal to employ or use solicitors (cappers or steerers).
- It is illegal to advertise professional services as being free or without cost.
- If costs of services are mentioned, they should be clearly identifiable. All variables and other material factors should be specifically disclosed.
- The price advertised for products should include charges for any related professional services, including dispensing and fitting services, unless the advertisement specifically and clearly indicates otherwise.

Source: Authors' review of state optometry laws, 2001.

---

regulations must be consulted to determine the specific restrictions in any particular jurisdiction.

Community Outreach

A community outreach program involves offering eye care and education. Among the most common and proven methods for community outreach are participation in eye care events and health fairs and the use of public speaking.

Eye Care Events

A well-organized special event can focus much attention on eye care in a short period, and it offers many opportunities to inform consumers about optometry.

There also are several national eye care events that provide optometrists with an ideal opportunity to build public exposure while offering a much-needed public service. The AOA-sponsored "Save Your Vision Week" is announced by presidential proclamation each year and takes place during the first full week of March. A major focal point of this event is "Give One Day," which promotes volunteer services for working individuals who are in need of eye care but not covered by insurance.

The AOA offers several tools to help practitioners participate in such events. Planning guides for national events, such as "Save Your Vision Week" and "Older Americans Month," are included periodically in the *AOA News*.

Especially effective are screenings for vision problems, cataracts, and glaucoma. Screenings attract positive attention from the media, as well as from potential patients. Target populations, such as high school athletes, children, or older adults, are excellent choices for screening programs. Good locations for vision screenings include schools, senior centers, banks, and shopping malls. Even though such screenings are wonderful opportunities to gain name recognition in a community, they should not be used as a source of patients. "Self-referral" may not be ethical in such an environment and may conflict with state law.

Different opportunities for exposure also arise at other times of the year. For example, an optometrist can volunteer to screen local high school football and basketball players. In many states, high school athletes must be given a physical examination before the start of the season. The optometrist might be able to work with local physicians and other health care providers in providing this service.

Health Fairs

Health fairs present excellent marketing opportunities for optometrists. Most health fairs are sponsored by at least one health-oriented group, such as a hospital or health organization. National Health Fair Week, which takes place in the spring, is supported by thousands of national, regional, and local groups that represent all levels of government; media; business and industry; and health, academic, and civic organizations.

Speaking Engagements

As a doctor of optometry, a practitioner is considered an expert in eye care in the community. As part of a public relations program, optometrists should endeavor to speak to as many groups as possible. To obtain speaking opportunities, practitioners can volunteer to be part of the speaker's bureau of a state or local optometric association.

Speaking engagements offer the advantage of a meeting with a large audience. The practitioner can promote optometry in an informal yet educational way that can result in new patients, while raising the level of consciousness about the need for eye care in the community. To help optometrists become effective speakers, the AOA has developed the *Optometric Speaker's Guidebook* (St. Louis, American Optometric Association 1978), which contains helpful statistics and guidelines for speech preparation.

In addition to public education, an aim of community outreach is to positively influence the way practitioners and the services provided by practitioners are perceived. This means enhancing the image of optometrists as providers of quality eye care.

Internal Marketing

Internal marketing involves the dissemination of information to an existing patient population to educate them about services, ophthalmic materials, new developments, and related matters that will motivate patients to return for further care.

Patient Perceptions

Patients can perceive changes. The most common and obvious change is when the practitioner decreases the time spent with patients. When this "quality time" begins to diminish, patients often remark, "When the doctor started the practice, he spent time with me. The doctor cared for his patients, but now the doctor is just too busy." The underlying message is that the practitioner is too busy to care anymore and, perhaps, is "chasing the dollar." Today, it is very common to hear patients openly complain about "greed among doctors" and how they miss their "old" doctor, "old" optometrist, or "old" dentist. They feel that these practitioners cared more about their patients, always had time, and showed compassion for them. What a sad commentary about our generation of health care providers—technically more skillful, but lacking in care and compassion for their patients.

The key to successful internal marketing is to adopt a philosophy that is committed to furthering the best interests of patients, to treating patients in the same manner as we would all wish to be treated, and to maintaining that philosophy.

Public opinion surveys regarding doctor-patient relationships come to the same conclusion again and again. Patients are most infuriated when practitioners convey an impression that they don't care. Such an attitude is indicated when patients comment that a practitioner does the following:

- "Doesn't care about the patient's feelings or personal comfort"
- "Is impressed with his or her own importance"
- "Is cold, distant, and patronizing"
- "Acts as though he or she knows everything"
- "Is a terrible listener"
- "Causes undue waiting, with no respect for the patient's time"
- "Is abrupt, rude, and rushed"
- "Turns patients over to a technician"
- "Has bad personal habits and mannerisms"
- "Gave the impression that I was just another patient and didn't remember my name"
- "Had an overcrowded waiting room"
- "Used too many technical terms"
- "Has inconvenient hours, parking, and location"
- "Speaks too fast or too slow, has pauses that go unnoticed, repeatedly clears the throat, speaks in a monotone; has a high-pitched voice, uses sloppy speech patterns; drops consonants, and slurs pronunciation"
- "Makes it seem like an assembly line—interest in money, not in patients"
- "Is disrespectful to patients and staff"
- "Didn't listen or give me enough time"
- "Belittled me and treated me like a child"

How to Obtain Patient Referrals

It has been said that a satisfied patient is one who gets what was bargained for—competent and skilled services—and that an enthusiastic patient is one who gets more than was expected—something "extra." Whenever a patient receives more in return than was given, that patient not only feels that something is owed in return but also feels motivated to reward the practitioner. An enthusiastic patient does this by providing the best form of "advertising"—recommending the practitioner to family and friends—which results in patient referrals.

Extras can make a big difference in the way people feel and respond. Common examples of this difference include the courteous waiter who supplies water, coffee, and other service without being asked and the hotel staff member who performs all the extras that make a stay or vacation a pleasant experience. Many success stories in business have been built on this concept of providing more than was expected. To provide extras, a practitioner should be creative. Being creative does not require genius. It means thinking of those little things that make a difference. For top-quality hotels, it means leaving a newspaper each morning outside the guest's door and allowing easy access to coffee service. For practitioners, it can include keeping a good supply of current magazines in the reception area, allowing patients to take home a magazine if they want to finish it, putting coins in the reception room with a sign reading, "For the parking meter," having the receptionist call patients to let them know that appointments are running late, and similar courtesies intended to provide that something extra.

A patient fully expects a professional examination. Even if a practitioner has the best technical skills, however, a patient is not competent to judge them. It also is difficult to impress a patient with professional skills because the patient is inevitably more aware of the results than the techniques. If all that is provided is a professional examination, the patient will not complain, but the patient will probably not become an active source of referrals. Taking that extra step makes for an enthusiastic patient. Because of this often subtle distinction, the line can be very thin that separates a successful practice from a mediocre practice.

To increase patient referrals, a practitioner must learn to reinforce services by adding psychological value. For example, if appreciation is shown to a patient for having made a referral, it will increase the likelihood that the patient will recommend the practitioner again. The more unique, personal, and individual a practitioner can make each "thank you," the more the patient will feel appreciated. One reason a "thank you" provides powerful reinforcement is that gratitude itself is an "extra," a bonus. Also, if a patient is a frequent source of referrals, something extra is truly required—such as flowers, a plant, or some other small gift that shows appreciation for the patient's support. It is important to send "thank you" notes to professional colleagues who provide referrals. In such cases, the practitioner should endeavor to turn the referred patient into an "enthusiastic" patient—the referring professional's reputation also is at stake.

Another way to increase referrals is by hiring friendly, outgoing assistants. This can help build referrals in two ways. First, the assistant is usually the first one to provide a greeting when the patient enters the office and the last one to say goodbye. Having a cheerful assistant can leave a good, lasting impression on patients. The cheerful assistant also helps others in the office become more cheerful and friendly. The second way the assistant helps is outside the office. When the assistant talks about the practice to family, neighbors, and friends, a positive message is conveyed about the practitioner and optometry.

Internal marketing involves sharing information with patients. Various means can be used to provide this information. The most common have already been identified—brochures, newsletters, personal letters, and the like. However, more personalized means of marketing involve the sharing of information and time with patients, often while the patient is in the office. Examples include the following:

- Showing consideration for a patient's time
- Providing a sympathetic and caring demeanor in direct ratio to the concerns and fears of each patient
- Being available to come to the telephone
- Giving what is free to give (pharmaceutical samples will be much more appreciated by patients than by family members or personal friends)
- Giving what is not free to give (e.g., a magazine that the patient did not get to finish reading)
- Charting a patient's personal interests and family situation
- Being effusive in acknowledging gifts from patients
- Having a duplicate set of patient education materials in each examination room and in the patient consultation room
- Keeping a suggestion box in the office for both patient and staff use
- Being on time
- Learning all that can be learned about the patient
- Impressing the patient with a cohesive team
- Taking the time to teach the patient habits for better health, even if not eye related
- Having a good physical appearance and dressing professionally
- Offering something more in the waiting room than old magazines (do not overlook a professional journal that is less technical)
- Avoiding patient surprises by explaining what is going to be done before it is attempted
- Communicating clearly and honestly
- Treating patients as equals
- Having the receptionist convey an attitude of appreciation (a patient needs to hear a sincere "thank you" after paying the bill)
- Touching patients (practitioners should make it a point to greet patients with a handshake or pat at the first and last encounter in the office)

Having a good bedside manner will result in a direct positive financial impact on the practice. Patients will be retained longer, and a higher rate of patient referrals will be generated.

Other suggestions for that something extra to increase patient enthusiasm include the following:

Before performing any procedure, explain in advance what is going to be done, why it is going to be done, and what the patient can expect to happen. Always explain the benefits of a procedure to the patient.

Provide an extra service. If it is late and if it is appropriate, ask where the patient is parked and offer to provide an escort. If there is an emergency in which the patient needs new glasses and lives near the office but cannot come in, offer to deliver the glasses to the patient.

The finishing touch of any eye examination or office visit is a "thank you!"

Today, most patients want information from their optometrists. They desire to take an active role and participate in their own well-being. They want a sense of control, which includes the use of options and alternatives. Many polls and surveys indicate that consumers feel that the "best doctors are those who explain in a manner that the consumer understands." It also is true that most patients who are dissatisfied will not return to complain.

In contemporary health care, decreases in reimbursement rates, decreases in "market share" due to competition, rising costs of operating a practice, costs of expensive technological instrumentation, economic recession, and other economic factors have forced many practitioners to decrease the time spent with patients. This can "dehumanize" the practice. In such practices, the practitioner allocates time to solve the patients' optometric, medical, or dental problems, but the time to "bond" with patients is significantly reduced or eliminated. The result is that the patient perceives the practitioner to have a "quantity" practice rather than a "quality" practice.

The major difference between a quality practice and a quantity practice is that in a quality practice, the range of services is emphasized to a limited number of patients, whereas in a quantity practice the emphasis is on patient volume, with limited services and procedures being provided. In a quality practice, growth results in an upward curve that accelerates at an increasingly faster rate until the demands on the practitioner reach a point of diminishing returns, resulting in a slowing and eventual flattening of growth. As the quality of services begins to deteriorate, there inevitably will be a decline in the number of referrals, and patients will begin to seek services from other practitioners. The reason will be the "dehumanization" of the practice, brought on by the demands of quantity and the resultant decreased time and attention for each patient.

Conclusion

Marketing is a useful tool to help build and maintain a patient base. Through the use of external and internal marketing techniques, the practitioner can communicate with patients, prospective and established, while conveying a positive image of the practice and the profession. The use of marketing plans is an accepted part of professional practice, and practitioners should make use of external and internal marketing techniques as appropriate for their setting and circumstances. It should never be forgotten, however, that the most successful practices are built on the basis of service and that such practices provide something extra that sets them apart from their competitors. There are no marketing techniques that can satisfy patients and motivate them to return for future care if this highly personal element, inherent in the doctor-patient relationship, is not provided.

Bibliography

Morrisey M, ed: *Managed care and changing health care markets.* Washington, DC, 1998, American Enterprise Institute Press.

Allergan, Inc: *Pathways in optometry.* Irvine, Calif, 1994, Author.

American Optometric Association: *Optometric speaker's Guidebook.* St. Louis, 1978, Author.

American Optometric Association: *Caring for the eyes of America—a profile of the optometric profession.* St. Louis, 2002, Author.

Bagdasar S, Chew I, Smith C, et al: *The relationship between practice characteristics of solo practices and amount spent on advertising: an analysis of the California survey of 1988.* Unpublished thesis. University of California at Berkeley, School of Optometry, 1991.

Berkowitz EN: *Essentials of health care marketing.* Gaithersburg, Md, 1996, Aspen Publishers.

Elmstrom G: *Advanced management for optometrists.* Chicago, 1974, Professional Press.

Pinto JB, Shepard DD: *Marketing your ophthalmic practice.* Thorofare, NJ, 1987, Slack.

www.aoa.org. Web site for the American Optometric Association and a source for AOA publications.

Section Six

Financial Aspects of Practice

Chapter 33

Financial Planning

Gary L. Moss and John G. Classé

I have been poor and I have been rich. Rich is better.
Sophie Tucker *Commenting on aging*

Personal financial planning should be considered a priority for all optometrists. A well thought out financial program can improve the choice of practice options after graduation, make it easier to repay student loans, ease the achievement of financial goals, and facilitate future decision making. Financial planning should not be a response to events, such as paying bills, reconciling a monthly bank statement, or filling out an annual tax return; these are examples of the results of previous financial dealings and are reactive in nature. Instead, financial planning should be proactive and anticipate future events; thus it is an ongoing, iterative process of identifying personal short-term, intermediate, and long-term goals and of creating a plan to accomplish them. Specific elements of personal plans can vary greatly. However, there are several key areas of planning that are essential to all optometrists' financial needs.

Budgeting. Planning begins with an analysis of the income derived from employment and of the cost of living, both current and anticipated. Key aspects of these costs include the purchase of a home and the accumulation of a cash reserve.
Tax planning. Because income can be significantly affected by taxes, knowledge of basic tax law, counsel from tax advisors, and appropriate use of tax benefits, write-offs, and strategies are essential.
Insurance. Adequate insurance protection involves life, disability, professional liability, and personal coverage that is sufficient to meet occupational and family needs, without the payment of premiums that are inappropriate, inadequate, or unduly costly.
Investments. The selection of investments requires a determination of the level of risk the investor is willing to undertake and a decision as to how much to

allocate to income-producing investments versus those with long-term potential growth.
Retirement income. Although retirement seems far away to beginning practitioners, it is a major aspect of personal financial planning. An anticipated retirement lifestyle can be adversely affected by inadequate retirement income, which can be eroded by inflation and increases in the cost of living.
Estate planning. The transfer of an estate to heirs can involve both lifetime giving (through gifts) and the use of wills to bequeath property at death. An understanding of gift and estate taxation is necessary to conserve assets for heirs and reduce estate taxes paid to government.
Special circumstances. Certain events may require special planning; these events may be short term (e.g., maternity leave) or long term (e.g., funding for a child's college education), one time (e.g., purchase of a second home) or ongoing (e.g., improving and enlarging a practice). An emerging area is long-term care of elderly parents, which can be financially devastating if proper planning does not take place.

During a professional career, optometrists make numerous financial decisions, many of which may not be viewed as being a part of financial planning, but which exert a significant effect on financial well-being. By developing an objective and comprehensive financial plan, however, the effects of these actions may be better anticipated and the goal of financial independence more readily attained.

Developing a Personal Financial Plan

There are five steps that a beginning practitioner should take to develop a financial plan. First, the practitioner's short-term, intermediate, and long-term goals and objectives need to be determined. Goals set the direction for the financial plan, whereas objectives define the desired endpoint. Goals can be open-ended, but objectives should be clearly focused. To create financial objectives, a practitioner should be *SMART*:

*S*pecific–the goals and objectives should fully describe the desired results and should be put in writing.

*M*easurable–financial objectives should be quantifiable so that progress can be measured at periodic assessments.

*A*chievable–the resources at hand should be quantified and compared with the resources required to achieve financial objectives, to ensure they are adequate.

*R*esults oriented–financial objectives must be considered outcomes, not just activities.

*T*ime bound–a defined time frame or milestone should be set for all financial objectives and monitored periodically to determine whether they should be revised.

Second, financial counselors should be selected. Tax attorneys, financial planners, and accountants can provide needed direction and advice. Attention should be paid to the advisor's approach to risk and how compatible it is with the practitioner's own: how aggressive or conservative is the advisor toward taxes and investing, and how comfortable is the practitioner with this approach?

Third, current personal, professional, and financial status must be assessed by the practitioner. This evaluation will involve both assets (things of value that can be used as collateral or for credit) and liabilities (short- or long-term debt that may impede investment). Cash flow also must be considered: can it be enhanced or augmented, or can it be abruptly ended? Are there constraints on income that will prevent access to the resources needed to achieve financial objectives? Insurance coverage must be analyzed to ensure that it is necessary, covers the appropriate eventualities, and is affordable. If there are investments, they too should be reviewed.

Fourth, financial goals and objectives need to be prioritized and a plan of action formulated to achieve them. This plan may require revision of the personal or family budget, the allocation of more funds to savings, the purchase of additional insurance, the liquidation of assets, the refinancing of debt, or an increase in the diversification of assets.

Fifth, progress should be reviewed on a periodic basis or whenever there is significant change in revenue, earning ability, or debt level. Periodical evaluations should be performed at least quarterly, and each year a comprehensive assessment should be undertaken to determine whether performance has been satisfactory or whether modifications are required.

As previously stated, key areas in the personal planning process that involve all practitioners and must be understood in the development of a personal financial plan are budgeting, tax planning, insurance, investments, retirement income, and estate planning.

Calculating Net Worth

After needs have been prioritized, the planning process begins with the calculation of net worth. A net worth statement is a "snapshot" of a graduate's financial status; net worth is determined by subtracting liabilities from assets. To calculate net worth, all assets are listed on the statement, at their fair market value. Assets include possessions that can be sold or otherwise converted into cash, such as savings and checking account balances, stocks, bonds, certificates of deposit (CDs), shares in mutual funds, the cash value of life insurance policies, home equity, individual retirement accounts, and investment-grade collectibles such as antiques, jewelry, fine art, or rare coins. From the sum of these assets, liabilities are deducted. Common liabilities include the mortgage on a home or other property; the balances due on car, educational, home improvement, or other personal loans; credit owed to stores or merchants; and amounts owed on credit cards. Net worth is often low for practitioners who have recently graduated from school and have accumulated significant debt. Any large, high-interest debt should be given priority to be paid off or reduced. To preserve essential assets, adequate life and disability insurance and a will should be obtained.

Developing a Budget

Personal financial planning demands that a budget be developed to limit spending and increase personal savings. Monthly cash flow needs to be monitored, and purchases and expenditures should be documented to see how money is spent. After a few months, an accurate picture will emerge of how much money is required for living expenses and where savings can be realized.

An income ledger should be maintained to keep track of salary, investment and rental income, interest earned, and any other money received. The sum of all income for the year thus can be determined. Fixed and discretionary expenses can be similarly monitored. Fixed expenses include mortgage or rent payments, property taxes, utilities, homeowner's expenses, automobile and life insurance, groceries, clothing and dry-cleaning costs, public transportation, gas and maintenance costs for motor vehicles, phone bills, household help, tax liabilities, credit card and bank payments, and similar living expenses. Discretionary expenses include meals at restaurants, movies, video rentals, baby-sitters, cellular telephones, rental cars, jewelry, vacations, sporting goods, tapes or compact discs, health club memberships, toys for children, and charitable contributions.

Monthly subtotals should be calculated for each expense category, then these figures should be used to determine an annual total. These expenses should be subtracted from the total income. If little remains, or if more has been spent than was taken in (with credit cards making up the difference), serious belt-tightening is in order. Even though fixed expenses are sometimes difficult to reduce without making sacrifices in living conditions, it is often easy to reduce expenses in the discretionary category. As a rule of thumb, discretionary expenditures should account for no more than 6% to 8% of net monthly income. Each month, projected expenses should be compared with actual expenses, and progress should be carefully evaluated on a quarterly and annual basis.

Once a school loan or a car note has been paid, the cash formerly paid for these expenses should be directed toward savings and investments rather than toward increasing the standard of living. The same approach should be followed with any windfalls or other money received. An emergency fund should be maintained, equal to at least 3 months of net income. These emergency funds should not be placed in a low-interest savings account but rather into liquid monetary instruments, such as a money-market account that permits 24-hour access to funds without penalty. In addition, all individuals should ensure that they are obtaining the maximum allowable tax deductions on federal and state tax returns.

A portion of monthly savings should be placed into specific investments. Personal financial goals and the amount of risk that one is willing to assume will determine the type of investment strategy to be used. When the time frame for a financial objective has been determined, the annual rate of return that is required to meet that objective can be estimated. Typically, stocks and Treasury bonds are used to finance long-term goals, whereas CDs are better suited for immediate

needs. The "Rule of 72" is a time-tested way to determine the period needed to double an investment for a given annual rate of return. To calculate the time needed, the rate of return is divided into 72. For example, if $1000 is invested at 12% interest, it will take 6 years to double the investment to $2000 ($72 \div 12 = 6$).

Insurance is a necessary expense to provide for families in the event of death or disability. Although life insurance usually is the first coverage purchased, statistically there is a greater probability of disabling injury or illness than of premature death. A disability policy usually provides 50% to 65% of income if the policyholder can no longer work. Individual disability policies tend to be expensive—as a rule, a young person has to spend 1% to 2% of salary on such a policy, an older person 3% to 4%—but group policies through national or state professional organizations can cost significantly less.

Investment Options

There are numerous investment choices for a young practitioner to choose from, ranging from conservative to aggressive. Many different names are given to these choices, including principal guaranteed; principal secure; growth, balanced, and income funds; international and emerging market funds; real estate; annuities; and stocks, bonds, and mutual funds. The risk of investment also is subject to terminology, such as "principal guaranteed," "principal secure," and "growth, balance, and income funds."

Principal Guaranteed

The term "principal guaranteed" generally means that 100% of the money invested is guaranteed to be returned at a future date. The guarantee may not apply to any fees that are deducted from the initial investment. The term is often confused with investments for which the interest rate is guaranteed but the principal is not. For this reason it is essential to determine whether the guarantee refers to principal or interest or both (the safest investment).

Principal Secure

"Principal secure" means that a large percentage of the investment is placed in cash, short-term money market securities, and government-backed securities. The investment return usually is equivalent to or slightly more than short-term interest rates. This investment choice is good for short-term returns or for security-conscious investors, but may not include a guarantee of the principal or interest.

Growth, Balanced, and Income Funds

These three types of investment funds are best suited for investors who are seeking higher returns over a medium to long term, 5 to 7 years at a minimum. With these funds the investor must be prepared to accept moderate market fluctuations during the short term because it is possible to experience negative returns during a 12-month period. However, the likelihood that there will be two or more consecutive years of negative returns is low. Thus these funds are not a good choice for short-term investors who are risk averse to market fluctuations. The main difference between the investments chosen is that "growth" funds usually are more aggressive than "balanced" or "income" funds.

Stocks, Bonds, and Mutual Funds

The main types of investments purchased today are stocks, bonds, and mutual funds. A *stock* is a share, or piece of ownership, of a company. When a publicly traded company wants to raise capital, it can either borrow money (from a bank on a short-term basis or from issuing bonds on a long-term basis) or issue stock. When a share of a corporation's common or preferred stock is sold, the buyer becomes one of the owners of that company. Publicly traded businesses sell stock to anyone who wants to buy it. Companies that are publicly traded are listed on stock exchanges, which are the places where stocks are bought and sold. To buy stock in a company, the services of a stockbroker are needed. The owners of stock in a company may receive dividends, which are profits that have been divided among the stockholders. Dividends may be paid in the form of money or as additional shares of stock.

Bonds are a more conservative type of investment than stocks. A bond is an interest-bearing security with a maturity date—or, more simply, it's a loan. Buying a bond is like lending money to a company instead of buying ownership in the company. When a bond is purchased, the seller promises to pay the purchaser back, with interest, after a stated period. There are several key elements that must be analyzed when evaluating the value and soundness of a bond, including the issuer (e.g., company, government), credit quality (e.g., Standard & Poor AAA rating), the interest rate (which varies in value for companies and governments), and the maturity date (which can vary from a few years to decades).

Local, state, and federal governments sell bonds, and government bonds generally are the safest choice. Corporate bonds often pay higher interest rates than do government bonds, but they can be riskier because the companies that issue them may not be able to make payment when the bond is due. Bonds usually pay higher interest rates than short-term investments such as stocks, but patience is required because the maturity date typically is many years in the future.

Another choice is to put money into a *mutual fund*. These funds can be low or high risk. Because they involve a variety of investments, mutual funds do not depend on the success of any one company. A mutual fund that invests in bonds and blue-chip stocks (valuable stocks that are unlikely to lose their value) is a safe, stable type of investment. A mutual fund that invests in small companies or technology is much riskier. A mutual fund's price per share, also called the *net asset value*, is calculated at the end of each trading day by dividing the total market value of all the securities owned by the fund by the number of outstanding shares.

Mutual funds offer a purchaser the ability to change money from one fund to another within the same "family" at a nominal fee. Also, mutual funds are very liquid (easily convertible) because the investment can be increased or withdrawn at any time. The volatility of a mutual fund is indicated by its standard deviation: the higher the standard deviation, the greater the range of returns and the more volatile the fund. Unlike past performance figures for stocks, which are rarely an indicator of future results, standard deviation is a reliable indicator of future volatility. Some examples of fund volatility are provided in Box 33-1. For example, growth funds which had an annual return of 14% for the past 5 years had a standard deviation of 12%. This means that for the next 2 out of 3 years, the range of returns expected from a growth fund is 26% to 2% (14%, its average annual return, plus or minus 12%). Money market funds are the most stable category by a wide margin, whereas precious metals are clearly the most volatile. "No-load" funds do not require the payment of commissions, and knowing which companies a mutual fund invests in can help an investor decide whether to choose that fund.

Annuities

An annuity is an investment purchased from an insurance company. Although annuities are offered only by the insurance industry, they have little in common

Box 33-1 Standard Deviation Indicators of Fund Volatility

FUND CATEGORY	STANDARD DEVIATION (%)
Money market	1
Government bonds	7
Growth	12
Utility bonds	13
International	17
Precious metals	41

with insurance coverage. Annuities are marketed and sold through brokerage firms, insurance agencies, banks, and savings and loan institutions. When an annuity is purchased, certain assurances are given by the insurance company. These promises depend on the company issuing the contract (the investment) and the type of annuity chosen. There are two main types of annuities, fixed-rate and variable. *Fixed-rate annuities* are similar to bank CDs. The investor (annuitant) makes a one-time investment (called a "single premium") and receives a guaranteed rate of return for the duration of the contract, which can be anywhere from 5 years to the life of the annuitant. Generally, the longer the period of time, the greater the rate of interest. *Variable annuities* are similar to mutual funds: the contract owner selects from one or more different investment portfolios, called "subaccounts." Usually a wide range of choices are offered, from ultraconservative (e.g., a money market account) to quite aggressive (e.g., Pacific Basin stocks). As with a mutual fund, the allocation of the investment can be changed at any time, and additional money can be added to the investment (called a "flexible premium"). A beneficiary also is necessary, in the event the contract owner does not live to receive the proceeds of the annuity.

International and Emerging Market Funds

Investment may involve the purchase of shares of stock in emerging companies. International market funds typically include shares of stock in companies from most economic regions. Investments may be divided between companies in North America, Europe, Japan, and Southeast Asia. The proportion allocated to each region will depend on the manager's views of how that region will fare in the future and also on the level of opportunity the manager envisions for companies

in that region. With international share investments, there is an added risk of currency fluctuation, and this risk must be carefully considered before making investments in this sector.

Real Estate and Real Estate Investment Trusts

Investments in real estate usually are listed properties and property trusts involved in residential, office, and industrial property markets. These real estate investment trusts own the properties, lease them to a variety of tenants, and pass the income (less costs) back to the investor. These investments are long term, with a minimum 3- to 5-year time frame.

Basic Investment Terminology

The *real rate of return* of an investment generally is described as being the gross yield (income plus growth), minus the rate of inflation. The real rate of return ignores taxes, whereas the "after-tax rate of return" ignores inflation. *Yield* is the income paid out as interest or dividends, divided by the current price of the investment. This figure usually is expressed as a percentage. Thus a 1-year CD annually paying 5% in interest has a yield of 5%. If interest is paid frequently during the year, however, and added to the original investment so that interest is earned on interest, there is an *effective* or compound yield. Money markets often report an effective yield.

Yield gets more complicated for stocks and bonds because, unlike a CD, stock prices change during the year. A stock selling at $100 and annually paying out $5 in dividends per share has a yield of 5%. If the stock price rises to $130, but the dividend remains $5, the yield drops to 3.84%. If a bond is held to maturity (when the bond principal is to be repaid to the bondholder), the yield is the same as its interest rate (assuming that interest payments are reinvested at the same rate of return). If the bond is sold before maturity, for a smaller or larger price than was paid for it, the yield will change.

Capital gains (or losses) measure in percentage terms how much an asset gains (or loses) in value over time. It also is referred to as price appreciation (or depreciation) and sometimes confusingly as annual return. A stock bought at $50 that rises in value to $60 a year later has appreciated 20%. Capital gains (or losses) also is a term that is applied to the tax consequences of the sale or other disposition of assets (like stock) that have been held for more than a year. Preferential tax treatment is given to the sale of these assets (see Chapter 38).

Total return generally is considered to be the best way to evaluate before-tax returns of similar or even dissimilar investments, since it compares apples with apples. However, inflation eats away at the purchasing power of total return. For example, if the total return for a year is 10% and inflation is 3%, then the real return actually received is 7%. Total return can be defined as yield plus or minus capital gains and losses. If a stock bought for $100 a share paid out $5 in dividends per share and gained $30 in value during the year, the total return is 35%. A $1000 bond that pays out $80 in interest but loses $5 in value during the year has a total return of 7.5%. The calculation can be more complicated than this because dividends and other income may be reinvested during the year. (Mutual funds that report the total return of the fund include reinvested dividends and capital gains and losses the fund may have realized during the year.) To compute an accurate total return, all buy and sell prices, dividends, and any other income from the investment must be factored into calculations.

Average return is a measure of total return over time. If an investor purchases a $50 stock that has a total return of 10% the first year and 20% the second, its average annual rate of return is 15%. The *average annual compound return* is a measure of how investment return grows faster over time due to compounding. For example, a $50 stock earning a 20% return for 2 years running actually has a compounded return of 44%, not 40% ($10 in gain the first year, and $12 the second year, for $22 in total gain, divided by the original $50 investment). Thus, its average annual compound return is 22%. On the other hand, the average annual compound return can be lower than the average return if, over the designated period (say 5 years), during the early years little gain or even a loss was experienced and during the later years performance was much better. An investment that loses 5% the first year, but gains 8% the second year and 40% the third year, has an average annual return of 9% but a compound return of 6.96%. This situation is more likely to occur with investments that experience a wide range of returns.

Dollar cost averaging is a popular technique that involves investing the same amount of money each month into the purchase of mutual fund shares. If the market is down this technique permits the investor to purchase more shares for the same amount. For example, if one share of stock is purchased the first month for $100, and another share for $100 the second month, and then both shares are sold in the third month for $150 each, the average cost of the shares was $100 and the profit was $2 \times $50 = 100. But if one share of stock is purchased the first month for $100,

and in the second month the share drops to $50, the investor can buy two shares for $100. If in the third month the stock goes up to $150, the investor has three shares at an average value of $66.66 per share, and if the stock is sold, the profit is $3 \times ($150 - $66.66) = 250. Dollar cost averaging is an investment technique that cushions an investor's long-term strategy from dramatic fluctuations in the market and value of stock.

Asset Allocation and Investments

Asset allocation is the process of allocating funds between stocks, bonds, and cash equivalents so that investment returns can be maximized for a given set of income sources, anticipated (and unanticipated) expenses, and retirement goals. Numerous books have been written on investments and asset allocation, but one does not need to be an investment expert to make sound decisions. When an investor is just starting out, it is necessary to understand the basics: the trade-off between risk, reward, and the time frame involved (how long funds are to be invested). The usual investments used at this stage are stocks, bonds, and cash or cash equivalents (such as CDs). As a general rule, stocks have historically outperformed bonds and cash equivalents over longer holding periods (10, 15, and 20 years). However, as with anything in life, additional risk accompanies efforts to obtain a higher reward. The stock market can be very volatile—especially if the time horizon involved is less than 7 or 8 years. After stocks, bonds generally outperform cash and cash equivalents over longer periods. However, the bond market also can be very volatile as interest rates rise and fall. Although an investor generally will receive the funds invested when the bond matures, this may not be true if the bond has to be sold before maturity. If it is expected that funds will be needed within a year or two, an investor may want to stick with cash and cash equivalents. Although some investment return may be lost, the investor will not have to worry about losing any of the funds that have been invested.

Developing an Investment Strategy

Starting out, it is essential to establish some short- and long-term goals. Initially, an investment strategy will be relatively simple. For example, until a sufficient amount of money has been placed into an emergency fund to cover 3 to 6 months of expenses, most excess income will be placed in investments that are liquid and risk-free. Because these funds need to be available for unexpected expenses, cash and cash equivalents are preferred. Examples of cash and cash equivalents are savings accounts, money market accounts, CDs, and U.S. Treasury bills.

At the other end of the spectrum is the investment strategy that an investor should develop for the funds in a retirement account. At the start of a career, an investor doesn't intend to use any of these funds for at least 10 to 20 years. Because of this long time frame, the investor can accept some risk because, at least historically, this risk should provide a greater reward over the long term. Thus an investor's retirement accounts should be more heavily weighted toward stocks and bonds as opposed to cash and cash equivalents.

Once an emergency fund has been created and maximum amounts are being contributed to any employer-provided retirement accounts, additional excess income should be deposited into an investment account (an investment reservoir). This is the point at which an investor must consider asset allocation: what portion of excess income should be invested in cash and cash equivalents? What portion in stocks? What portion in bonds or mutual funds?

An investor's asset allocation will depend on that investor's particular facts and circumstances (e.g., age, goals). Typically, asset allocation should be more heavily weighted toward cash and cash equivalents and bonds in the beginning—especially if there are multiple short-term goals. As an investor accumulates more savings, a higher percentage can be invested in stocks.

If an investor establishes a long-term goal to retire at age 65 and to maintain the same standard of living in retirement as while working, the amount of income needed to satisfy this goal can be quantified. If ordinary living expenses are currently $40,000, the investor will have to make an assumption as to whether this amount, adjusted for inflation, will be sufficient for retirement. Certain expenses are bound to be reduced (e.g., work clothing, home mortgage) but others may be increased (e.g., travel, medical expenses). Financial planners frequently assume that a retiree will need 80% to 100% of current ordinary living expenses adjusted for inflation at retirement. For example, if an investor requires $40,000 in today's dollars at retirement in 20 years, and the assumed inflation rate is 4%, the investor will need approximately $88,000 to cover ordinary living expenses. This process allows retirement goals to be quantified: the investor needs resources (retirement income, savings) sufficient to provide $88,000 (adjusted for inflation) during each of the investor's retirement years.

This process also allows the investor to determine whether there will be a "retirement gap." A retirement gap is the projected annual shortfall that an investor would have at retirement because projected savings and income are insufficient. To make this calculation, all retirement income sources must be converted to an annual income stream. For example, if the projected annual income stream in retirement was $85,000 and the annual retirement expenses were $88,000, there would be a retirement gap of $3000. The investor would need to take one or more of the following actions:

- Re-evaluate retirement needs to consider which, if any, projected costs can be reduced.
- Modify current cash flow to build additional savings in retirement plans.
- Adjust the investment mix to try to increase the return of assets available for retirement.
- Delay the projected retirement date.

If a retirement gap is not projected, the investor will need to evaluate whether there is a sufficient cushion to add short- or long-term goals or to "leave well enough alone" and continue with the same assumptions until projections can be updated. Generally, the farther from retirement an investor is, the more the investor should consider any excess income projected in retirement as a cushion. Projections should be updated, or at least verified, periodically to make sure that there have been no material changes in retirement assumptions.

Retirement Accounts

One of the benefits of self-employment is the opportunity to create a retirement account that addresses long-term personal financial needs. There are numerous choices, and a practitioner needs to consider the differences between plans and determine which is most compatible with the financial goals that have been set. Over time, just as goals may change, plans may change as well, necessitating revision in the retirement plan or the addition of other plans. For a young practitioner, however, financial planning for retirement begins with the fate of Social Security.

Social Security

Social Security is a government-administered retirement, disability, family, and survivors benefits plan. Because of changes in the Social Security law made in 1983, the full retirement age for persons born in 1960 or later will increase to age 67 (although reduced benefits still will be available at age 62). There is skepticism about the long-term viability of Social Security unless the program undergoes substantial modification because in 30 years there will be twice as many older Americans drawing benefits. In fact, many financial planners do not consider Social Security in their sources of retirement income for young individuals who are just entering the workforce. A conservative approach to planning, therefore, would be to develop a retirement plan and projected budget without including Social Security. If Social Security remains economically viable over the years, there will be an opportunity to change goals, investment strategy, or retirement income projections. Social Security payments are never available in a lump sum, and, as a general rule, the maximum annual amount payable is much smaller than the amount provided under an employer-provided pension plan.

Traditional Individual Retirement Accounts

Traditional individual retirement accounts (IRAs) can be used advantageously by young practitioners who understand the value of long-term investment for retirement. There are various types of IRAs, with slightly different rules and limits for contributions. The oldest is the traditional IRA, which can be used by both self-employed and employed individuals. The annual contribution that can be made to a traditional IRA is limited in amount but will gradually increase over a period of years (Table 33-1). This contribution is tax deductible if the individual also does not contribute to an employer-maintained retirement plan (such as an individual practitioner who is self-employed). For individuals who also participate in an employer-maintained retirement plan, the deductibility of contributions is based on income, with different levels of income used for individuals who are single or who are married filing a joint tax return (Table 33-2). Contributions also can be made for a nonworking spouse if the income requirements are met.

Over time an IRA account increases in value because the annual contributions are invested and provide a return. This growth in the IRA is tax deferred, with taxes paid by the contributor only when withdrawals are made at retirement. There is no mandatory withdrawal age, but withdrawals without penalty cannot be made until age 59½ (with some exceptions, including death, disability, eligible higher education expenses, unreimbursed medical expenses, and the purchase or construction of a first home). An individual must begin withdrawing funds from an IRA by age 70½ to avoid penalties.

Traditional IRAs demonstrate the value of establishing a retirement plan while young (Table 33-3). If a practitioner were to begin placing $2000 a year into an IRA at age 25 and kept doing so for 35 years, assuming there was an 8% annual return, the fund would be worth $315,000 at age 60. If $2000 was put into the IRA starting at age 35, at age 60 the account would be worth only $146,000. In fact, if an IRA was begun at age 25, contributions could have been stopped entirely at age 35, and there would be far more in the IRA ($198,000) than if contributions were started at 35 and continued to 60. Because of the benefit of compound interest, beginning the account early allows contributions of 40% less to still yield 35% more money.

Roth Individual Retirement Accounts

Roth IRAs differ from traditional IRAs in that there is no age restriction for contributions, and contributions to a Roth IRA cannot be deducted from income. However, the Roth account grows tax free, and—unlike a traditional IRA—withdrawals from a Roth IRA at retirement are not taxed. The annual contribution limits for a Roth IRA are the same as for a traditional IRA (see Table 33-1).

There is an income ceiling to be eligible to contribute to a Roth IRA, which is based on marital status and income (Table 33-4). Contributions can be made for a nonworking spouse as long as the income requirements are met. Both self-employed and employed practitioners may easily reach this ceiling, however, which is a limitation for this type of IRA. These income limits are periodically adjusted upwards to compensate for economic changes. The age requirements for withdrawals without penalty are the same as those for a traditional IRA, and early withdrawals without penalty are permitted for death, disability, or a

Table 33-1 Annual Contribution Limits for Traditional and Roth IRAs, 2002-2006

YEAR	AGE	CONTRIBUTION LIMIT
2002-2004	Under 50	$3000
	50 and older	$3500
2005	Under 50	$4000
	50 and older	$4500
2006	Under 50	$4000
	50 and older	$5000

Source: Taxpayer Relief Acts of 1997 and 2000.

Table 33-2 Traditional IRA Tax Deductions, 2003

STATUS	ADJUSTED GROSS INCOME	DEDUCTION
Single with no other retirement plan	No limit	Full
Married with no other retirement plan and spouse has no other retirement plan	No limit	Full
Single with another retirement plan	$0–$40,000	Full
	$40,000–$50,000	Partial
	Over $50,000	None
Married with another retirement plan	$0–$60,000	Full
	$60,000–$70,000	Partial
	Over $70,000	None
Married with no other retirement plan but spouse has a retirement plan	$0–$150,000	Full
	$150,000–$160,000	Partial
	Over $160,000	None

Source: Taxpayer Relief Acts of 1997 and 2000.
These limits are adjusted periodically.

qualified special purpose (e.g., to buy or build a first home).

Simplified Employee Pension IRA

A Simplified employee pension (SEP) IRA is a tax-deferred retirement plan that can be established for self-employed individuals and for employees who are eligible to participate. The employer can contribute up to 20% of total income, subject to an earnings ceiling (Table 33-5). Because of the higher contribution limits, the amount that can be placed annually into an SEP IRA far exceeds that of a traditional or Roth IRA. For employees, contributions are made by the employer, up to 20% of the employee's total compensation, again subject to an earnings ceiling. With the exception of the higher contribution limits, SEP IRAs are subject to the same rules as for a regular IRA.

In a SEP IRA, as with other types of IRA, both contributions and investment earnings grow tax-deferred until withdrawal (age limits are the same as those for traditional IRAs), at which time they are taxed as ordinary income. Early withdrawals without penalty are permitted for death, disability, and qualified special purpose.

Savings Incentive Match Plan for Employees IRA

The savings incentive match plan for employees (SIMPLE) IRA is a tax-deferred retirement plan provided by self-employed individuals or other small businesses (fewer than 100 employees) that do not maintain or contribute to any other retirement plan. Contributions are made not only by employees but also by the employer, who may choose to make matching contributions or nonelective contributions (Table 33-6).

Table 33-3 Contributions to an IRA: Projected Growth*

PERIOD	AT 5% GROWTH	AT 10% GROWTH	AT 15% GROWTH
After 5 years	$11,603	$13,431	$15,507
After 10 years	$26,410	$35,899	$46,698
After 15 years	$45,308	$69,899	$109,434
After 20 years	$69,428	$126,005	$235,620
After 25 years	$100,213	$216,363	$489,423

Contributions are $2000 per year, made each year.

Table 33-4 Roth IRA Income Limits, 2003

STATUS	ADJUSTED GROSS INCOME	CONTRIBUTION
Single	$0–$95,000	Full
	$95,000–$110,000	Partial
	Over $110,000	None
Married	$0–$150,000	Full
	$150,000–$160,000	Partial
	Over $160,000	None

Source: Taxpayer Relief Act of 1997.
These limits are adjusted periodically.

Table 33-5 Simplified Employee Pension (SEP) IRA Annual Contribution Limits, 2003*

ANNUAL PERCENTAGE	MAXIMUM INCOME	MAXIMUM CONTRIBUTION
Up to 20% of income	$200,000	$40,000

Source: Tax Relief Act, 2000.
*Percentage contribution limits are set by the employer but must be the same for both employer and employees. For example, the annual contribution for a 10% SEP IRA for an employer earning $100,000 would be $10,000, and for an employee earning $20,000 would be $2000.

As with other types of IRA, both contributions and investment earnings grow without taxation until they are withdrawn (which is ordinarily at retirement), at which time they are taxed as ordinary income. There are maximum annual employee contribution limits, and there are percentage limits for the employer's contribution. The employer's contributions can be made even if the employee does not contribute to the plan. With the exception of the higher contribution limits, SIMPLE IRAs are subject to the same rules as those for a traditional IRA.

Keogh Plans

A Keogh plan is a flexible tax-deferred plan designed to help self-employed individuals and eligible employees establish a retirement savings program. There are two different types of Keogh plans, called defined contribution and defined benefit plans (Table 33-7). *Defined contribution* plans involve profit sharing and money purchase plans. Under Keogh regulations, the *money purchase* contributions are mandatory, and the same percentage contribution must be made for both employer and employees each year (whether there are profits or not). The amount to be contributed is a percentage of annual income, established by the employer. *Profit sharing* contributions are much more flexible, being set by the employer from year to year, and based on profits. Thus annual contributions may fluctuate significantly. It also is permissible for contributions to be made to both money purchase and profit sharing plans in the same year. *Defined benefit* plans are set up to pay a fixed income during retirement, and contributions are based on an actuarial determination of the amounts that must be contributed annually to fund the plan. Defined benefit plans allow larger annual contributions than do defined contribution plans and are largely based on salary and years of service.

Table 33-6 Savings Incentive Match Plan for Employees (SIMPLE) IRA Annual Contributions, 2002-2005*

EMPLOYEE CONTRIBUTIONS

YEAR	AGE	CONTRIBUTION LIMIT
2002	Under 50	$7000
	50 and older	$7500
2003	Under 50	$8000
	50 and older	$9000
2004	Under 50	$9000
	50 and older	$10,500
2005	Under 50	$10,000
	50 and older	$12,000

EMPLOYER CONTRIBUTIONS

YEAR	AGE	CONTRIBUTION LIMIT
2002-2005	None	Matching contributions may be made, from 1% to 3% of income, or nonelective contributions of 2% may be made, up to $3200.

Source: Taxpayer Relief Acts of 1997 and 2000.
*Contributions are made by both employee and employer; for example, assuming in 2002 an employee under 50 years of age earning $20,000 contributed $7000 to the SIMPLE IRA, if the employer made a matching contribution of 3% the amount would be $600 ($20,000 × 3%), or if the employer chose to make a nonelective contribution the amount would be $400 ($20,000 × 2%), so that the total contributed to the employee's SIMPLE IRA for 2002 would be $7600 or $7400.

The most attractive feature of Keogh plans is the high maximum contribution they allow. Contributions and the investment earnings grow tax-deferred until withdrawal (assumed to be at retirement), at which time they are taxed as ordinary income. All contributions are made pre-tax, reducing taxable income or salary. Even if individuals participate in a Keogh plan, they still may invest in traditional IRAs.

Currently, Keogh plans are for self-employed individuals or partnerships, but eligible employees also must be included in the plan. The right of employees to their contributions is based on the plan's *vesting period*. Employers may require employees to work for a minimum number of years (5 or 7) before they are eligible to receive 100% of the benefits in the plan. Employees who leave before being fully vested forfeit a percentage of the income their contributions have earned, but they keep the contributions that they have made to the plan.

Table 33-7 Limits for Defined Contribution and Defined Benefit Plans, 2003

TYPE OF PLAN	MAXIMUM ANNUAL CONTRIBUTION LIMITS
Money purchase, profit sharing, or a combination of both	20% of income up to a $200,000 ceiling, for a maximum of $40,000
Defined benefit	The smaller of $160,000 or the average compensation for the three highest consecutive calendar years

Source: Tax payer Relief Act of 2000.

Pension Plans

A pension plan is a retirement plan, usually offered by large employers, that pays a set amount each year during retirement. As with Keogh plans, there are both defined contribution and defined benefit plans (see Table 33-7). *Defined benefit* plans provide a specific retirement benefit to employees, calculated using a formula that typically includes final salary, years of service, and a fixed percentage rate. An actuary is needed to calculate the annual contributions that are needed to fund the benefit. *Defined contribution* plans establish the amount to be contributed to the pension plan as a percentage of income, rather than by the amount to be received at retirement (as in a defined benefit plan). Contributions to both types of plans are subject to certain limits, but the annual contributions to a defined benefit plan can be significantly more than those to a defined contribution plan.

Most pension plans are insured by the Pension Benefit Guaranty Corporation, a federal agency that protects employer-sponsored defined benefit plans. Eligibility for a pension plan requires fulfillment of the vesting period (either 5 or 7 years). However, not all workers or all jobs may be eligible to participate in the plan. Most pension plan benefits are paid out in the form of an *annuity*, which is a fixed monthly payment for a period of years or for the rest of the individual's life. Pension plan benefits can be distributed as a lump sum or paid over the life of the retiree or the joint lives of the retiree and the retiree's beneficiary. In most cases, a 10% early withdrawal penalty is applied for withdrawals before age 59½, unless the plan allows early withdrawal for hardship.

401(k) Plans

A 401(k) plan is a personal pension plan offered by an employer. The employee decides the amount to be deducted (called "salary reduction"), which reduces income before federal taxes are imposed; an employer may offer a "matching amount." Both contributions are subject to certain income limits (Table 33-8). The employee chooses how to invest contributions, depending on the choices offered by the plan. At retirement, the employee receives the contributions made, plus the earnings of these contributions, minus income taxes. One benefit of a 401(k) over a traditional or Roth IRA is the employee's ability to contribute a much higher amount annually to the retirement account.

A "pension plan," when broadly defined, includes company 401(k) plans; however, a pension plan is different from a 401(k) plan in the following ways:

Benefits. If a defined benefit plan is used, pension plan benefits at retirement are known in advance. In a 401(k) plan, benefits are dependent on individual contribution levels and portfolio performance and thus are not determined until retirement.

Transferability. A company pension plan cannot be transferred if an employee's employment ends.

Table 33-8 401(k) Plan Contribution Limits, 2002-2006

YEAR	AGE	CONTRIBUTION LIMIT
2002	Under 50	$11,000
	50 and older	$12,000
2003	Under 50	$12,000
	50 and older	$13,000
2004	Under 50	$13,000
	50 and older	$15,000
2005	Under 50	$14,000
	50 and older	$17,000
2006	Under 50	$15,000
	50 and older	$20,000

Source: Taxpayer Relief Act of 1997.

A 401(k) account can be rolled over into another 401(k) plan or an IRA.

Investment allocation decisions. A plan administrator makes the decisions for the future "pensioners" in a company pension plan, whereas in a 401(k) plan each participant manages his or her individual portfolio.

Funding. Funding is provided by employers only in a pension plan and is optional for employers in a 401(k) plan.

To a limited extent, 401(k) plans fall under the provisions of the Employee Retirement Income Security Act (ERISA), and individuals responsible for the administration of 401(k) plans are considered "fiduciaries," which means they must comply with requirements described in ERISA related to the selection of investments, monitoring of performance, reasonableness of expenses, and various other matters.

Although contribution limits are less for a 401(k) plan compared with those of defined contribution or defined benefit pension plans, 401(k) plans offer the following:

Matching funds. Many employers offer to match a percentage or set dollar amount of the money that is put into a 401(k).

Instant savings. Employees are forced to save for retirement because 401(k) contributions are automatically deducted.

Built-in dollar-cost averaging. Because contributions usually are a percentage of salary, the same amount is deducted from every paycheck. This is, in effect, dollar-cost averaging, a staple of successful investing.

Tax-deferred contributions and earnings. Before being taxed, money is contributed and allowed to grow along with earnings; at retirement, taxes are paid on withdrawals, when the individual usually is in a lower tax bracket.

Reduced taxes. Federal, state, and local taxes are taken out of salary only after 401(k) contributions have been deducted, so taxes are lower.

403(b) Plans

These plans were established by the federal government to encourage employees of certain tax-exempt organizations to establish retirement savings. These plans allow the employees of hospitals, educational institutions, and other nonprofit organizations to save and invest for retirement. Depending on the program, employees authorize pretax payroll deductions to be invested in a tax-sheltered annuity contract or in a custodial account made up of mutual funds offered by the organization. Both the contributions and the investment earnings grow tax-deferred until withdrawal (typically at retirement), at which time they are taxed as ordinary income.

Employees choose whether to participate. If the employer is involved in setting up the plan and selecting the financial services vendor or vendors, the plan must offer a number of different investment options, which means that employees can select their investments, based on individual time horizons, degree of risk aversion, and financial risk tolerance. 403(b) investments also are portable. When an employee changes jobs, the 403(b) plan can be "rolled over" into an account in another organization's 403(b) plan or into an IRA. 403(b) plans are popular among the employees of certain 501(c)(3) nonprofit institutions, including hospitals and health care organizations, charitable foundations, religious organizations, scientific and research organizations, and educational institutions.

403(b) plans are often called "401(k) plans for nonprofit institutions." Although this is generally true, some differences are apparent:

Employer involvement. In a 403(b) plan, employer involvement is not mandatory (beyond deduction of contributions). However, it is mandatory in a 401(k) plan for setting up, administering, and performing discrimination testing on the plan.

Subject to ERISA regulations. Unlike a 401(k) plan, a 403(b) plan is only subject to ERISA regulations if there is employer involvement in setting up the program.

Vesting schedule. In most cases, vesting is automatic for a 403(b) plan, whereas in most 401(k) plans vesting occurs over a 3- to 5-year period.

Type of account. A 403(b) plan is a custodial account, whereas a 401(k) plan is a trust.

Withdrawals from 403(b) plans are often referred to as *distributions*. Assets in a 403(b) account can be withdrawn without penalty after age 59½, and withdrawals must begin by 70½ (unless the individual is still working). Distributions must be taken annually.

Conclusion

Financial goals often are not achieved without the guidance of a well-conceived financial plan and consistent, regular contributions to savings and investments. Effort must be expended to determine and monitor changes in net worth, redefine financial goals as necessary, and develop a savings and investment program. An early commitment to financial planning is essential. The power of compound interest, combined with an early start to contributions, will make a significant difference in the ultimate results to be enjoyed at retirement.

Bibliography

Bach D: *Smart women finish rich*. New York, 1999, Broadway Books.

Baum S: Educational debt and professional school students. *Optom Education* 25(2):54, 2000.

Eisesnson M, Detweiler J, Castleman N: *Invest in yourself.* New York, 2001, John Wiley & Sons.

Farber L: Money management (personal financing tips). *Med Economics* 75(23):192, 1998.

Fisher S: *The complete idiot's guide to personal finance in your 20's and 30's*. New York, 1999, Alpha Books.

Garner RJ, Arnone WJ, Pape GM, et al: *Ernst & Young's retirement planning guide*. New York, 1999, John Wiley & Sons.

Godin S: *If you're clueless about financial planning and want to know more*. Chicago, 1998, Dearborn.

Hallman G, Rosenbloom J: *Personal financial planning*. New York, 2000, McGraw-Hill Professional Publishing.

Mason SG: Rethinking student loan debt: tools and strategies for debt management. *Optom Education* 26(2):52, 2001.

McClure LH: Student indebtedness: the challenge of financing an optometric education. *Optom Education* 25(2):45, 2000.

Rye D: *1,001 Ways to save, grow, and invest your money*. Franklin Lakes, NJ, 1999, Career Press.

Wurman RS, Siegel A, Morris KM: *The Wall Street Journal guide to understanding money and markets*. New York, 1990, Access Press.

www.opted.org. Web site for the Association of Schools and Colleges of Optometry.

Chapter 34

Setting Fees

John G. Classé

Money makes the world go around.
Fred Ebb *Cabaret*

Before the publication of Charles Percival's enlightening work, *Medical Ethics,* in 1803, physicians routinely charged for services based on the ability of patients to pay rather than on a fixed fee schedule. His ideas on the ethics of payment for services exerted a profound influence on medicine in America, in time representing the prevailing point of view, that each patient should be charged the same amount for the same service.

Optometry has followed a similar evolutionary process in the setting of fees. Practitioners working in commercial environments at the start of the 20th Century were subjected to "free examination" promotions by the businesses employing them, and it was common practice to "charge for glasses" in a lump sum rather than to separate fees into amounts for services and for materials. Gradually, the use of fee schedules and the separation of fees for services from materials by professional optometrists exerted an effect on the profession, causing the value of services to be given greater emphasis. Even so, a survey of practitioner attitudes conducted by the American Optometric Association in 1966 found that optometrists:

- Lacked confidence in fee schedules
- Could not effectively answer questions asked by patients about fees
- Believed fees were inconsistent from one group of services to another
- Considered fees to have no rational relationship to the cost of services and materials
- Believed these inconsistencies were widespread throughout the profession

At this time, another influence on fee setting began to be experienced by the profession: third-party reimbursement, principally by the government. Through Medicare and Medicaid, fees were established for services rendered to the elderly and to indigent children and adults. For other individuals, private insurance plans offering reimbursement for examinations and, to a lesser degree, for ophthalmic materials, established the fees that could be charged. The effect of these programs was to change the traditional mode of payment (from patient to practitioner), inserting a third party into the process, and to take the ability to set fees out of the hands of practitioners.

Medicare, in particular, has wielded considerable influence on fee schedules. After the Medicare "parity" amendment was enacted by the U.S. Congress in 1986, optometrists examining Medicare-eligible patients were able to receive reimbursement for services within the scope of licensure that led to the diagnosis or treatment of disease. Reimbursement levels were established by determining a fee "profile" for the optometrist's area of practice. The fees charged by all the practitioners in the area were used to establish this profile, and reimbursement levels were set at 70% of the mean fee. Optometrists who charged more than the 70% level were limited to this amount, but optometrists who charged less than the 70% level received the lesser amount. However, fees charged to Medicare patients for services could not be more than the fees charged to patients younger than 65 years old for these same services. As a result, fees for services received a considerable amount of revision, for patients of all ages.

Charges for ophthalmic materials have been less subjected to regulation because few insurance plans provide complete reimbursement for spectacles or contact lenses, offering instead a partial payment or credit toward purchase. The difference is paid by the patient. Under Medicare, the only ophthalmic materials for which reimbursement is provided are the initial spectacles or contact lenses used for the correction of aphakia or pseudophakia. The setting of charges for ophthalmic materials has been an ongoing problem for optometry, one that is confounded by the ethical obligation to separate charges for services from those for materials.

Ethically, a professional has the responsibility to inform patients of the charges for care and how they were determined. Abuses such as "free" examinations hid the practitioner's fee for services in the charge for spectacles, and "bait and switch" tactics lured patients to practitioners for the purpose of selling eyewear at high markup rather than the inexpensive eyewear advertised. Even worse, "rebates" paid to a prescribing practitioner for ophthalmic materials sold by a dispenser kept from the patient the practitioner's financial incentive to "steer" the patient to the dispenser. These and other unsavory practices led to a demand for reform within optometry and to the passage of rules of practice that emphasized the obligation to set uniform fees, separate charges for materials from fees for services, and avoid economic discrimination in patient care.

Within this historical context, contemporary practitioners still struggle to determine the amount to charge for services, the proper pricing of ophthalmic materials, the fair apportionment of charges between services and materials, and the ethical presentation of fees to patients. The most fundamental of these problems, particularly for a beginning practitioner, is determining a fee schedule.

Determining a Fee Schedule

The determination of a fee schedule must be divided into two parts: setting fees for services and establishing charges for ophthalmic materials. Because optometrists not only provide vision services but also dispense a product, two different methods of setting the fee schedule must be used. As recounted, in the past the services of the optometrist were frequently undervalued, often amounting to less than the chair cost (i.e., the cost per patient of keeping the office open and operating), while the price of the materials was increased twofold to fourfold for purposes of sale, so that a reasonable profit could be realized. In addition, the fee for both examination and spectacles was presented as one charge, usually being described as "the cost of the glasses." Much of the effort to promote professionalism during the past 2 decades has been directed toward the elimination of the "single charge" concept. This effort has been aided by the Federal

Trade Commission's "Eyeglasses Rules," which granted to patients an unfettered right to the spectacle prescription, allowing them to take the prescription from an optometrist charging a low fee for services to a less expensive dispenser to be filled. Aid also was received from Medicare "parity" legislation because its fee "profiles" for services caused optometrists charging lower fees than those described on the profile to recognize that their services were undervalued. The result of this reconsideration was an increase in the relative value of professional services and a devaluation of the charge for ophthalmic materials. As a result, the emphasis today is on fees for services.

Fees for Services

Although fees for services have become the key consideration in optometric reimbursement, the ability of optometrists to establish a reasonable return for their professional skill has been significantly influenced by the steady emergence of vision care as an insurance benefit. Because of the success of managed care programs such as health maintenance organizations and preferred provider organizations and the dictates of companies providing vision care benefits to workers, fees for services increasingly have been determined not by practitioners but by these entities. If many workers enrolled in an insurance program are the patients of an optometrist or would likely become the patients of an optometrist, the reimbursement offered by the insurer must be accepted by the optometrist or these patients will be lost. The fee paid by the insurer is often well below the optometrist's usual and customary fee, but it is accepted by the optometrist in return for the prospect of serving a sizeable population of patients. The optometrist's autonomy over fee setting is lost in such an arrangement, but the ramifications extend beyond fees to include ethical concerns, such as the time to be allocated for examination. Since the optometrist receives less compensation for each examination, there is a natural tendency to attempt to increase the number of examinations within the same unit of time. Such a development may result in less-thorough examinations, to the potential detriment of patients. This effect is certainly not what patients had in mind when the insurance program was initiated.

The determination of fees to be charged for services are complicated, therefore, by the erosion of the traditional payment philosophy of health care, in which the practitioner set the fee to be paid and the payment was received directly from the patient. The intrusion of third parties—government and the insurance industry—

has created a complication, in which the fee to be received by the practitioner is most often set and paid by the third party. As a result, true "fee for service" has rapidly diminished as the most common payment mechanism for optometric health care services.

Given these developments, when optometrists do establish fees to be charged for professional services, several factors must be considered: the optometrist's "chair cost"; the fees for like services charged by other practitioners in the community; the fees paid by third parties (most notably in the Medicare program) for like services; and the optometrist's determination of the value of individual experience, skill, and knowledge.

Determining "Chair Cost." If an optometrist determines the overhead costs for patient examinations and divides this amount by the time spent by the practitioner performing these examinations, the cost of services can be calculated (see Chapter 41). The "chair cost" is the expense incurred by the optometrist to perform examinations, usually expressed as an hourly amount. If the hourly fee derived from patient fees is less than this figure, the optometrist is operating at a loss. An optometrist must know the "chair cost" because it exerts an obvious effect on the fee to be charged for services. The examination fee must be at least this amount, or the optometrist will not be able to operate an economically viable practice. The "chair cost," therefore, represents a minimum fee for services, below which the optometrist cannot operate the practice (or at least continue to operate the practice at its current level).

Comparison With Other Practitioners. Within the group of optometrists in any community there is a range of fee schedules, from which a minimum, a maximum, and a mean charge may be derived. A new practitioner entering a community to start a practice should be familiar with this range of fees and should consider it when attempting to establish the fee schedule for the new practice. In general, it is preferable to be neither the lowest nor the highest in such a situation. For an established practitioner seeking to alter fees, this information also is valuable and should be considered during the decision-making process, along with the other factors previously enumerated. It also can be useful to determine the fee schedules for ophthalmologists in the community, particularly if optometrists work with them. This information allows the fee schedule finally chosen to fit within the economic boundaries of the community's ophthalmic marketplace, and for the practitioner to understand where within that marketplace the fees may rank.

Fees Paid by Third Parties. A practitioner cannot determine fees for services without being cognizant of the fee schedules established by third parties such as government and insurance companies. Because of the growing use of optometric services by Medicare-eligible patients, the influence of government reimbursement schedules is obvious. Practitioners cannot charge more for the same service to patients who are not Medicare-eligible than to patients who are Medicare-eligible, so the reimbursement allowed to Medicare providers must be considered when establishing a fee schedule or changing fees. One particularly important influence is the determination of level of skill involved in the service. Because of the requirements of Medicare, the fee to be charged must reflect the skill exercised during the examination. As a result, fee schedules are organized to reflect these differences, not only for Medicare patients but for patients of all ages (Table 34-1). The definition of these different levels of service is described elsewhere, as are the payment schemes used by third-party providers (see Chapters 36 and 37).

Individual Experience, Skill, and Knowledge. Every practitioner should consider individual capacity when pondering the fees to be charged for services. Generally speaking, as a practitioner grows in experience and skill, fees are adjusted to reflect the additive effect of the knowledge acquired in these years of practice. This individual factor should be tempered, however, by the economic realities of the ophthalmic marketplace, the prevailing fees in the community, and the other considerations previously described.

An optometrist must evaluate all these factors when deciding on a fee schedule for services or the alteration of an existing fee schedule. A different set of influences is exerted on the decision making necessary to determine the charges for ophthalmic materials.

Pricing of Ophthalmic Materials

Historically, ophthalmic materials have not only been supplied by optometrists but also have been provided by opticians, optical companies, and other retail establishments. Because of this wealth of competition, it is wise for optometrists to be familiar with the pricing strategies used in the marketing of goods and services. Marketing is the process of studying the wants and needs of a target population and satisfying those needs with quality goods and services at competitive prices (see Chapter 32). Once a specific need has been identified, the marketing process involves the following four factors:

Table 34-1 Office and Other Outpatient Services for Medicare[a]

SUB-CATEGORY	HISTORY	EXAM	MEDICAL DECISION MAKING	COUNSELING	COORDINATION OF CARE	NATURE OF PRESENTING PROBLEM	TIME[b]
New Patient							
	All three components required						
99201	Problem focused	Problem focused	Straight forward	Contributory	Contributory	Self-limited or minor	10 min
99202	Expanded problem focused	Expanded problem focused	Straight forward	Contributory	Contributory	Low to moderate severity	20 min
99203	Detailed	Detailed	Low complexity	Contributory	Contributory	Moderate severity	30 min
99204	Comprehensive	Comprehensive	Moderate complexity	Contributory	Contributory	Moderate to high severity	45 min
99205	Comprehensive	Comprehensive	High complexity	Contributory	Contributory	Moderate to high severity	60 min
Established Patient							
99211	Requires physician's supervision only					Minimal	5 min
	2 of 3 components required						
99212	Problem focused	Problem focused	Straight forward	Contributory	Contributory	Self limited or minor	10 min
99213	Expanded problem focused	Expanded problem focused	Low complexity	Contributory	Contributory	Low to moderate severity	15 min
99214	Detailed	Detailed complexity	Moderate	Contributory	Contributory	Moderate to high severity	25 min
99215	Comprehensive	Comprehensive	High complexity	Contributory	Contributory	Moderate to high severity	40 min

Source: Procedure codes and definitions are copyrighted by the American Medical Association.
Shaded areas = required.
[a]*Counseling/coordination of care must be documented in record. Please refer to CPT definitions/guidelines.*
[b]*Time is only pertinent in determining the level of service when it constitutes more than 50% of the face-to-face physician encounter.*

- Design a product that satisfies the need
- Place the product where people will purchase it
- Promote the product
- Set a price for the product

These four factors are interdependent in terms of both real and perceived value to the consumer of the product. For the practitioner of optometry, the "need" that has been identified is quality vision and eye health care, including ophthalmic materials. To satisfy the need for ophthalmic materials, optometrists offer a quality "product": the determination of the prescription and the fitting and dispensing of eyewear from a single source. The optometrist's dispensary serves as the place where the eyewear can be purchased. To ensure that patients are aware of the availability of these services and materials, marketing is used, both to existing patients and the public. The pricing of the ophthalmic materials is based on the following three fundamental business strategies:

Neutral pricing. The price is based on the product's value to the average consumer, so that the price equals the worth of the product.
Skim pricing. The price is set to obtain the highest participation from the segment of the market that is

insensitive to price, so that the price is more than the product's value to the average consumer.

Penetration pricing. The price is set at a low level to obtain and hold a large share of the price-sensitive segment of the market, so that the price is less than the product's value to the average consumer.

In the ophthalmic marketplace all three strategies are used. In the discussion of fees for services, a neutral strategy was presented, with consideration given to the cost of delivering services, the external influence of third-party payers, and the perception of value that is based on individual skill and knowledge. A skimming strategy may be found in the pricing of new surgical techniques such as LASIK. Services for refractive care have long been subjected to penetration pricing, to the extent that even "free" examinations have been offered to capture and hold market share.

Because of the great variety of competitors and strategies within eye care, it cannot be said that there is one best way to price ophthalmic materials. Each practitioner has to assess the patient population, the location, and the competition in the marketplace. Even so, it should be emphasized that the pricing of ophthalmic materials is not to be determined by the low prices inherent in penetration strategies. The dispensing of ophthalmic materials in a professional office is quite different from the retail sale of eyewear in an optical shop. Patients appreciate the unified quality service that can be obtained in a professional office and expect a consistent value—not the lowest value—for the materials purchased.

When establishing a neutral strategy the optometrist must assess the cost of purchasing and maintaining an inventory of frames; the expense involved in the use of staff members for the selection, dispensing, and repair of eyewear; and the proportionate cost of operating an in-office dispensary. To offset these expenses, the practitioner should consider the contribution to profit that can be made by the sale of frames and lenses. Using this approach, a practitioner can determine a "cost per unit" for eyewear, much in the same manner that "chair cost" can be calculated for professional services. The amount so calculated becomes the minimum mark-up to be added to the cost of the ophthalmic materials. This amount is often referred to as a "materials service fee"; under some insurance plans this amount must be used for the pricing of ophthalmic materials. Because the costs of maintaining an inventory of frames (and providing related services) increases with more expensive materials, the mark-up for ophthalmic materials is usually two to two and a half times the cost of the materials. Ophthalmic

lenses usually are priced in the same manner. If discounted materials costs are required by some vision care plans, this factor must be built into the minimum materials service fee charged by the practice.

The price of ophthalmic materials must be organized and presented in a coherent way to patients. Spectacle frames, ophthalmic lenses, and contact lenses must be categorized in some practical manner, and charges must be set for each category. For lenses, the results are typically described on a fee schedule, which lists the various categories and charges to be applied. Spectacle frames are priced on an individual basis, and the price is often attached to the frame with a small sticker or other means of identifying differences.

Contact lenses have become a very competitive part of the ophthalmic materials market. There has been a gradual decrease in the mark-up for lenses and an accompanying increase in the professional fees charged for fitting and follow-up. Disposable lenses usually are priced at one and a half to two times their cost, whereas other lenses are usually priced at two times their cost. Prepaid service agreements and planned lens replacement programs have been used to support the cost of providing services and materials to contact lens wearers. These approaches also join together the pricing of services and materials, for the convenience of the patient.

In response to consumer demands for faster delivery of spectacles by ophthalmic providers, many optometrists have obtained in-office equipment to edge and dye lenses or apply lens coatings. The purchase price of this equipment, the cost of its operation and maintenance, the value of the time expended by employees to operate it, and other factors must be considered by the optometrist in setting the charge to patients for edging, tinting, and coating services. The prevailing charges for these services in the community also must be considered. These ancillary services can be an important source of income and can add to patient satisfaction by reducing the amount of time needed to provide eyewear after examination.

Fees for services and materials also may be influenced by the method of payment chosen by the patient.

Methods of Payment

Payment may be immediate or deferred. The usual methods of immediate payment are cash, check, or credit card. If cash is paid, the optometrist receives full value for the amount charged. If a check is used, the same result usually is obtained, but a small percentage of patients will have insufficient funds in their checking account. The optometrist will be required to spend time and, occasionally, money in an effort to collect the amount owed. The result is less than full value for the amount charged. Credit cards allow payment to be received, but at a discount. The credit card companies customarily receive 2% to 6% of the amount charged on the card for insuring payment, and thus the optometrist will not receive full value for the services rendered.

If payment is deferred, it is because the payment is to be made by a third party or credit has been extended to the patient. In both situations, the optometrist will not receive full value for the amount billed. Third-party claims for reimbursement are subject to approval by the third party before payment; not infrequently reimbursement is delayed or payment is disallowed. If the claim is denied, the optometrist may turn to the patient for payment, but the collection of the amount due is achieved in less than 100% of cases. The same is obviously true in situations in which credit is extended to patients. Even though billing and collections efforts may be used, some payments inevitably will not be received. Again, the end result is less than complete payment for the amount charged.

Optometrists must consider carefully the method of payment to be permitted (particularly the credit policy to be used), attend scrupulously to the billing requirements of third parties providing vision and eye care benefits, and organize workable procedures for the collection of accounts receivable. The setting of fees and their method of payment are intimately related problems that cannot be separated from one another.

One other essential consideration is the accounting system used to document the charges made and payments received for services and materials.

Accounting System

The ideal accounting system would be simple, accurate, and require little time to use. Computers seem to fulfill these requirements, for they can be used to bill patients and track accounts with great efficiency and accuracy. Software programs can be purchased that permit individual payment schedules to be set for patients, calculate interest on unpaid accounts, and provide preprinted receipts to be mailed to the practice with payment. Tracking of accounts payable also can be efficiently performed by the computer, as can the financial productivity of the office. This versatility gives the computer an edge over other methods of financial recordkeeping.

Personal computers are used by the majority of optometrists in private practice. Software programs have been designed for use in optometric offices and offer many features that provide time-saving steps in the scheduling of appointments, recording of patient information, tracking of orders for ophthalmic materials, entering and analysis of financial records, completion and submission of insurance claims, and preparing of communications with patients.

Scheduling of Appointments

Computers allow appointments to be easily scheduled or rescheduled, with a set of related information (such as telephone numbers) that allow for patients to be contacted by mail or telephone to verify appointment dates and times. Appointment entries usually can be linked to computerized billing for services and materials and to the recall system.

Recording of Patient Data

Some software systems permit "paperless" records to be maintained, and to provide security for entries some systems prevent changes to be made to the record after the passage of a certain period (to prevent alteration or destruction of data). The computer will print the information on a specialized form or a personalized letter or transfer it electronically to another computer. Computers also can be linked to instruments such as automatic refractors and lensometers to record patient data automatically.

Ophthalmic Materials

Computer programs can send orders for lenses and frames to optical laboratories, track the status of orders, keep track of frame and lens inventories, track frame and lens usage, use bar code scanning, and perform helpful analyses of ophthalmic materials costs and usage.

Financial Records

Software programs can be used to perform a variety of financial management functions, including the completion of daysheets, statements for patients, deposit slips for payments, bills and accounts receivables, and even to prepare the checks for employees, maintain payroll accounts, and issue annual W-2 forms for employees.

Insurance Claims

There are programs that enable forms to be completed and printed for various health insurance plans, including the HCFA 1500 form (used for most medical insurance plans and Medicare) and the form for Vision Service Plan.

Communications With Patients

Cards and letters can be printed through computerized programs that generate recall notices, service agreements for contact lens patients, referral letters, thank you letters, and vision analyses. The use of computer programs allows these communications to be personalized, making them more effective with patients.

It is this versatility that makes computer programs favored over other means of data management. Regardless of the system used, the opportunity always exists for manipulation of the system by a dishonest employee and for loss of funds through embezzlement to result. No system is foolproof, and it is appropriate for practitioners to take steps intended to improve their familiarity with the system while at the same time hopefully discouraging dishonesty on the part of an employee.

Inspection and Evaluation of Financial Records

There are several steps that a practitioner should take to reduce the likelihood of loss from embezzlement. One is to obtain insurance protection. Although employees who handle substantial amounts of money may be bonded (a process whereby a company guarantees reimbursement to the employer for loss in return for the payment of a fee to the company), the experience that employees must go through to obtain the bond usually makes it a less desirable alternative to insurance coverage. A rider can be purchased by the optometrist, as part of professional liability insurance protection, usually at a nominal fee.

Employees should be hired only after references have been verified and questioned. Employees who manage money should be informed that their work will be periodically checked. If possible, more than one employee should be assigned to bookkeeping tasks. Vigilance on the part of the practitioner can be an important deterrent to this unfortunate but too often encountered downside of practice.

Conclusion

Although the setting of fees for services and of charges for materials is a personal act that must be performed by the individual practitioner, considerable influence is exerted on the practitioner by outside factors. The fees charged by competitors; the economic status of the community; and the practitioner's skill, experience, and knowledge are among the factors exerting that influence. However, the greatest influence on professional fees is the trend toward increasing use of third-party reimbursement plans.

The reimbursement "parity" achieved by optometrists under Medicare was a great legislative achievement for the profession. However, it significantly changed the economic relationship between optometrists and their patients and even the manner in which optometrists regard the issue of charging for services. Added to the influence of Medicare is the growing use of vision care plans and the use of optometrists as providers under eye health plans, which have substituted insurance reimbursement for the traditional method of payment. Despite these changes, the earnings of optometrists continue to rise and patient loads continue to increase, offering a suggestion that the profession is adapting well to these changes in health care reimbursement mechanisms.

Acknowledgement

The authors of this chapter in the first edition of *Business Aspects of Optometry* were John G. Classé and Donald H. Lakin.

Bibliography

American Medical Association: *Physicians current procedural terminology*, ed 4 (CPT-4). Chicago, 2001, Author.

American Optometric Association: *Handbook for assistants.* St. Louis, 1989, Author.

American Optometric Association: *Manual on completion of insurance claim forms*, ed 4. St. Louis, 1994, Author.

American Optometric Association: *Managed care resource guide.* St. Louis, 1997, Author.

American Optometric Association: *Codes for optometry.* St. Louis, 2003, Author.

Barresi BJ, Brooks RE: Full-scope optometry meets managed care. *Optom Economics* 4(6):10-3, 1994.

Beebe K, Hoffer D: Give insurers the slip. *Optom Management* 27(3):43-6, 1992.

Cleinman A: How to guard your margin. *Optom Management* 28(5):17-20, 1993.

Coleman DL: Watch for these booby traps in managed care contracts. *Optom Economics* 4(7):14-7, 1994.

Elmstrom G: *Advanced management strategies for optometrists.* Chicago, 1982, Professional Press.

Everett S: Don't undercharge for medical services. *Rev Optom* 128(12):25, 1991.

Gailnard NB: Cracking the codes: how to use CPT-4 codes to get prompt payment. *Rev Optom* 132(3):33, 1995.

Hayes J: The fearless way to raise fees. *Optom Management* 26(6):14-20, 1991.

Hayes J: How to guarantee a higher net. *Optom Management* 28(1):16, 1993.

Irving F: Are your fees in line? *Optom Management* 28(10): 22-5, 1993.

Lahr J: A no-nonsense guide to third-party plans. *Optom Management* 26(10):29-32, 1991.

Lee J: Set your fees for a fair profit. *Optom Management* 28(9):26-9, 1993.

Lookabaugh R: Double your patient-pleasing power. *Optom Management* 27(3):16-20, 1992.

Maino DM: Personal finance programs tell you where it all went. *Rev Optom* 130(11):25-7, 1993.

Muellerleile J: Fix your prices without price fixing. *Optom Economics* 4(3):19-22, 1994.

Shuldiner R: Total recall. *Optom Management* 26(9):14-22, 1991.

Tlachac CA: Fees for difficult fits. *Optom Economics* 4(6):24-7, 1994.

www.optometric.com. Online version of *Optometric Management* magazine, which offers surveys and other information on fees.

www.revoptom.com. Online version of *p* magazine, which offers surveys and other information on fees.

Chapter 35

Credit and Collections

John G. Classé

Ah, take the Cash and let the Credit go.
Edward FitzGerald *The Rubaiyat of Omar Khayyam*

Even for practitioners on the cash system, it is inevitable that billing of patients will be required, and for the majority of practitioners the collection of accounts receivable is a constant problem, one directly related to the necessity of billing for fees. The time, manpower, and money expended on billing and collection efforts can be considerable, particularly in practices that do not have a well-organized and coordinated system for these efforts. If billing and collections practices are inadequate, a financial loss will be incurred, one that could have been prevented if proper planning and procedures had been instituted. For these reasons, it is important for practitioners to consider the related issues of billing and collections, which may be divided into three topics: payment for services, methods of billing, and methods of collection. All of these issues should be considered and decided on by the practitioner before beginning a billing and collections program.

This discussion concerns only the billing and collection of fees for service; it does not describe the remediation of disputes with third-party providers such as insurance companies and government agencies. For the collection of debts from third parties, practitioners must consult the guidelines established by these parties for the remediation of disputes.

Payment for Services

There are five basic methods of payment (Box 35-1). Practitioners may be required to use many of these methods or relatively few, depending on the services offered and preferences of the practitioner.

Advance Payment

This method requires that payment be made before services are rendered or materials are obtained. The most common examples are prepaid service agreements for contact lens patients, in which the fee is paid at the start of the covered period of services, and payments for contact lenses that are required in full before the lenses will be ordered.

Step Payments

This method permits the patient to make serial payments as services or materials are received. An example would be a planned replacement program for contact lenses, in which periodic replacement of lenses is a feature of the program.

Deposit and Balance

This traditional method of payment for optometrists requires the patient to pay a percentage of the amount due after services have been rendered and to pay the balance when ophthalmic materials are received. An example situation would be to require payment of 50% of the cost of services and spectacles after the examination and the remaining 50% at the dispensing of the spectacles.

Credit and Billing

If no payment is required, credit is extended to the patient and billing is used to obtain payment of the amount credited. For example, the patient is billed for the cost of the examination and ophthalmic materials, with no payment required until the bill is received.

347

Box 35-1 Methods of Payment for Services

1. Advance payment
2. Step payments
3. Deposit and payment of balance
4. Credit and billing
5. Installment payments

Installment Payments

This method requires payment in stated amounts or over a fixed period. An example would be to allow payment in three fixed installments, paid during a 3-month period.

Of all these methods, only the first and second do not result in the extension of credit to the patient. The third, deposit and balance, has been relied on by optometrists because the deposit can be used to cover the cost of ophthalmic materials, thereby preventing financial loss to the optometrist if the patient should fail to pay the balance. The last two methods are true credit transactions because they do not obligate the patient to make payment until after services and materials have been received. Billing of the patient is necessary to collect the amount due. If credit and billing are used, it has been determined that approximately 70% of patients will pay upon receipt of the first statement; approximately 25% will require extra billings or special arrangements; and the remaining 5% cannot or will not pay. In a well-run practice, the percentage of unpaid accounts should not exceed 3% to 5% of the patients billed.

The billing of patients requires that a statement be prepared and mailed. If a computerized system is used, the amount due can be posted in the patient's file, for transfer to a statement at the time of billing. With computerized systems, it is relatively easy for accounts receivable to be monitored.

The unpaid accounts control sheet lists the patient accounts that are 30, 60, 90, and 120 days in arrears. It not only permits the practitioner to keep track of the accounts that remain unpaid and the period that they have been due, but also allows in-office collection efforts to be documented. These efforts must be organized by the practitioner in a manner that is in keeping with the practitioner's philosophy toward collections.

If billing is to be used, collections will become necessary. If bills remain unpaid beyond a reasonable period, the practitioner must decide whether an effort will be made to collect the amount due, and if such an effort is instituted, whether the practitioner will collect the account or allow a third party to serve as the collection agent. This decision is an important one and must be given due consideration by the practitioner because it will dictate the manner in which the office is organized to initiate collections efforts. It also will have ramifications outside the office because the method chosen by the practitioner for the collection of unpaid accounts can adversely affect the practitioner's reputation if it is poorly done. It is advisable to discuss methods of collection with other practitioners before instituting a policy and to seek legal counsel as well so that ill-advised policies or efforts will not be incorporated into the procedures of the practice.

Legal Considerations

Several legal issues are of importance when credit is extended to patients: first, the decision to deny credit to an individual is regulated by federal law; second, the Truth-in-Lending Act can be imposed on certain credit practices; and third, the collection of unpaid fees by collections agencies and attorneys is subject to both federal and state regulation, which has ramifications for the optometrist employing the agency or attorney.

Equal Credit Opportunity

If an optometrist extends credit to patients, it must be awarded on a nondiscriminatory basis. Credit cannot be refused because of a patient's race, color, religion, national origin, sex, marital status, age, or because the patient receives public assistance. If an optometrist refuses credit to a patient, the proper basis for the denial should be documented. Violation of this federal law is punishable by both civil and criminal penalties.

Truth-in-Lending

Practitioners who permit credit and subsequently bill patients for amounts due should be careful to structure the billing program so as to avoid the voluminous disclosure and reporting requirements of Truth-inLending. This federal law, which is applicable in all jurisdictions, requires creditors to provide certain information when extending credit to individuals, even when the creditor is a health care professional such as an optometrist. To fall under the obligations of Truth-in-Lending, an optometrist must merely apply a finance charge to unpaid accounts or structure payment from patients in more than four installments (not including a down payment). To avoid the complications of Truth-in-Lending, therefore, an optometrist should not use finance charges and should allow patients either to make payments in four or fewer installments or allow payments to be made by the patient on an unstructured basis (i.e., not on a fixed schedule). Penalties for violation of this act are both civil and criminal in nature.

Fair Debt Collections

Federal law regulates the collections practices of collections agencies and attorneys. In-office collections efforts by an optometrist to collect unpaid fees are not subject to federal requirements. All states have enacted statutes that regulate the harassment of debtors, however, and the collections efforts of optometrists would be subject to those laws.

Because of legal regulations, the awarding of credit and the collection of unpaid fees should be carefully organized and scrupulously managed. The first step in structuring a practice to meet these demands is to prepare a written contract for services.

Contract for Services

To prevent misunderstanding between practitioner and patient and to provide a legal basis for the resolution of disputes with patients regarding the payment of fees for services and materials, a printed contract should be used. This form should contain three parts: a section requesting certain patient information; a section devoted to the practitioner's payment policy; and a statement concerning collections efforts (Figure 35-1).

Patient Information

The patient's name, birth date, address, place of work, and other basic information should be requested, as should vital information concerning the patient's spouse.

Payment Policy

The method of payment chosen by the practitioner (e.g., deposit and balance) should be described, as should the manner in which payment may be tendered by the patient (e.g., cash, check, credit card).

Collections Policy

If the practitioner has decided to collect unpaid accounts, information should be provided to the patient concerning the method of collection. It also is essential to put the patient on notice that, if an attorney's services are required or if it is necessary to resort to small claims court, the patient will be required to pay the attorney's fees and the costs of court in addition to paying the amount due or ordered by the court. Only if this language is included in the agreement can the practitioner collect the full amount due and have legal and court costs borne by the patient.

This contract is signed by the patient and retained in the patient's record of care. If legal action becomes necessary, this contract may be used as evidence of the agreement between the parties. The patient contract should be updated at each annual examination to ensure that the patient information is current and to provide documentation of the agreement.

If a patient does not pay as agreed and collections become necessary, the usual resort of practitioners is an in-office collections effort that involves the use of letters. Telephone collections efforts should not be attempted because of the vulnerability of such efforts to charges that they constitute harassment under state laws regulating debt collections. A three-letter sequence is the preferable means of encouraging payment, with the first letter serving as a reminder that payment has not been received (Figure 35-2); the second letter requesting that contact be made with the office to arrange payment (Figure 35-3); and the third letter asserting that alternative action is imminent unless payment or an explanation is forthcoming (Figure 35-4). These letters generally are sent after the bill has been unpaid for 30, 60, and 90 days, respectively.

If payment is not received despite these in-office efforts, the practitioner must decide whether to pursue the matter further or to dismiss the claim as a bad debt. If the practitioner is on the cash system of accounting, the bad debt cannot be claimed as a tax deduction; if the practitioner is on the accrual system, it can be written off because it already has been claimed as income. If the practitioner decides to pursue the collections effort, there are two alternatives available: collect it in small claims court or turn it over to an attorney or collections agency for further disposition.

Methods of Collection

If an optometrist is in a community that has a small claims court and is willing to invest the time and effort

---

Optometry Eye Group

111 Main Street
Anytown, US 12345

PATIENT INFORMATION

PATIENT'S NAME_____ BIRTHDATE____/____/____ AGE_____

HOME ADDRESS_____ CITY_____ STATE_____ ZIP_____

IF PATIENT IS A CHILD, SHOW PARENT'S NAME_____
HOME
PHONE_____

Provide the following information for the RESPONSIBLE party:

NAME OF PERSON RESPONSIBLE FOR THIS ACCOUNT_____

ADDRESS_____ CITY_____ STATE_____

SOC SEC #____/____/____ EMPLOYED BY_____ BUSINESS PHONE_____

SPOUSE'S NAME_____ EMPLOYED BY_____
BUSINESS
PHONE_____

IN CASE OF EMERGENCY, NOTIFY_____PHONE_____

STATEMENT OF FINANCIAL POLICY

As a service to you, this office offers several means of payment for the services and materials that you may require:

- It is customary to pay the examination fee at the time of the examination.
- 50% of the cost of spectacles and contact lenses must be paid when ordered, and the balance when dispensed.
- Payment for follow-up examinations is required at each visit.

To ensure that we understand how you wish your account to be handled, please check the payment plan that you prefer and sign in the place indicated. If you have any questions, please ask the receptionist before you make your choice.

☐ CASH   ☐ PERSONAL CHECK   ☐ CREDIT CARD (select one)   __ American Express
__ Discover
__ Mastercard
__ Visa

The doctor, at the doctor's discretion, may place an UNPAID account with an attorney for collection. In the event the account is referred to an attorney for collection of unpaid charges, the patient or person responsible for the account agrees to pay an attorney's fee, court costs, and any other reasonable costs of collection.

DATE_____ SIGNATURE OF RESPONSIBLE PARTY_____

Figure 35-1 Sample contract for services.

involved to file, process, and collect a legal claim, then small claims court is a viable option. If the optometrist wishes to turn the matter over to a third party, either an attorney or a collections agency should be consulted. The choice is left to the practitioner, based on individual preferences and attitudes. Each option has its own strengths and weaknesses.

Small Claims Court

These courts, which settle disputes involving relatively small claims, do not require an attorney, use relatively informal rules, and are not expensive. The procedures of these courts vary somewhat from community to community, but the general requirements are as fol-

---

Optometry Eye Group

**111 Main Street
Anytown, US 12345**

Date

Mr. Unpaid Account
123 Central Avenue
Anytown, US 12345

Dear Mr. Account:

We have not heard from you with regard to our recent statement concerning your account with this office.

If the enclosed account is in error, please contact us so that we may make the appropriate adjustment.

If it is correct, we would enjoy hearing from you soon.

Sincerely,

Accounts Manager

AM/ab
Enclosure

Figure 35-2 Sample "first letter" for in-office collections.

lows. To file a claim, the optometrist must file a complaint, allege a legal cause of action (i.e., breach of contract), and pay a filing fee. The address of the defendant must be known so that the complaint can be served. (If the optometrist's contract specifies that the patient is responsible for the costs of collection, an attorney may be hired to file the claim and collect the debt, with the attorney's fees charged to the patient.) A date and time will be set for the trial, which is held before a judge. At the trial, strict rules of evidence are not followed, but the optometrist will need documentation of the examination, services rendered, and reasonable fees charged. Once this evidence is presented, the defendant may offer a defense. After the presentation of evidence is completed, the judge issues a ruling; if it favors the optometrist, the defendant will be ordered to pay a judgment and court costs. If the defendant pays the judgment, the matter is concluded.

Although the defendant has the right to appeal the judgment to a trial court, the amount of money in question virtually always precludes this alternative. If the defendant does not pay the judgment within a

reasonable period, the optometrist can obtain an order from the court, allowing the judgment to be satisfied by the seizure and sale of the defendant's assets, the taking of money from the defendant's bank account, or periodic payment from the defendant's salary.

Occasionally, a defendant will not answer the complaint or appear in court. At the time set for trial the optometrist can ask the judge to award a default judgment. After the passage of a certain period, the judgment will be deemed final, and the optometrist will be able to seek the remedies previously described for the satisfaction of the judgment.

Collections Attorney

An attorney hired to manage the collection of unpaid accounts should be instructed by the optometrist in the methods to be used. For example, an optometrist may not want the attorney to file suit or may not be willing to have the patient's assets sold to satisfy a judgment awarded in small claims court.

Optometry Eye Group

111 Main Street
Anytown, US 12345

Date

Mr. Unpaid Account
123 Central Avenue
Anytown, US 12345

Dear Mr. Account:

We are disappointed in the fact that we have not received a response to the letter and statement mailed to you last month.

However, we are aware that unexpected developments can make it difficult to meet financial obligations from time to time.

Please consider how you wish to take care of the enclosed statement of account, and contact this office within the next few days so that we may discuss this matter with you.

Sincerely,

Accounts Manager

AM/ab
Enclosure

Figure 35-3 Sample "second letter" for in-office collections.

The practitioner should establish the bounds of the attorney's efforts. If an attorney is to be used, however, it is advisable to require patients to sign a written contract and to include the clause requiring payment of attorneys fees and courts costs if legal action must be instituted against the patient to collect the amount owed (see Figure 35-1). The reason for this language is that a collections attorney will charge the optometrist 33% to 50% of the amount collected for professional services. If the clause is used, the optometrist may collect the full amount owed, and the patient pays for the attorney and other legal costs of collection.

Collections Agency

Before a collections agency is hired to collect overdue fees, the optometrist should evaluate the reputation of the agency and assess the collections efforts that it uses. Collections agencies are subject to federal and state laws that regulate debt collections practices, and aggressive or dubious collections practices could result in undesirable ramifications for the optometrist, ranging from injury to the optometrist's reputation to legal action involving the optometrist. The optometrist should be comfortable with the collection agency's practices because they will represent the optometrist in the community.

A second consideration is payment of the collections agency. The preferred method of payment is based on the debts actually collected; the usual fee is 33% to 50% of the amount collected for the optometrist. The less desirable method is one in which the optometrist is charged for collections efforts, whether successful or not. This situation can become very expensive, with little return, and should be avoided. The optometrist should have a clear understanding of how the agency will charge for its services before entering into a contract for collections.

Optometry Eye Group

111 Main Street
Anytown, US 12345

Date

Mr. Unpaid Account
123 Central Avenue
Anytown, US 12345

Dear Mr. Account:

In our previous efforts to contact you concerning your overdue account, we have evidently failed to make it clear that this is a matter requiring your immediate attention.

Much to our regret, unless we hear from you about the enclosed statement, we will be compelled to take an alternative course of action.

Please contact this office immediately so that we may resolve this matter.

Sincerely,

Accounts Manager

AM/ab
Enclosure

Figure 35-4 Sample "third letter" for in-office collections.

Conclusion

If an optometrist chooses to provide credit to patients, billing and collections are an integral part of the process and must be planned for by the optometrist. The optometrist must determine the following:
- The type of payment plan to use
- How to keep track of the accounts receivable
- How to prepare and use a written contract for patient services
- The philosophy of the office with respect to collections
- In-office billing procedures (including "past due" letters)
- How past due accounts will be collected

In making these decisions, the optometrist should consult with other practitioners, practice management advisors, and legal counsel to ensure that efforts are legal, tasteful, and within the bounds of professional conduct.

Bibliography

Classé JG: *Legal aspects of optometry*. Boston, 1989, Butterworth.
Consumer Credit Protection Act, 15 USC §1601 et seq.
Elmstrom G: *Advanced management strategies for optometrists*. Chicago, 1982, Professional Press.
Equal Credit Opportunity Act, 15 USC §1691 et seq.
Fair Credit Reporting Act, 15 USC §1681 et seq.
Fair Debt Collection Practices Act, 15 USC §1692 et seq.
Truth-in-Lending Act 102(a), 12 CFR §226.
Regulation Z, Truth-in-Lending, 12 CFR §226.
www.optometric.com. Online version of *Optometric Management* magazine, which offers information on credit and collections methods.
www.revoptom.com. Online version of *Review of Optometry* magazine, which offers information on credit and collections methods.

Chapter 36

Managed Care and Third-Party Reimbursement

Roger D. Kamen, Mark R. Wright, and Ronald S. Rounds

Oh, I get by with a little help from my friends.
John Lennon and Paul McCartney *With a Little Help from My Friends*

During the past 50 years, the financing of health care in the United States has changed drastically. Before the mid-20th Century, patients paid their health care providers directly "out of pocket." There was little, if any, involvement of employers or government in the paying of fees. Providers set fees, and patients paid them.

In the mid-20th Century, because of the impetus of unions, employers began to offer health insurance to employees as a low-cost alternative to salary increases. Insurance companies, which had handled traditional life and property insurance, began offering health coverage. Health insurance programs were modeled after the casualty insurance these companies were accustomed to handling. This type of insurance was an indemnity plan, used to protect against catastrophic loss. Health insurance assumed this same indemnity format, at a very low cost to employers.

The federal government in 1965 became a major player in financing health care with the introduction of Medicare and Medicaid (see Chapter 37). Health insurance became more comprehensive as employers and the federal government added additional benefits for their employees. Over time the low-cost health benefit became a high-cost item. This high cost became burdensome for businesses competing in a global market and a federal government struggling with sizable deficits.

In an attempt to counter the spiraling cost of health care, during the late 20th century, the United States turned to managed care. This chapter explores third-party reimbursement in this context. Managed care has become widespread throughout the country and is still growing rapidly. It is imperative that optometrists understand managed care to function and flourish in the U.S. health care environment.

Health Care Plans

Third-party reimbursement occurs when someone other than the patient pays directly for the health care provided. (Patients pay indirectly in the form of premiums, taxes, and benefits.) Managed care is a health care system that controls the use, cost, and quality of care. It includes both the delivery and financing of health care.

There are various types of health care plans, including traditional indemnity insurance, health maintenance organizations (HMOs), preferred provider organizations (PPOs), and service plans. In the past, particularly during the period of spiraling increases in health care costs (in the 1970s and continuing into the early 1990s), traditional indemnity insurance was the primary health care plan. Most indemnity plans were fee-for-service plans. For every service provided, a fee was paid. In this system, providers are actually rewarded financially for performing more and more procedures for patients. There are no controls on cost or use. As long as the patient has a medical problem, the services are covered. One can see how this system promotes increased health care costs.

In this environment, managed care blossomed. HMOs and PPOs are the major types of managed care systems.

Health Maintenance Organizations

HMOs incorporate the delivery and financing of health care. Traditionally, HMOs offered a prepaid system to deliver care to an enrolled group at a predetermined rate; this is known as the *per member per month (PMPM) rate*. It covers all services provided to the member (patient). Currently there are five types of HMOs:

Staff. The HMO owns the facility, and the providers are employees.

Group. The HMO contracts with one medical group for member services.

Network. The HMO contracts with more than one medical group to provide services at various locations.

Independent practice association (IPA). The HMO contracts with a provider association, a network of providers who work in their own personal offices.

Point of service (POS). A hybrid HMO that allows members the option of going outside the HMO for a particular needed service, but at higher personal cost. The POS HMO has overcome the main complaint of HMO members—the inability to go outside the HMO for care when the member believes it is in his or her best interest.

Preferred Provider Organizations

The second type of managed care organization is a PPO. A PPO is a network of select providers (panel) operating under utilization management and negotiated fee schedules. Patients might use nonpanel providers, but at a higher personal cost. Another difference with a PPO is the money trail. The provider bills the PPO, the PPO bills the employer, the employer pays the PPO, and then the PPO pays the provider, according to the contractual fee schedule. PPO programs generally are more costly to employers than HMO plans.

A type of PPO is the *specialty PPO*, which consists of one specialty or type of provider. Many vision plans are examples of specialty PPOs.

Service plans can be part of a managed care organization. Service plans pay providers set fees for covered services but might or might not involve utilization management and quality control. A provision of the plan is that the provider must accept the fee schedule as payment in full (i.e., no balance billing).

As managed care has evolved, the distinction among the various systems has become blurred. Traditional indemnity insurance has added utilization management and is more appropriately labeled managed indemnity. PPOs and HMOs have taken on common features, some of which include permitting patients access to outside providers (at higher personal cost), utilization management, and the passing of financial risk to the provider. The provider needs to look closely at the plan organization and not just at the label or classification of the health plan to determine its actual status.

Currently, health plans are turning to an integrated system of health care delivery. This system involves the integration of many types of providers or a hospital/provider network. Integration allows for greater cost reduction, better efficiency, and more convenience for patients. Examples of integration include the following:

- Independent practice association
- Group practice without walls
- Group practice
- Physician hospital organization

Optometrists can be included in these networks, joining with ophthalmologists and other physicians to offer the convenience of "one-stop" health care.

Compensation Methods

Health care plans reimburse for patient care through different methods. It is essential for the provider to understand how the plan reimburses for services. Examples of compensation methods include fee for service, discounted fee for service, fee allowance schedule, relative value scale, and capitation.

Fee for Service

Under fee for service, providers are compensated for services rendered. Compensation is determined by a "usual and customary" fee. Usual and customary compensation is based on the provider's fee record as it equates to that of different providers in the region. The "usual fee" is the standard fee that is charged by the provider for a given procedure to private paying patients. Usual fees are determined by the provider and are on record with the health care plan as the provider's fee profile.

"Customary fees" for each particular procedure are set by the health care plan. The health care plan determines the customary fee as a percentile of the usual fees charged by providers in the same general area (e.g., 90th percentile).

Under *fee-for-service* programs, providers are paid the actual amount of their usual fees, if those fees fall within the range of customary fees. If the provider charges more than the customary fee, the provider will be paid only the customary fee (in essence, writing off the difference). On the other hand, if the provider charges less than the customary fee, the provider will be paid the usual fee. Under *discounted fee for service*, providers receive their usual and customary fee, minus a certain discount (e.g., 25%). Another common variation is for the third party to pay a percentage of the Medicare allowable fee (e.g., 70% of Medicare allowable). It is important to recognize that the Medicare allowable fee is a discounted program, so a plan offering a percentage of Medicare as a fee schedule is a discounted discount plan.

Fee Allowance Schedule (Fee Schedule)

Under a fee allowance schedule, providers are compensated based on a schedule of fees for each procedure. The fee schedule is not correlated to the provider's usual and customary fees.

Relative Value Scale

Under a *relative value scale*, the health care program assigns a numeric score to each procedure plan (described by a current procedural terminology [CPT] code) that indicates the "value" of the procedure. For example, the intermediate eye examination, new patient (92002) can be assigned a relative value of 1.1, whereas a comprehensive eye examination, new patient (92004) can be assigned a relative value of 1.7. Reimbursed amounts are determined by multiplying the relative value of the procedure by a predetermined negotiated number (the multiplier). If the multiplier were $30, then the reimbursement for the just mentioned relative values would be $33 for 92002 and $51 for 92004. Medicare uses a form of this method, called a *resource-based relative value scale* (see Chapter 37).

Capitation

Capitation is a prepayment program that pays the provider a fixed amount for each member (patient) per month. The amount paid covers all provided health care services for the member regardless of the number of visits or the associated cost of the services. If the patient is healthy and requires little service, then the provider is in a positive financial status. On the other hand, if the patient is sickly and requires many services, the provider might be in a negative financial status. It is assumed that the overall mix of members will result in a positive income status for the provider. With the capitation method, the provider assumes financial risk.

Optometrists participate in health care plans that might use any of the aforementioned compensation methods. In fact optometrists deal with patients who can have two kinds of insurance—vision and medical.

Medical or Vision Insurance

A confusing issue for many patients, and for some optometrists, is the case of a patient with separate vision and medical plans.

Vision Insurance

Coverage usually provides for basic periodic vision examinations, ophthalmic lenses, eyeglass frames, and contact lenses. Often the cycle of covered services is different than the cycle for covered materials (e.g., vision examination once per year, spectacles every two years). Vision claim forms can request information about the vision examination procedures performed, refractive diagnosis, visual acuities, lens prescription details, and frame data.

Medical Insurance

Coverage is limited to medical services and supplies. Regardless of the final diagnosis, a medical sign or symptom is needed as the initial reason for the examination for reimbursement to be allowed. Medical necessity is needed to bill major medical plans for services and supplies rendered. A medical diagnosis has to be included on the claim form to substantiate medical necessity. Examples of medical diagnoses include headaches, hypertensive retinopathy, blepharitis, glaucoma, and conjunctivitis.

The optometrist must first decide which plan (vision or medical) to bill for services rendered. This decision is based on the reason for the office visit. If the reason for the office visit is refractive, the vision plan, not the medical plan, should be billed. However, if there is a medical reason for the office visit, the medical plan should be billed.

Vision plans lack uniformity and standardization in claim forms and submitting requirements. Most plans have their own unique claim forms with unique codes (if any) for procedures. This diversity makes it very difficult for the optometrist to process vision claims efficiently and makes office computer systems less effective in the billing process.

Medical insurance has become more standardized, and there is uniformity of claim forms, with most major medical plans using the HCFA 1500 form. Additionally, over time various systems have been developed to improve the efficiency of handling third-party claims. These improvements include diagnostic and procedural codes.

Diagnostic Codes. To indicate diagnoses and diseases for third-party reimbursement, the *International Classification of Diseases (9th edition) Clinical Modification (ICD-9-CM) System* (Washington, DC, 2001, U.S. Department of Health and Human Services) must be used. The ICD system is required by the U.S. Public Health Services and the Center for Medicare and Medicaid (formerly the Health Care Financing Administration renamed in 2001) and most medical third-party programs. Codes are published in two volumes; one provides a tabular list, and the other provides an alphabetical list.

For each patient, the code should be used that is appropriate for the diagnosis, whether it is visual or medical in nature.

The number of digits for each code varies from 3 to 5. The more digits used, the more specific the diagnosis. Three-digit codes are the basic subdivision of the disease classification. Four-digit codes are a subdivision of the primary three-digit codes. Five-digit codes are the most precise and specific of the subdivisions. Examples of three-, four- and five-digit vision and medical codes are provided in Box 36-1. Under current coding rules a practitioner must code to the highest level of specificity possible or the claim will be rejected.

ICD codes and titles are all listed in bold type. "Includes" are notes that additionally clarify or give samples of the contents of the category. "Excludes," which are printed in italics, list items that are not included in this code and must be coded elsewhere. An example of "includes" and "excludes" can be found in Box 36-2.

Codes should be as specific as possible, and the five-digit category should be used whenever obtainable. If there are no further subdivisions, four- and three-digit codes can be used. "Includes" and "excludes" need to be monitored and evaluated as they relate to billing procedures. A diagnosis code should not be used if the diagnosis is uncertain or supported only by intuition or suspicion. In this case, signs or symptoms should be used to describe the condition. The practitioner should only code to the level of certainty.

Procedural Codes. The American Medical Association has published a book containing medical and visual diagnostic procedures and treatment service codes. The book is titled *Current Procedural Terminology (4th edition) (CPT-4)* (Chicago, 2001). These codes are used to report to third parties the services provided to patients regarding the examination, treatment, and patient management plans. The *CPT-4* has been adapted by HCFA for use in Medicare programs and by most other third-party programs. Examples of *CPT-4* codes are provided in Box 36-3.

Format of the Terminology. *CPT* procedure terminology has been developed as a stand-alone description of medical procedures. Stand-alone descriptions are self-contained and ready to use.

Some of the procedures in *CPT* are not printed in their entirety. They refer to the common portion of the procedure listed in the preceding entry. For example, in Box 36-4 it can be seen that code 92226 is not printed in its entirety and refers back to code 92225, which is termed an "add-on" description. Add-on entries are used to conserve space.

Box 36-1 Examples of Medical Diagnoses

CODE	DESCRIPTION
367	Disorders of refraction and accommodation
367.2	Astigmatism
367.22	Irregular astigmatism
370	Keratitis
370.2	Superficial keratitis without conjunctivitis
370.22	Macular keratitis

Box 36-2 Sample "Includes" and "Excludes" for Diagnostic Coding

372.04	Pseudomembranous conjunctivitis
Includes	Membranous conjunctivitis
Excludes	*Diphtheritic* conjunctivitis (032.281)

Box 36-3 Examples of Medical Procedures Codes

CODE	PROCEDURES
99201	Office or outpatient visit for the evaluation and management of a new patient that requires three key components: a problem-focused history, a problem-focused examination, and straightforward medical decision making.
92081	Visual field examination, unilateral or bilateral, with interpretation and report; limited examination (e.g., tangent screen, arc perimeter on single stimulus level automated test)

Table 36-1 Examples of Procedural Modifiers

CODE	MODIFIER	PROCEDURE
—	-50	Bilateral procedure
—	-51	Multiple procedure
—	-52	Reduced services
92283	-51	Color vision examination, extended (e.g., anomaloscope or equivalent [including Farnsworth-Munsell 100 Hue test and Edridge-Green color perception lantern test])

Modifiers. A modifier provides the ability to report that a procedure or service has been altered by some specific circumstance but has not changed in its definition or code. When there is something unusual about a procedure, the appropriate modifier should be used to report the change. Modifiers are found in Appendix A of the *CPT*. Examples of modifiers can be found in Table 36-1.

The modifier is listed on the claim form next to the procedure code. Space is allowed to explain further unusual circumstances. An example of a procedure code with modifier also is included in Table 36-1.

Modifiers are required on some claims such as post-operative cataract co-management or punctal plug insertion. As a general rule of thumb, if possible, modifiers should be avoided unless they are required.

Evaluation and Management Service Codes. Evaluation and management (E/M) service codes are used to report the length and type of care provided to the patient. E/M codes are broken down into major categories that describe the location where the service

was provided (e.g., practitioner's office, hospital, nursing facility, emergency room). These categories are further broken down into subcategories (e.g., new or established patient for the office setting).

It is important to stress that these codes cannot be determined before the patient's visit nor can they be assigned by the office staff. Only after providing the care to the patient can the practitioner determine the proper level for the service rendered. The purpose of this coding system is to accurately reflect (and identify for reimbursement) the nature of the services the practitioner has provided the patient. Higher levels of service yield greater reimbursements.

Most of the care provided by optometrists is in the office setting. Codes available for the office setting are divided into two subgroups: new patient or established patient. An established patient is one who has been seen in the practice in the preceding 3 years for any examination reason by any doctor of the same specialty type. There are five levels of codes (Box 36-5).

The selection of the proper level is based on seven components: history, examination, medical decision making, counseling, coordination of care, nature of

Box 36-4 Example "Add On" Procedural Code

CODE	PROCEDURE
92225	Ophthalmoscopy, extended with retinal drawing (e.g., for retinal detachment, melanoma), with interpretation and report; initial
92226	Subsequent

Box 36-5 Sample E/M Codes

New patient	Established patient
99201	99211
99202	99212
99203	99213
99204	99214
99205	99215

presenting problem, and time. Of the seven components, three are particularly important: history, examination, and medical decision making. These three key components normally determine the proper level of service provided. The *CPT-4* specifically describes these three key components and divides each into four types (Box 36-6). The *CPT* manual discusses the specific description and documentation requirements for each type of history, examination, and medical decision making.

Table 36-2 illustrates the key component requirements for each level of service. For a new patient, all three key components must meet or exceed the requirements for a particular level of E/M code. For an established patient (one seen in the practice within the past 3 years), two of the three key components must meet or exceed the requirements for a particular level of service. For example, the proper E/M level is 99213 if it is determined that, for an established patient, the key components are as follows:

• History–problem focused
• Examination–expanded problem focused
• Medical decision making–low complexity

These codes only cover the evaluation and management of the patient and do not include independent diagnostic and treatment procedures, if clinically indicated (e.g., visual fields–99081). Both the E/M code and the independent procedure code should be reported on the claim form, along with the proper diagnosis.

General Ophthalmologic Service Codes. In addition to the E/M codes, the following four codes cover general ophthalmologic services:

Box 36-6 Types of History, Examination, and Medical Decision Making

History
  Problem focused
  Expanded problem focused
  Detailed
  Comprehensive
Examination
  Problem focused
  Expanded problem focused
  Detailed
  Comprehensive
Medical decision making
  Straightforward
  Low complexity
  Moderate complexity
  High complexity

• 92002–Intermediate medical examination, new patient
• 92012–Intermediate medical examination, established patient
• 92004–Comprehensive medical examination, new patient
• 92014–Comprehensive medical examination, established patient

Intermediate and comprehensive ophthalmologic services constitute integrated services, which do not permit medical diagnostic evaluations to be separated from the examining techniques used. Itemization of service com-

---

Table 36-2 Sample Examination Codes

CODE	HISTORY	EXAMINATION	DECISION MAKING
New Patients (three components required)			
99201	Problem focused	Problem focused	Straightforward
99202	Expanded problem focused	Expanded problem focused	Straightforward
99203	Detailed	Detailed	Low complexity
99204	Comprehensive	Comprehensive	Moderate complexity
99205	Comprehensive	Comprehensive	High complexity
Established Patients (two components required)*			
99211	Physical supervision only	–	–
99212	Problem focused	Problem focused	Straightforward
99213	Expanded problem focused	Expanded problem focused	Low complexity
99214	Detailed	Detailed	Moderate complexity
99215	Comprehensive	Comprehensive	High complexity

Two of the three components must meet or exceed the requirements for a particular level of service.

ponents such as slit lamp examination, keratometry, ophthalmoscopy, retinoscopy, tonometry, and oculomotor evaluation are not applicable. If a complete eye examination was performed as described by these codes, the appropriate code could be used. The office examination E/M codes can be used as necessary to provide reimbursement for other levels of care.

It is important to understand that documentation drives coding. No matter what tests were performed, if they were not documented in the patient record, from an auditor's perspective they were never done. If additional testing is required, the patient record needs to reflect the medical necessity. A sentence in the record, such as "the field loss discovered during screening fields created the medical necessity for a threshold visual field," satisfies the auditor's search for documented medical necessity.

Another area that is subject to poor documentation is medical decision making. The patient record should reflect the medical decision making, using terminology described in the *CPT* code definitions.

Because the *CPT* codes are frequently modified, the American Medical Association annually publishes an updated book containing the newest procedure codes. Each update contains hundreds of changes, and it is important to use the most current edition. Improper coding will cause delays in reimbursement and can result in the claim being paid at a lower level.

The American Optometric Association publishes *Codes for Optometry* (St. Louis, 2003). This manual consists of the following four parts:
- Procedural codes (*CPT-4*)
- Diagnostic codes (*ICD-9-CM*)
- Codes for materials (Health care Common Procedure Coding System *(HCPCS)*)
- Pharmaceutical codes (American Hospital Formukry Service *(AHFS)*)

This manual reprints the appropriate information for the optometrist and displays it in an easy-to-use format. The manual is updated annually by the association.

Cost Sharing

One aspect of third-party reimbursement is cost control through cost sharing. To achieve this goal, third-party health plans use two important concepts: deductibles and copayments.

Deductible

A *deductible* is a specified sum that the beneficiary must pay toward the cost of care before the benefits of the health plan go into effect. Deductible amounts can range from $0 to $2000, with $100 to $300 common. Deductibles might be required for each individual covered by the plan or for the family. If a patient has not paid the deductible, the provider should collect the deductible from the patient at the end of the examination. This is a complicated process because many patients do not know whether they have paid their deductible. The provider's office often will have to call the plan to obtain this information.

Copayment

A *copayment* is the patient's share of cost for covered materials and services. It usually is set as a fixed dollar amount per visit. Another term, *co-insurance,* is used to describe a sharing of cost when the amount is a percentage of the covered materials and services. Common major medical insurance plans are termed 80/20 plans. After the patient has met the deductible, the plan pays 80% of covered services and the patient is responsible for the remaining 20%. An example of an 80/20 payment can be found in Box 36-7.

Other cost-sharing measures include maximums and exclusions.

Maximums

Health care plans can stipulate a maximum amount paid for a given year or for a lifetime. For example, Medicare pays a set maximum for an eyeglass frame once in a lifetime (one for each eye) for a patient with a diagnosis of pseudophakia.

Exclusions

Health plans can exclude payment for certain services and materials. Examples of exclusions include the following:
- Preexisting conditions
- Cosmetic contact lenses
- Orthoptics

Box 36-7 Example Copayment

Procedure: Gonioscopy (90020)
   Total charge = $35.00
   Insurance coverage (80%) = $28.00
   Patient portion (20%) = $7.00

Individual plan provisions will have to be consulted to determine the requirements for a particular patient.

Claim Form

The most widely used claim form is the HCFA-1500 (Figure 36-1), which is used in billing for medical conditions. Like most claim forms, it has two primary information sections. Patient and subscriber information is found on the top half of the form in sections 1 through 13. Physician information is recorded on the bottom half of the form in sections 14 through 33.

Sections 1 through 13 can be completed by insurance staff after the information has been reported by the patient on the registration form. It is important to have the patient sign line 13, regarding release of information. Information about the patient's diagnosis and treatment is confidential and can be released only with the patient's permission. The patient's signature on line 12 gives the practitioner authorization to disclose details regarding medical or vision care to the insurance company.

Item 13 provides an assignment of benefits and should be signed by the patient if the practitioner prefers to collect benefits from the insurance company directly. The patient's signature authorizes the insurance company to pay allowable benefits directly to the practitioner. If the patient does not sign box 13, the insurance payment will go directly to the patient.

If benefits are assigned to the practitioner, financial settlements of the patient's share (deductibles, co-payments) of the costs usually are made at the end of the visit. If benefits are not assigned to the practitioner, financial arrangements are made for the total fee to be paid directly by the patient. When benefits are not assigned, it is as if the patient had no insurance. Then the patient pays the practitioner directly for the materials and services.

Signature on File

It is important to have patients review and sign statements authorizing release of information and payment of benefits on a patient registration form. The registration form should have wording similar to the wording in boxes 12 and 13 of the HCFA-1500 form. If the patient is not available to sign an insurance claim form, it is permissible to type "signature on file," since that authorization is provided on the registration form.

Physician Information

Items 14 through 33 are to be completed by office personnel. Most of the boxes are self-explanatory, and additional instructions can be found in the provider manuals for each health plan. Line 21 requires a diagnosis listed by *ICD* code—carried out to two decimal points if possible. The first diagnosis listed should be chiefly responsible for the patient's visit that day. This should be followed by additional codes describing any current coexisting conditions.

Box 24D requires a (*CPT*) procedure or (HCPCS) material code. Box 24E should list the diagnosis (referenced by line number) that corresponds to the billing procedure or materials.

Item 24B requires a code for place of service. "Place of service" refers to the practitioner's office, hospital, nursing home, and so forth. Type of service (item 24C) refers to medical care, surgery, consultation, or other service. A sample form with completed information can be found in Figure 36-1.

Third parties are moving toward electronic claims submission. It is helpful if the office practice management software can arrange the patient data and communicate directly with the third party for claims submission.

Processing Procedures for Claims

Because of the current environment of managed care, practitioners first need to determine whether care can be provided to the patient. Many health care delivery systems use a closed network or panel of providers (e.g., HMOs and PPOs). If the practitioner is not a member of the panel, the practitioner may not provide the care. Even if the provider is a member of the panel, there still can be utilization requirements and controls, including a primary care physician as a gatekeeper who authorizes all care. The provider needs to understand the structure and organization of the health plan.

If the practitioner determines that care can be provided, several issues still must be addressed, including eligibility, patient information, processing steps, and computerization of claims.

Eligibility

The provider needs to determine whether a patient is entitled to benefits under the health plan or the vision plan. A patient can be eligible for a vision examination only once every year. If it has been 11 months since the last vision examination, the plan might not pay for the

APPROVED OMB-0938-0008

PLEASE
DO NOT
STAPLE
IN THIS
AREA

CARRIER

PICA

HEALTH INSURANCE CLAIM FORM

PICA

1. MEDICARE   MEDICAID   CHAMPUS   CHAMPVA   GROUP HEALTH PLAN   FECA BLK LUNG   OTHER   1a. INSURED'S I.D. NUMBER (FOR PROGRAM IN ITEM 1)
[X] (Medicare #) [ ] (Medicaid #) [ ] (Sponsor's SSN) [ ] (VA File #) [ ] (SSN or ID) [ ] (SSN) [ ] (ID)   **12345678A**

2. PATIENT'S NAME (Last Name, First Name, Middle Initial)
VISION JOSEPH A

3. PATIENT'S BIRTH DATE   MM 01 DD 02 YY 31   SEX M [X] F [ ]

4. INSURED'S NAME (Last Name, First Name, Middle Initial)

5. PATIENT'S ADDRESS (No., Street)
2020 REFRACTION LANE

6. PATIENT RELATIONSHIP TO INSURED
Self [ ] Spouse [ ] Child [ ] Other [ ]

7. INSURED'S ADDRESS (No., Street)

CITY
ANYTOWN   STATE MI

8. PATIENT STATUS
Single [ ]   Married [ ]   Other [ ]

CITY   STATE

ZIP CODE 49000   TELEPHONE (Include Area Code) (616) 5551221

Employed [ ]   Full-Time Student [ ]   Part-Time Student [ ]

ZIP CODE   TELEPHONE (INCLUDE AREA CODE) (   )

9. OTHER INSURED'S NAME (Last Name, First Name, Middle Initial)

10. IS PATIENT'S CONDITION RELATED TO:

11. INSURED'S POLICY GROUP OR FECA NUMBER
NONE

a. OTHER INSURED'S POLICY OR GROUP NUMBER

a. EMPLOYMENT? (CURRENT OR PREVIOUS)
[ ] YES [X] NO

a. INSURED'S DATE OF BIRTH   MM DD YY   SEX M [ ] F [ ]

b. OTHER INSURED'S DATE OF BIRTH   MM DD YY   SEX M [ ] F [ ]

b. AUTO ACCIDENT?   PLACE (State)
[ ] YES [X] NO

b. EMPLOYER'S NAME OR SCHOOL NAME

c. EMPLOYER'S NAME OR SCHOOL NAME

c. OTHER ACCIDENT?
[ ] YES [X] NO

c. INSURANCE PLAN NAME OR PROGRAM NAME

d. INSURANCE PLAN NAME OR PROGRAM NAME

10d. RESERVED FOR LOCAL USE

d. IS THERE ANOTHER HEALTH BENEFIT PLAN?
[ ] YES   [ ] NO   *If yes*, return to and complete item 9 a-d.

READ BACK OF FORM BEFORE COMPLETING & SIGNING THIS FORM.

12. PATIENT'S OR AUTHORIZED PERSON'S SIGNATURE I authorize the release of any medical or other information necessary to process this claim. I also request payment of government benefits either to myself or to the party who accepts assignment below.

SIGNED   SIGNATURE ON FILE   DATE

13. INSURED'S OR AUTHORIZED PERSON'S SIGNATURE I authorize payment of medical benefits to the undersigned physician or supplier for services described below.

SIGNED   SIGNATURE ON FILE

14. DATE OF CURRENT: MM DD YY   ILLNESS (First symptom) OR INJURY (Accident) OR PREGNANCY(LMP)

15. IF PATIENT HAS HAD SAME OR SIMILAR ILLNESS. GIVE FIRST DATE   MM DD YY

16. DATES PATIENT UNABLE TO WORK IN CURRENT OCCUPATION   FROM MM DD YY   TO MM DD YY

17. NAME OF REFERRING PHYSICIAN OR OTHER SOURCE

17a. I.D. NUMBER OF REFERRING PHYSICIAN

18. HOSPITALIZATION DATES RELATED TO CURRENT SERVICES   FROM MM DD YY   TO MM DD YY

19. RESERVED FOR LOCAL USE

20. OUTSIDE LAB? $ CHARGES
[ ] YES [ ] NO

21. DIAGNOSIS OR NATURE OF ILLNESS OR INJURY. (RELATE ITEMS 1,2,3 OR 4 TO ITEM 24E BY LINE)
1. 373 . 02
2. ___ . ___
3. ___ . ___
4. ___ . ___

22. MEDICAID RESUBMISSION CODE   ORIGINAL REF. NO.

23. PRIOR AUTHORIZATION NUMBER

24. A DATE(S) OF SERVICE						B Place of Service	C Type of Service	D PROCEDURES, SERVICES, OR SUPPLIES (Explain Unusual Circumstances) CPT/HCPCS | MODIFIER	E DIAGNOSIS CODE	F $ CHARGES	G DAYS OR UNITS	H EPSDT Family Plan	I EMG	J COB	K RESERVED FOR LOCAL USE
From MM	DD	YY	To MM	DD	YY										
11	30	95	11	30	95	11		99213	1	28 00	001				013
11	30	95	11	30	95	11		92015	1	10 00	001				013

25. FEDERAL TAX I.D. NUMBER   SSN [ ] EIN [X]

26. PATIENT'S ACCOUNT NO. 531

27. ACCEPT ASSIGNMENT? (For govt. claims, see back)   [X] YES [ ] NO

28. TOTAL CHARGE $ 38 00

29. AMOUNT PAID $

30. BALANCE DUE $

31. SIGNATURE OF PHYSICIAN OR SUPPLIER INCLUDING DEGREES OR CREDENTIALS (I certify that the statements on the reverse apply to this bill and are made a part thereof.)
Jim Smith OD
SIGNED   DATE 12/1/95

32. NAME AND ADDRESS OF FACILITY WHERE SERVICES WERE RENDERED (If other than home or office)

33. PHYSICIAN'S, SUPPLIER'S BILLING NAME, ADDRESS, ZIP CODE & PHONE # 6165552020
SMITH JIM OD
455 BROOK AVE
HAPPY MI 49307
PIN#   GRP# 0E123456789

PATIENT AND INSURED INFORMATION

PHYSICIAN OR SUPPLIER INFORMATION

(APPROVED BY AMA COUNCIL ON MEDICAL SERVICE 8/88)   **PLEASE PRINT OR TYPE**   FORM HCFA-1500 (12-90)
FORM OWCP-1500   FORM RRB-1500
#19423 — #29423 — Medical Arts Press
Use with Envelope #14145 (gummed) or #14146 (self-seal)

Mfd. by Medical Arts Press
Call toll-free: 1-800-328-2179

Figure 36-1 Sample HCFA-1500 form.

visit. Other plans may pay for the visit but only if a preauthorization request is filed before the examination occurs.

It is important to verify that spouses and children are covered under the plan. If questions arise regarding eligibility, it is best to call the plan to determine who is eligible for services and materials. Most plans have authorization cards that provide a telephone number to verify coverage. It is prudent to verify coverage before substantial fees are charged because payment can be lost if there is a misunderstanding.

Patient Information

Information is needed to provide details about plan beneficiaries and the plan that supplies reimbursement. It is best to obtain patient information on a registration form (Figure 36-2). This information must be correct and complete because a claim will be rejected

---

PATIENT REGISTRATION FORM

PLEASE COMPLETE THE FOLLOWING INFORMATION SO THAT YOUR VISION RECORD WILL BE COMPLETE. ALL INFORMATION IS NECESSARY.

NAME _____
                    FIRST   MIDDLE   LAST

ADDRESS _____
                 NUMBER AND STREET   CITY   ZIP

HOME PHONE (   )_____, WORK PHONE (   )_____

SOCIAL SECURITY NUMBER_____

BIRTHDATE_____.   SEX   (   ) MALE   (   ) FEMALE

DRIVER'S LICENSE NUMBER_____

REFERRED BY_____

OCCUPATION_____

NAME OF EMPLOYER_____

WORK ADDRESS_____

ARE YOU COVERED BY MEDICARE?   (   ) YES   (   ) NO

ARE YOU COVERED BY MEDI-CAID?   (   ) YES   (   ) NO

ARE YOU ENROLLED IN AN HMO SUCH AS KAISER, FHP, CIGNA OR OTHERS?
                                        (   ) YES   (   ) NO
VISION INSURANCE COMPANY_____

MEDICAL INSURANCE COMPANY_____

NOTIFY IN CASE OF EMERGENCY_____

RELATIONSHIP_____ TELEPHONE NUMBER_____

I consent to optometric evaluation and treatment by Dr._____

                                    _____
                                                    (signature)

I authorize the release of any medical information necessary to process my insurance claims. I also request payment of my insurance benefits to Dr._____

                                    _____
                                                    (signature)

Figure 36-2 Sample patient registration form.

without proper facts. If information is incorrect, the claim will be returned for correction. Payment will be delayed, and extra work will be created.

Processing Steps

As patients schedule appointments, the receptionist should request that all insurance forms, identification cards, and benefits information be brought to the appointment. With so many different carriers and policy provisions, it is helpful to have trained staff review and explain coverage to patients.

When the patient arrives, the registration form should be completed and the patient's identification card should be reviewed to confirm coverage. It is wise to photocopy the identification card for the patient's record and for future reference.

The patient should be informed of the benefits, deductibles, and co-insurance. At the end of the visit, the patient's share of the services and material fees should be collected.

Claims should be mailed or electronically transferred to the plan at a suitable time. Unprocessed claims represent money owed to the practice. All claims should be complete and legible. A copy of the claim should be kept in a "claims pending" file for review until payment is received.

If claims have not been paid within 4 weeks, it is advisable to call the carrier to determine whether a problem exists. Most states now have laws that set time limits on third parties to either deny or pay claims. Practitioners should know what the law is for the state in which they practice. If a claim is returned because of an error, corrections should be made and the claim resubmitted in a timely manner. Many carriers can deny claims if they are not submitted within a specified period. That time may be as short as 30 days for some carriers.

Computerization of Claims

Many of the computer software packages for office management include the ability to complete claim forms such as the HCFA-1500. The computer templates match the claim form, and the information can automatically be transferred. It is important to enter the correct diagnosis, procedures, fees, patient insurance information, and any additional information required.

"Electronic claims submission" refers to the ability to send claims to the insurance company through telephone lines. The office's computer links with the carrier's computer through a modem, and information is downloaded to the carrier. Sending claims by modem speeds up processing time by eliminating the need to mail them. It also reduces errors since the data do not have to be re-entered by the carrier into the computer. Payment is often faster because of the time saved in processing claims. It is anticipated that, in the future, electronic transfer might be required by some third-party payers, such as Medicare.

Conclusion

Health care financing is in a state of flux. The pace of change is exponential, with no sign of slowing down. All practitioners need to understand the basics of managed care and third-party reimbursement. Managed care is spreading throughout the country, and no region or area will escape. The knowledgeable practitioner will likely flourish in this environment, whereas the uninformed practitioner will likely struggle and perhaps not survive.

Acknowledgement

The authors of this chapter in the first edition of *Business Aspects of Optometry* were Roger D. Kamen, David L. Park, and Craig Hisaka.

Bibliography

American Medical Association: *Physicians' current procedural terminology,* ed 4 (CPT-4). Chicago, 2001, Author.

American Optometric Association: *Manual on completion of insurance claim forms,* ed 4. St. Louis, 1994, Author.

American Optometric Association. *Managed care resource guide.* St. Louis, 1997, Author.

American Optometric Association: *Codes for optometry.* St. Louis, 2003, Author.

Kamen RD: Are you ready for your Medicare audit. *Mich Optom* 78(4):3-5, 1999.

Kamen RD: Evaluation and management coding. *Mich Optom* 78(7):12-5, 1999.

Knight K: *Managed care: what it is and how it works.* Gaithersburg, Md, 1998, Aspen.

Kongstvedt PR: *Essentials of managed health care,* ed 2. Gaithersburg, Md, 1997, Aspen.

Krefman A (ed): Managed care and contracting. A primer for the practicing optometrist. *Optom Today* (Suppl);2(9): 1-30, 1994.

McGreal JA: Coding higher for success, part 1. *Optom Management* 34(3):42-8, 1999.

McGreal JA: Coding higher for success, part 2. *Optom Management* 34(4):53-6, 1999.

McGreal JA: Coding higher for success, part 3. *Optom Management* 34(5):45-54, 1999.

Rosenthal J, Soroka M: *Managed vision benefits*, ed 2. Brookfield, Wis, 1998, International Foundation of Employee Benefit Plans.

Sultz HA, Young KM: *Health care USA*, ed 2. Gaithersburg, Md, 1999, Aspen.

Wright M: *Reimbursement and managed care*, ed 2, Columbus, Ohio, 1998, Anadem.

www.cms.hhs.gov. U.S. government Web site for the Medicare and Medicaid programs.

Chapter 37

Medicare and Medicaid

Roger D. Kamen and Mark R. Wright

You can be young without money
but you can't be old without it.
Tennessee Williams *Cat on a Hot Tin Roof*

The government executes and finances numerous third-party insurance plans that involve optometric participation. These plans include programs such as Medicare; Medicaid; Civilian Health and Medical Program of the Uniformed Services (CHAMPUS); the Veterans Administration; the Department of Defense; the Public Health Service; health departments; Vocational Rehabilitation; the Developmental Disabilities Program; and Maternal, Child Health, and Crippled Children's Services. This chapter focuses on the two most commonly used programs—Medicare and Medicaid.

Although this chapter describes government as a third-party financier, it is important to understand that much overlap exists between government (or public sector) and private sector (nongovernment) programs. For example, health maintenance organizations (HMOs) are private sector programs with significant government involvement, especially with regard to grants. Medicare and Medicaid are government programs managed, in many states, by private insurance companies.

Medicare

The Medicare program was authorized by the U.S. Congress in 1965 as Title XVIII of the Social Security Act. Medicare originally provided hospital and medical insurance benefits to persons age 65 and older. Throughout the years, the Medicare program has expanded to include care for people younger than 65 who are blind, or disabled, or who suffer from chronic renal disease.

Medicare benefits include basic hospital insurance (Part A) and medical insurance for physicians' services (Part B). Part A is financed by universal compulsory contributions. Part B is obtainable on an elective basis. It is half-financed by the government and half-financed by premium payments from the enrollees.

Eligibility

The Social Security Administration determines who is eligible for Medicare. To be eligible for Part B, the person must be one of the following:
- 65 years old or older
- Younger than age 65, with permanent kidney inadequacy
- Younger than age 65 and permanently disabled

The Social Security Administration issues a card to all patients entitled to Medicare benefits. To determine whether a patient is eligible for medical benefits (Part B), it is necessary to review the patient's Medicare card. The card identifies the Medicare recipient and contains the following details:
- Name
- Medicare health insurance claim number
- Enrollee's signature
- Date of entitlement
- Kind of benefits for which the beneficiary is entitled under the Medicare policy (Part A, Part B, or both)

It is critical to check the Medicare card at least once a year. Medicare numbers and suffixes can change according to the beneficiary's record of entitlement. Changes are particularly significant in the case of marriage or remarriage.

On claim forms, the name and health insurance claim numbers (HICNs) should be entered exactly as shown on the Medicare card. All claim forms are transmitted to one of nine host sites, where records regarding Medicare eligibility and deductible status are kept. Any mistake in entering the name and HICN on the Medicare Request for Payment form (HCFA-1500) will cause the claim to be rejected because it will not agree with the Social Security register.

Claim Submission

Medicare requires the use of the HCFA-1500 claim form (Figure 37-1) for the submission of paper claims. The claim form is available in a single sheet, a two-part snapout, and a two-part computer pin-feed continuous form. Optometrists are responsible for purchasing their own claim forms, which can be obtained through the U.S. Government Printing Office or through commercial outlets. Commercial forms must contain the information required by the Centers for Medicare and Medicaid (formerly known as the Health Care Financing Administration [HCFA]) on both the front and back of the form. The current version (12/90) has been in use since 1992. Claim forms must be printed in "drop-out red." (See Chapter 36 for information on completing the form.)

Diagnostic Codes. All Medicare providers must use the Healthcare Common Procedure Coding System (HCPCS) Levels I, II, and III procedures codes for claim submission.

Level I codes are the procedures contained in the *Current Procedural Terminology, 4th edition* (*CPT-4*), which is revised periodically (Chicago, 2001, American Medical Association) (see Chapter 36 for a description of these codes).

Level II codes are national alphanumeric codes that supplement the *CPT-4* codes. These five-digit codes include services such as audiology, physical therapy, and vision care and supplies such as drugs and durable medical equipment (including frames, lenses, contact lenses, and prosthetic devices). The codes start with a letter (A through V) and are followed by four numbers.

Level III codes are local codes assigned by the local carrier for Medicare. These codes cover procedures not included in the first two levels. The codes begin with a letter (W through Z) followed by four numbers.

Time Limits for Filing Medicare Claims. Claims must be filed by the end of the calendar year after the year in which services are provided. Services provided during the last 3 months of the calendar year are con-

sidered, for billing purposes, to be provided in the next calendar year.

Covered Services

Eye examinations by an optometrist (or physician) for the purpose of determining or changing the prescription for eyeglasses or contact lenses are not covered under Medicare. Eye examinations are covered in the following situations:

When performed in conjunction with the fitting and prescribing of postsurgical lenses when the lens of the eye has been removed (aphakia or pseudophakia). (Refractive services are excluded from coverage, even with the diagnosis of aphakia or pseudophakia.)

When performed for a medical condition, diagnosis, sign, or symptom.

Therefore, eyeglasses or contact lenses that are required to replace a lens removed as a result of intraocular surgery or to replace congenitally missing lenses are covered benefits. Corneal bandage contact lenses are a covered benefit when used as a moist bandage to aid corneal healing, relieve pain, reduce erosion, and improve vision.

Independent procedures are covered benefits when billed with an appropriate diagnosis but require a medical sign or symptom as the initial reason for the examination. A sampling of independent procedures includes gonioscopy, extended ophthalmoscopy, external photography, retinal photography, color vision testing, contrast sensitivity testing, ultrasonography, and electrodiagnostic testing.

Claim Payment

Every Medicare carrier is charged with processing claims in accordance with Medicare regulations. No payment may be made for any items or services that are not reasonable or necessary for the diagnosis or treatment of an illness or injury.

During each calendar year a $100 deductible must be satisfied before payment can be made. Bills for services are applied toward the deductible on the basis of incurred medical expenses. The deductible is applied to the approved charge. Noncovered services do not count toward the deductible.

Expenses are allocated to the deductible in the order in which the bills are received by Medicare. Enrollees must satisfy the deductible–regardless of when during

PLEASE
DO NOT
STAPLE
IN THIS
AREA

CARRIER →

HEALTH INSURANCE CLAIM FORM

PICA | | PICA

| | 1. MEDICARE | MEDICAID | CHAMPUS | CHAMPVA | GROUP HEALTH PLAN (SSN or ID) | FECA BLK LUNG (SSN) | OTHER | 1a. INSURED'S I.D. NUMBER (FOR PROGRAM IN ITEM 1) |

X (Medicare #) | (Medicaid #) | (Sponsor's SSN) | (VA File #) | | | (ID) | 12345678A

2. PATIENT'S NAME (Last Name, First Name, Middle Initial)
Vision Joseph A

3. PATIENT'S BIRTH DATE MM 01 DD 02 YY 31 SEX M X F

4. INSURED'S NAME (Last Name, First Name, Middle Initial)

5. PATIENT'S ADDRESS (No., Street)
2020 Refraction Lane

6. PATIENT RELATIONSHIP TO INSURED
Self [ ] Spouse [ ] Child [ ] Other [ ]

7. INSURED'S ADDRESS (No., Street)

CITY
Anytown

STATE
MI

8. PATIENT STATUS
Single [ ] Married [ ] Other [ ]
Employed [ ] Full-Time Student [ ] Part-Time Student [ ]

CITY | STATE

ZIP CODE
49000

TELEPHONE (Include Area Code)
( )

ZIP CODE | TELEPHONE (INCLUDE AREA CODE) ( )

9. OTHER INSURED'S NAME (Last Name, First Name, Middle Initial)

10. IS PATIENT'S CONDITION RELATED TO:

11. INSURED'S POLICY GROUP OR FECA NUMBER
None

a. OTHER INSURED'S POLICY OR GROUP NUMBER

a. EMPLOYMENT? (CURRENT OR PREVIOUS)
[ ] YES X NO

a. INSURED'S DATE OF BIRTH MM DD YY
SEX M [ ] F [ ]

b. OTHER INSURED'S DATE OF BIRTH MM DD YY SEX M [ ] F [ ]

b. AUTO ACCIDENT? PLACE (State)
[ ] YES X NO

b. EMPLOYER'S NAME OR SCHOOL NAME

c. EMPLOYER'S NAME OR SCHOOL NAME

c. OTHER ACCIDENT?
[ ] YES X NO

c. INSURANCE PLAN NAME OR PROGRAM NAME

d. INSURANCE PLAN NAME OR PROGRAM NAME

10d. RESERVED FOR LOCAL USE

d. IS THERE ANOTHER HEALTH BENEFIT PLAN?
[ ] YES [ ] NO *If yes*, return to and complete item 9 a-d.

READ BACK OF FORM BEFORE COMPLETING & SIGNING THIS FORM.
12. PATIENT'S OR AUTHORIZED PERSON'S SIGNATURE I authorize the release of any medical or other information necessary to process this claim. I also request payment of government benefits either to myself or to the party who accepts assignment below.

SIGNED Signature on File DATE 9/1/96

13. INSURED'S OR AUTHORIZED PERSON'S SIGNATURE I authorize payment of medical benefits to the undersigned physician or supplier for services described below.

SIGNED Signature on File

14. DATE OF CURRENT: ILLNESS (First symptom) OR INJURY (Accident) OR PREGNANCY(LMP) MM DD YY

15. IF PATIENT HAS HAD SAME OR SIMILAR ILLNESS. GIVE FIRST DATE MM DD YY

16. DATES PATIENT UNABLE TO WORK IN CURRENT OCCUPATION
FROM MM DD YY TO MM DD YY

17. NAME OF REFERRING PHYSICIAN OR OTHER SOURCE

17a. I.D. NUMBER OF REFERRING PHYSICIAN

18. HOSPITALIZATION DATES RELATED TO CURRENT SERVICES
FROM MM DD YY TO MM DD YY

19. RESERVED FOR LOCAL USE

20. OUTSIDE LAB? $ CHARGES
[ ] YES [ ] NO

21. DIAGNOSIS OR NATURE OF ILLNESS OR INJURY. (RELATE ITEMS 1,2,3 OR 4 TO ITEM 24E BY LINE)
1. 250 .50
2. ___ . ___
3. ___ . ___
4. ___ . ___

22. MEDICAID RESUBMISSION CODE ORIGINAL REF. NO.

23. PRIOR AUTHORIZATION NUMBER

24. A DATE(S) OF SERVICE From MM DD YY	To MM DD YY	B Place of Service	C Type of Service	D PROCEDURES, SERVICES, OR SUPPLIES (Explain Unusual Circumstances) CPT/HCPCS MODIFIER	E DIAGNOSIS CODE	F $ CHARGES	G DAYS OR UNITS	H EPSDT Family Plan	I EMG	J COB	K RESERVED FOR LOCAL USE
9 1 96	9 1 96	11	3	99245	1	175 00	001				013

25. FEDERAL TAX I.D. NUMBER SSN EIN
123-45-6789 [ ] X

26. PATIENT'S ACCOUNT NO.
531

27. ACCEPT ASSIGNMENT? (For govt. claims, see back)
X YES [ ] NO

28. TOTAL CHARGE
$ 175 00

29. AMOUNT PAID
$

30. BALANCE DUE
$

31. SIGNATURE OF PHYSICIAN OR SUPPLIER INCLUDING DEGREES OR CREDENTIALS (I certify that the statements on the reverse apply to this bill and are made a part thereof.)
SIGNED John O'Dee OD DATE 9/1/91

32. NAME AND ADDRESS OF FACILITY WHERE SERVICES WERE RENDERED (If other than home or office)

33. PHYSICIAN'S, SUPPLIER'S BILLING NAME, ADDRESS, ZIP CODE & PHONE # 616-555-2020
O'Dee John OD
2020 Vision Street
Insight MI 49000
PIN# OE GRP# 123-45-6789

(APPROVED BY AMA COUNCIL ON MEDICAL SERVICE 8/88) **PLEASE PRINT OR TYPE**

FORM HCFA-1500 (12-90)
FORM OWCP-1500 FORM RRB-1500

PATIENT AND INSURED INFORMATION

PHYSICIAN OR SUPPLIER INFORMATION

Figure 37-1 Sample HCFA-1500 form used for billing a Medicare claim.

the calendar year they became eligible–before they can receive any medical benefits.

After the Part B deductible has been satisfied, Medicare reimburses 80% of the approved charge incurred during the calendar year. The remaining 20% is the responsibility of the patient, as co-insurance.

For services rendered on or after Jan. 1, 1992, Medicare payments are based on physician payment reform. The payment methodology reform contains the following three major elements:

National fee schedule. For dates of service on or after Jan. 1, 1992, reimbursement for physician services is based on a fee schedule. The fee schedule is based on a resource-based, relative value scale adjusted by geographic cost differences.

Medicare volume performance standard (MVPS). MVPS is a mechanism for limiting growth in Medicare Part B expenditures.

Beneficiary protection. Under physician payment reform, the new limiting charge caps the amount that non-participating physicians may bill Medicare patients above the fee schedule.

The fee schedule is a relative value scale (described in Chapter 36) that is resource-based. A relative value unit is assigned to each procedure and is based on the relative amount of provider work (time and intensity), overhead expenses, and malpractice expense for the procedure. This unit value (adjusted for geographic location) is then multiplied by a conversion factor (multiplier) to obtain the reimbursement amount.

Medicare Assignment Agreement

Under Medicare law, the physician who accepts *assignment* is one who accepts the carrier's allowable (approved) charge as the full charge. Medicare will reimburse 80% of this allowable amount if the deductible has been met. The beneficiary is responsible to the physician for the remaining 20%. The beneficiary also is responsible for any portion of the unmet deductible and the full charge for services not covered by Medicare.

For services covered under the assignment agreement, the physician cannot bill the patient the difference between the allowable amount and the actual charge. Medicare law also requires that for an assigned claim, the physician must make an effort to collect from the beneficiary any deductible amount as well as the co-insurance. Repeated, willful violations of the

assignment agreement can result in fines of $2000, up to 6 months of imprisonment, or both.

Medicare rules require that the patient be informed in writing of any noncovered fees before the service or material is provided. If this is not documented in the record with the patient's signature, then the provider cannot bill the patient.

Participating or Nonparticipating Provider

Providers are either participating ("par") or non-participating ("nonpar"). The par provider must accept assignment for all covered services on all claims. The nonpar provider can accept assignment on a claim-by-claim basis. There are incentives given to providers to become par providers. Examples of these incentives include the following:

• Reimbursement that is 5% more than for nonpar providers
• A listing in the directory of providers
• Exemption from limiting charges
• Direct payments (reimbursement) from Medicare
• "One stop" billing for Medigap coverage

Even if the nonpar provider accepts assignment, reimbursement will be based on a 5% lower fee schedule. If a nonpar provider does not accept assignment, the charge for the procedure is subject to a limiting charge. This charge is the maximum amount the nonpar provider is allowed to bill the patient. Currently this amount is 115% of the nonpar fee schedule amount.

The Medicare carrier issues an Explanation of Medicare Benefits (EOMB) as the final step in the processing of a Medicare claim. The EOMB is sent to the beneficiary. A copy is not provided to the physician if assignment was not accepted. When assignment is accepted, the original EOMB is sent to the physician, and the beneficiary also receives a copy. If benefits cannot be paid for a claim or if all the benefits are applied to the deductible, the EOMB still will be issued, advising the beneficiary and the physician of the disposition of the claim.

The EOMB gives detailed information on the action taken on the claim. It shows the name of the physician, dates of service, amount billed, amount approved, and total payable amount. It also provides the beneficiary with the current deductible status.

For assigned claims, Medicare uses the Remittance Notice for settlement of assigned Medicare claims. The check sent to the provider often includes payment for several patients. This helps reduce paperwork. Claims are processed on a weekly basis. If there is no reimbursable amount due on the summary statement, the statement is still issued, and it provides detailed information on every claim listed. Each claim line shows the date of service, type and place of service, procedure code, amount billed, and amount approved for payment.

Medigap and Crossover Claims

Medigap is a private, supplemental insurance that is used to fill the "gaps" in Medicare benefits—in particular the 20% co-insurance. Only par providers can take advantage of the single claim submission to Medicare and the Medigap company. With single-claim submission, neither the provider nor the beneficiary needs to file a secondary claim. After the Medicare carrier finishes processing the Medicare benefit, a payment record is sent to the Medigap carrier for the payment of supplemental insurance benefits.

Crossover claims involve an automated process in which Medicare sends an electronic EOMB to the supplemental insurance carrier. This service applies to both par and nonpar providers. The crossover carriers have a contract (fee per claim) to receive this information for their insurees. Medicare and Medicaid crossover claims are an example of this process.

A Medicare and Medicaid *crossover claim* is a claim for services covered under two separate programs. Crossover claims must contain covered Medicare services provided to a Medicare patient who is also eligible under the state Medicaid program. Benefits are paid by both programs on the basis of a single claim. The claim is first submitted to the Medicare carrier and then transferred, or crossed over, to the Medicaid program.

Medicare determines the approved charge for the service, which is established if an annual deductible has been met, and Medicare pays 80% of the approved charge. Medicaid considers payment of any unmet deductible and the remaining 20% of the approved charge.

Medicare and Medicaid crossover claims must clearly identify that the patient is covered by Medicaid in order for the claim to be crossed over. Many claims do not cross over because the provider does not indicate that the patient is covered under the Medicaid program. The patient should be identified on the HCFA-1500 form as covered by Medicaid, and a copy of the Medicaid identification card, proof of eligibility label, or eligibility number should be included (Figure 37-2).

For claims to cross over, the provider must accept assignment and the assignment must be checked on the claim form. The claim must include positive identification of the patient's Medicaid eligibility. The claim must have paid at least one covered item or must have applied at least one covered item on the claim to the patient's deductible.

Medicare and Medicaid crossover claims should be submitted to the Medicare carrier on the customary HCFA-1500 claim form. Separate billing to the Medicare carrier and to the Medicaid carrier is required when services included on the crossover claim do not automatically transfer for payment. For example, dual billing requirements for eyewear might be required.

Services that are denied or not covered under Medicare but that are Medicaid benefits will not automatically cross over. These services can be billed to the Medicaid program. For example, eyeglasses for a patient who has not had cataract surgery is a noncovered service under Medicare. If the patient is eligible for Medicaid, the eyeglasses should be billed to the Medicaid program. If the provider did not know that the patient was eligible for Medicaid at the time of Medicare billing, the billing will not cross over. Another important example is the fee for refraction. Medicare does not cover a refraction; however, Medicaid does. If the refraction is submitted on the Medicare claim, when it is denied it will cross over and Medicaid will reimburse the fee. This also is true for any spectacle dispensing fees. The Medicare EOMB should be attached to a Medicaid form to bill for deductible and co-insurance amounts that did not cross over.

Services and supplies not covered by Medicare, but payable by Medicaid, should be billed separately to the Medicaid program, indicating they are not Medicare-covered services. These services can be billed directly to the Medicaid program.

Medicare and Managed Care

Managed care has expanded into the Medicare program because the federal government hopes to control the high cost of health care for Medicare patients. The Tax Equity and Fiscal Responsibility Act of 1982, implemented in 1985, provided the means for managed care to become involved with Medicare. Since then, other laws have strengthened the ties between managed care organizations and Medicare.

In the past there were three basic types of managed care contracts with the government for Medicare: risk contracts, cost contracts, and Medicare demonstration programs.

Risk Contracts

Federally qualified HMOs and competition medical plans contract with Medicare on a prepaid basis to

APPROVED OMB-0938-0008

PLEASE
DO NOT
STAPLE
IN THIS
AREA

HEALTH INSURANCE CLAIM FORM

PICA   PICA

| 1. MEDICARE | MEDICAID | CHAMPUS | CHAMPVA | GROUP HEALTH PLAN | FECA BLK LUNG | OTHER | 1a. INSURED'S I.D. NUMBER (FOR PROGRAM IN ITEM 1) |

(Medicare #) [X] (Medicaid #) (Sponsor's SSN) (VA File #) (SSN or ID) (SSN) (ID)   12345678A

2. PATIENT'S NAME (Last Name, First Name, Middle Initial)
Vision Joseph A

3. PATIENT'S BIRTH DATE MM 01 DD 02 YY 31 SEX M [X] F

4. INSURED'S NAME (Last Name, First Name, Middle Initial)

5. PATIENT'S ADDRESS (No., Street)
2020 Refraction Lane

6. PATIENT RELATIONSHIP TO INSURED
Self [ ] Spouse [ ] Child [ ] Other [ ]

7. INSURED'S ADDRESS (No., Street)

CITY
Anytown   STATE MI

8. PATIENT STATUS
Single [ ] Married [ ] Other [ ]

CITY   STATE

ZIP CODE 49000   TELEPHONE (Include Area Code) (616) 555-1212

Employed [ ] Full-Time Student [ ] Part-Time Student [ ]

ZIP CODE   TELEPHONE (INCLUDE AREA CODE) ( )

9. OTHER INSURED'S NAME (Last Name, First Name, Middle Initial)

10. IS PATIENT'S CONDITION RELATED TO:

11. INSURED'S POLICY GROUP OR FECA NUMBER
None

a. OTHER INSURED'S POLICY OR GROUP NUMBER
Medicaid 45678910

a. EMPLOYMENT? (CURRENT OR PREVIOUS) YES [ ] NO [X]

a. INSURED'S DATE OF BIRTH MM DD YY SEX M [ ] F [ ]

b. OTHER INSURED'S DATE OF BIRTH MM DD YY SEX M [ ] F [ ]

b. AUTO ACCIDENT? PLACE (State) YES [ ] NO [X]

b. EMPLOYER'S NAME OR SCHOOL NAME

c. EMPLOYER'S NAME OR SCHOOL NAME

c. OTHER ACCIDENT? YES [ ] NO [X]

c. INSURANCE PLAN NAME OR PROGRAM NAME

d. INSURANCE PLAN NAME OR PROGRAM NAME

10d. RESERVED FOR LOCAL USE
MCD

d. IS THERE ANOTHER HEALTH BENEFIT PLAN? YES [ ] NO [ ] *If yes, return to and complete item 9 a-d.*

READ BACK OF FORM BEFORE COMPLETING & SIGNING THIS FORM.

12. PATIENT'S OR AUTHORIZED PERSON'S SIGNATURE I authorize the release of any medical or other information necessary to process this claim. I also request payment of government benefits either to myself or to the party who accepts assignment below.

SIGNED Signature of File   DATE 9/1/96

13. INSURED'S OR AUTHORIZED PERSON'S SIGNATURE I authorize payment of medical benefits to the undersigned physician or supplier for services described below.

SIGNED Signature on File

14. DATE OF CURRENT: ILLNESS (First symptom) OR INJURY (Accident) OR PREGNANCY(LMP) MM DD YY

15. IF PATIENT HAS HAD SAME OR SIMILAR ILLNESS. GIVE FIRST DATE MM DD YY

16. DATES PATIENT UNABLE TO WORK IN CURRENT OCCUPATION FROM MM DD YY TO MM DD YY

17. NAME OF REFERRING PHYSICIAN OR OTHER SOURCE

17a. I.D. NUMBER OF REFERRING PHYSICIAN

18. HOSPITALIZATION DATES RELATED TO CURRENT SERVICES FROM MM DD YY TO MM DD YY

19. RESERVED FOR LOCAL USE

20. OUTSIDE LAB? YES [ ] NO [ ] $ CHARGES

21. DIAGNOSIS OR NATURE OF ILLNESS OR INJURY. (RELATE ITEMS 1,2,3 OR 4 TO ITEM 24E BY LINE)
1. 373 . 02
2. ____ . ____
3. ____ . ____
4. ____ . ____

22. MEDICAID RESUBMISSION CODE   ORIGINAL REF. NO.

23. PRIOR AUTHORIZATION NUMBER

24. A DATE(S) OF SERVICE From MM DD YY To MM DD YY	B Place of Service	C Type of Service	D PROCEDURES, SERVICES, OR SUPPLIES (Explain Unusual Circumstances) CPT/HCPCS MODIFIER	E DIAGNOSIS CODE	F $ CHARGES	G DAYS OR UNITS	H EPSDT Family Plan	I EMG	J COB	K RESERVED FOR LOCAL USE
9 1 96 9 1 96	11		99213	1	28 00	001				013
9 1 96 9 1 96	11		92015	1	10 00	001				013

25. FEDERAL TAX I.D. NUMBER SSN EIN
123-45-6789 [X]

26. PATIENT'S ACCOUNT NO.
531

27. ACCEPT ASSIGNMENT? (For govt. claims, see back) YES [X] NO [ ]

28. TOTAL CHARGE $ 38 00

29. AMOUNT PAID $

30. BALANCE DUE $

31. SIGNATURE OF PHYSICIAN OR SUPPLIER INCLUDING DEGREES OR CREDENTIALS (I certify that the statements on the reverse apply to this bill and are made a part thereof.)
SIGNED John O'Dee OD DATE 9/1/96

32. NAME AND ADDRESS OF FACILITY WHERE SERVICES WERE RENDERED (If other than home or office)

33. PHYSICIAN'S, SUPPLIER'S BILLING NAME, ADDRESS, ZIP CODE & PHONE # 616-555-2020
O'Dee John OD
2020 Vision Street
Insight MI 49000
PIN#   GRP#   OE 123-45-6789

(APPROVED BY AMA COUNCIL ON MEDICAL SERVICE 8/88)   **PLEASE PRINT OR TYPE**   FORM HCFA-1500 (12-90) FORM OWCP-1500 FORM RRB-1500

Mfd. by Medical Arts Press
Call toll-free: 1-800-328-2179

#19423 – #29423 – Medical Arts Press
Use with Envelope #14145 (gummed) or #14146 (self-seal)

CARRIER — PATIENT AND INSURED INFORMATION — PHYSICIAN OR SUPPLIER INFORMATION

Figure 37-2 Sample HCFA-1500 form used for billing a crossover claim.

provide covered services to eligible patients under risk contracts.

Cost Contracts

Federally qualified HMOs and health care prepayment plans contract with Medicare to provide covered services on a cost recovery basis. This contract is less advantageous to Medicare than risk contracts.

Medicare Demonstration Programs

In the past there were two Medicare demonstration programs:

Medicare insured group (MIG). An entity (corporation or union) contracts with Medicare to provide both the Medicare benefits and supplemental coverage for the beneficiary.

Medicare select. Medicare supplemental insurance carriers are allowed to offer a preferred provider organization for basic Medicare coverage and supplemental benefits.

All of these programs were optional for the Medicare beneficiary. However, there were some advantages for patients to forgo the fee-for-service Medicare plan in favor of these managed care plans. Possible incentives include the waiving of the 20% co-insurance and the use of additional benefits not normally covered by Medicare (e.g., prescription drugs). Currently, managed care has been fully integrated in Medicare.

Medicare+Choice

The Medicare managed care carveout plans are called Medicare+Choice. (Sometimes these plans are called Medicare C.) Medicare+Choice plans present as:

- PPOs (preferred provider organizations)
- HMOs with a POS (point of service)
- PSOs (provider sponsored organizations)
- PFFSPs (private fee-for-service plans)
- MSAs (medical savings accounts)

Individuals could enroll or withdraw in these plans on a monthly basis until the year 2002. During that year they could make a special election to change plans. After 2003 Medicare+Choice plans can be changed only during the first 3 months of the year.

Fraud and Abuse

Abuse refers to practices by Medicare providers that are not consistent with accepted sound medical,

business, or fiscal practices. Examples include the following:
- Excessive charges for services or supplies
- Claims for services that are not medically necessary
- Breach of assignment agreements
- Exceeding the limiting charges
- Submission of bills to Medicare instead of to the primary insurer
- Routine waiver of copayment and deductible

Fraud is an intentional deception by the provider that results in some unauthorized benefit to the provider. Examples include the following:
- Billing for services not provided
- Altering claim forms to obtain a higher payment amount
- Soliciting, offering, or receiving a kickback
- Claims for noncovered services billed as covered services

The Medicare carrier is responsible for identifying and investigating incidents of suspected fraud or abuse. These cases can then be referred to the Office of the Inspector General for further investigation and possible criminal, civil, or administrative sanctions.

Medicaid

Medicaid is a joint federal-state program that provides funding of health care for the poor. Title XIX, an amendment of the Social Security Act known as Medicaid, became effective Jan. 1, 1966. Although Medicaid operates under federal guidelines, it is administered by individual states. Funding is provided by both federal and state governments.

Each state develops a single comprehensive medical care program. Twenty-one services are permissible under the federal act. States are given broad authority in the determination of eligibility requirements and covered services, but federal guidelines require the inclusion of the following seven services in any plan:
- Inpatient hospital services
- Outpatient hospital services
- Laboratory and x-ray services
- Skilled nursing home services
- Physician's services
- Home health services
- Early and periodic screening, diagnosis, and treatment (EPSDT)

The other services are optional and can be included if the state desires. Vision care is an optional service. Nevertheless, a 1992 survey conducted by the

American Optometric Association found that optometrists were used to provide periodic vision examinations to Medicaid-eligible individuals in all states but that significant variations existed among the states in covered services. The survey reported the following:

In 11 states, the approval of gatekeepers or prior approval from the Medicaid carrier is needed before contact lenses, low vision therapy, and vision therapy can be provided.

In 13 states, contact lenses, low vision devices, and vision therapy cannot be provided.

In 12 states, spectacles cannot be provided to adults.

Significant limits exist in all states with respect to spectacle lenses and frames. Restrictions include the cost of ophthalmic materials, the dioptric changes in prescriptions needed before eyewear can be changed, and the limited availability of frame styles.

EPSDT screenings typically are performed by optometrists or nurses. There are only three states in which physicians are used for vision screenings.

Reimbursement in the vast majority of states is based on a fixed fee schedule. *CPT-4* codes are used in all but nine of the states.

The screenings, required by EPSDT for eligible individuals younger than 21 years, must include vision testing. If vision deficits are discovered during the screening, the patient must be referred for diagnosis and treatment, at Medicaid's expense. In this manner, eye examinations, eye appliances, visual therapy, and other visual treatments can be covered in a state that does not offer vision care services.

Billing Information

Because of the great variance that exists from state to state, it is not possible to address the issue of billing in any detail. The 1992 American Optometric Association survey found that fees for vision examinations under Medicaid ranged from $16 to $55. Individual state vision care provider manuals must be consulted for information on billing.

Medicaid and Managed Care

Medicaid program costs have significantly increased for the state and federal governments during the past few decades. The states and Centre for Medicare and Medicaid are encouraging managed care organizations to become involved with Medicaid in the hope that costs can be controlled. The following three plans are available:

Risk contract. Federally qualified or state-qualified HMOs contract with the state on a prepaid basis for providing covered services to eligible patients.

Prepaid health plan. This is an organization that contracts with the state to provide care for covered services on a risk and noncomprehensive basis.

Primary care case management plan. A primary care case management plan contracts with the state to provide services on a fee-for-service basis, with an additional fee for case management.

There is a wide variety of managed care plans available, and individual states will have to be surveyed to obtain information on the services provided.

Conclusion

Medicare and Medicaid are the two major federal third-party plans. Optometrists are intimately involved in both programs. An understanding of these programs is essential to a practitioner's financial and professional well-being. Because managed care has become more pervasive in these programs, optometrists need to remain vigilant about changes in eligibility and reimbursement.

Acknowledgement

The authors of this chapter in the first edition of *Business Aspects of Optometry* were Roger D. Kamen, David L. Park, Thomas Sandler, and W. Howard McAlister.

Bibliography

American Optometric Association: *Manual on completion of insurance claim forms,* ed 4. St. Louis, 1994, Author.

American Optometric Association: *Managed care resource guide.* St. Louis, 1997, Author.

American Optometric Association: *Physician's current procedural terminology,* ed 4, (CPT-4) Chicago, 2001 Author.

American Optometric Association. *Codes for optometry.* St. Louis, 2003, Author.

Boland P: *Making managed health care work, a practical guide to strategies and solutions.* Gaithersburg, Md, 1993, Aspen.

Kongstvedt PR: *Essentials of managed health care,* ed 2. Gaithersburg, Md, 1997, Aspen.

Newcomb RD, Marshall EC: *Public health and community optometry*, ed 2. Stoneham, Mass, 1990, Butterworth.

Vision Service Plan: *Vision Service Plan—doctor's procedure manual*. Rancho Cordova, Calif, 1995, Author.

Wright M: *Reimbursement and managed care*, ed 2. Columbus, Ohio, 1998, Anadem.

www.cms.hhs.gov. Web site of the Centers for Medicare and Medicaid (CMS), formerly the Health Care Financing Administration (HCFA); the name change was effective July 1, 2001. This Web site provides access to the rules for Medicare and Medicaid, documentation guidelines for the E/M codes, and information on fraud and abuse.

Chapter 38

Individual Income Tax

John G. Classé

The Congress shall have power to lay and collect taxes on income, from whatever source derived, without apportionment among the several states, and without regard to any census or enumeration.

Sixteenth Amendment *Constitution of the United States*

At the time of the birth of the United States, the English government drew the ire of those in the colonies through the use of an import tariff, the purpose of which was to create a favorable balance of trade (i.e., exports were not subject to the tariff, but imports were charged a duty that was, ultimately, paid by the American consumer). The Boston Tea Party was a result of the perception by the citizens of the colonies that the tariff was unfair. Yet, one of the first acts of the new U.S. Congress was to impose an internal tariff on imports to America! Thus began a widespread system of duties on imports rather than a true tax, because of the provisions of the U.S. Constitution, which limited the ability of the federal government to tax the U.S. citizenry.

The general taxing power permitted to Congress by the Constitution was that "The Congress shall have power to lay and collect taxes, duties, imports and excises, to pay the debts and provide for the common defense and general welfare of the United States." But as far as internal revenue was concerned, there were only two sources of income provided for in the Constitution:

- Duties, imports, and excise taxes were permitted, but could not be higher in one part of the country than in another.
- No direct tax could be levied on the income of individual citizens unless it was applied in proportion to the population of the states, so that each state would have a different tax rate, a cumbersome and impractical system that made the collection of direct taxes a slow and grossly unequal operation.

Attempts during the 1800s and early 1900s to impose an income tax met with limited success, with the most important development being a 1% tax on income of more than $5000 earned by corporations organized for profit. In 1913 the U.S. Congress proposed an amendment to the Constitution that would allow a tax on all incomes without apportionment. Its ratification allowed an income tax to be levied on individual citizens. The tax consisted of two parts: a normal tax, which was a flat 1% of the net income in excess of the personal exemption, and a surtax that was a progressive tax levied on net incomes in excess of $20,000 (for which another 1% was collected) up to a maximum of $500,000 (for which a 6% maximum was imposed). Thus, a married man with a net income of $80,000 in 1913 paid a total tax of $1710. Subsequent changes in the rates and system of taxation have created dramatic differences in the tax burden incurred by American citizens; by 1980, this same married man would have to pay an income tax of $26,914. Of such things is tax reform born, and the result has been decade after decade of unceasing tax reform acts passed by the federal Congress.

In fact, tax reform has become such a favorite pastime of the federal government that tax counsel often must be consulted when significant financial decisions are made. One year's tax laws rapidly give way to another's, and the wise optometrist always will seek professional advice before making personal or business decisions that have tax ramifications. Even so, it is necessary for optometrists to possess a reasonable understanding of the tax process. Given the significance of taxes as an item of both personal and business expense, contemporary practitioners can ill afford to live in ignorance of the basic provisions of tax law. Once these fundamental concepts are understood, the process of revision becomes less confusing and the significance of proposed changes more apparent.

Determination of Income Tax

The tax base to which the income tax rates are applied is called the taxable income. To determine a person's taxable income (Figure 38-1), the *gross income* must be calculated, from which allowable *deductions* are subtracted, resulting in an intermediary sum called the *adjusted gross income (AGI)*. From this there are certain *itemized deductions* allowed, which may be used to further reduce the AGI. *Exemptions* from income are then subtracted, resulting in the *taxable income*. From this amount the tax table tax can be determined. *Credits* are taken from the tax table tax, resulting in the actual tax owed.

The income tax rates for individuals are graduated, which means they increase as the level of taxable income increases. The current tax rates, authorized by federal tax reform in 2003, consist of six brackets, unless further modified by Congress. The stepwise application of this tax to income may be found on Internal Revenue Service (IRS) Form 1040 (Figure 38-2).

Filing Status

Taxes are reported based on the status of the taxpayer, who has the following five choices:
- Single
- Married filing jointly
- Married filing separate returns
- Head of household
- Qualifying widow/widower with dependent child

The choice of filing status is left to the taxpayer; the tax rates that will be applied to the taxpayer's income are based on the choice made. However, the milestone tax reform act enacted in 2003 has altered the tax brackets for the "married filing jointly" category, reducing the tax imposed on individuals choosing this status (and thereby eliminating the marraige "tax penalty").

Gross Income

Every income tax return begins with gross income, which is defined in the federal tax code as "all income from whatever source derived." This all-inclusive phrase embraces such diverse means of income as compensation for services (including those of an optometrist); business income; gains from the sale or exchange of property; interest; rent; royalties; divi-

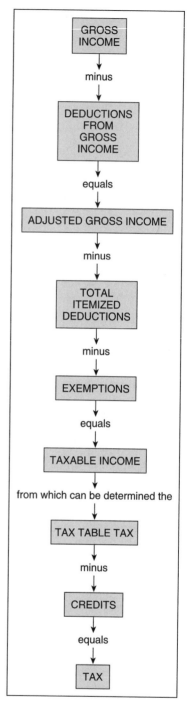

Figure 38-1 Schematic representation of the income taxation process.

dends; annuities; pensions; partnership income; income from an estate or trust; prizes; winnings from gambling; alimony; and illegally obtained windfalls such as embezzlement, theft, fraud, and related offenses.

Form **1040** Department of the Treasury—Internal Revenue Service
U.S. Individual Income Tax Return 2002 (99) IRS Use Only—Do not write or staple in this space.

For the year Jan. 1–Dec. 31, 2002, or other tax year beginning , 2002, ending , 20 | OMB No. 1545-0074

Label
(See instructions on page 21.)

Use the IRS label. Otherwise, please print or type.

Your first name and initial: John G | Last name: O'Dee
Your social security number: 123 45 6789

If a joint return, spouse's first name and initial: June B | Last name: O'Dee
Spouse's social security number: 987 65 4321

Home address (number and street). If you have a P.O. box, see page 21.: 321 Main Street | Apt. no.

City, town or post office, state, and ZIP code. If you have a foreign address, see page 21.: Anytown, ST 12345

▲ **Important!** ▲ You **must** enter your SSN(s) above.

Presidential Election Campaign (See page 21.)
Note. Checking "Yes" will not change your tax or reduce your refund.
Do you, or your spouse if filing a joint return, want $3 to go to this fund? ►
You: ☑ Yes ☐ No Spouse: ☐ Yes ☑ No

Filing Status
Check only one box.

1 ☐ Single
2 ☑ Married filing jointly (even if only one had income)
3 ☐ Married filing separately. Enter spouse's SSN above and full name here. ►
4 ☐ Head of household (with qualifying person). (See page 21.) If the qualifying person is a child but not your dependent, enter this child's name here. ►
5 ☐ Qualifying widow(er) with dependent child (year spouse died ►). (See page 21.)

Exemptions

6a ☑ **Yourself.** If your parent (or someone else) can claim you as a dependent on his or her tax return, **do not** check box 6a
b ☑ **Spouse**

c **Dependents:**

(1) First name	Last name	(2) Dependent's social security number	(3) Dependent's relationship to you	(4) ✔ if qualifying child for child tax credit (see page 22)
Junior	O'Dee	234 56 7890	child	☐
				☐
				☐
				☐
				☐

If more than five dependents, see page 22.

No. of boxes checked on 6a and 6b: 2
No. of children on 6c who:
• lived with you: 1
• did not live with you due to divorce or separation (see page 22)
Dependents on 6c not entered above
Add numbers on lines above ► 3

d Total number of exemptions claimed

Income

Attach Forms W-2 and W-2G here. Also attach Form(s) 1099-R if tax was withheld.

If you did not get a W-2, see page 23.

Enclose, but do not attach, any payment. Also, please use Form 1040-V.

7 Wages, salaries, tips, etc. Attach Form(s) W-2 | 7 | 6,200
8a **Taxable** interest. Attach Schedule B if required | 8a | 400
b **Tax-exempt** interest. **Do not** include on line 8a | 8b
9 Ordinary dividends. Attach Schedule B if required | 9
10 Taxable refunds, credits, or offsets of state and local income taxes (see page 24) | 10
11 Alimony received | 11
12 Business income or (loss). Attach Schedule C or C-EZ | 12 | 139,925
13 Capital gain or (loss). Attach Schedule D if required. If not required, check here ► ☐ | 13
14 Other gains or (losses). Attach Form 4797 | 14
15a IRA distributions | 15a | b Taxable amount (see page 25) | 15b
16a Pensions and annuities | 16a | b Taxable amount (see page 25) | 16b
17 Rental real estate, royalties, partnerships, S corporations, trusts, etc. Attach Schedule E | 17
18 Farm income or (loss). Attach Schedule F | 18
19 Unemployment compensation | 19
20a Social security benefits | 20a | b Taxable amount (see page 27) | 20b
21 Other income. List type and amount (see page 29) | 21
22 Add the amounts in the far right column for lines 7 through 21. This is your **total income** ► | 22 | 141,925

Adjusted Gross Income

23 Educator expenses (see page 29) | 23
24 IRA deduction (see page 29) | 24
25 Student loan interest deduction (see page 31) | 25
26 Tuition and fees deduction (see page 32) | 26
27 Archer MSA deduction. Attach Form 8853 | 27
28 Moving expenses. Attach Form 3903 | 28
29 One-half of self-employment tax. Attach Schedule SE | 29 | 9,885
30 Self-employed health insurance deduction (see page 33) | 30 | 2,800
31 Self-employed SEP, SIMPLE, and qualified plans | 31 | 10,000
32 Penalty on early withdrawal of savings | 32
33a Alimony paid b Recipient's SSN ► | 33a
34 Add lines 23 through 33a | 34 | 22,685
35 Subtract line 34 from line 22. This is your **adjusted gross income** ► | 35 | 119,240

For Disclosure, Privacy Act, and Paperwork Reduction Act Notice, see page 76. Cat. No. 11320B Form **1040** (2002)

Figure 38-2 Sample Form 1040.

Continued

Form 1040 (2002)   Page **2**

Tax and Credits	36	Amount from line 35 (adjusted gross income)	36	119,240

Standard Deduction for—
- People who checked any box on line 37a or 37b **or** who can be claimed as a dependent, see page 34.
- All others:

Single, $4,700

Head of household, $6,900

Married filing jointly or Qualifying widow(er), $7,850

Married filing separately, $3,925

37a	Check if: ☐ **You** were 65 or older, ☐ Blind; ☐ **Spouse** was 65 or older, ☐ Blind. Add the number of boxes checked above and enter the total here . . . . ▶ 37a	
b	If you are married filing separately and your spouse itemizes deductions, or you were a dual-status alien, see page 34 and check here . . . . . . ▶ 37b ☐	

38	**Itemized deductions** (from Schedule A) **or** your **standard deduction** (see left margin) . .	38	35,608
39	Subtract line 38 from line 36	39	83,632
40	If line 36 is $103,000 or less, multiply $3,000 by the total number of exemptions claimed on line 6d. If line 36 is over $103,000, see the worksheet on page 35 . . .	40	9,000
41	**Taxable income.** Subtract line 40 from line 39. If line 40 is more than line 39, enter -0-	41	74,632
42	**Tax** (see page 36). Check if any tax is from: **a** ☐ Form(s) 8814 **b** ☐ Form 4972 . .	42	13,945
43	**Alternative minimum tax** (see page 37). Attach Form 6251	43	
44	Add lines 42 and 43 . . . . ▶	44	13,945

45	Foreign tax credit. Attach Form 1116 if required	45	
46	Credit for child and dependent care expenses. Attach Form 2441	46	
47	Credit for the elderly or the disabled. Attach Schedule R .	47	
48	Education credits. Attach Form 8863	48	
49	Retirement savings contributions credit. Attach Form 8880 .	49	
50	Child tax credit (see page 39)	50	600
51	Adoption credit. Attach Form 8839	51	
52	Credits from: **a** ☐ Form 8396 **b** ☐ Form 8859 . .	52	
53	Other credits. Check applicable box(es): **a** ☐ Form 3800 **b** ☐ Form 8801 **c** ☐ Specify _____	53	

54	Add lines 45 through 53. These are your **total credits**	54	600
55	Subtract line 54 from line 44. If line 54 is more than line 44, enter -0- . . ▶	55	13,345

Other Taxes				
	56	Self-employment tax. Attach Schedule SE	56	19,770
	57	Social security and Medicare tax on tip income not reported to employer. Attach Form 4137 . .	57	
	58	Tax on qualified plans, including IRAs, and other tax-favored accounts. Attach Form 5329 if required .	58	
	59	Advance earned income credit payments from Form(s) W-2	59	
	60	Household employment taxes. Attach Schedule H	60	
	61	Add lines 55 through 60. This is your **total tax** . . . . ▶	61	33,115

Payments					
	62	Federal income tax withheld from Forms W-2 and 1099 . .	62	33,000	
If you have a qualifying child, attach Schedule EIC.	63	2002 estimated tax payments and amount applied from 2001 return	63		
	64	**Earned income credit (EIC)**	64		
	65	Excess social security and tier 1 RRTA tax withheld (see page 56)	65		
	66	Additional child tax credit. Attach Form 8812 . . .	66		
	67	Amount paid with request for extension to file (see page 56)	67		
	68	Other payments from: **a** ☐ Form 2439 **b** ☐ Form 4136 **c** ☐ Form 8885 .	68		
	69	Add lines 62 through 68. These are your **total payments** . . . . . ▶	69	33,000	

Refund				
Direct deposit? See page 56 and fill in 71b, 71c, and 71d.	70	If line 69 is more than line 61, subtract line 61 from line 69. This is the amount you **overpaid**	70	
	71a	Amount of line 70 you want **refunded to you** . . . . ▶	71a	
▶ b	Routing number ☐☐☐☐☐☐☐☐☐ ▶ c Type: ☐ Checking ☐ Savings			
▶ d	Account number ☐☐☐☐☐☐☐☐☐☐☐☐☐☐☐☐☐			
	72	Amount of line 70 you want **applied to your 2003 estimated tax** ▶	72	

Amount You Owe				
	73	**Amount you owe.** Subtract line 69 from line 61. For details on how to pay, see page 57 ▶	73	115
	74	Estimated tax penalty (see page 57)	74	

Third Party Designee	Do you want to allow another person to discuss this return with the IRS (see page 58)? ☐ **Yes.** Complete the following. ☐ **No**

Designee's name ▶   Phone no. ▶ ( )   Personal identification number (PIN) ▶ ☐☐☐☐☐

Sign Here	Under penalties of perjury, I declare that I have examined this return and accompanying schedules and statements, and to the best of my knowledge and belief, they are true, correct, and complete. Declaration of preparer (other than taxpayer) is based on all information of which preparer has any knowledge.

Joint return? See page 21.
Keep a copy for your records.

Your signature	Date	Your occupation	Daytime phone number
JE O'Dee	4-15-03	Optometrist	(111) 222-3456
Spouse's signature. If a joint return, **both** must sign. *June H V Dee*	Date 4-15-03	Spouse's occupation	

Paid Preparer's Use Only	Preparer's signature	Date	Check if self-employed ☐	Preparer's SSN or PTIN
	Firm's name (or yours if self-employed), address, and ZIP code ▶		EIN	
			Phone no. ( )	

Form **1040** (2002)

Figure 38-2, Cont'd

Exclusions from Income

There are *exclusions from income* that permit certain types of gross income to escape taxation. These exempt classes of income should not be confused with deductions from gross income. Some of the more important exclusions include the following:

Life insurance death proceeds. The proceeds of life insurance policies, if paid by reason of the death of the insured, are excluded from the gross income of the beneficiary. The manner in which the policy proceeds is paid is of no consequence (i.e., whether in a lump sum or in installments). If the proceeds of a life insurance contract are paid for reasons other than the death of the insured, however, the insured is entitled to recover tax-free only what was paid for the contract.

Gifts, bequests, and devises. The amount of cash or the value of property received by gift or inheritance is excluded from gross income. However, income derived from property received by gift is taxable as income to the recipient.

Retirement income. Social Security benefits are not subject to taxation as gross income.

Interest on government securities. State and local bonds produce interest income that is not included as gross income. Obligations of the federal government are subject to federal taxation, and the interest on U.S. Savings Bonds (Series E) is fully taxable.

Compensation for injuries or sickness. Compensation awarded for personal rights, such as workman's compensation, damages for personal injury, damages for defamation, and damages for other legal actions intended to "make the person whole again" are excluded from gross income. A like exclusion is permitted for accident and health benefits received under a policy purchased by the policyholder.

Employee's accident and health benefit plans. Amounts received by an employee as reimbursement for medical care; payments for permanent injuries or loss of bodily function; and to a limited extent, wages or payments in lieu of wages during a period of absence from work as a result of permanent and total disability are excluded from gross income.

Employer's educational assistance plans. Amounts paid by an employer for an employee's education, pursuant to a plan meeting certain requirements, are excluded from gross income. Amounts received that may be excluded include tuition and fees, books, supplies, and equipment. For an educational assistance program to qualify, it must be in writing, limited to providing employees with education assistance, and not discriminatory in favor of certain employees or a certain class of employees.

Scholarship and fellowship grants. Scholarships and fellowship grants are tax exempt for degree candidates but only to the extent that amounts are paid for tuition, books, and supplies; room and board and other expenses that are paid by the scholarship or fellowship are not excluded from income.

Sale of main residence. A single homeowner who sells a main residence that has been lived in for 2 years and realizes a profit may exclude $250,000 of the gain from the sale; if the sale is by a married couple filing a joint tax return, the exclusion is $500,000.

Capital Gains

Not all gross income will be taxed the same because there is an important distinction between ordinary income and capital gains. *Ordinary income* includes money earned as salary, benefits that are subject to taxation, income earned through the providing of services or the sale of products (as in optometry), bonuses, exchanges, and gains realized on the sale of items owned for a year or less. *Capital gains* are limited only to gains earned on certain assets that are held for more than a year. These assets—which must be owned and used for personal purposes, pleasure or investment—are termed *capital assets* and include stocks, bonds, homes, household furnishings, coins, stamps, jewelry, art, and similar items. When capital assets are sold for a gain after being held for more than a year, a capital gain is realized.

The tax rate to which these assets are subject varies, depending on the asset, and ranges from 5% to 15%, which is less than the tax rates for ordinary income, which as of 2003 ranged from 10% to 35%. (There also are special rates that apply to assets held for 5 years.) The tax on capital gains is calculated differently than the tax on ordinary income, and the calculation is performed on Schedule D. If there is a capital loss (e.g., capital assets held for more than a year and sold for a loss), it can be used to offset a capital gain. The computation of these gains can become quite complicated, requiring an accountant's expertise. Capital gains also must be included in gross income and reported on Form 1040.

Once gross income has been determined, the next step is to consider the deductions available to the taxpayer.

Deductions

There are certain expenses that may be subtracted from gross income to arrive at the AGI. Both business and nonbusiness expenses are included, but they are limited in number. As of 2003, the nonbusiness deductions were:

Contributions to an individual retirement account (IRA). Contributions to a traditional IRA can be deducted by taxpayers who meet certain qualifications (see Chapter 33); contributions to a Roth IRA are not deductible.

Student loan interest deduction. Any loan taken out to pay for qualified higher education expenses incurred by a taxpayer or taxpayer's spouse or dependent may be claimed in part as a deduction. The deduction is limited but gradually has been increased throughout the years ($2500 in 2003).

Medical savings accounts. These accounts are a combination of a high-deductible insurance plan and tax-deferred savings account like an IRA. Tax-deductible contributions may be made to the account, the amounts contributed are invested and grow on a tax-deferred basis, and tax-free withdrawals may be made for medical expenses. Tax deductions for medical savings accounts are figured on Form 8853.

Moving expenses. The cost of moving to another location to start a new job may qualify as a deduction if certain conditions are met; the most important are that the move be connected with employment, within a year of starting a new job, and that the distance be at least 50 miles (the distance is measured between the old home and the new place of employment). The actual costs of the move may be deducted, but pre-move expenses, temporary living expenses, and expenses for the sale, purchase, or lease of a residence are not deductible. Allowable expenses must be calculated on Form 3903.

Self-employment tax. Self-employed individuals must contribute to Social Security and Medicare, and one-half of the tax paid (which is calculated on Schedule SE for individual practitioners) may be claimed as a deduction (see Chapter 40 for a discussion of the tax).

Self-employed health insurance deduction. The cost of health insurance premiums for a self-employed individual, spouse, and dependents may be deducted if the insurance plan was established by the individual's business. If the spouse is employed and also has insurance coverage that includes the self-employed individual, however, the premium costs for the self-employed individual cannot be deducted.

Contributions to a simplified employee pension IRA, Keogh plan, pension plan, or other tax-deductible retirement

plan. Self-employed individuals or partners who participate in tax-deferred retirement plans may deduct their contributions from gross income (see Chapter 33 for a discussion of these plans).

Penalties for early withdrawal of savings. Premature withdrawals of funds from a time savings account or deposit are subject to penalty; the amount paid as a penalty may be deducted as an exclusion from gross income.

Alimony. Alimony and separate maintenance payments are deductible from gross income by the one paying them if the following four criteria are met: they must be made under a written decree or agreement; they must qualify as periodic payments (i.e., payments that are uncertain in amount, or for an indefinite period, or for more than 10 years); they must not be specifically designated for the support of minor children; and they must not be in the form of a lump sum or settlement. Child support is not deductible.

These deductions, when subtracted from the gross income, produce the AGI. This amount has relevance to certain expenses that may be claimed when determining itemized deductions, a calculation that is performed on Schedule A. To figure itemized deductions, however, the concept of the standard deduction must be understood.

The Standard Deduction

The lowest bracket for each category of taxpayer (e.g., single, married filing jointly) has a tax of zero; these brackets are referred to as the standard deduction (Box 38-1). Additional deductions are allowed for individuals 65 years of age and older and for individuals who are blind. Thus, a single taxpayer who is both 65 and blind could claim two additional deductions, in addition to the standard deduction.

For purposes of claiming the deduction for blindness, the taxpayer must get a statement certified by the "eye doctor or registered optometrist" that verifies either of the following:

• Visual acuity is less than 20/200 in the better eye with glasses or contact lenses
• The field of vision is 20 degrees or less

The statement also must assert that the acuity or field of vision is "not likely to improve."

Only income in excess of the standard deduction (plus exemptions, to be discussed) is subject to taxation. Any taxpayer may claim the standard deduction, but as income increases, this deduction fails to yield the best

Box 38-1 Standard Deduction, 2003

The standard deduction increases from year to year, but for purposes of illustration the 2003 amounts were:
- $4750 for single taxpayers
- $9500 for married couples filing jointly
- $4750 for married taxpayers filing separately
- $7000 for heads of household

In 2003 an additional $1150 was allowed for individuals 65 years of age and older ($950 if married filing jointly) and for individuals who were blind. Thus, a single taxpayer who was both 65 and blind could claim an additional $2300 ($1900 if married filing jointly).

Source: Internal Revenue Service publication 17, Your income tax.

tax benefit. This is because taxpayers are permitted to claim certain personal deductions to ascertain whether these *itemized deductions* provide a better tax benefit than the standard deduction (but the extra deductions for elderly and blind taxpayers cannot be claimed when itemizing). The calculation is performed on Schedule A.

An illustration of how the itemized deductions are calculated on Schedule A may be found in Figure 38-3.

Itemized Deductions

There are eight categories of expenses that are commonly incurred by taxpayers and recognized as itemized deductions which are calculated on Schedule A:

Medical, dental, and optometric expenses. The deduction allowed for these expenses is limited in several respects. First, a taxpayer may not claim a deduction for any expenses for which there was reimbursement by insurance. Second, the deduction is limited to the amount that is in excess of 7½ % of the AGI. For example, if the AGI is $100,000, and $8000 of expenses (unreimbursed by insurance) were incurred, only $500 would be deductible. Amounts paid for medicine and drugs may be deducted, but drugs are defined as prescription drugs and insulin only. Premiums for health care are included as deductions, as are transportation costs for health care (as of 2003, 13 cents a mile and up to $50 a night for lodging).

Taxes. Certain taxes may be deducted, including state, local, and foreign real property taxes; state and local personal property taxes (e.g., an automobile tag tax);

and state, local, and foreign income taxes. State and local sales taxes, however, are not deductible.

Interest. Only limited interest expenses paid by a taxpayer are deductible, with the most important example being mortgage interest payments. (Student loan interest is deductible as an expense to reduce gross income and does not have to be claimed on Schedule A).

Charitable contributions. Charitable contributions are allowed for money or property contributed to qualified organizations, which include a state, a possession of the United States, or any subdivision of these; a corporation, trust, or other organization that is operated exclusively for religious, charitable, scientific, literary, or educational purposes; posts or organizations of war veterans, or an auxiliary unit or society of, or trust or foundation for, any such post or organization; or a domestic fraternal society, order, or association, operating under the lodge system (if the contribution is made for charitable purposes). The amount of a contribution in property other than money is its fair market value at the time of the contribution. To determine this value, it is advised that IRS publication 526, *Charitable Contributions*, be consulted.

Casualty and theft losses. A taxpayer may deduct a limited amount for casualty losses to nonbusiness property that are due to fire, storm, shipwreck, or other casualties not covered by insurance. Such a loss is limited, however, to the extent by which it exceeds 10% of the taxpayer's AGI. For example, if the AGI were $100,000 and the loss were $12,000, the deduction would be limited to $2000.

Job expenses and most miscellaneous deductions. For employed individuals, most job-related expenses for which there is no reimbursement by the employer will be claimed in this category. Miscellaneous personal expenses also may be claimed (Box 38-2). These expenses provide a tax deduction, however, only to the extent that they exceed 2% of the taxpayer's AGI. For example, for an employed optometrist with an AGI of $50,000, only expenses in excess of $1000 would be deductible.

Other miscellaneous deductions. Examples of miscellaneous deductions that may be claimed in the "other" category include gambling losses, casualty and theft losses from income-producing property, and impairment-related work expenses of a disabled individual.

If itemized deductions exceed a certain amount, which is adjusted annually, they are reduced. Careful record-keeping is necessary to document Schedule A expenses.

SCHEDULES A&B (Form 1040)	Schedule A—Itemized Deductions	OMB No. 1545-0074

Department of the Treasury Internal Revenue Service (99)

(Schedule B is on back)

2002

Attachment Sequence No. **07**

► **Attach to Form 1040.** ► **See Instructions for Schedules A and B (Form 1040).**

Name(s) shown on Form 1040

John G & June B O'Dee

Your social security number

123 : 45 : 6789

Medical and Dental Expenses	**Caution.** Do not include expenses reimbursed or paid by others.			
	1 Medical and dental expenses (see page A-2)	1	2,765	
	2 Enter amount from Form 1040, line 36 ⌐2⌐ 119,240			
	3 Multiply line 2 by 7.5% (.075)	3	8,943	
	4 Subtract line 3 from line 1. If line 3 is more than line 1, enter -0-	4		Ø
Taxes You Paid (See page A-2.)	5 State and local income taxes	5	5,906	
	6 Real estate taxes (see page A-2)	6	4,282	
	7 Personal property taxes	7	466	
	8 Other taxes. List type and amount ►	8		
	9 Add lines 5 through 8	9		10,654
Interest You Paid (See page A-3.) Note. Personal interest is not deductible.	10 Home mortgage interest and points reported to you on Form 1098	10	20,123	
	11 Home mortgage interest not reported to you on Form 1098. If paid to the person from whom you bought the home, see page A-3 and show that person's name, identifying no., and address ►	11		
	12 Points not reported to you on Form 1098. See page A-3 for special rules	12		
	13 Investment interest. Attach Form 4952 if required. (See page A-3.)	13		
	14 Add lines 10 through 13	14		20,123
Gifts to Charity If you made a gift and got a benefit for it, see page A-4.	15 Gifts by cash or check. If you made any gift of $250 or more, see page A-4	15	4,000	
	16 Other than by cash or check. If any gift of $250 or more, see page A-4. You **must** attach Form 8283 if over $500	16	831	
	17 Carryover from prior year	17		
	18 Add lines 15 through 17	18		4,831
Casualty and Theft Losses	19 Casualty or theft loss(es). Attach Form 4684. (See page A-5.)	19		Ø
Job Expenses and Most Other Miscellaneous Deductions (See page A-5 for expenses to deduct here.)	20 Unreimbursed employee expenses—job travel, union dues, job education, etc. You **must** attach Form 2106 or 2106-EZ if required. (See page A-5.) ►	20		
	21 Tax preparation fees	21		
	22 Other expenses—investment, safe deposit box, etc. List type and amount ► Investment 500 box 50	22	550	
	23 Add lines 20 through 22	23	550	
	24 Enter amount from Form 1040, line 36 ⌐24⌐ 119,240			
	25 Multiply line 24 by 2% (.02)	25	2,384	
	26 Subtract line 25 from line 23. If line 25 is more than line 23, enter -0-	26		Ø
Other Miscellaneous Deductions	27 Other—from list on page A-6. List type and amount ►	27		Ø
Total Itemized Deductions	28 Is Form 1040, line 36, over $137,300 (over $68,650 if married filing separately)? ☐ **No.** Your deduction is not limited. Add the amounts in the far right column for lines 4 through 27. Also, enter this amount on Form 1040, line 38. ☐ **Yes.** Your deduction may be limited. See page A-6 for the amount to enter. ►	28		35,608

For Paperwork Reduction Act Notice, see Form 1040 instructions.

Cat. No. 11330X

Schedule A (Form 1040) 2002

Figure 38-3 Sample Schedule A.

Box 38-2 Miscellaneous Expenses Deductible on Schedule A

EMPLOYEE EXPENSES

License fees
Dues to professional societies
Employment-related education (i.e., continuing education)
Expenses of looking for a job in the same field
Malpractice insurance premiums
Subscriptions to professional journals and magazines
Work clothes or uniforms
50% of unreimbursed business-related entertainment or meal expenses
Business-related travel and transportation expenses in excess of reimbursement by the employer

PERSONAL EXPENSES

Legal and accounting fees
Fees paid to investment counsel
Fees paid to the custodian of an IRA
Custodial fees paid for income-producing property
Cost of safety deposit box rental
Cost of tax services, periodicals, or return preparation
Appraisal fees for establishing a casualty loss or charitable contribution

Receipts, checks, and other evidence of these expenditures should be retained and stored so that proof of claimed deductions will be readily available should the IRS audit the taxpayer's return.

Exemptions

A certain amount of income is deemed to be exempt from taxation. The amount exempt from taxation is based on filing status, with one exemption allowed to each of the following:

• Taxpayer
• Taxpayer's spouse (if filing jointly)
• Each dependent

Therefore, for a married couple filing jointly with two children, there would be four exemptions (Box 38-3). Although this amount is claimed after the standard or itemized deduction has been subtracted from the AGI, the determination of the number of exemptions is made on the first page of Form 1040, under the category "Exemptions."

There is an income test for exemptions, and if a taxpayer's AGI exceeds a certain amount, the exemption begins to be reduced.

Computing the Tax

The computation of individual income tax is based on the tax tables prepared by the IRS. The tables are constructed according to the tax status of the taxpayer: single, married couple filing jointly, married person filing separately, head of household, and widow/widower with dependent child.

As of 2003 there were six tax rates: 10%, 15%, 25%, 28%, 33%, and 35%. Each rate applies to a certain bracket of income, which is different for single taxpayers and for married persons filing jointly (Table 38-1). Both the tax rates and the

Box 38-3 Exemptions, 2003

Exemptions from income are modest in amount and increase slightly each year; examples for 2003 are:
• $3050 for the taxpayer
• $3050 for the taxpayer's spouse (if filing jointly)
• $3050 for each dependent

For taxpayers filing jointly with two dependents, the amount to be claimed in 2003 would be 4 × $3050, or $12,200. There is an income test for exemptions, and if a taxpayer's adjusted gross income exceeds the allowable amount, the exemption begins to be reduced. The exemption is phased out completely when the taxpayer's income exceeds an income ceiling.

Source: Internal Revenue Service publication 17, Your income tax.

Table 38-1 Income Tax Rates and Brackets, 2003

Income tax is determined by the income tax rate and the bracket to which it is applied; under the tax reform act passed in 2003, rates were reduced and brackets were changed. The brackets vary for single, married filing jointly, and other classifications of taxpayers. As an example, the rates and brackets for single and joint return taxpayers in 2003 were:

	SINGLE	MARRIED FILING JOINTLY
10% Bracket	$0 to $7000	$0 to $14,000
15% Bracket	$7001 to $28,400	$14,001 to $56,800
25% Bracket	$28,401 to $68,800	$56,801 to $114,650
28% Bracket	$68,801 to $143,500	$114,651 to $174,700
33% Bracket	$143,501 to $311,950	$174,701 to $311,950
35% Bracket	$311,951 and up	$311,951 and up

brackets have been affected by the 2003 federal tax law changes.

The determination of the tax due from the tax tables does not conclude the tax computation process; once the actual tax is figured, any credits may be deducted.

Tax Credits

Whereas deductions and exemptions reduce the amount of income that the taxpayer must report for purposes of computing the tax owed, tax credits actually reduce the tax that must be paid, by being deducted dollar-for-dollar from the tax. For example, $10,000 of tax owed–based on taxable income of $56,000–would be reduced to $8000 by a $2000 tax credit. Some credits are nonrefundable (i.e., they cannot be refunded to the extent that they exceed the income tax owed by the taxpayer).

The credits likely to be of most importance to optometrists are described in the following:

Credit for child and dependent care expenses. A credit may be claimed for expenses incurred to have someone take care of a child younger than 13 years of age or a dependent or spouse who cannot care for himself or herself. As of 2003, the maximum allowable credit was $3000 per child or dependent, and the total credit that may be claimed annually was $6000. However, because of income limitations, optometrists are likely to be eligible to claim only 20% of the credit. Computation of the credit is performed on Form 2441.

Credit for the elderly and the disabled. This credit may be claimed by individuals age 65 and older (younger than 65 if a government retiree) and by individuals who are permanently and totally disabled. The credit is reported on Schedule R.

Education credits. The Hope credit may be claimed for expenses paid for a taxpayer, spouse, or child to enroll in and attend the first 2 years of college or vocational education. The student must be enrolled in a degree-earning program and must carry at least a half-academic load. As of 2003, the allowable credit was up to $1500 per student (for 2 years). The lifetime earning credit does not require enrollment in a degree program and permits a credit of up to $1000 to be claimed per family (for an unlimited number of years). These credits are not allowed if the AGI exceeds an income ceiling, which differs for single individuals and married persons filing jointly. The credit must be computed on Form 8863.

Child tax credit. A tax credit may be claimed for a child who is a dependent and is younger than 17 years at the end of the tax year. As of 2003, to receive the $1000 credit the taxpayer's AGI could not exceed an income ceiling, which differed based on whether the person claiming the credit was single or married filing jointly.

Adoption credit. A credit may be claimed for expenses incurred in adopting a child. There is a maximum allowable amount, but unused credit may be carried forward for 5 years. The credit must be figured on Form 8839.

Some credits are refundable and can be refunded to the extent that they exceed the tax owed by the taxpayer, being treated as payments of taxes. These credits generally are not applicable to optometrists.

Self-Employment Tax

There are additional taxes that may have to be paid by an individual taxpayer, including taxes imposed on IRAs and other types of retirement plans, and household employment taxes (which are imposed on wages paid to employees working in a home). For a self-employed individual, however, the most significant tax that must be paid is the self-employment tax.

This tax is the Social Security and Medicare tax paid by self-employed individuals, and it represents their contributions to these programs. The calculation and payment of this tax, which is performed on Schedule SE, are described in Chapter 40.

Because this tax must be paid quarterly and submitted to the IRS before the calculation of the annual tax return by the taxpayer, it is subtracted from the tax due.

Income Tax

Taxpayers must have income taxes calculated, withheld, and submitted to the IRS at least quarterly (Chapter 40). For employed individuals, the amount that has been withheld is reported to the IRS on Form W-2, which lists the total annually income taxes for the employee. This amount is reported in the "Payments" section of the taxpayer's Form 1040. For self-employed individuals, the income tax is submitted quarterly to the IRS on Form 941; the total amount withheld is also reported on Form 1040 in the "Payments" section.

If the amount withheld exceeds the total tax indebtedness calculated on the return, the taxpayer is due a refund. If the amount withheld is less than the total amount owed, the taxpayer must pay an additional sum to the IRS.

Filing Requirements

Taxpayers need not file a return if their gross income is less than the standard deduction plus the personal exemption (Box 38-4). These amounts are relatively modest, and optometrists are likely to exceed them.

A child with unearned income (such as investment income) who can be claimed as a dependent must file a return if the unearned income is $750 or more. Earned income of a child is taxable to the child, and the child must file a tax return; the parents should not report the child's earnings on their return. The child will be permitted to use a standard deduction (which is less than that for adults) to shield earned income from taxes.

Individuals' returns must be filed by the 15th day of the fourth calendar month after the close of the taxable year—April 15 for a calendar year. The IRS has an electronic filing system that may be used in lieu of the traditional paper system.

Although taxpayers will be granted an automatic 2-month extension for the filing of income tax returns if they file Form 4868 on or before the due date of the return, they also must pay a tentative estimate of the income tax due at the time of making the extension application. Applications for further extensions of time for filing must be made in writing and will be granted only in hardship cases. There are penalties for failure to file and for failure to pay by the due date. In addition, there is a penalty for substantially understating the tax due, which will be applied if the unpaid amount is more than 10% of the final tax liability or is more than $5000, whichever is larger.

Any taxpayer may revise a previous return to claim a refund of taxes or pay additional taxes by filing Form 1040X.

Penalties

In addition to the penalty for underpaid tax, there is a penalty that may be imposed on frivolous returns. If any part of the deficiency in tax is due to the negligence or intentional disregard of IRS regulations, a penalty of 5% of the total amount of the deficiency, plus an additional penalty of 50% of the interest due, will be assessed. If there is fraud, the penalty is 75% of the underpayment due to fraud and 50% of the interest payable on the underpayment. Fraud also may be the basis for a criminal action against the taxpayer, which can result in a jail sentence of up to 5 years and a $10,000 fine. The period within which criminal prosecution may be started is generally 3 years after the commission of the offense but may be longer in many circumstances.

Box 38-4 Income Levels Not Subject to Tax, 2003

There is a minimum income that is not subject to income taxation. This minimum income level is composed of:
- The standard deduction
- The personal exemption

For example, in 2003 the standard deduction for single taxpayers younger than 65 years was $4750 and the personal exemption was $3050, for a total of $7800. Single taxpayers earning less than this amount did not have to file a return. For a married couple younger than 65 years filing jointly in 2003, the total was $15,600.

Tax returns are examined by the IRS through several programs. A computer system known as the Discrimination Function System selects most returns that are examined, by evaluating selected entries and giving the return a score, which is then reviewed by IRS personnel. Returns deemed to have the highest probability of error are selected for audit.

Returns also may be analyzed through the Taxpayer Compliance Measurement Program, which is a random selection system that is used to determine correct tax liability and measure and evaluate taxpayer compliance characteristics. The information obtained through Taxpayer Compliance Measurement Program audits is used to update and improve the Discrimination Function System program.

Returns also may be examined directly by IRS personnel, by assessing claims for credit or refunds of previously paid taxes or by matching tax documents, such as Form W-2 or 1099. The place and method of examination are determined by the IRS and may be no more than an exchange of correspondence, a more formal hearing at the taxpayer's office, or at the office of the IRS. Most taxpayers represent themselves at these meetings, and many disagreements are settled at this level. If the taxpayer does not agree with the changes proposed by the examiner, the taxpayer may appeal through the IRS or proceed to tax court. See IRS publication 5, *Appeal Rights and Preparation of Protests for Unagreed Cases*, and Publication 556, *Examination of Returns, Appeal Rights, and Claims for Refund*.

Bibliography

Classé JG: *Legal aspects of optometry.* Boston, 1989, Butterworth.

Internal Revenue Service publication 1, *Your rights as a taxpayer.*

Internal Revenue Service publication 4, *Student's guide to federal income tax.*

Internal Revenue Service publication 5, *Appeal rights and preparation of protests for unagreed cases.*

Internal Revenue Service publication 15, *Employer's tax guide (circular E).*

Internal Revenue Service publication 17, *Your income tax.*

Internal Revenue Service publication 334, *Tax guide for small business.*

Internal Revenue Service publication 463, *Travel, entertainment, gift and car expenses.*

Internal Revenue Service publication 505, *Tax withholding and estimated tax.*

Internal Revenue Service publication 509, *Tax calendars for 2002.*

Internal Revenue Service publication 533, *Self-employment tax.*

Internal Revenue Service publication 535, *Business expenses.*

Internal Revenue Service publication 538, *Accounting periods and methods.*

Internal Revenue Service publication 541, *Partnerships.*

Internal Revenue Service publication 542, *Corporations.*

Internal Revenue Service publication 544, *Sales and other dispositions of assets.*

Internal Revenue Service publication 551, *Basis of assets.*

Internal Revenue Service publication 553 *Tax highlights of 2000 tax changes.*

Internal Revenue Service publication 553, *Tax highlights of 2001 tax changes.*

Internal Revenue Service publication 556, *Examination of Service returns, appeal rights, and claims for refund.*

Internal Revenue Service publication 560, *Retirement plans for small business (SEP, Keogh, and SIMPLE plans).*

Internal Revenue Service publication 583, *Starting a business and keeping records.*

Internal Revenue Service publication 587, *Business use of your home.*

Internal Revenue Service publication 929, *Tax rules for children and dependents.*

Internal Revenue Service publication 946, *How to depreciate property.*

www.irs.gov/formspubs. Web site for the Internal Revenue Service, which contains forms and publications that can be downloaded.

Chapter 39
Business Taxes

John G. Classé

The more things change, the more they remain the same.
Alphonse Karr *Les Guepes*

A business is an activity carried on for profit, and for an activity to be considered a business, a profit motive must be involved. An activity is presumed to be engaged in for-profit activities if it produces a profit in any 3 out of 5 consecutive years.

One of the most important decisions made when entering into business is the form of organization to use. Tax considerations are a key aspect of the decision-making process, as each type of business entity offers different tax advantages and disadvantages. Although the individual proprietorship has been the historical backbone of optometry, economic and sociological factors have combined to make partnerships and group practices grow in popularity. For purposes of illustration, however, the computation of business taxes for an individual proprietor is described in this chapter. Legal counsel and accounting advisors will be required when beginning a business enterprise to ascertain the appropriate type of organization and tax reporting requirements.

A business must have its own unique identification, and so each business is required to have an employer identification number, which must be provided on all business tax returns. Personal tax returns, with Schedule C attached, must include the individual's Social Security number. If a sole proprietorship is incorporated or merged with another sole proprietorship to form a limited liability company (LLC) or partnership, then a new employer identification number is needed for the resulting corporation, LLC, or partnership. To apply for an employer identification number, Form SS-4, *Application for Employer Identification Number*, must be completed and submitted to the Internal Revenue Service (IRS) (Figure 39-1).

When organizing a business, there are three important income-related considerations: books and records, accounting periods, and accounting methods.

Books and Records

When starting a business, a system of recordkeeping that is suitable for the business should be established. The tax year and the accounting method must be determined because the recordkeeping system must show the income for the accounting period that is the tax year. Computerized bookkeeping is the preferred method to use for financial records (see Chapter 20).

All business receipts should be deposited in a separate bank account established for that purpose, and all disbursements should be made by check from this account. This permits the documentation of both income and expenses. Checks payable to one's self should be written only when making withdrawals of income from the business for one's own use; checks payable to "cash" should be avoided.

A petty cash fund should be established for minor expenses, and all business expenses paid for by cash should be supported by documents showing their business purpose. To document recordkeeping, the following rules should be observed:

Support all entries. Cancelled checks, paid bills, duplicate deposit slips, and other items that support entries in the practice accounts should be kept in an orderly manner.

Keep all records. Business records should be kept available for review as needed; backup computer records should be scrupulously maintained; these records

Form **SS-4**

(Rev. December 2001)

Department of the Treasury
Internal Revenue Service

Type or print clearly.

Application for Employer Identification Number

(For use by employers, corporations, partnerships, trusts, estates, churches, government agencies, Indian tribal entities, certain individuals, and others.)

▶ See separate instructions for each line.   ▶ Keep a copy for your records.

EIN

OMB No. 1545-0003

1 Legal name of entity (or individual) for whom the EIN is being requested
John G O'Dee, OD

2 Trade name of business (if different from name on line 1)

3 Executor, trustee, "care of" name

4a Mailing address (room, apt., suite no. and street, or P.O. box)
321 Main Street

5a Street address (if different) (Do not enter a P.O. box.)

4b City, state, and ZIP code
Anytown, ST   12345

5b City, state, and ZIP code

6 County and state where principal business is located
County, State

7a Name of principal officer, general partner, grantor, owner, or trustor
John G O'Dee

7b SSN, ITIN, or EIN
123 45 6789

8a Type of entity (check only one box)
☑ Sole proprietor (SSN) *123 45 6789*
☐ Partnership
☐ Corporation (enter form number to be filed) ▶
☐ Personal service corp.
☐ Church or church-controlled organization
☐ Other nonprofit organization (specify) ▶
☐ Other (specify) ▶

☐ Estate (SSN of decedent)
☐ Plan administrator (SSN)
☐ Trust (SSN of grantor)
☐ National Guard   ☐ State/local government
☐ Farmers' cooperative   ☐ Federal government/military
☐ REMIC   ☐ Indian tribal governments/enterprises
Group Exemption Number (GEN) ▶

8b If a corporation, name the state or foreign country (if applicable) where incorporated

State

Foreign country

9 Reason for applying (check only one box)
☑ Started new business (specify type) ▶ *Optometry*

☐ Hired employees (Check the box and see line 12.)
☐ Compliance with IRS withholding regulations
☐ Other (specify) ▶

☐ Banking purpose (specify purpose) ▶
☐ Changed type of organization (specify new type) ▶
☐ Purchased going business
☐ Created a trust (specify type) ▶
☐ Created a pension plan (specify type) ▶

10 Date business started or acquired (month, day, year)
1 Jan 2003

11 Closing month of accounting year
December

12 First date wages or annuities were paid or will be paid (month, day, year). Note: *If applicant is a withholding agent, enter date income will first be paid to nonresident alien. (month, day, year)* . . . . ▶ *31 Jan 2003*

13 Highest number of employees expected in the next 12 months. Note: *If the applicant does not expect to have any employees during the period, enter "-0-."* . . . . ▶

Agricultural	Household	Other
		1

14 Check **one** box that best describes the principal activity of your business.
☐ Construction ☐ Rental & leasing ☐ Transportation & warehousing ☑ Health care & social assistance ☐ Wholesale–agent/broker
☐ Real estate ☐ Manufacturing ☐ Finance & insurance ☐ Accommodation & food service ☐ Wholesale–other ☐ Retail
☐ Other (specify)

15 Indicate principal line of merchandise sold; specific construction work done; products produced; or services provided.
Optometry

16a Has the applicant ever applied for an employer identification number for this or any other business? . . . . ☐ Yes ☑ No
Note: *If "Yes," please complete lines 16b and 16c.*

16b If you checked "Yes" on line 16a, give applicant's legal name and trade name shown on prior application if different from line 1 or 2 above.
Legal name ▶   Trade name ▶

16c Approximate date when, and city and state where, the application was filed. Enter previous employer identification number if known.

Approximate date when filed (mo., day, year)	City and state where filed	Previous EIN

Third Party Designee

Complete this section **only** if you want to authorize the named individual to receive the entity's EIN and answer questions about the completion of this form.

Designee's name

Designee's telephone number (include area code)
(   )

Address and ZIP code

Designee's fax number (include area code)
(   )

Under penalties of perjury, I declare that I have examined this application, and to the best of my knowledge and belief, it is true, correct, and complete.

Name and title (type or print clearly) ▶ *John G O'Dee, OD*

Applicant's telephone number (include area code)
(123) 456-7890

Signature ▶ *J O'Dee*   Date ▶ *1 Dec 2002*

Applicant's fax number (include area code)
(123) 456-7899

For Privacy Act and Paperwork Reduction Act Notice, see separate instructions.   Cat. No. 16055N   Form **SS-4** (Rev. 12-2001)

Figure 39–1 Sample Form SS–4.

should be kept for a period that exceeds the statute of limitations for liability and contract actions.

Retain copies. Supporting records for tax returns should be kept until the statute of limitations for tax returns runs out (3 years after the return is due or 2 years from the date the tax is paid, whichever occurs later).

Keep comprehensive employee records. All records on employment taxes (e.g., income tax withholding, Social Security, Medicare, federal unemployment tax) should be kept for at least 4 years after the due date of the return or the date the tax is paid, whichever is later; business records always should contain the employer identification number, copies of the returns filed, and the dates and amounts of tax deposits made.

Withholding and submission of employment taxes are described in Chapter 40.

Accounting Periods

Every taxpayer must calculate taxable income and file a tax return on the basis of an annual accounting period, called a *tax year*. A tax year usually is 12 consecutive months. It may be a calendar year or a fiscal year; under certain circumstances, it may be less than 12 months, a partial year.

A *calendar year* is 12 consecutive months ending Dec. 31. A *fiscal year* is either 12 consecutive months ending on the last day of any month other than December, or a 52- to 53-week year. To report on a fiscal basis, the practice books must be kept on that basis. A short tax year, or *partial year*, is a tax year of less than 12 months, but a short tax year return is treated as a return for a full tax year. A short tax year usually results when a taxpayer is not in business for an entire tax year. Most optometrists and other small businesses are on a calendar year accounting period.

Accounting Methods

Taxable income is determined by using a fixed accounting period and a set of rules to decide when and how to report income and deductions. There are two types of accounting methods, cash and accrual, for income and expenses of business activities.

Cash Method

The cash method of accounting is used by most individuals and many small businesses with no inventories. With the cash method, all items of income actually or constructively received during the year are included in gross income. Both property and services received must be included as income at their fair market value. Constructive receipt of income occurs when an amount is credited to the practice account or made available to the practice without restriction as to the time and manner of payment.

For example, an optometrist on the cash method of accounting renders services to a patient on Dec. 31 but does not receive a check as payment until Jan. 1. The payment is income reportable in the year beginning Jan. 1.

Accrual Method

Under the accrual method all items of income are included in gross income when earned, even though payment may be received in another tax year. All events that fix the right to receive the income must have occurred and the amount must be able to be determined with reasonable accuracy.

For example, an optometrist on the accrual method of accounting renders services to a patient Dec. 31 but does not receive payment until Jan. 1. The payment is income reportable in the year ending Dec. 31.

An accountant should be consulted before making any decision as to the most appropriate type of book-keeping, accounting period, and method of accounting for a given business enterprise.

Business Assets

Ophthalmic instruments have obvious value to the practice of optometry because they contribute directly to earning the income that supports the practice. Such property is termed a *business asset*.

A business asset can be tangible real estate, such as a building or a parking lot, or tangible personal property, such as furniture or examination room equipment. It also can be intangible property, such as goodwill or a covenant not to compete.

The amount paid for a business asset usually is a *capital expenditure* rather than a deductible expense. This distinction has important tax ramifications. The cost of capital expenditures cannot be deducted all at once but rather must be recovered through the use of depreciation or amortization, which permits recovery over a period of years. Some business assets cannot be depreciated or amortized (e.g., land), and the cost of these assets can be recovered only when the asset is sold or otherwise disposed of. A *deductible expense*, on the other hand, may be claimed in full for the tax year in which it was incurred. Examples of deductible expenses include office supplies, drugs and solutions, and repairs.

A capital expenditure actually is an investment of capital, either to acquire property with a useful life of more than 1 year or to make permanent improvements that increase the value of property or appreciably prolong its life. Thus purchases of equipment, instruments, and other capital assets incur long-term tax ramifications that must be taken into account when the purchases are being considered.

Business assets have to be classified for tax purposes; the tax accounting for a practice must distinguish between the types of capital expenditures because the depreciation period varies for different types of property. The tax ramifications of this classification system also are important when purchasing a practice or the assets of a practice (see Chapter 3).

Tax Basis for Business Property

The tax *basis* of business property is used to figure the gain or loss from the sale or other disposition of the property. It also is used for determining tax deductions for depreciation or amortization. When property is purchased, its original basis is the cost. (If the property is received in some other manner, such as by gift or inheritance, then a basis other than cost is used.) If an asset is used for business purposes and depreciation or amortization deductions are claimed by the taxpayer, then these deductions are used to calculate the adjusted basis of the asset. In addition, this information may be needed to determine the taxable income of the taxpayer's business. The adjusted basis also is necessary for determining gain or loss when business property is sold or exchanged. Such transactions are a common part of the decisions made by a small business owner such as an optometrist.

For example, if an optometrist purchases a computer for $5000 and uses it for a year, it will have a depreciated value (adjusted basis) of $4000. If the optometrist sells it for $3000, there will be a $1000 loss; if it is sold for $5000 there will be a $1000 gain.

As this example illustrates, cost serves as a beginning point for basis determination in many cases. Another important aspect of basis is fair market value, which is the price at which property would change hands between a willing buyer and seller.

For example, an automobile used exclusively for business purposes by an optometrist has been depreciated so that it has an adjusted basis of $13,000, but it has a fair market value of $14,500. The optometrist decides to trade it for a truck that also has a fair market value of $14,500. The basis in the truck after the sale is $13,000, the same as the traded automobile.

If the optometrist decides to trade the truck for a new automobile that has a fair market value of $15,000, and pays $1000 in addition to the trade-in, the basis in the new car becomes $14,000 (the $13,000 basis of the old truck plus the $1000 cash).

The effect of basis on a contemplated sale or exchange of equipment or other business assets always should be carefully considered. It is important to retain a competent accountant or tax attorney so that advice concerning the tax consequences of a business transaction can be ascertained before entering into the transaction.

Although the preceding examples have used tangible assets for purposes of illustration, intangible assets also have a basis that may be adjusted as required. Typical examples include the following:

Goodwill. The basis of goodwill is its cost when the purchase of a practice is involved.
Covenant not to compete. Usually, the basis of a covenant not to compete is what is paid for it; if a covenant is part of a sales agreement for the purchase of a practice, its cost must be listed in the contract.
Franchise. The basis of a franchise is its cost.

The determination of basis can become complicated, but each purchase and sale or exchange of a business asset has tax consequences, and nowhere is this more important than in the purchase of a practice: it is not the price paid but the value allocated to the various types of assets being purchased that determines the tax ramifications (see Chapter 3).

Determining Net Profit From a Business

The determination of profit (or loss) for an individual practitioner is calculated on Schedule C (Figure 39-2). Schedule C is divided into two parts: income and deductions. Information concerning the type of business activity being reported and the accounting method (cash or accrual) being used also must be provided. A review of the calculation of income and business deductions for Schedule C is provided to illustrate how income is determined for an optometrist in private practice and to describe the various types of business deductions that typically may be claimed in the practice of optometry.

Income

The principal activity of an optometry practice is to provide personal services. All compensation received

SCHEDULE C
(Form 1040)

Department of the Treasury
Internal Revenue Service   (99)

Profit or Loss From Business
(Sole Proprietorship)

▶ Partnerships, joint ventures, etc., must file Form 1065 or 1065-B.

▶ Attach to Form 1040 or 1041.   ▶ See Instructions for Schedule C (Form 1040).

OMB No. 1545-0074

2002

Attachment
Sequence No. **09**

Name of proprietor   *John G O'Dee*

Social security number (SSN)   *123 : 45 : 6789*

A Principal business or profession, including product or service (see page C-1 of the instructions)   *Optometrist*

B Enter code from pages C-7, 8, & 9   ▶ | | | 9 2 9 0

C Business name. If no separate business name, leave blank.   *John G O'Dee, OD*

D Employer ID number (EIN), if any   8 7 6 5 4 3 2 1

E Business address (including suite or room no.) ▶ *321 Main Street*
City, town or post office, state, and ZIP code   *Anytown, ST 12345*

F Accounting method: (1) ☑ Cash   (2) ☐ Accrual   (3) ☐ Other (specify) ▶ ....

G Did you "materially participate" in the operation of this business during 2002? If "No," see page C-3 for limit on losses   ☑ Yes   ☐ No

H If you started or acquired this business during 2002, check here . . . . ▶ ☐

Part I   Income

1	Gross receipts or sales. **Caution.** If this income was reported to you on Form W-2 and the "Statutory employee" box on that form was checked, see page C-3 and check here . . . . . . ▶ ☐	**1**	*353,940*
2	Returns and allowances	**2**	
3	Subtract line 2 from line 1	**3**	*353,940*
4	Cost of goods sold (from line 42 on page 2)	**4**	*120,000*
5	**Gross profit.** Subtract line 4 from line 3	**5**	*233,940*
6	Other income, including Federal and state gasoline or fuel tax credit or refund (see page C-3) . .	**6**	
7	**Gross income.** Add lines 5 and 6 . . . . ▶	**7**	*233,940*

Part II   Expenses. Enter expenses for business use of your home **only** on line 30.

8	Advertising	**8**		**19**	Pension and profit-sharing plans	**19**	
9	Bad debts from sales or services (see page C-3) . .	**9**		**20**	Rent or lease (see page C-5):		
10	Car and truck expenses (see page C-3)	**10**	*3,285*		**a** Vehicles, machinery, and equipment .	**20a**	*16,000*
11	Commissions and fees . .	**11**			**b** Other business property . .	**20b**	
12	Depletion	**12**		**21**	Repairs and maintenance . .	**21**	*1,500*
13	Depreciation and section 179 expense deduction (not included in Part III) (see page C-4) .	**13**	*14,600*	**22**	Supplies (not included in Part III) .	**22**	
				23	Taxes and licenses	**23**	*6,515*
				24	Travel, meals, and entertainment:		
14	Employee benefit programs (other than on line 19) . . .	**14**	*4,500*		**a** Travel	**24a**	*1,360*
15	Insurance (other than health) .	**15**	*3,200*		**b** Meals and entertainment *700*		
16	Interest:				**c** Enter nondeductible amount included on line 24b (see page C-5) . *350*		
	a Mortgage (paid to banks, etc.) .	**16a**	*11,700*		**d** Subtract line 24c from line 24b	**24d**	*350*
	b Other	**16b**		**25**	Utilities	**25**	*10,200*
17	Legal and professional services	**17**	*1,250*	**26**	Wages (less employment credits) .	**26**	*18,000*
18	Office expense	**18**	*1,555*	**27**	Other expenses (from line 48 on page 2)	**27**	

28	**Total expenses** before expenses for business use of home. Add lines 8 through 27 in columns . ▶	**28**	*94,015*
29	Tentative profit (loss). Subtract line 28 from line 7	**29**	*139,925*
30	Expenses for business use of your home. Attach **Form 8829**	**30**	
31	**Net profit or (loss).** Subtract line 30 from line 29.		
	• If a profit, enter on **Form 1040, line 12,** and **also** on **Schedule SE, line 2** (statutory employees, see page C-6). Estates and trusts, enter on Form 1041, line 3. • If a loss, you **must** go to line 32.	**31**	*139,925*
32	If you have a loss, check the box that describes your investment in this activity (see page C-6).		
	• If you checked 32a, enter the loss on **Form 1040, line 12,** and **also** on **Schedule SE, line 2** (statutory employees, see page C-6). Estates and trusts, enter on Form 1041, line 3. • If you checked 32b, you **must** attach **Form 6198.**	**32a** ☐ All investment is at risk. **32b** ☐ Some investment is not at risk.	

For Paperwork Reduction Act Notice, see Form 1040 instructions.   Cat. No. 11334P   Schedule C (Form 1040) 2002

Figure 39–2   Sample Schedule C.

Continued

Schedule C (Form 1040) 2002   Page **2**

Part III   **Cost of Goods Sold** (see page C-6)

33 Method(s) used to
value closing inventory: **a** ☑ Cost   **b** ☐ Lower of cost or market   **c** ☐ Other (attach explanation)

34 Was there any change in determining quantities, costs, or valuations between opening and closing inventory? If
"Yes," attach explanation . . . . ☐ Yes   ☑ No

35 Inventory at beginning of year. If different from last year's closing inventory, attach explanation . . | **35** | 11,000 |

36 Purchases less cost of items withdrawn for personal use . . . . | **36** | |

37 Cost of labor. Do not include any amounts paid to yourself . . . . | **37** | |

38 Materials and supplies . . . . | **38** | 121,000 |

39 Other costs . . . . | **39** | |

40 Add lines 35 through 39 . . . . | **40** | 132,000 |

41 Inventory at end of year . . . . | **41** | 12,000 |

42 **Cost of goods sold.** Subtract line 41 from line 40. Enter the result here and on page 1, line 4 . . | **42** | 120,000 |

Part IV   **Information on Your Vehicle.** Complete this part **only** if you are claiming car or truck expenses on
line 10 and are not required to file Form 4562 for this business. See the instructions for line 13 on page
C-4 to find out if you must file.

43 When did you place your vehicle in service for business purposes? (month, day, year) ▶ . . . . . . / . . . . / . . . .

44 Of the total number of miles you drove your vehicle during 2002, enter the number of miles you used your vehicle for:

a Business . . . .   **b** Commuting . . . .   **c** Other . . . .

45 Do you (or your spouse) have another vehicle available for personal use? . . . . ☐ Yes   ☐ No

46 Was your vehicle available for personal use during off-duty hours? . . . . ☐ Yes   ☐ No

47a Do you have evidence to support your deduction? . . . . ☐ Yes   ☐ No

b If "Yes," is the evidence written? . . . . ☐ Yes   ☐ No

Part V   **Other Expenses.** List below business expenses not included on lines 8–26 or line 30.

. . . .	
. . . .	
. . . .	
. . . .	
. . . .	
. . . .	
. . . .	
. . . .	
. . . .	

48 **Total other expenses.** Enter here and on page 1, line 27 . . . . | **48** | |

                                                                        ✸   Schedule C (Form 1040) 2002

Figure 39–2, Cont'd

for personal services, no matter what the form of payment, must be included in gross income and must be reported in the year received (if on the cash basis) or in the year earned (if on the accrual basis). Such income is ordinary income and is taxable whether earned by a sole proprietor, owner of an LLC, shareholder in a subchapter S corporation, or partner in a partnership.

For the majority of optometrists there is another source of income: the sale of ophthalmic materials. An optometrist who dispenses eyewear, contact lenses, solutions, ophthalmic devices (such as magnifiers), and similar items must report the income derived from their sale. Thus "goods sold" usually are a significant part of the income earned by an optometrist.

In some states a sales tax is imposed on the sale of ophthalmic materials and other items by optometrists, and the optometrist collects the tax from the patient-purchaser. These taxes should be included as income, but because they must be paid to the state they are also deducted as a business expense, so the net effect is zero.

In addition, business-related gains from dealings in property, bartering of property or services, or distributive shares of partnership income also are "income" that must be reported by an optometrist-taxpayer.

Income from services is reported as "gross receipts and sales" in Part I of Schedule C, as is income from the sale of ophthalmic materials and other items. To determine the profit from the sale of materials, however, the "cost of goods sold" must be known (i.e., from the price paid by patients for these materials, the cost of the materials must be deducted to calculate profit). To make this calculation, inventories must be conducted at the start of the tax year. To arrive at a dollar amount for an inventory, a method for identifying inventory items (such as frames) and a basis for valuing each item in the inventory must be established. Next, the cost of materials, supplies, labor, or other expenses incurred during the tax year must be added to the inventory. From this amount, the value of the inventory at the end of the tax year must be subtracted. The result is the "cost of goods sold," which is the sum entered on Schedule C.

"Returns and allowances" also may be included as income. For example, cash discounts from invoice price may be awarded to an optometrist by an ophthalmic laboratory or frame manufacturer for the optometrist's good record of prompt payment during the year or for buying in volume. Either of two methods may be used to account for these refunds: they can be deducted directly from the purchases made during the year, or they can credited to a discount income account and reported at the end of the tax year. If the latter method is used, they are credited as "returns and allowances."

The sum total of all these sources of income results in the "gross income" for the tax year. From this amount, deductions may be taken, so that the "net income" for the year can be determined.

Business Deductions

Capital expenditures are not deductible as ordinary business expenses. To be deductible, a business expense must be ordinary in the business and necessary to its operation. *Ordinary* refers to expenses that are common and an accepted practice within optometry; *necessary* expenses are those that are appropriate and helpful in developing and maintaining an optometric practice.

If property is used both for business and for personal purposes (such as an automobile), then it must be determined which part of the expenses are for business and which part are for personal matters. Only the business expenses are deductible.

There are numerous business deductions that may be claimed; the major categories are:

- Salaries, wages, and related payments
- Rent expense
- Repairs, improvements, and replacements
- Bad debts
- Travel, entertainment, and gift expenses
- Business interest
- Insurance premiums
- Taxes
- Utility costs
- Profession-related expenses
- Miscellaneous business expenses

Salaries, Wages, and Related Expenses. Compensation paid to employees, in its various forms, is deductible as a business expense.

Salaries. A sole proprietor (or partner) may not deduct his or her salary or any withdrawal for personal use, but salaries paid to the employees of a sole proprietorship (or partnership) are a deductible business expense; salaries paid by a professional corporation or association to its employees (including optometrists) are similarly deductible.

Bonuses. Payment of money or of other items of value are deductible if they are intended as additional compensation rather than as a gift (e.g., a turkey given to an employee as a gift at Christmas).

Education expenses. Tuition expenses paid for employees under a qualified educational assistance program related to their employment are not considered gross income for the employees and are deductible by the business.

Interview expense allowances. Payments made to prospective employees to compensate them for the costs of an interview are deductible by the business and are not income for the interviewees.

Moving expenses. Payments to employees as an allowance or reimbursement for the cost of moving to a new job site can be deducted if the employee is eligible for a tax deduction for the move.

Meals and lodging. The cost of meals, lodging, and inventoriable items, (i.e., lenses and frames) furnished to employees as part of their compensation, is deductible by the business.

Fringe benefits. There are numerous forms of indirect compensation that may be provided to employees, such as health or accident insurance, life or disability insurance, reimbursement for medical care, medical savings accounts, reimbursement for business-related use of an automobile, fees for membership in professional organizations, licensure fees, and reimbursement for expenses related to continuing education; these fringe benefits are deductible as business expenses and are not taxable as income for the employee.

Rent Expense. If business property is leased, the rental amount generally may be deducted. Certain other expenses also may be deducted as rent.

Rent is the amount that is paid for the use of property that is not owned. In general, rent may be deducted as an expense only if the rent is for property that is used in the practice of optometry. If the renter has or will have equity in or title to the property, the rent is not deductible. If an optometrist leases business property, any taxes that must be paid for or to the lessor may be deducted. If a building is leased and an addition or other permanent improvement is made to it, the optometrist may be able to either depreciate or amortize the improvements.

Repairs, Improvements, and Replacements. The cost of repairing, improving, or replacing property used in the practice of optometry is either a deductible expense or a capital expenditure. An expenditure necessary to keep property in a normal and efficient operating condition is a deductible expense. However, if the expenditure adds to the value of the property or significantly increases its life, the cost must be capitalized rather than deducted and recovered through the use of depreciation.

Repairs do not add to the value or the usefulness of property, nor do they appreciably lengthen its life (e.g., repairs to floors, painting). Thus they are deductible expenses and not capital expenditures.

Improvements add to the value of property, lengthen its life, or adapt it to a different use. The cost of an improvement is a capital expenditure. Examples are a new floor, lighting renovations, and altering an office as part of a general restoration plan.

Replacements, such as the amount paid to replace parts of an instrument that only keep it in a normal operating condition, do not add to life and are deductible expenses. A replacement that stops deterioration and adds to the life of the property has to be capitalized and depreciated.

Bad Debts. If money is owed but the debt cannot be collected, it is known as a bad debt. Under certain circumstances, the bad debt may qualify as a business deduction. For the debt to qualify, there must be a true creditor-debtor relationship between the creditor and the person who owes the money. Optometrists using the accrual method of accounting report income that is due them as soon as it is earned. Therefore, they may take a bad debt deduction when they are unable to collect what is owed. If the bad debt is later recovered, all or in part, it must be reported as income in the year that it is collected. Cash method optometrists do not report income that is due until payment is received. For this reason, they may not take a bad debt deduction on payments they have not received or cannot collect.

Travel, Entertainment, and Gift Expenses. Important deductions for a business are the travel, entertainment, and gift expenses that are related to the conduct of the business. This is an area that is carefully scrutinized by the IRS, so meticulous recordkeeping, documentation, and planning are essential.

Travel expenses. Travel expenses are those ordinary and necessary expenses of foreign and domestic travel away from home for the practice of optometry. These expenses include meals and lodging, transportation and baggage charges, the cost of maintaining and operating a car, cleaning and laundry expenses, telephone and other communications expenses, and similar costs related to qualified travel, including tips incidental to any of these expenses.

The general rule is that if a trip was entirely for business, then the ordinary and necessary travel expenses may be deducted, but if the trip was primarily personal, no travel expenses may be deducted, even if there was some business activity at the destination. If the trip was primarily for business and while at the business destination the trip was extended for vacation or other nonbusiness activities, then the expenses of travel to and from the destination may be deducted. Whether the primary purpose of the trip was business or pleasure, the expenses incurred at the destination that were related to business may be deducted.

Travel expenses that an optometrist incurs in attending an optometric convention or seminar may be deducted. A spouse or other family member accompanying an optometrist on such a trip cannot be included in the deduction unless it can be shown that there is a business purpose and need for the other person's attendance.

Transportation expenses for business purposes may be deducted even though the optometrist is not away from home. Transportation expenses include such items as air, train, bus, and cab fares and the expenses of driving or maintaining a car or other vehicle. Meals and lodging are not considered in computing transportation expenses, and commuting expenses between the home and the usual place of business are not deductible. Special rules involved in the use of an automobile or other vehicle for business purposes are described in a subsequent section of this chapter.

Business entertainment. Business entertainment expenses are deductible only if they are ordinary and necessary expenses of carrying on the practice of optometry and can be documented. This deduction may be taken only if the amounts spent are directly related to or associated with the active conduct of optometry or directly precede or follow a substantial business discussion related to the practice of optometry. Furthermore, only 50% of business-related entertainment expenses may be deducted.

For example, an optometrist wishing to establish a cooperative for the purpose of purchasing spectacle frames at discount may take a prospective member of the co-op to dinner, at which they discuss the details of such a business association. If the cost of the meal is $100, the optometrist may deduct $50 as a business deduction.

Entertainment includes any activity generally considered to provide entertainment, amusement, or recreation. This covers entertaining guests at night clubs; social, athletic and sporting clubs; theaters; sporting events; on yachts; or hunting, fishing, or vacation trips. It also may include satisfying the personal, living, or family needs of any individuals, such as furnishing food and beverages, hotel accommodations, or an automobile. However, expenses cannot be deducted for entertainment that is lavish or extravagant. Dues and fees paid to a club organized for business, pleasure, recreation, or other social purposes are not deductible as a business expense.

Business gifts. Business gifts may be deducted, but the total cost of such gifts made directly or indirectly to any person during the tax year cannot be more than $25. If a gift is not intended for the eventual personal use or benefit of a particular person or limited class of people, the gift will not be allowed.

The proof necessary to establish travel, entertainment, and business gift expenses should be kept in an account book, diary, statement of expense, or similar record, supported by adequate documentary evidence, that together will support each element of an expense. For example, entries on a desk calendar, not supported by evidence, are not considered to be proper proof.

Employee travel expenses. Expenses reimbursed to employees for travel expenses are deductible by the business. Employee travel expenses that are unreimbursed by the employer may be claimed only as itemized deductions (under the "miscellaneous" category on Schedule A) to the extent that they exceed 2% of adjusted gross income (see Chapter 38).

Employee entertainment expenses. Entertainment expenses reimbursed to employees are deductible. Employee entertainment expenses that are not reimbursed by the employer are deductible, but the deduction is limited to 50% of these costs. They must be claimed on Schedule A and thus may be realized as deductions only to the extent they exceed 2% of adjusted gross income.

Interest. Interest is the charge made for the use of money. All interest paid or accrued in the tax year on a debt that is related to business may be deducted. The interest must be on a debt for which there is a valid obligation to pay a fixed or determinable sum of money.

Generally, the amount agreed on by the lender and the borrower as interest may be deducted when paid or accrued. Examples of deductible interest include the following:

• Interest on business loans used to purchase instruments or equipment (or for other business purposes)

- Mortgages on real property or personal property ("chattel mortgages")
- Interest on loans taken out on insurance policies
- Interest on business-related credit card charges

If a taxpayer uses the cash method of accounting, interest may be deducted only in the year in which it was paid. If the taxpayer uses the accrual method of accounting, the interest may be deducted in the year it accrued.

Insurance. The cost of insuring a business may be deducted as an expense, but generally the cost of life insurance cannot be deducted. Premiums paid on business insurance policies such as the following may be deducted:

- Fire, theft, flood, or other casualty insurance
- Merchandise and inventory insurance
- Employees' group hospitalization and medical plans
- Employer's liability insurance
- Malpractice insurance
- Public liability insurance covering liability for bodily injury to persons who are not employees
- Worker's compensation insurance
- State unemployment insurance
- Office overhead insurance
- Employee performance bonds
- Car and other vehicle insurance

Premiums on a life insurance policy covering an employer are not deductible if the employer is directly or indirectly a beneficiary of the policy. Thus, a sole proprietor cannot deduct the cost of his or her life insurance policy, and if a partner in a partnership purchases life insurance on the partner's life, naming the other partners as beneficiaries, the premiums are not deductible. However, there are some exceptions. For example, group term life insurance purchased by a professional association or corporation for its employees (including shareholder optometrists) is deductible. The same is true for a subchapter S corporation.

Taxes. Various taxes imposed by federal, state, local, and foreign governments may be deducted if they are incurred in the ordinary course of business. Federal income, estate, gift, state, inheritance, legacy, and succession taxes are not deductible. Deductible taxes may be categorized as the following:

Real property taxes. All taxes imposed on real estate that is owned and used for business purposes may be deducted.

Income taxes. State income taxes imposed on a professional corporation are deductible; state income taxes cannot be deducted by an individual proprietor as a business expense (but may be claimed on Schedule A as an itemized deduction).

Employment taxes. If an employer has one or more employees, Social Security and Medicare taxes, and federal (or state) unemployment taxes will have to be withheld; the employer's share of the Social Security and Medicare taxes and the federal (or state) unemployment taxes may be claimed as a tax deduction.

Sales taxes. State and local sales taxes imposed on the sale of ophthalmic materials and other goods by an optometrist may be deducted if the taxes also were credited as income; if equipment or instruments were purchased, and a sales tax was imposed, the tax is considered part of the cost of the items purchased and is depreciated rather than deducted as an expense.

Other taxes. There are other taxes that may be deducted as a business expense, including personal property taxes (e.g., automobiles), gasoline taxes (for vehicles used for business purposes), and corporate franchise taxes.

The tax accounting of personal tax items (such as the tax on a home) is performed on Schedule A when itemizing deductions.

Utility Costs. Utility charges, such as those for heat, light, power, or water expenses for an office; the costs of telephones or telephone services; Internet access or similar costs that are incurred for the operation of a business are deductible.

Profession-related Expenses. The ordinary and necessary expenses of conducting a private practice can be deducted and include numerous items, such as the following:

- Membership in professional organizations or societies
- Subscriptions to journals
- Professional texts or books
- Business-related supplies and materials
- Equipment that has a useful life of less than 1 year
- Legal and accounting fees
- Licenses or regulatory fees
- Advertising
- Costs of attending continuing education (but only 50% of expenses for meals is deductible)

These expenses are deducted in the year they are incurred.

Expenses of Looking for a New Job. An individual in an occupation who travels for the purpose of finding employment elsewhere may deduct the expenses of job-seeking trips, including travel costs, meals (limited to 50%), and lodging, even if the trips do not result in an employment offer. The individual must be able to establish, however, that the trips were taken primarily for the purpose of finding employment and have documentation to support this purpose. In determining the purpose of the trip, the amount of time spent on personal activity compared with the amount of time spent looking for employment is the key issue.

Miscellaneous Business Expenses. There are other types of expenses that may qualify for business deductions. Among these are payments to charitable, religious, educational, or scientific organizations (but the expenses claimed must not be charitable contributions) and the amounts spent to purchase a franchise, trademark, or trade name.

The business expenses are totaled on the "Expenses" section of Schedule C and subtracted from gross business income to provide a tentative profit. For most optometrists, this amount will in fact be the net profit, but if a home is used as a business office, certain expenses also may be deducted.

Expenses for the Business Use of a Home Office

Space in a home may qualify as a deduction if it is used regularly and exclusively for business purposes; the home office must be:
- The principal place of business
- Used to meet with patients in the normal course of business

To claim the deduction, the number of square feet used for the office must be determined as a percent of the total square feet of the house. This percentage is then multiplied by the mortgage interest expense, home taxes, insurance, utilities, repairs, maintenance, and allowable depreciation for the home. The calculation is performed on Form 8829.

The total home expenses are subtracted from the tentative profit to yield the net profit for the business.

One other deduction that may be included on Schedule C, but must be discussed separately because of its complexity, is depreciation.

Depreciation, Amortization, and Expensing Deductions

Depreciation is one of the most important business deductions available to an optometrist. To a lesser extent, amortization can be used to reduce taxable income as a claimed deduction.

Depreciation

If business property that has a useful life of more than 1 year is purchased, its cost cannot be deducted as an expense when business income is determined for tax purposes. Instead, the cost must be spread over more than 1 year and deducted a portion at a time. This process is called *depreciation* and is a means of allowing the recovery of the cost over a period of years.

Depreciable property may be classified as either real or personal. Personal property is anything that is not real estate, whereas real property is the land and anything that is erected on, growing on, or attached to it. The land itself cannot be depreciated, only the structures or other things on it.

Property is depreciable if it meets the following three requirements:
- It must be used in business or held for the production of income
- It must be something that wears out, decays, gets used up, becomes obsolete, or loses value from natural causes
- It must be expected to last more than 1 year

In general, if property does not meet these requirements, it is not depreciable.

Depreciation may only be deducted on property that is used for business purposes or held for the production of income; depreciation cannot be claimed on nonbusiness property such as a car that is used for commuting, vacations, or other nonbusiness activities. If property is used for both business and nonbusiness purposes, however, depreciation may be deducted for business use. Automobiles often are used for both purposes and are eligible for depreciation, but only for the percent of use that is related to business.

For example, if an automobile used both for personal reasons and for the practice of optometry is driven 20,000 miles during the year, and 12,000 of these miles are for business purposes, the optometrist is entitled to use 60% (12,000 of 20,000) of the costs of operating the car for purposes of claiming a business deduction.

Depreciable property includes the following:
- Ophthalmic instruments and equipment
- Motor vehicles
- Furniture and furnishings
- Computers and other electronic equipment
- Computer software
- An office building

- Professional libraries
- Repairs or improvements to property that lengthen its life, make it more useful, or increase its value
- Patents and copyrights
- Restrictive covenants
- Franchises

Property that cannot be depreciated includes land, rented property, inventory, goodwill, and trademarks or trade names that already are in existence when purchased.

To calculate depreciation, three things must be known about the property: its basis, the date it was placed in service, and the method of depreciation to be applied.

Basis. For property that is purchased, the original basis is its cost. Events often will change the basis of a piece of property to a value called the adjusted basis. Some events (e.g., permanent repairs or improvements) improve basis; others (e.g., casualty losses) decrease basis. If basis is adjusted, the depreciation deduction also may be affected.

Date of Service. Property is considered to be placed in service when it is in a condition or state of readiness and availability for a specifically assigned function in a business. Depreciation begins when the property is first ready for service.

Method of Depreciation. There are several types of depreciation that may be used for business property. Tangible property used by optometrists (automobiles, computers, furniture, instruments, and ophthalmic equipment) must be depreciated under the modified Accelerated Cost Recovery System (ACRS) unless another allowable method is elected. Because the modified ACRS does not include intangible property (goodwill, covenant not to compete, trade names), this type of property must be amortized. A special first-year depreciation deduction for tangible property, known as the section 179 deduction, also may be claimed.

Modified Accelerated Cost Recovery System

In general, the method of depreciation that is used for tangible business property is the modified ACRS. This system requires that property be depreciated over a 3-, 5-, 7-, 10-, 15-, or 20-year period. There is no distinction made between new and used property; rather, the difference is between classes of assets. The 5- and 7-year periods include the types of assets that are most likely to be found in the practice of optometry (Box 39–1).

Box 39-1 Property Eligible for 5- and 7-Year Recovery Periods Under the Modified Accelerated Cost Recovery System

5-YEAR PROPERTY	7-YEAR PROPERTY
Automobiles and other vehicles used for business	Office furniture and fixtures (e.g., desks, chairs, eyeglass display cabinets)
Computers and peripheral equipment	Ophthalmic equipment and instruments
Office machinery (e.g., calculators)	

Data From: Internal Revenue Service publication 946, How to depreciate property.

Deductions under the modified ACRS are calculated by multiplying the original basis in the property by a certain percentage that varies from year to year during the recovery period. The annual percentages for 5- and 7-year property are listed in Table 39–1. (It should be noted that the actual write-off periods are 6 and 8 years in length.)

For example, computers and peripheral equipment purchased for $5000 fall under 5-year property, with an original basis of $5000. The modified ACRS deduction for the first year is 20%, or $1000; for the second year the depreciation deduction is increased to 32%, or $1600. If computer software also is purchased for $600,

---

Table 39-1 Annual Percentages for 5- and 7-Year Property Under The Modified Accelerated Cost Recovery System

5-YEAR PROPERTY		7-YEAR PROPERTY	
YEAR	PERCENT DEDUCTIBLE	YEAR	PERCENT DEDUCTIBLE
1	20.00	1	14.29
2	32.00	2	24.49
3	19.20	3	17.49
4	11.52	4	12.49
5	11.52	5	8.93
6	5.76	6	8.92
		7	8.93
		8	4.46

Data From: Internal Revenue Service publication 946, How to depreciate property.

it has to be depreciated by the straight line method for 3 years ($200 a year).

Amortization

Intangible business assets of most significance to the practice of optometry cannot be depreciated under the modified ACRS and instead are subject to amortization.

Amortization provides for equal deductions over a period of years. Goodwill and covenants not to compete are intangible business assets and must be deducted over 15 years. For example, if $45,000 of goodwill is part of the purchase price of an optometric practice, the purchaser may claim a $3000 deduction for 15 years.

Patient records, even though they are tangible assets, also are required to be deducted in equal installments over a 15-year period. For example, if patient records are valued at $60,000 in the same purchase of an optometric practice, the tax deduction allowed the purchaser would be $4000 per year for 15 years.

The recovery period for nonresidential real property is 39 years, and if an office building is purchased by an optometrist, the tax deduction for the purchase must be claimed over this period.

Expensing

A taxpayer may choose to treat the cost of depreciable property as an expense rather than as a capital expenditure. If the taxpayer elects to deduct the property as an expense—known as a *section 179 deduction*—a sizable write-off may be claimed in the year the property is placed in service. This deduction may be claimed only once, in the first year of service, and the amount claimed must be subtracted from the basis of the property, thereby reducing the depreciation available in later years. The maximum amount that may be claimed, as of 2003, was $25,000. (This amount is adjusted annually.)

For example, if an optometrist purchases $50,000 worth of ophthalmic equipment and puts it into service, the optometrist may elect to claim the section 179 deduction. If the optometrist elects to expense the maximum amount available, this $25,000 reduces the taxable business income reported on Schedule C by that amount. The next tax year, the adjusted basis in the equipment becomes $25,000 (the cost, $50,000, less the section 179 amount claimed, $25,000). The basis in the property is adjusted to $25,000. Because ophthalmic equipment is 7-year property, the second-

year depreciation is 25% of $25,000, or $6250. There are limits on the amount of a section 179 deduction that can be claimed for automobiles (discussed later).

Special Rules for Motor Vehicles

There are special rules that apply to depreciation deductions for automobiles or other motor vehicles used for business purposes. Motor vehicles are termed "listed property," and although they are considered 5-year property depreciable under the modified ACRS, there are special "caps" for write-offs that limit the amount of allowable depreciation. The dollar caps for automobiles are listed in Box 39-2. These caps are further reduced, however, if the business use of the automobile is less than 100%, which is a certainty for an optometrist.

For example, if a self-employed optometrist buys a $20,000 automobile that is used 60% for business purposes, the depreciable basis for the first year will be $12,000 (60% of $20,000). The first year cap is $3060, or 20%, of the depreciable basis, whichever is less. The allowable deduction is $2400 (20% of $12,000), which is less than the cap. If a vehicle is purchased for $40,000, however, and used 60% of the time for business purposes, the depreciable basis is $24,000 (60% of $40,000), and the allowable deduction is $3060 (because 20% of $24,000 is $4800).

If qualified use for business purposes does not exceed 50%—which is likely for an optometrist—then the modified ACRS cannot be used and the vehicle's depreciable basis must be recovered over 5 years using a straight line depreciation method, which is similar to amortization. For example, if a vehicle is purchased for $30,000 and used 25% for business purposes, the basis in the vehicle is $7500. The deduction

Box 39-2 Depreciation Caps for Automobile Deductions Under the Modified Accelerated Cost Recovery System, 2003	
1st year limit	$3060
2nd year limit	$4900
3rd year limit	$2950
4th year limit	$1775
5th and later year limit	$1775

Data From: Internal Revenue Service publication 463, Travel, entertainment, gift and car expenses.

must be claimed in equal amounts over a 5-year period ($1500 a year).

If the modified ACRS is originally claimed for a vehicle and during the recovery period business use decreases to 50% or less, part of the depreciation claimed in prior years is "recaptured," and the taxpayer must switch to a straight line depreciation thereafter.

Determining Expenses for Business Use of a Motor Vehicle

To obtain an accurate tax write-off, an optometrist should maintain an automobile log that records the miles traveled for business purposes. This mileage must be compared with the total miles traveled to determine the percent of business use. This percent is then applied to the actual costs of operating the vehicle (Box 39-3).

Instead of the actual costs of operating a vehicle, a taxpayer may deduct a flat amount, known as the *standard mileage rate*, based on the miles traveled for business purposes. This rate is changed every year (36 cents in 2003). In addition to this rate, the taxpayer may include parking fees and tolls, loan interest, and state and local taxes (other than gas tax) that are related to business use of the vehicle. Ordinarily, the standard mileage deduction will not be as large as the write-off for depreciation and actual operating expenses, but for some taxpayers it may be the best option. It should be noted, however, that the standard mileage rate must be chosen in the first year to be claimed in subsequent years.

The calculation of the depreciation deduction is performed on Form 4562 (Figure 39-3). The total depreciation deduction is then transferred to Schedule C, where it is listed as a business expense.

Payments to Independent Contractors

Optometrists often employ individuals to assist them in private practice. If the individuals are in fact employees, the optometrist will be required to withhold income, Social Security, and Medicare taxes from their wages (see Chapter 40). If the individuals are not employees, however, the optometrists do not incur this obligation. These individuals are referred to as independent contractors.

The question as to whether an individual is an employee or an independent contractor is a legal one. It is generally held that an individual who performs services that are subject to the control of the employer—where the employer has the legal right to determine what duties are to be performed and how they are to be performed—is an employee. Whether the employer chooses to exercise this right is not the determining factor, nor is the description given to the individual (e.g., partner, agent, employee, independent contractor), nor even how the individual is paid (i.e., for full-time or part-time employment). The determinative characteristic is the right of control, two especially important aspects of which are the right to discharge the individual and the supplying of equipment and a place to work. If an individual is deemed to be an independent contractor, the wages paid to the individual are reported to the IRS on Form 1099, and there is no tax withholding.

Income Tax, Social Security and Medicare, and Unemployment Taxes

An employer must withhold income, Social Security, and Medicare taxes from the wages of employees. In addition, the employer must pay unemployment taxes. For self-employed individuals (like an optometrist in private practice), his or her income, Social Security, and Medicare taxes also must be withheld and submitted periodically as required. These important business expenses and the system for withholding and paying them are described in Chapter 40.

This discussion omits the topic of payment of state and local taxes, which are too numerous and varied for inclusion. Tax counsel should be consulted to make sure that tax reporting is performed correctly to federal and state governments.

Box 39-3 Actual Costs of Operating a Motor Vehicle

- Gas and oil and tires
- Repairs
- Insurance
- Depreciation
- Interest on a loan taken out to buy the car
- Taxes
- Licenses and tags
- Garage rent and parking fees and tolls

Data From: Internal Revenue Service publication 463, Travel, entertainment, gift and car expenses.

Form **4562**	**Depreciation and Amortization**	OMB No. 1545-0172
Department of the Treasury / Internal Revenue Service	**(Including Information on Listed Property)** ▶ See separate instructions. ▶ Attach to your tax return.	**20**02 / Attachment Sequence No. **67**

Name(s) shown on return John G O'Dee	Business or activity to which this form relates Optometry	Identifying number 123 45 6789

Part I **Election To Expense Certain Tangible Property Under Section 179**

Note: *If you have any listed property, complete Part V before you complete Part I.*

1	Maximum amount. See page 2 of the instructions for a higher limit for certain businesses	**1**	$24,000
2	Total cost of section 179 property placed in service (see page 2 of the instructions)	**2**	20,000
3	Threshold cost of section 179 property before reduction in limitation	**3**	$200,000
4	Reduction in limitation. Subtract line 3 from line 2. If zero or less, enter -0-	**4**	0
5	Dollar limitation for tax year. Subtract line 4 from line 1. If zero or less, enter -0-. If married filing separately, see page 2 of the instructions	**5**	24,000

(a) Description of property	(b) Cost (business use only)	(c) Elected cost	
6 Ophthalmic equipment	20,000	10,000	

7	Listed property. Enter the amount from line 29 **7** 0		
8	Total elected cost of section 179 property. Add amounts in column (c), lines 6 and 7	**8**	10,000
9	Tentative deduction. Enter the **smaller** of line 5 or line 8	**9**	10,000
10	Carryover of disallowed deduction from line 13 of your 2001 Form 4562	**10**	0
11	Business income limitation. Enter the smaller of business income (not less than zero) or line 5 (see instructions)	**11**	24,000
12	Section 179 expense deduction. Add lines 9 and 10, but do not enter more than line 11	**12**	10,000
13	Carryover of disallowed deduction to 2003. Add lines 9 and 10, less line 12 ▶ **13** 0		

Note: *Do not use Part II or Part III below for listed property. Instead, use Part V.*

Part II **Special Depreciation Allowance and Other Depreciation (Do not** include listed property.**)**

14	Special depreciation allowance for qualified property (other than listed property) placed in service during the tax year (see page 3 of the instructions)	**14**	0
15	Property subject to section 168(f)(1) election (see page 4 of the instructions)	**15**	0
16	Other depreciation (including ACRS) (see page 4 of the instructions)	**16**	0

Part III **MACRS Depreciation (Do not** include listed property.**)** (See page 4 of the instructions.)

Section A

17	MACRS deductions for assets placed in service in tax years beginning before 2002	**17**	0
18	If you are electing under section 168(i)(4) to group any assets placed in service during the tax year into one or more general asset accounts, check here ▶ ☐		

Section B—Assets Placed in Service During 2002 Tax Year Using the General Depreciation System

(a) Classification of property	(b) Month and year placed in service	(c) Basis for depreciation (business/investment use only—see instructions)	(d) Recovery period	(e) Convention	(f) Method	(g) Depreciation deduction
19a 3-year property						
b 5-year property						
c 7-year property						
d 10-year property						
e 15-year property						
f 20-year property						
g 25-year property			25 yrs.		S/L	
h Residential rental property			27.5 yrs.	MM	S/L	
			27.5 yrs.	MM	S/L	
i Nonresidential real property			39 yrs.	MM	S/L	
				MM	S/L	

Section C—Assets Placed in Service During 2002 Tax Year Using the Alternative Depreciation System

20a Class life					S/L	
b 12-year			12 yrs.		S/L	
c 40-year			40 yrs.	MM	S/L	

Part IV **Summary** (see page 6 of the instructions)

21	Listed property. Enter amount from line 28	**21**	4,600
22	**Total.** Add amounts from line 12, lines 14 through 17, lines 19 and 20 in column (g), and line 21. Enter here and on the appropriate lines of your return. Partnerships and S corporations—see instr.	**22**	14,600
23	For assets shown above and placed in service during the current year, enter the portion of the basis attributable to section 263A costs **23**		

For Paperwork Reduction Act Notice, see separate instructions.	Cat. No. 12906N	Form **4562** (2002)

Figure 39-3 Sample Form 4562.

Continued

Form 4562 (2002)   Page **2**

Part V — Listed Property (Include automobiles, certain other vehicles, cellular telephones, certain computers, and property used for entertainment, recreation, or amusement.)

Note: *For any vehicle for which you are using the standard mileage rate or deducting lease expense, complete **only** 24a, 24b, columns (a) through (c) of Section A, all of Section B, and Section C if applicable.*

Section A—Depreciation and Other Information (Caution: *See page 8 of the instructions for limits for passenger automobiles.*)

24a Do you have evidence to support the business/investment use claimed? ☑ **Yes** ☐ **No**   24b If "Yes," is the evidence written? ☑ **Yes** ☐ **No**

(a) Type of property (list vehicles first)	(b) Date placed in service	(c) Business/ investment use percentage	(d) Cost or other basis	(e) Basis for depreciation (business/investment use only)	(f) Recovery period	(g) Method/ Convention	(h) Depreciation deduction	(i) Elected section 179 cost
25 Special depreciation allowance for qualified listed property placed in service during the tax year and used more than 50% in a qualified business use (see page 7 of the instructions)						25	0	
26 Property used more than 50% in a qualified business use (see page 7 of the instructions):								
automobile	1-2002	60 %	15,000	9,000	5	MCRS	1,500	
equipment	1-2002	100 %	20,000	20,000	7	MCRS	2,800	
		%						
27 Property used 50% or less in a qualified business use (see page 7 of the instructions):								
		%				S/L –		
		%				S/L –		
		%				S/L –		

28 Add amounts in column (h), lines 25 through 27. Enter here and on line 21, page 1 . .   **28** | 4,600

29 Add amounts in column (i), line 26. Enter here and on line 7, page 1 . . . .   **29** | 0

Section B—Information on Use of Vehicles

Complete this section for vehicles used by a sole proprietor, partner, or other "more than 5% owner," or related person.
If you provided vehicles to your employees, first answer the questions in Section C to see if you meet an exception to completing this section for those vehicles.

		(a) Vehicle 1		(b) Vehicle 2		(c) Vehicle 3		(d) Vehicle 4		(e) Vehicle 5		(f) Vehicle 6	
30	Total business/investment miles driven during the year (do not include commuting miles— see page 2 of the instructions)	9,000											
31	Total commuting miles driven during the year	6,000											
32	Total other personal (noncommuting) miles driven												
33	Total miles driven during the year. Add lines 30 through 32	15,000											
		Yes	No	Yes	No	Yes	No	Yes	No	Yes	No	Yes	No
34	Was the vehicle available for personal use during off-duty hours?	✓											
35	Was the vehicle used primarily by a more than 5% owner or related person?	✓											
36	Is another vehicle available for personal use?	✓											

Section C—Questions for Employers Who Provide Vehicles for Use by Their Employees

Answer these questions to determine if you meet an exception to completing Section B for vehicles used by employees who **are not** more than 5% owners or related persons (see page 8 of the instructions).

		Yes	No
37	Do you maintain a written policy statement that prohibits all personal use of vehicles, including commuting, by your employees?		
38	Do you maintain a written policy statement that prohibits personal use of vehicles, except commuting, by your employees? See page 8 of the instructions for vehicles used by corporate officers, directors, or 1% or more owners		
39	Do you treat all use of vehicles by employees as personal use?		
40	Do you provide more than five vehicles to your employees, obtain information from your employees about the use of the vehicles, and retain the information received?		
41	Do you meet the requirements concerning qualified automobile demonstration use? (See page 9 of the instructions.) . .		

Note: *If your answer to 37, 38, 39, 40, or 41 is "Yes," do not complete Section B for the covered vehicles.*

Part VI — Amortization

(a) Description of costs	(b) Date amortization begins	(c) Amortizable amount	(d) Code section	(e) Amortization period or percentage	(f) Amortization for this year
42 Amortization of costs that begins during your 2002 tax year (see page 9 of the instructions):					

43 Amortization of costs that began before your 2002 tax year . . . .   **43** | 0

44 **Total.** Add amounts in column (f). See page 9 of the instructions for where to report . . . .   **44** | 0

✱   Form **4562** (2002)

Figure 39–3, Cont'd

Bibliography

Classé JG. *Legal aspects of optometry*. Boston, 1989, Butterworth.

Internal Revenue Service publication 1, *Your rights as a taxpayer*.

Internal Revenue Service publication 4, *Student's guide to federal income tax*.

Internal Revenue Service publication 15, *Employer's tax guide (circular E)*.

Internal Revenue Service publication 334, *Tax guide for small business*.

Internal Revenue Service publication 463, *Travel, entertainment, gift and car expenses*.

Internal Revenue Service publication 509, *Tax calendar for 2002*.

Internal Revenue Service publication 553, *Tax highlights of 2000 tax changes*.

Internal Revenue Service publication 505, *Tax withholding and estimated tax*.

Internal Revenue Service publication 533, *Self-employment tax*.

Internal Revenue Service publication 535, *Business expenses*.

Internal Revenue Service publication 538, *Accounting periods and methods*.

Internal Revenue Service publication 541, *Partnerships*.

Internal Revenue Service publication 542, *Corporations*.

Internal Revenue Service publication 544, *Sales and other dispositions of assets*.

Internal Revenue Service publication 551, *Basis of assets*.

Internal Revenue Service publication 556, *Examination of returns, appeal rights, and claims for refund*.

Internal Revenue Service publication 560, *Retirement plans for small business (SEP, Keogh, and SIMPLE plans)*.

Internal Revenue Service publication 583, *Starting a business and keeping records*.

Internal Revenue Service publication 587, *Business use of your home*.

Internal Revenue Service publication 946, *How to depreciate property*.

Internal Revenue Service publication 972, *Child tax credit*.

Internal Revenue Service publication 1518, *Tax calendar for small business*.

Internal Revenue Service publication 1976, *Independent contractor or employee?*

www.irs.gov/formspubs. Web site for the Internal Revenue System, which contains forms and publications that can be downloaded.

Chapter *40*

Tax Reporting

John G. Classé

Laws are like cobwebs, which may catch small flies, but let wasps and hornets break through.

Jonathan Swift *A Critical Essay upon the Faculties of the Mind*

O ne of the inviolable obligations of the practice of optometry is the payment of taxes to federal and state governments. Taxes must be paid for income, to the Social Security system, and–in many states–to the unemployment compensation system. In some respects this system is two-tiered, requiring payment to both federal and state governments, and the tax reporting itself is periodic, demanding both quarterly and annual payments from the practitioner. The purpose of this chapter is to clarify these obligations and to describe the applicable tax deadlines that must be met to satisfy reporting requirements.

This discussion considers the tax reporting obligations of self-employed practitioners in private practice. Optometrists who serve as independent contractors, however, are subject to these same requirements. Only employees do not have these obligations, since the withholding of taxes and the payment of these taxes are the responsibility of the employer. The employee receives a W-2 form at the conclusion of the tax year, describing the withholding of income for federal and state income taxes, Social Security taxes, and county or local taxes, if applicable. (For a sample form, see Chapter 5.)

The most important tax reporting requirements are for income, Social Security, and unemployment compensation. These obligations, which are summarized in Table 40-1, are described in terms of current reporting requirements. Tax counsel always should be consulted when preparing to report and pay taxes because tax law is among the most ephemeral legislations of government, and changes are common.

Tax Reporting for Business Organizations

Before a self-employed practitioner begins the practice of optometry, there are several important steps that must be taken, which depend in part on the type of business organization being used–individual proprietorship, partnership, limited liability company (LLC), professional association or corporation (PA or PC), or S corporation–and on state requirements for the initiation of a new business (see Chapters 2 and 6). For the purpose of tax reporting, it is necessary for the practitioner to secure a federal tax identification number, which will be used for the payment of both federal and state business income taxes. This number may be obtained by completing Form SS-4, *Application for Employer Identification Number*, and submitting it to the Internal Revenue Service (IRS) (for an example form, see Chapter 39). The employer identification number is used only for the reporting of business income; any business tax return or reporting schedule should contain the employer identification number of the optometrist.

Sole Proprietorship

Form 1040 is used for the reporting of income and the calculation of taxes (see Chapter 38). If an optometrist is in practice as an individual proprietor, the business income and allowable deductions are computed on a separate form (Schedule C). The business profit or loss calculated on this schedule is entered on Form 1040 and used for the determination of the optometrist's income tax. Therefore, the tax

Table 40-1 Federal Tax Reporting Deadlines

YOU MAY BE LIABLE FOR	IF YOU ARE	USE FORM	DUE ON OR BEFORE
Income Tax	Sole proprietor	Schedule C (Form 1040)	Same day as Form 1040
	Individual who is a partner, LLC owner, or S corporation shareholder	1040	15th day of fourth month after end of tax year
	Corporation	1120 or 1120-A	15th day of third month after end of tax year
	S corporation	1120S	15th day of third month after end of tax year
Self-employment tax	Sole proprietor or individual who is a partner	Schedule SE (Form 1040)	Same day as Form 1040
Estimated tax	Sole proprietor or individual who is a partner or S corporation shareholder	1040-ES	15th day of fourth, sixth, and ninth months of tax year, and 15th day of first month after the end of tax year
	Corporation	1120-W	15th day of fourth, sixth, ninth, and 12th months of tax year
Annual return of income	Partnership or LLC	1065	15th day of fourth month after end of tax year
Social security (FICA) tax and the withholding of income tax	Sole proprietor, corporation, LLC, S corporation, or partnership	941 / 8109 (to make deposits)	4-30, 7-31, 10-31, and 1-31
Providing information on Social Security (FICA) tax and the withholding of income tax	Sole proprietor, corporation, LLC, S corporation or partnership	W-2 (to employee)	1-31
		W-2 and W-3 (to the Social Security Administration)	Last day of February
Federal unemployment (FUTA) tax	Sole proprietor, corporation, LLC, S corporation, or partnership	940 / 8109 (to make deposits)	1-31, 4-30, 7-31, 10-31, and 1-31, but only if the liability for unpaid tax is more than $100
Information returns	Sole proprietor, corporation, LLC, S corporation, or partnership transactions with other persons	Form 1099—to the recipient by 1-31	For payments to non-employees and to the Internal Revenue Service by February 28

Data From: Internal Revenue Service. Tax guide for small business. Washington, DC, 2001, U.S. Government Printing Office.

reporting for an individual proprietor is the most straightforward for any type of business organization.

Partnership

If an optometrist is in partnership, the partnership must determine its income and the distributive share of profit or loss received by the partners on a separate return, Form 1065. The profit or loss received by the partners from the partnership is reported on Schedule K-1, which is attached to each partner's individual Form 1040.

Income tax is not paid by the partnership, only by the partners, who are taxed on the profit or loss they receive.

Limited Liability Company

A one-practitioner LLC is considered a sole proprietorship for tax purposes; the LLC pays no tax, but profits are calculated on Schedule C, which is attached to the owner's Form 1040. Multiple-owner LLCs are partnerships, and the LLC submits a Form 1065 that reports income and the distribution of profit or loss and provides a Schedule K-1 for each of the owners, who file individual Form 1040s.

Professional Association or Corporation

If an optometrist is a shareholder in a PA or PC, the association or corporation is regarded as a separate, tax-paying entity, which must report all business income and claim all business deductions on Form 1120. The optometrist-shareholder also is the employee of the association or corporation, which withholds the optometrist's income tax and issues the optometrist a W-2 form at the conclusion of the tax year, just as for any other employee. The optometrist reports this income on Form 1040; claims allowable personal adjustments, exemptions, or deductions; and calculates the additional tax payment or refund. With a PA or PC, therefore, both the association or corporation and the optometrist may pay income taxes (the "double tax").

S Corporation

Although an S corporation pays no taxes, it must file a return on Form 1120S, reporting income, expenses, and profit or loss distributions to shareholders. Each shareholder receives a Schedule K-1, which reports that individual's share of the S corporation income and is attached to Form 1040.

Because of the complexity of these various reporting requirements and because the most common type of business organization used by optometrists is the individual proprietorship, the tax reporting described in this chapter emphasizes the obligations of an individual proprietor.

Income Tax Reporting for Individuals

Federal income tax reporting for an individual proprietor requires quarterly payments to the federal government. Payments must be made both for the optometrist's income and for the income of employees. To determine the appropriate withholding of taxes, the optometrist must consult IRS publication 15, *Employer's Tax Guide (Circular E)*. This publication provides guidelines and tables that can be used to determine the amount of withholding to be forwarded to an authorized federal bank. The deadlines for payment of these taxes are, for practitioners on a calendar year, April 15, June 15, Sept. 15, and Jan. 15 (see Table 40-1). At each quarterly payment, the optometrist must submit the proper amount of income taxes, for both employer and employees; failure to make payment, or submission of an improper payment, results in a stiff penalty. Thus this system obligates the optometrist to forward income taxes to the federal government every few months, rather than send the entire sum at the conclusion of the tax year.

The forms that are used for income tax reporting are Form 1040-ES, *Estimated Tax for Individuals*, which contains a worksheet that allows self-employed optometrists to estimate their income and Social Security taxes (Figure 40-1), and Form 941, *Employer's Quarterly Tax Return*, which is used to describe the income tax withholding for employees (Figure 40-2).

These quarterly payments are estimates of the annual income tax. At the conclusion of the tax year, the optometrist is obligated to calculate the exact amount of income tax owed. The optometrist's business income and any necessary and ordinary business deductions are described on Schedule C (for an example form, see Chapter 39), and the profit or loss so determined is then entered on Form 1040. After adjustments, exemptions, and deductions are calculated and subtracted, the income tax is determined. The estimated income taxes that have been paid quarterly are then subtracted from the income tax owed, and if the result is less than the amount owed, an additional payment must be made to the IRS. If the taxes paid exceed the amount actually owed, the optometrist receives a refund.

State business income tax for individual proprietors usually is determined by the profit or loss calculated on Schedule C. The optometrist lists the profit or loss on the state income tax return; computes the allowable adjustments, exemptions and deductions; and determines the tax due. From this amount the optometrist may subtract the quarterly estimated taxes paid to the federal government. If payment is less than the income tax owed, additional payment must be made; if it is more, a refund may be collected.

The payment of income tax is intimately connected to the payment of Social Security taxes, which must be forwarded to the federal government in much the same manner as income taxes.

Social Security Tax Reporting

The Federal Insurance Contributors Act was established by the federal government to ensure that employers and employees would have at least some income at retirement, for disability, or as a survivor's benefit at the death of a working spouse. To fund the Social Security system, taxes are imposed on both employers and employees. The collection and submission of these taxes to the

2002 Estimated Tax Worksheet (keep for your records)

1	Enter amount of adjusted gross income you expect in 2002 (see instructions)	1	120,000
2	• If you plan to itemize deductions, enter the estimated total of your itemized deductions. **Caution:** *If line 1 above is over $137,300 ($68,650 if married filing separately), your deduction may be reduced. See Pub. 505 for details.* • If you do not plan to itemize deductions, see **Standard Deduction** on page 2 and enter your standard deduction here.	2	34,100
3	Subtract line 2 from line 1	3	85,900
4	Exemptions. Multiply $3,000 by the number of personal exemptions. If you can be claimed as a dependent on another person's 2002 return, your personal exemption is not allowed. **Caution:** *See Pub. 505 to figure the amount to enter if line 1 above is over: $206,000 if married filing jointly or qualifying widow(er); $171,650 if head of household; $137,300 if single; or $103,000 if married filing separately* . . .	4	9,000
5	Subtract line 4 from line 3	5	76,900
6	**Tax.** Figure your tax on the amount on line 5 by using the **2002 Tax Rate Schedules** on page 2. **Caution:** *If you have a net capital gain, see Pub. 505 to figure the tax*	6	15,840
7	Alternative minimum tax from Form 6251	7	
8	Add lines 6 and 7. Also include any tax from Forms 4972 and 8814 and any recapture of the education credits (see instructions)	8	15,840
9	Credits (see instructions). **Do not** include any income tax withholding on this line	9	200
10	Subtract line 9 from line 8. If zero or less, enter -0-	10	15,640
11	Self-employment tax (see instructions). Estimate of 2002 net earnings from self-employment $...120,000...... ; if **$84,900 or less,** multiply the amount by 15.3%; if **more than $84,900,** multiply the amount by 2.9%, add $10,527.60 to the result, and enter the total. **Caution:** *If you also have wages subject to social security tax, see Pub. 505 to figure the amount to enter* . .	11	11,545
12	Other taxes (see instructions)	12	∅
13a	Add lines 10 through 12	13a	27,185
b	Earned income credit, additional child tax credit, and credit from **Form 4136**	13b	
c	**Total 2002 estimated tax.** Subtract line 13b from line 13a. If zero or less, enter -0- ▶	13c	27,185

14a	Multiply line 13c by 90% (66⅔% for farmers and fishermen) . . .	14a	24,466		
b	Enter the tax shown on your 2001 tax return (112% of that amount if you are not a farmer or fisherman and the adjusted gross income shown on line 34 of that return is more than $150,000 or, if married filing separately for 2002, more than $75,000)	14b	23,500		
c	**Required annual payment to avoid a penalty.** Enter the **smaller** of line 14a or 14b . . ▶		14c	23,500

Caution: *Generally, if you do not prepay (through income tax withholding and estimated tax payments) at least the amount on line 14c, you may owe a penalty for not paying enough estimated tax. To avoid a penalty, make sure your estimate on line 13c is as accurate as possible. Even if you pay the required annual payment, you may still owe tax when you file your return. If you prefer, you may pay the amount shown on line 13c. For details, see Pub. 505.*

15	Income tax withheld and estimated to be withheld during 2002 (including income tax withholding on pensions, annuities, certain deferred income, etc.)	15	∅
16	Subtract line 15 from line 14c. (**Note:** *If zero or less or line 13c minus line 15 is less than $1,000, stop here. You are not required to make estimated tax payments.*)	16	23,500
17	If the first payment you are required to make is due April 15, 2002, enter ¼ of line 16 (minus any 2001 overpayment that you are applying to this installment) here, and on your payment voucher(s) if you are paying by check or money order. (**Note:** *Household employers, see instructions.*) . .	17	5,875

Page 4

Figure 40-1 Sample Estimated Tax Worksheet from Form 1040-ES.

government, however, are the responsibility of the employer. To determine the amount to withhold, employers use IRS publication 15, *Employer's Tax Guide (Circular E)*, which describes the computation of both income and Social Security taxes. The Social Security tax is expressed as a percentage of taxpayers' income and has two components: a retirement tax and a Medicare tax.

Retirement Tax

The percentage of retirement tax that must be paid to Social Security by employees is 6.2%, which is imposed on wages up to an earnings ceiling that changes annually (Table 40-2). If income exceeds the earnings ceiling, no tax is applied to the excess amount. The Social Security law requires the employer also to contribute 6.2% of wages, however, which means that an optometrist who is an employer contributes an equal amount to the Social Security system on behalf of the employee. Therefore, the total that must be paid as Social Security retirement taxes for each employee is 12.4% of the employee's wages, with the employee contributing 50% and the employer contributing 50%.

Form 941 (Rev. January 2003) — Department of the Treasury, Internal Revenue Service (99)

Employer's Quarterly Federal Tax Return

▶ See separate instructions revised January 2003 for information on completing this return.

Please type or print.

Enter state code for state in which deposits were made **only** if different from state in address to the right ▶ (see page 2 of separate instructions).

Name (as distinguished from trade name): John G O'Dee

Trade name, if any:

Address (number and street): 321 Main Street

Date quarter ended: 31 March 2003

Employer identification number:

City, state, and ZIP code: Anytown, ST 12345

OMB No. 1545-0029

T / FF / FD / FP / I / T

If address is different from prior return, check here ▶

IRS Use: 1 1 1 1 1 1 1 1 1 1 2   3 3 3 3 3 3 3   4 4 4   5 5 5 / 6 7 8 8 8 8 8 8 8   9 9 9 9 9   10 10 10 10 10 10 10 10 10 10

A If you **do not have to file** returns in the future, check here ▶ ☐ and enter date final wages paid ▶

B If you are a seasonal employer, see **Seasonal employers** on page 1 of the instructions and check here ▶ ☐

1	Number of employees in the pay period that includes March 12th ▶	1	
2	Total wages and tips, plus other compensation	2	5,775
3	Total income tax withheld from wages, tips, and sick pay	3	720
4	Adjustment of withheld income tax for preceding quarters of **this calendar year**	4	
5	Adjusted total of income tax withheld (line 3 as adjusted by line 4)	5	720

6	Taxable social security wages	6a	5,775	× 12.4% (.124) =	6b	716
	Taxable social security tips	6c		× 12.4% (.124) =	6d	
7	Taxable Medicare wages and tips	7a	5,775	× 2.9% (.029) =	7b	167

8	Total social security and Medicare taxes (add lines 6b, 6d, and 7b). **Check here if wages are not subject to social security and/or Medicare tax** ▶ ☐	8	883
9	Adjustment of social security and Medicare taxes (see instructions for required explanation) Sick Pay $_____ ± Fractions of Cents $_____ ± Other $_____ =	9	
10	Adjusted total of social security and Medicare taxes (line 8 as adjusted by line 9)	10	883
11	**Total taxes** (add lines 5 and 10)	11	1,603
12	Advance earned income credit (EIC) payments made to employees (see instructions)	12	
13	Net taxes (subtract line 12 from line 11). If $2,500 or more, this must equal line 17, column (d) below (or line D of Schedule B (Form 941))	13	1,603
14	Total deposits for quarter, including overpayment applied from a prior quarter	14	
15	**Balance due** (subtract line 14 from line 13). See instructions	15	1,603
16	**Overpayment.** If line 14 is more than line 13, enter excess here ▶ $_____		

and check if to be: ☐ Applied to next return **or** ☐ Refunded.

- **All filers:** If line 13 is less than $2,500, **do not** complete line 17 or Schedule B (Form 941).
- **Semiweekly schedule depositors:** Complete Schedule B (Form 941) and check here ▶ ☐
- **Monthly schedule depositors:** Complete line 17, columns (a) through (d), and check here ▶ ☑

17	Monthly Summary of Federal Tax Liability. (Complete **Schedule B (Form 941)** instead, if you were a semiweekly schedule depositor.)

(a) First month liability	(b) Second month liability	(c) Third month liability	(d) Total liability for quarter
535	534	535	1,603

Third Party Designee Do you want to allow another person to discuss this return with the IRS (see separate instructions)? ☐ **Yes. Complete the following.** ☐ **No**

Designee's name ▶   Phone no. ▶ (   )   Personal identification number (PIN) ▶

Sign Here Under penalties of perjury, I declare that I have examined this return, including accompanying schedules and statements, and to the best of my knowledge and belief, it is true, correct, and complete.

Signature ▶ JG O'Dee   Print Your Name and Title ▶ John G O'Dee owner   Date ▶ 1 April 2003

For Privacy Act and Paperwork Reduction Act Notice, see back of Payment Voucher.   Cat. No. 17001Z   Form **941** (Rev. 1-2003)

Figure 40-2 Sample Form 941.

Table 40-2 Social Security and Medicare Tax Rates and Earnings Ceilings, 1993-2002

	YEAR	EARNINGS CEILING FOR TAX	TAX RATE	MAXIMUM CONTRIBUTIONS
		EMPLOYER OR EMPLOYEE CONTRIBUTIONS*		
Social Security	1993	$57,600	6.20%	$3517
Medicare		$135,000	1.45%	$1957
Social Security	1994	$60,600	6.20%	$3757
Medicare		No ceiling	1.45%	No limit
Social Security	1995	$61,200	6.20%	$3794
Medicare		No ceiling	1.45%	No limit
Social Security	1996	$62,700	6.20%	$3887
Medicare		No ceiling	1.45%	No limit
Social Security	1997	$65,400	6.20%	$4054
Medicare		No ceiling	1.45%	No limit
Social Security	1998	$68,400	6.20%	$4240
Medicare		No ceiling	1.45%	No limit
Social Security	1999	$72,600	6.20%	$4501
Medicare		No ceiling	1.45%	No limit
Social Security	2000	$76,200	6.20%	$4724
Medicare		No ceiling	1.45%	No limit
Social Security	2001	$80,400	6.20%	$4985
Medicare		No ceiling	1.45%	No limit
Social Security	2002	$84,900	6.20%	$5263
Medicare		No ceiling	1.45%	No limit

*These payments represent one half of the annual tax; both employer and employee contribute equal amounts. For example, an employee receiving a salary of $50,000 would contribute $3825 ($50,000 × 7.65%), and the employer also would contribute $3825. The total paid would be $7650.

Medicare Tax

As of 1991, a specific percentage of the Social Security tax has been payable to Medicare, which provides health care benefits to persons 65 years and older. Like its retirement tax counterpart, the Medicare portion is calculated as a percentage, but unlike the retirement tax there is no earnings ceiling. The percentage imposed for Medicare payments is 2.9% of wages, regardless of the amount earned. Employer and employee contribute equally to the tax.

Therefore, the Social Security system requires a total payment of 15.3% of an employee's wages, with the employer contributing half, or 7.65%, to a specific ceiling amount for the Social Security tax and without a ceiling for the Medicare tax. Payments for employees are made quarterly, at the same times and with the same form (Form 941) used for income taxes (see Figure 40-2). This amount may be listed on the employer's Schedule C and claimed as a business deduction.

The Social Security tax for self-employed individuals is calculated in a slightly different manner.

Self-Employment Tax

The Social Security payments of an individual practitioner are based on the income or loss reported on Schedule C. This amount must exceed $400 or no Social Security tax need be paid. If the amount is in excess of $400, the Social Security tax must be determined on Schedule SE, *Self-employment Tax* (Figure 40-3). The calculation is again dependent on the use of a percentage, but there is an earnings ceiling for the retirement tax, which changes annually. As with employees, the total percentage contributed to Social Security is 12.4%, up to the earnings ceiling. The Medicare tax is 2.9%, but without a ceiling. Thus an individual practitioner pays to Social Security 15.3% of income, up to the earnings ceiling, and 2.9% thereafter (Table 40-3).

The payment of Social Security taxes is made quarterly by self-employed optometrists, based upon the estimated tax figured on the worksheet for Form 1040-ES. At the end of the tax year, when the optometrist completes Form 1040, Schedule SE is used to calculate the exact amount of Social Security tax owed, and that

SCHEDULE SE
(Form 1040)

Department of the Treasury
Internal Revenue Service (99)

OMB No. 1545-0074

Self-Employment Tax

▶ **Attach to Form 1040.** ▶ **See Instructions for Schedule SE (Form 1040).**

20**02**

Attachment
Sequence No. **17**

Name of person with **self-employment** income (as shown on Form 1040)

John F O'Dee

Social security number of person
with **self-employment** income ▶   123 : 45 : 6789

Who Must File Schedule SE

You must file Schedule SE if:

● You had net earnings from self-employment from **other than** church employee income (line 4 of Short Schedule SE or line 4c of Long Schedule SE) of $400 or more **or**

● You had church employee income of $108.28 or more. Income from services you performed as a minister or a member of a religious order **is not** church employee income. See page SE-1.

Note. Even if you had a loss or a small amount of income from self-employment, it may be to your benefit to file Schedule SE and use either "optional method" in Part II of Long Schedule SE. See page SE-3.

Exception. If your only self-employment income was from earnings as a minister, member of a religious order, or Christian Science practitioner **and** you filed Form 4361 and received IRS approval not to be taxed on those earnings, **do not** file Schedule SE. Instead, write "Exempt–Form 4361" on Form 1040, line 56.

May I Use Short Schedule SE or Must I Use Long Schedule SE?

Did You Receive Wages or Tips in 2002?

No / **Yes**

Are you a minister, member of a religious order, or Christian Science practitioner who received IRS approval **not** to be taxed on earnings from these sources, **but** you owe self-employment tax on other earnings? — **Yes** ▶

No ↓

Are you using one of the optional methods to figure your net earnings (see page SE-3)? — **Yes** ▶

No ↓

Did you receive church employee income reported on Form W-2 of $108.28 or more? — **Yes** ▶

No ↓

Was the total of your wages and tips subject to social security or railroad retirement tax **plus** your net earnings from self-employment more than $84,900? — **Yes** ▶

No ↓

Did you receive tips subject to social security or Medicare tax that you **did not** report to your employer? — **Yes** ▶

No ◀

You May Use Short Schedule SE Below

You Must Use Long Schedule SE on the Back

Section A—Short Schedule SE. Caution. Read above to see if you can use Short Schedule SE.

1	Net farm profit or (loss) from Schedule F, line 36, and farm partnerships, Schedule K-1 (Form 1065), line 15a	**1**	
2	Net profit or (loss) from Schedule C, line 31; Schedule C-EZ, line 3; Schedule K-1 (Form 1065), line 15a (other than farming); and Schedule K-1 (Form 1065-B), box 9. Ministers and members of religious orders, see page SE-1 for amounts to report on this line. See page SE-2 for other income to report	**2**	139,925
3	Combine lines 1 and 2	**3**	139,925
4	**Net earnings from self-employment.** Multiply line 3 by 92.35% (.9235). If less than $400, **do not** file this schedule; you do not owe self-employment tax . . . . ▶	**4**	129,220
5	**Self-employment tax.** If the amount on line 4 is: ● $84,900 or less, multiply line 4 by 15.3% (.153). Enter the result here and on **Form 1040, line 56.** ● More than $84,900, multiply line 4 by 2.9% (.029). Then, add $10,527.60 to the result. Enter the total here and on **Form 1040, line 56.**	**5**	19,770
6	**Deduction for one-half of self-employment tax.** Multiply line 5 by 50% (.5). Enter the result here and on **Form 1040, line 29**	**6**	9,885

For Paperwork Reduction Act Notice, see Form 1040 instructions.

Cat. No. 11358Z

Schedule SE (Form 1040) 2002

Figure 40–3 Sample Schedule SE.

Table 40-3 Social Security and Medicare Tax Rates and Earnings Ceilings, 1993-2002

	YEAR	EARNINGS CEILING FOR TAX	TAX RATE	MAXIMUM CONTRIBUTIONS
		SELF-EMPLOYED CONTRIBUTIONS*		
Social Security	1993	$57,600	12.4%	$7142
Medicare		$135,000	2.9%	$3915
Social Security	1994	$60,600	12.4%	$7514
Medicare		No ceiling	2.9%	No limit
Social Security	1995	$61,200	12.4%	$7588
Medicare		No ceiling	2.9%	No limit
Social Security	1996	$62,700	12.4%	$7774
Medicare		No ceiling	2.9%	No limit
Social Security	1997	$65,400	12.4%	$8109
Medicare		No ceiling	2.9%	No limit
Social Security	1998	$68,400	12.4%	$8481
Medicare		No ceiling	2.9%	No limit
Social Security	1999	$72,600	12.4%	$9002
Medicare		No ceiling	2.9%	No limit
Social Security	2000	$76,200	12.4%	$9448
Medicare		No ceiling	2.9%	No limit
Social Security	2001	$80,400	12.4%	$9969
Medicare		No ceiling	2.9%	No limit
Social Security	2002	$84,900	12.4%	$10,526
Medicare		No ceiling	2.9%	No limit

*These payments represent the Social Security and Medicare taxes paid by a self-employed practitioner. For example, an optometrist earning $100,000 in 2002 contributed $10,526 ($84,900 × 12.4%) to Social Security and $2900 ($100,000 × 2.9%) to Medicare. The total paid was $13,426.

amount is entered on Form 1040. Quarterly payments are deducted from the total tax owed; if less tax has been paid than is owed, the balance must be remitted to the IRS. If more has been paid than is owed, a refund may be collected.

Social Security taxes do not have to be paid to state government. Failure to pay Social Security taxes on time or payment made in improper amounts is punishable by sizable fines, both for the employer's payments and for those made on behalf of employees.

Unemployment Tax Reporting

The federal government, in concert with the states, has devised a system of unemployment compensation for unemployed workers under the Federal Unemployment Tax Act (FUTA). The system is funded exclusively by employers, most of whom must pay taxes to both federal and state governments; some states do not require unemployment tax, and payment must be made exclusively to the federal government.

The tax is paid for each employee, with the amount being a percentage of the employee's wages, to a stated ceiling. The federal unemployment tax is 6.2% of wages, to a maximum of $7000. Thus, for an employee earning $7000 or more, the employer must contribute $434. This tax is not taken from the wages of the employee; rather, it is paid exclusively from the earnings of the employer. The federal government allows a credit for unemployment taxes paid by an employer to the state, up to 5.4% of wages. In such a case, the employer must pay to the federal government only the balance. If the employer pays the maximum, 5.4% of wages, to the state, only 0.8% of wages must be paid to the federal government.

The reporting of federal unemployment taxes is performed on Form 940, *Employer's Annual Federal Unemployment Tax Return* (Figure 40-4). Payment must be made quarterly, unless the tax owed is less than $100, in which case the quarterly deposit does not have to be submitted until the amount owed exceeds $100. Form 940 is submitted with the final payment, which must be sent to the IRS within a month of the end of the tax year (Jan. 31 if the tax year is a calendar year).

State unemployment tax deposits usually must be made on a quarterly basis, and a form must be submit-

Form **940**	Employer's Annual Federal Unemployment (FUTA) Tax Return	OMB No. 1545-0028
Department of the Treasury Internal Revenue Service (99)	► See separate Instructions for Form 940 for information on completing this form.	2002

You must complete this section. ►

T		
FF		
FD		
FP		
I		
T		

Name (as distinguished from trade name)
John G O'Dee

Calendar year
2002

Trade name, if any
321 Main Street

Address and ZIP code
Anytown, ST 12345

Employer identification number
09 : 8765432

A Are you required to pay unemployment contributions to only one state? (If "No," skip questions B and C). ☑ **Yes** ☐ **No**

B Did you pay all state unemployment contributions by January 31, 2003? ((1) If you deposited your total FUTA tax when due, check "Yes" if you paid all state unemployment contributions by February 10, 2003. (2) If a 0% experience rate is granted, check "Yes." (3) If "No," skip question C.) . . . . ☑ **Yes** ☐ **No**

C Were all wages that were taxable for FUTA tax also taxable for your state's unemployment tax? . . . . . ☐ **Yes** ☑ **No**

If you answered "No" to any of these questions, you must file Form 940. If you answered "Yes" to all the questions, you may file Form 940-EZ, which is a simplified version of Form 940. (Successor employers, see **Special credit for successor employers** on page 2 of the instructions.) You can get Form 940-EZ by calling 1-800-TAX-FORM (1-800-829-3676) or from the IRS Web Site at **www.irs.gov.**

If you will not have to file returns in the future, check here (see **Who Must File** in separate instructions) **and complete and sign the return** . . . . ► ☐

If this is an Amended Return, check here (see **Amended Returns** on page 2 of the separate instructions) . . . . ► ☐

Part I   Computation of Taxable Wages

1	Total payments (including payments shown on lines 2 and 3) during the calendar year for services of employees	**1**	18,000	
2	Exempt payments. (Explain all exempt payments, attaching additional sheets if necessary.) ►	**2**	0	
3	Payments of more than $7,000 for services. Enter only amounts over the first $7,000 paid to each employee. (see separate instructions) Do not include any exempt payments from line 2. The $7,000 amount is the Federal wage base. Your state wage base may be different. **Do not use your state wage limitation**.	**3**	11,000	
4	Add lines 2 and 3	**4**	11,000	
5	Total taxable wages (subtract line 4 from line 1) . . . . ►	**5**	7,000	

Be sure to complete both sides of this form, and sign in the space provided on the back.

For Privacy Act and Paperwork Reduction Act Notice, see separate instructions.   ▼ **DETACH HERE** ▼   Cat. No. 11234O   Form **940** (2002)

Form **940-V**	Form 940 Payment Voucher	OMB No. 1545-0028
Department of the Treasury Internal Revenue Service	Use this voucher only when making a payment with your return.	2002

Complete boxes 1, 2, and 3. Do not send cash, and do not staple your payment to this voucher. Make your check or money order payable to the "United States Treasury." Be sure to enter your employer identification number, "Form 940," and "2002" on your payment.

1 Enter your employer identification number.	2 Enter the amount of your payment. ►	Dollars	Cents
09 : 8765432		108	50

3   Enter your business name (individual name for sole proprietors).
John G O'Dee, OD
Enter your address.
321 Main Street
Enter your city, state, and ZIP code.
Anytown, ST 12345

Figure 40–4 Sample Form 940.

Continued

Form 940 (2002)   Page **2**

Part II   **Tax Due or Refund**

1	Gross FUTA tax. (Multiply the wages from Part I, line 5, by .062)		1	434
2	Maximum credit. (Multiply the wages from Part I, line 5, by .054) . .	2		
3	Computation of tentative credit (**Note:** All taxpayers must complete the applicable columns.)			

(a) Name of state	(b) State reporting number(s) as shown on employer's state contribution returns	(c) Taxable payroll (as defined in state act)	(d) State experience rate period		(e) State experience rate	(f) Contributions if rate had been 5.4% (col. (c) x .054)	(g) Contributions payable at experience rate (col. (c) x col. (e))	(h) Additional credit (col. (f) minus col.(g)) If 0 or less, enter -0-.	(i) Contributions paid to state by 940 due date
			From	To					

3a	Totals . . . ▶	
3b	**Total tentative credit** (add line 3a, columns (h) and (i) only—for late payments, also see the instructions for Part II, line 6) . . . . ▶	3b Ø
4		
5		
6	**Credit:** Enter the smaller of the amount from Part II, line 2 or line 3b; or the amount from the worksheet on page 5 of the separate instructions	6 Ø
7	**Total FUTA tax** (subtract line 6 from line 1). If the result is over $100, also complete Part III . .	7 434
8	Total FUTA tax deposited for the year, including any overpayment applied from a prior year . .	8 325 50
9	**Balance due** (subtract line 8 from line 7). Pay to the "United States Treasury." If you owe more than $100, see **Depositing FUTA Tax** on page 3 of the separate instructions . . . . . . ▶	9 108 50
10	**Overpayment** (subtract line 7 from line 8). Check if it is to be: ☐ **Applied to next return** or ☐ **Refunded** . . . . ▶	10

Part III   **Record of Quarterly Federal Unemployment Tax Liability** (Do not include state liability.) **Complete only if line 7 is over $100.** See page 6 of the separate instructions.

Quarter	First (Jan. 1–Mar. 31)	Second (Apr. 1–June 30)	Third (July 1–Sept. 30)	Fourth (Oct. 1–Dec. 31)	Total for year
Liability for quarter	108.50	108.50	108.50	108.50	434

Third Party Designee	Do you want to allow another person to discuss this return with the IRS (see instructions page 6)? ☐ **Yes.** Complete the following. ☐ **No**		
	Designee's name ▶	Phone no. ▶ ( )	Personal identification number (PIN) ▶

Under penalties of perjury, I declare that I have examined this return, including accompanying schedules and statements, and, to the best of my knowledge and belief, it is true, correct, and complete, and that no part of any payment made to a state unemployment fund claimed as a credit was, or is to be, deducted from the payments to employees.

Signature ▶ *JF O'Dee*   Title (Owner, etc.) ▶ *owner*   Date ▶ 4 Jan 03

Form **940** (2002)

Figure 40–4 Cont'd

ted annually by April 15 if the employer's tax year is a calendar year. The employer receives a business tax deduction for the unemployment tax paid to the state or federal government. This deduction is claimed on Schedule C if the employer is an individual proprietor.

Federal Tax Penalties

Because an individual practitioner must file Schedules C and SE along with Form 1040 and because most individual practitioners will use a calendar year as the tax year, the deadline for the submission of the annual tax return will be April 15. An automatic 2-month extension will be granted if a Form 4868 is filed on or before this date; payment of the estimated tax must accompany the request for an extension. Application for further extensions will be granted only if there is hardship. There are penalties for failure to pay by the due date and for substantially underpaying the tax due, and these penalties will be applied if the unpaid amount is more than 10% of the final tax owed, or more than $5000. These penalties also are applicable if quarterly income tax and Social Security tax payments are not filed by the due date or are substantially underpaid. The employer is responsible for the collection and payment of these taxes and will be held liable for any amounts due.

Bibliography

Classé JG: *Legal aspects of optometry.* Boston, 1989, Butterworth.

Internal Revenue Service publication 15, *Employer's tax guide (circular E).*

Internal Revenue Service publication 15-A, *Employer's supplemental tax guide.*

Internal Revenue Service publication 17, *Your federal income tax (for individuals)*.

Internal Revenue Service publication 334, *Tax guide for small businesses*.

Internal Revenue Service publication 463, *Travel, entertainment, and gift expenses*.

Internal Revenue Service publication 505, *Tax withholding and estimated tax*.

Internal Revenue Service publication 533, *Self-employment tax*.

Internal Revenue Service publication 535, *Business expenses*.

Internal Revenue Service publication 538, *Accounting periods and methods*.

Internal Revenue Service publication 541, *Tax information on partnerships*.

Internal Revenue Service publication 542, *Tax information on corporations*.

Internal Revenue Service publication 583, *Starting a business and keeping records*.

Internal Revenue Service publication 589, *Tax information on S corporations*.

Internal Revenue Service publication 917, *Business use of a car*.

Internal Revenue Service publication 946, *How to depreciate property*.

www.irs.gov/formspubs. Web site for the Internal Revenue System, which contains forms and publications that can be downloaded.

Chapter *41*

Analysis of Practice Economics and Growth

C. Thomas Crooks III and Craig Hisaka

Living well is the best revenge.
George Herbert *Jacula Prudentum*

The ability to develop a systematic, universal method for determining the economic status of a professional practice is essential for survival in today's competitive atmosphere. Optometric practice economics is the process of data gathering, formulation, and analysis of all financial information related to the running of a professional practice. It is the basis from which one can derive pertinent information to determine the economic status of a business. Without the ability to formulate and analyze financial data, the practicing optometrist would not be able to survive in the business world.

There is a specialized vocabulary that is used in financial transactions, and this vocabulary must be understood. Just as the language of clinical care is learned, so also must the language of business be learned to better communicate with business professionals, colleagues, and other individuals in the business world. Box 41-1 provides a limited list of basic terms that are the foundation for many of the business financial statements used in the day-to-day operations of a professional practice.

The day-to-day recordkeeping of financial transactions in a professional practice can be a nightmare for the poorly organized optometrist. If an accurate means of tracking income and expenses is not used, a practitioner cannot manage the practice profitably. Optometrists have developed sophisticated methods for maintaining patient records to ensure that proper care is rendered and to provide protection from potential liability. Yet all too often the average optometrist does not maintain an accurate, efficient method of financial recordkeeping. This deficiency obviously leads to poor financial management and increases the risk of incurring financial liability. Documentation of financial records is an essential component of a successful practice. Greater profitability, enhanced financial security, and reduced risk of financial liability are all benefits of proper financial management.

Basic Financial Statement Construction

In organizing the financial records of a practice, the optometrist should prepare a balance sheet and an income statement (see also Chapter 15).

The Balance Sheet

The balance sheet is a financial document that summarily depicts a company's or an individual's financial status at a specific point in time. It balances the amount of assets a business has against its liabilities and the owner's equity. In simple terms it shows how much a company owns versus how much a company owes. The difference between the two is the net worth of the company.

The balance sheet is composed of four basic areas: title, assets, liabilities, and net worth (Figure 41-1).

Title. In this area is contained the name of the business, the title of the financial document, and the specific date that the information was valid.

Box 41-1 Common Business Terms

Accounts payable: Money owed by the business to some other business or individual for goods and services already received by the business.

Accounts receivable: Money owed to the business by patients or customers for goods and services they have already received.

Accrual basis of accounting: A form of accounting that incorporates accounts receivables, accounts payable, depreciation, and inventory.

Amortization schedule: A financial statement that summarizes a loan by showing the principal borrowed, the interest rate charged, the payment frequency, and the payment-by-payment allocation of principal and interest throughout the term of the loan.

Assets: Items of value owned by a business, including cash and bank accounts, material inventory, equipment, buildings, and land. Fixed assets are items of value that have a lifetime of greater than 1 year. Current assets are items of value that have a lifetime of less than 1 year.

Balance sheet: A financial statement that shows a business assets, liabilities, and the owner's equity at a particular point in time. A balance sheet provides a snapshot in time of the company's asset-to-debt status.

Business: A series of activities that are coordinated and integrated toward the production of goods or services, the end purpose being the generation of profit.

Cash basis of accounting: A form of accounting that is strictly determined by the amount of cash received and cash paid out.

Cash flow: A term that refers to the flow of funds within a company, reflecting actual funds received and actual funds expended for a specific time period. Cash flow is usually calculated on a daily or monthly basis.

Co-signer: An individual who assumes liability for a debt in the event of a default by the primary borrower.

Credit risk: The rating factor used by lenders to judge a borrower for the purpose of determining credit terms for that borrower. If an individual or business is a high risk, the loan terms will be less favorable; the lower the risk, the more favorable the loan terms will be.

Credit terms: The terms by which money is either owed to or by a business. Terms include principal amount, interest rate, and the time period in which the money is due.

Effective interest rate: The actual interest rate calculated by incorporating the associated services fees into the total cost of borrowing the principal amount. The effective service rate generally differs from the stated interest rate of a loan.

Income statement: A financial statement that summarizes all the revenue and expense transactions that will result in a profit or loss over a specific period of time. The income statement provides an assessment of the company's financial profitability status over time.

Interest rate: The percentage rate fee that is charged by a lender for the funds that are borrowed. Legal requirements obligate lenders to express the interest rate as an annual percentage rate.

Liabilities: Claims of creditors against the assets of a business. Fixed liabilities are claims of creditors that last for longer than 1 year. Current liabilities are claims of creditors that last for less than 1 year.

Loan term: The time period that is allowed for repayment of the principal. This is not always the time period used to calculate the allocation of interest and principal per payment.

Owner's equity: Items of value or money contributed that the owner or owners have invested in the business.

Points: A service fee charged by the lender to process a loan that is usually expressed in the form of a percentage based on the principal amount of the loan.

Principal: When borrowing or loaning money, the principal is the amount of money either borrowed or loaned.

Profit and loss statement: A financial analysis related to the income statement that shows total received income compared against total actual expenditures for a given period. The profit and loss statement does not take into consideration non-cash expenditures that are included in an income statement.

Assets. The asset area usually is on the left side of the document or on the top. The asset section is defined by subsections that itemize "fixed" and "current" assets. These two subsections list the specific items within each category. At the bottom of the asset section is the sum total of all fixed and current assets for the business.

Liabilities. The liabilities area is located either on the right side of the balance sheet or under the asset section. Like the asset section the liability section is broken into two subsections, which consist of "fixed" and "current" liabilities. These subsections are again further subdivided by individual components that constitute the total. The subtotals for fixed and current

Acme Vision Clinic, P.C.
30-Jun-2002
Balance Sheet

ASSETS			LIABILITIES		
Current Assets			**Current Liabilities**		
Bank Accounts	$ 12,000.00		Accounts Payable	$ 27,500.00	
Cash On Hand	2,000.00		Contracts Payable	4,000.00	
Merchandise Inventory	35,000.00		Short-Term Note Payable	5,000.00	
Accounts Receivable	30,000.00				
Total Current Assets		$ 79,000.00	**Total Current Liabilities**		$36,500.00
Fixed Assets			**Fixed Liabilities**		
Store fixtures	$ 47,500.00		Personal notes payable	$ 56,000.00	
Office furniture	25,000.00		Equipment notes payable	25,000.00	
Optometric equipment	87,000.00		Line of credit payable	5,000.00	
Computer equipment	15,000.00				
			Total Fixed Liabilities		$86,000.00
Total Fixed Assets		$ 174,500.00			
			Total Liabilities		$122,500.00
Total Assets		$ 253,500.00			
			Net Worth		
			Owners Equity		$131,000.00
			Total Liabilities & Net Worth		$253,500.00

Figure 41-1 Balance sheet—assets and liabilities.

liabilities are added together at the bottom of this section to provide a sum for total liabilities.

Net Worth. This area also is referred to as the *owner's equity*. The net worth figure represents the financial contribution the owner or owners have made to the business. It is determined by calculating the mathematical difference between the total assets and the total liabilities. If a business owns more than it owes, it has a positive net worth. If a business has incurred more debt than it owns in assets, it has a negative net worth. Therefore, the sum of the total liabilities and the net worth must equal the total assets of the business. This relationship is why the document is called a balance sheet.

The Income Statement

The income statement, or *profit and loss statement*, is one of the most informative of all financial statements. It provides a summary of all revenues and expenses that occur in a business that ultimately will result in a profit or loss. The construction of this statement is signifi-

cantly more complex than that of the balance sheet, but when properly constructed can offer a wealth of information at a glance. The income statement is divided into four major sections: income, operating expenses, profit and loss statement, and break-even analysis.

Income. In the practice of optometry, income is derived from the services provided and the materials sold. It is important to specify which income is generated by services and which is generated by materials. Services revenue and materials revenue are both subsections of the category termed *gross sales revenue* (Figure 41-2). When services and materials revenues for a given month are added together, the total gross income for the specified time period is obtained. The credits and adjustments are then subtracted from this figure to obtain the "*net sales revenue.*" This figure represents the actual amount of income that was earned after all credits and adjustments to gross income were made.

The next item incorporated into the income statement is the *cost of goods sold*, which represents the actual

Acme Vision Clinic, P.C.
2002 Income Statement
1 January - 31 March 2002
Quarterly Report

GROSS SALES REVENUE:

Practice Revenue	January	February	March	Quarterly Grand Total	Percentage of Gross Income
Services:	$22,000.00	$23,500.00	$24,750.00	$70,250.00	56.09%
Materials:	$15,000.00	$18,000.00	$22,000.00	$55,000.00	43.91%
Subtotal	$37,000.00	$41,500.00	$46,750.00	$125,250.00	100.00%
Less credit/adjust	$2,405.00	$2,697.50	$3,038.75	$8,141.25	6.50%
Net Sales Revenue	$34,595.00	$38,802.50	$43,711.25	$117,108.75	93.50%
Cost of Goods Sold	$12,210.00	$13,695.00	$15,427.50	$41,332.50	33.00%
Gross Margin on Sales	$22,385.00	$25,107.50	$28,283.75	$75,776.25	60.50%

OPERATING EXPENSES:
Fixed Expenses:

	January	February	March	Quarterly Grand Total	Percentage of Gross Income
Advertising Yellow Pages	$500.00	$500.00	$500.00	$1,500.00	1.20%
Depreciation	$1,200.00	$1,200.00	$1,200.00	$3,600.00	2.87%
Dues AOA	$100.00	$100.00	$100.00	$300.00	0.24%
Dues Employees	$0.00	$0.00	$0.00	$0.00	0.00%
Dues Business Club	$75.00	$75.00	$75.00	$225.00	0.18%
Dues Athletic Club	$75.00	$75.00	$75.00	$225.00	0.18%
Insurance Basic Overhead	$100.00	$100.00	$100.00	$300.00	0.24%
Insurance Disability	$50.00	$50.00	$50.00	$150.00	0.12%
Insurance Major Medical	$250.00	$250.00	$250.00	$750.00	0.60%
Insurance Property/Liability	$100.00	$100.00	$100.00	$300.00	0.24%
Insurance Worker's Compensation	$50.00	$50.00	$50.00	$150.00	0.12%
Lease Professional Equipment	$548.00	$548.00	$548.00	$1,644.00	1.31%
Lease Office Equipment	$200.00	$200.00	$200.00	$600.00	0.48%
Licenses	$6.67	$6.67	$6.67	$20.00	0.02%
Plant Service	$65.00	$65.00	$65.00	$195.00	0.16%
Rent (including utilities)	$3,000.00	$3,000.00	$3,000.00	$9,000.00	7.19%
Salary Dr. Acme	$5,000.00	$5,000.00	$5,000.00	$15,000.00	11.98%
Salary Staff #1	$1,239.58	$1,239.58	$1,239.58	$3,718.75	2.97%
Salary Staff #2	$1,097.92	$1,097.92	$1,097.92	$3,293.75	2.63%
Taxes Federal Income	$900.00	$900.00	$900.00	$2,700.00	2.16%
Taxes State Income	$400.00	$400.00	$400.00	$1,200.00	0.96%
Taxes Personal Property	$395.00	$395.00	$395.00	$1,185.00	0.95%
Taxes Payroll Federal	$3,283.75	$3,283.75	$3,283.75	$9,851.25	7.87%
Taxes Payroll State	$798.75	$798.75	$798.75	$2,396.25	1.91%
Telephone Basic Service	$65.00	$65.00	$65.00	$195.00	0.16%
Telephone Cellular	$50.00	$50.00	$50.00	$150.00	0.12%
Telephone Long Distance	$35.00	$35.00	$35.00	$105.00	0.08%
Telephone Maintenance	$29.00	$29.00	$29.00	$87.00	0.07%
Total Fixed Expenses:	$19,613.67	$19,613.67	$19,613.67	$58,841.00	46.98%

Variable Expenses:

	January	February	March	Quarterly Grand Total	Percentage of Gross Income
Accounting	$100.00	$100.00	$100.00	$300.00	0.24%
Advertising General	$0.00	$0.00	$0.00	$0.00	0.00%
Attorney/Legal	$0.00	$0.00	$0.00	$0.00	0.00%
Automotive	$80.00	$80.00	$80.00	$240.00	0.19%
Bank Card Discount	$130.00	$130.00	$130.00	$390.00	0.31%
Bank Charges	$40.00	$40.00	$40.00	$120.00	0.10%
Continuing Education Staff	$20.00	$20.00	$20.00	$60.00	0.05%
Continuing Education O.D.'s	$50.00	$50.00	$50.00	$150.00	0.12%
Entertainment	$150.00	$0.00	$0.00	$150.00	0.12%
Equipment Purchase Dispensary	$0.00	$0.00	$0.00	$0.00	0.00%
Equipment Purchase Front Office	$0.00	$0.00	$0.00	$0.00	0.00%
Equipment Purchase Professional	$0.00	$0.00	$0.00	$0.00	0.00%
Equipment Purchase Lab	$0.00	$0.00	$0.00	$0.00	0.00%
Equipment Repairs	$0.00	$0.00	$0.00	$0.00	0.00%
Furnishings	$0.00	$0.00	$0.00	$0.00	0.00%
Miscellaneous	$60.00	$60.00	$60.00	$180.00	0.14%
Office Supplies	$75.00	$75.00	$75.00	$225.00	0.18%
Optometric Supplies	$50.00	$50.00	$50.00	$150.00	0.12%
Postage	$250.00	$250.00	$250.00	$750.00	0.60%
Postage Meter Reset Fees	$7.50	$7.50	$7.50	$22.50	0.02%
Printing	$0.00	$0.00	$0.00	$0.00	0.00%
Publication	$0.00	$0.00	$0.00	$0.00	0.00%
Refunds	$150.00	$150.00	$150.00	$450.00	0.36%
Shipping	$30.00	$30.00	$30.00	$90.00	0.07%
Subscriptions Front Office	$8.33	$8.33	$8.33	$25.00	0.02%
Subscriptions Professional	$4.17	$4.17	$4.17	$12.50	0.01%
Temporary Services	$0.00	$0.00	$0.00	$0.00	0.00%
Tenant Improvements	$0.00	$0.00	$0.00	$0.00	0.00%
Travel	$200.00	$150.00	$175.00	$525.00	0.42%
Tuition	$0.00	$0.00	$0.00	$0.00	0.00%
Uncollectable Debt	$185.00	$207.50	$233.75	$626.25	0.50%
Total Variable Expense:	$1,590.00	$1,412.50	$1,463.75	$4,466.25	3.57%
Total Expenses	$21,203.67	$21,026.17	$21,077.42	$63,307.25	50.54%
Net Income On Operations	$1,181.33	$4,081.33	$7,206.33	$12,469.00	9.96%

DEBT SERVICE

	January	February	March	Quarterly Grand Total	Percentage of Gross Income
Line of Credit Interest	$50.00	$50.00	$50.00	$150.00	0.12%
Line of Credit Principal	$43.00	$43.00	$43.00	$129.00	0.10%
Term Note Interest	$200.00	$200.00	$200.00	$600.00	0.48%
Term Note Principal	$195.00	$195.00	$195.00	$585.00	0.47%
Total Debt Service:	$488.00	$488.00	$488.00	$1,464.00	1.17%
Net Cash Available:	$693.33	$3,593.33	$6,718.33	$11,005.00	8.79%

Figure 41–2 Income statement—quarterly report.

costs of all items purchased for retail sales in the practice. In a typical practice, these expenditures would represent optical laboratory bills, purchases of contact lenses, frame inventory purchases, purchases of ophthalmic solutions, and any accessory items. This figure is particularly important. The difference between net sales revenue and the cost of goods sold is called the *gross margin on sales*. This figure represents the amount of income that remains after payments for material costs have been made. The gross margin on sales is the last figure in the income section of the income statement.

Operating Expenses. The operating expenses area of the financial statement is broken down into two subsets, called fixed and variable expenses (see Figure 41-2). *Fixed expenses* are defined as those expenses that are independent of the number of patients seen or amount of business done. *Variable expenses* are those expenses that are dependent on the number of patients seen or the volume of business done. Typical examples of fixed expenses are rent, salaries, and insurance premiums. Typical examples of variable expenses are laboratory bills, supplies, and commissions. Both the fixed and variable expenses are listed, and a total for the two categories is obtained, called *total expenses*. The mathematical difference between the gross margin on sales and the total operating expenses yields the *net income on operations*.

In a practice without debt this figure is the bottom line net income (see Figure 41-2). However, most practices have incurred some debt, which is described in a different section, termed *debt service*. This section breaks down the principal and interest portion of each payment according to the amortization schedule that is created for the loan. It is important that the interest portion is itemized separately because of its tax deductibility. The sum of the principal and interest should equal the *total debt service*.

The difference between the net income on operations and the total debt service will result in the true net income of the business.

Cash Flow Statement

The cash flow statement is a condensation of the income statement, sharing most of the same information (Figure 41-3), but the profit and loss statement provides a more timely and dollar relevant picture of the financial status of the company. Definitively, this statement reveals the cash flow status of the company, recording only the amount of actual payments received by the company and the actual paid expenses of the company. It specifically does not include noncash expenditures such as depreciation, credits and adjustments, or uncollectable debts. Thus it reveals a true cash picture of the profitability of a business and aids management in determining whether adjustments are needed in collections policies or spending habits.

The cash flow statement strictly compares cash in and cash out. There is no differentiation between fixed and variable expenses. The cost of goods sold and the debt service are considered ordinary expenses just like any others. It does not make any difference if the amount varies with the amount of business done or if it is fixed, because only the actual income received and actual dollars spent for a particular time period need to be measured to derive the profitability (or loss) for the business.

A cash flow statement generally is produced on a monthly basis for most businesses. However, the frequency with which this information is needed is highly individualized for each particular practice and often is based on the degree of management that is needed or desired.

Break-even Analysis

Having the ability to perform a break-even analysis for day-to-day situations is highly desirable in the private practice of optometry. Whether a practice is started cold or purchased from a practitioner, costs are incurred to purchase assets, finance inventory, and fund operating expenses. The need for seeing how quickly the revenues generated can satisfy the overhead costs and cause the practice to become profitable is essential for effective financial management and prudent fiscal planning. Optometrists, like other health care providers, must face the financial burden of having to keep offices technologically current. This cost of new equipment and the supporting technology is significant. It thus becomes very important to be able to show that the cost of this equipment can be justified by the revenue the equipment can generate. These simple concepts show the necessity of needing to be able to quickly calculate or graphically produce a break-even analysis. It is important to remember that the definition of the break-even point is "total revenues equal to total expenses," which means that no profit or loss has been incurred. In fact, the entire purpose of performing a break-even analysis is to determine the point in time at which, or the number of procedures performed after which, the first dollar of profit will be generated.

Acme Vision Clinic, P.C.
2002 Profit & Loss Statement
1 January - 31 March 2002
Quarterly Report

GROSS SALES REVENUE:	January	February	March	Quarterly Grand Total	Percentage of Gross Income
Practice Revenue					
Net Sales Revenue	$34,595.00	$38,802.50	$43,711.25	$117,108.75	100.00%

OPERATING EXPENSES:

	January	February	March	Quarterly Grand Total	Percentage of Gross Income
Accounting	$100.00	$100.00	$100.00	$300.00	0.26%
Advertising General	0.00	0.00	0.00	0.00	0.00%
Advertising Yellow Pages	500.00	500.00	500.00	1,500.00	1.28%
Attorney/Legal	0.00	0.00	0.00	0.00	0.00%
Automotive	80.00	80.00	80.00	240.00	0.20%
Bank Card Discount	130.00	130.00	130.00	390.00	0.33%
Bank Charges	40.00	40.00	40.00	120.00	0.10%
Continuing Education O.D.'s	50.00	50.00	50.00	150.00	0.13%
Continuing Education Staff	20.00	20.00	20.00	60.00	0.05%
Cost of Goods Sold	12,210.00	13,695.00	15,427.50	41,332.50	35.29%
Dues AOA	100.00	100.00	100.00	300.00	0.26%
Dues Athletic Club	75.00	75.00	75.00	225.00	0.19%
Dues Business Club	75.00	75.00	75.00	225.00	0.19%
Dues Employees	0.00	0.00	0.00	0.00	0.00%
Entertainment	150.00	0.00	0.00	150.00	0.13%
Equipment Purchase Dispensary	0.00	0.00	0.00	0.00	0.00%
Equipment Purchase Front Office	0.00	0.00	0.00	0.00	0.00%
Equipment Purchase Lab	0.00	0.00	0.00	0.00	0.00%
Equipment Purchase Professional	0.00	0.00	0.00	0.00	0.00%
Equipment Repairs	0.00	0.00	0.00	0.00	0.00%
Furnishings	0.00	0.00	0.00	0.00	0.00%
Insurance Basic Overhead	100.00	100.00	100.00	300.00	0.26%
Insurance Disability	50.00	50.00	50.00	150.00	0.13%
Insurance Major Medical	250.00	250.00	250.00	750.00	0.64%
Insurance Property/Liability	100.00	100.00	100.00	300.00	0.26%
Insurance Worker's Compensation	50.00	50.00	50.00	150.00	0.13%
Lease Office Equipment	200.00	200.00	200.00	600.00	0.51%
Lease Professional Equipment	548.00	548.00	548.00	1,644.00	1.40%
Licenses	6.67	6.67	6.67	20.01	0.02%
Line of Credit　Principal	43.00	43.00	43.00	129.00	0.11%
Line of Credit　Interest	50.00	50.00	50.00	150.00	0.13%
Miscellaneous	60.00	60.00	60.00	180.00	0.15%
Office Supplies	75.00	75.00	75.00	225.00	0.19%
Optometric Supplies	50.00	50.00	50.00	150.00	0.13%
Plant Service	65.00	65.00	65.00	195.00	0.17%
Postage	250.00	250.00	250.00	750.00	0.64%
Postage Meter Reset Fees	7.50	7.50	7.50	22.50	0.02%
Printing	0.00	0.00	0.00	0.00	0.00%
Publication	0.00	0.00	0.00	0.00	0.00%
Refunds	150.00	150.00	150.00	450.00	0.38%
Rent (including utilities)	3,000.00	3,000.00	3,000.00	9,000.00	7.69%
Salary Dr. Acme	5,000.00	5,000.00	5,000.00	15,000.00	12.81%
Salary Staff #1	1,239.58	1,239.58	1,239.58	3,718.75	3.18%
Salary Staff #2	1,097.92	1,097.92	1,097.92	3,293.75	2.81%
Shipping	30.00	30.00	30.00	90.00	0.08%
Subscriptions Front Office	8.33	8.33	8.33	24.99	0.02%
Subscriptions Professional	4.17	4.17	4.17	12.51	0.01%
Taxes Federal Income	900.00	900.00	900.00	2,700.00	2.31%
Taxes Payroll Federal	3,283.75	3,283.75	3,283.75	9,851.25	8.41%
Taxes Payroll State	798.75	798.75	798.75	2,396.25	2.05%
Taxes Personal Property	395.00	395.00	395.00	1,185.00	1.01%
Taxes State Income	400.00	400.00	400.00	1,200.00	1.02%
Telephone Basic Service	65.00	65.00	65.00	195.00	0.17%
Telephone Cellular	50.00	50.00	50.00	150.00	0.13%
Telephone Long Distance	35.00	35.00	35.00	105.00	0.09%
Telephone Maintenance	29.00	29.00	29.00	87.00	0.07%
Temporary Services	0.00	0.00	0.00	0.00	0.00%
Tenant Improvements	0.00	0.00	0.00	0.00	0.00%
Term Note　Interest	200.00	200.00	200.00	600.00	0.51%
Term Note　Principal	195.00	195.00	195.00	585.00	0.50%
Travel	200.00	200.00	200.00	600.00	0.51%
Tuition	0.00	0.00	0.00	0.00	0.00%
Uncollectable Debt	185.00	207.50	233.75	626.25	0.53%
Total Expenses	$32,701.67	$34,059.17	$35,817.92	$102,578.76	87.59%
Net Income From Operations	$1,893.33	$4,743.33	$7,893.33	$14,529.99	12.41%

Figure 41-3 Cash flow statement—quarterly report.

The essential elements for constructing a break-even analysis are the total revenues, total expenses, total fixed expenses, and total variable expenses. These values are derived from the income statement. Non-cash expenditures such as depreciation should not be included in the total fixed expenses or the total expenses because such expenditures will artificially raise or increase the break-even point. By eliminating these items from the break-even analysis, only the actual income generated and actual expenses incurred or paid out are considered. (For the calculation of a break-even analysis, see Chapter 3.)

When constructing the break-even graph it is important to establish some standards for comparison (Figure 41-4). The Y axis always represents the income values generated. The X axis represents either the amount of time passed or the number of procedures performed until break-even is reached. Total revenues are placed on the graph, with the starting point at the origin. Thus if the time is zero or if the number of procedures performed is zero, total revenue is zero. Total fixed costs will start at some income level on the Y axis, but will be at zero on the X axis. These costs will be the same regardless of time or number of procedures performed. Total costs (the total fixed costs added to the total variable costs) will use the intersection of the

fixed cost line and the Y axis as its starting point. The slope of the total costs line represents the variable costs incurred. The area between the total costs line and the fixed costs line represents the total variable costs. The point at which the total costs line and the total revenue line intersect is the break-even point ($14,000 in Fig. 41-4). The area between the total costs line and the total revenue line before the break-even point represents the loss incurred. The area between the total costs line and the total revenue line after the break-even point represents the profit gained. An optometrist can use this form of analysis very easily in the day-to-day operations of a practice to gain insightful financial information that is crucial to the planning it takes to make a practice successful.

Financial Statement Analysis

Analysis of these financial statements is critical for the assessment of a practice's financial status. It is not only important to assess the performance of the practice for the time period in question but also to analyze the financial history of the practice, which enables the optometrist to predict and plan the practice's financial future. Determining the financial status, or health of a practice, can be approached by using methodology

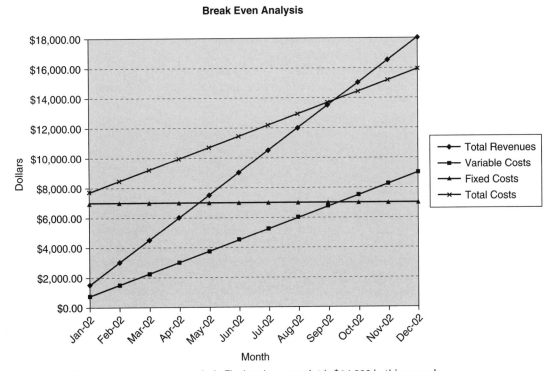

Break Even Analysis

Figure 41-4 Graph illustrating a break-even analysis. The break-even point is $14,000 in this example.

that is similar to the approach taken to patient care. A practitioner takes a case history, gathers data, performs some form of data analysis, determines a diagnosis, and prescribes a plan for treatment. In financial terms, when a practitioner takes a case history of a business, information that is relevant to the business is gathered from various sources. How many patients did the practice see? What was the gross income of the practice? What was the inventory turnover? What was the recall percentage? These are but a few of the many questions a business owner needs to ask. Gathering the data is fairly simple once it is determined what one needs to know. Obtaining the financial statements in the proper format is essential to learning necessary information about the practice. Standardization of financial statements and the information they contain is somewhat lacking in optometric practices, thus analysis can be more difficult until the information is placed into a format in which industry standards can be compared. Unless the practitioner is comparing "apples to apples," the analysis performed and conclusions reached will not be valid.

Ratio Analysis

To determine whether a business is healthy there are different ratios that can be applied to a balance sheet to determine the relationships between different variables of assets, liabilities, and net worth, or owner's equity. When the ratios are applied, it is important to use them as a means of answering questions about a business. This goal can best be accomplished by comparing the business's current data to past performance, as well as to industry standards. Standard ratios used for analysis include balance sheet ratios and various income statement ratios.

Balance Sheet Ratios

Standard balance sheet ratios that are considered useful include the current ratio, the quick ratio, and the estimate of working capital.

Current Ratio. The current ratio shows the relationship between current assets and current liabilities. Current assets are those presumed to be convertible into cash within 90 days. Current liabilities are those debts due within 1 year. The current ratio measures the business's liquidity or cash position. It is used to measure the business's ability to satisfy short-term debt. Standard accounting norms indicate that a sound current ratio would be 2:1. Interpreting this ratio means that a business has twice as many current or liquid assets as it has current debts.

Quick Ratio. This ratio compares the business's available cash plus receivables to current liabilities. The quick ratio is commonly known as the "acid test" of liquidity. It compares only the most liquid assets with current liabilities. As can be seen, only available cash and accounts receivable are used as assets in this case. A desirable quick ratio is 1:1.

Working Capital. Working capital is the mathematical difference between current assets and current liabilities, expressed in dollars. In everyday business operations it is the net working capital that provides the ability of the business to meet all obligations as they become due.

Income Statement Ratios

There are various income statement figures that can be analyzed. Among the most important are the gross margin percentage, inventory turnover, and income as a percentage of gross sales.

Gross Margin Percentage. This is the difference between the cost of products sold and their sales price. This important figure is used to determine whether the difference between the purchase cost and the selling price is adequate.

Inventory Turnover. This ratio is determined by dividing the cost of goods sold by the average inventory. To calculate the average inventory, the beginning and ending inventory for the period in question are added and this sum is divided by two. Inventory turnover allows the practitioner to compare the turnover of the practice with that of industry standards.

Income as a Percentage of Gross Sales. This is probably the most important ratio that can be obtained from an income statement. It is calculated by subtracting total expenses from total sales and dividing this figure by total sales. It shows, on a percentage basis, the portion of every dollar of sales that results in profit. It also allows the practitioner to derive, on a line item basis, what percentage of every sales dollar goes to operational expenses. This figure is very helpful because it enables the practitioner to see how and where practice dollars are spent.

Contribution Margin. This ratio is the amount by which revenue exceeds the variable cost of producing revenue. It indicates the marginal income after variable cost is covered. It is calculated by subtracting variable costs from total sales and dividing the resulting figure by total sales. This ratio can be quite helpful in determining the income necessary to cover the purchase price for equipment or the cost of additional employees (Figure 41-5).

These ratios are a few of many figures that financial analysts work with when analyzing a practice. These relationships are not inclusive, and there are many others that exist that can be applied to analyze different financial relationships within a business.

Analysis of Chair Cost

Although most optometrists have heard about or seen calculations on chair cost, many do not realize that this is the most effective method of establishing professional fees. This concept is used in many industries, yet is seldom used by optometrists due to lack of understanding, misinterpretation of results, and reluctance to change existing financial methods.

Chair cost by definition is a formula that is based on analyzing a practice's overhead, as it relates to professional services, and the number of practitioner production hours. This concept is hard for many practitioners to understand because optometry as a profession has historically relied much too heavily on the retail sale of frames, lenses, and contact lenses as the major source of practice revenue. In these changing times practitioners must be able to determine what it actually costs to produce service revenues only, without the sale of retail items. True profitability in the service portion of a practice would then be able to be accurately analyzed and prices for services accurately determined. Figure 41-6 provides an example of how chair cost is analyzed.

From this example it can be seen that chair cost is one financial tool that a practitioner simply cannot do without. With increasing third-party involvement in optometry, it also becomes the best analytical tool to use when evaluating professional service fees for profitability and for determining whether an optometrist can afford to participate in a vision service plan offered by a third-party carrier.

Productivity Statistics

One important application of economic analysis is the generation of productivity statistics. The purpose of these statistics may be to provide a financial goal for the practice or to analyze the financial performance of the practice. In the former case a goal worksheet can be prepared, which describes the productivity desired for a specific period. For example, the practice productivity goal for a month can be described in terms of the daily, weekly, and monthly revenues needed to meet the goal (Figure 41-7). The financial performance of the practice also can be analyzed over a period to evaluate the productivity of the practitioner and staff and the costs of

---

Use of Contribution Margin

An optometrist purchases a corneal topography unit for $18,000. What utilization is needed in terms of additional gross income to cover the unit's cost?

The contribution margin is the amount by which the revenue derived from the use of the unit exceeds the cost of its use.

If the contribution margin is .55 or 55%, then $\frac{\$18,000}{.55} = \$32,727$ of additional gross income.

If the contribution margin is .40 or 40%, then $\frac{\$18,000}{.40} = \$45,000$ of additional gross income.

Figure 41-5 Use of contribution margin to analyze the purchase of a corneal topography unit.

Example Calculation of Chair Cost

There are several assumptions made in this example:

• Sole practitioner

• Yearly gross income	$400,000.00
• Monthly gross income	$33,333.33
• Cost of goods sold	$9,999.99 @ 30% of gross income
• Gross margin on sales	$23,333.33 @ 70% of gross income
• Operating costs	$11,666.66 @ 35% of gross income
• Pre-tax net income	$9,999.99 @ 30% of gross income

• Comprehensive examination fee $55.00

• Monthly prorated operating expenses

       70% professional = $8,166.66

       30% dispensary   = $3,499.99

• Professional overhead/hours

       Doctor hours per month = 160 hours

       5 days per week

       250 days per year

       20 days per month

       160 hours per month

Chair Cost Calculation

$$\text{Chair Cost} = \frac{\text{Professional overhead per month}}{\text{Practitioner hours per month}}$$

$$\text{Chair Cost} = \frac{\$8,166.66}{160} = \$51.04 \text{ per hour}$$

Profit Margin on the Services Provided

$55.00 - $51.04 = $3.96 per examination or a 7.75% profit margin on services alone.

If the doctor needs to have a higher profit margin, then it should be calculated appropriately. For example, if a 20% margin is desired then the appropriate examination fee would be $61.25.

Figure 41–6 Example calculation of chair cost.

October Productivity				
2002				
Work Days In Month	Goal for Month			
23	$ 63,000.00			
Week Ending	10/6/02	10/13/02	10/20/02	10/31/02
# of Days Past:	5	10	15	23
Gross Charges	$21,039.69	$43,038.09	$56,555.00	$66,537.29
Total Receipts	$23,057.83	$43,208.55	$55,428.66	$61,484.06
Net Charges	$19,121.83	$39,283.37	$42,879.61	$63,448.93
Gross Charges/Day	$4,207.94	$4,303.81	$3,770.33	$2,892.93
Total Receipts/Day	$4,611.57	$4,320.86	$3,695.24	$2,673.22
Net Charges/Day	$3,824.37	$3,928.34	$2,858.64	$2,758.65
Monthly Projections				
Gross Charges	$96,782.57	$98,987.61	$86,717.67	$66,537.29
Total Receipts	$106,066.02	$99,379.67	$84,990.61	$61,484.06
Net Charges	$87,960.42	$90,351.75	$65,748.74	$63,448.93
Daily Billing Requirement				
To Reach Goal	$2,437.68	$1,824.36	$2,515.05	($448.93)

Figure 41-7 Example productivity goals for one month.

operation and to calculate the chair cost, contribution margin, and other economic issues of significance (Figure 41-8). Practitioners should use this information to assess the financial performance of the practice and to identify where change or improvement is needed.

Conclusion

Providing a practice with the proper financial documentation and observing sound financial practices will allow the practitioner of optometry to be able to manage and properly assess the financial condition of the practice at any given time. It also will allow financial comparisons to be made to industry-wide norms. If a practitioner is to be an effective manager, he or she must have the proper reporting methods and financial information available and must use that information to best advantage. U.S. health care has become a very competitive environment, and if survival is the rule and numbers are the playing field, then optometrists

Acme Vision Clinic, P.C.					
Productivity Statistics					
Calendar Year 2002					ANNUAL
	Q1	Q2	Q3	Q4	TOTAL RECEIPTS
Gross Receipts per Quarter	$129,583.49	$134,338.00	$168,492.00	$177,762.00	$610,175.49
Total Variable Costs per Quarter	$48,384.00	$45,260.00	$61,528.00	$62,420.00	$217,592.00
Operating Costs per Quarter	$60,385.00	$57,544.00	$66,093.00	$80,985.00	$265,007.00
Professional Costs per Quarter	$ 42,269.50	$ 40,280.80	$ 46,265.10	$ 56,689.50	$185,504.90
Dispensing Costs per Quarter	$ 18,115.50	$ 17,263.20	$ 19,827.90	$ 24,295.50	$79,502.10
	Q1	Q2	Q3	Q4	ANNUAL TOTALS
Doctor Hours per Quarter	571.56	571.56	571.56	571.56	2286.24
Full Time Staff per Quarter	3	3	3	3	
Part Time Staff per Quarter	0.5	0.5	0.5	0.5	
					ADJUSTED
2002 Examination Fee = $89.00	Quarter 1	Quarter 2	Quarter 3	Quarter 4	YEARLY AVERAGE
Chair Cost per Quarter	$73.95	$70.48	$80.95	$99.18	$81.14
Contribution per Quarter	$81,199.49	$89,078.00	$106,964.00	$115,342.00	$98,145.87
Contribution Margin per Quarter	62.66%	66.31%	63.48%	64.89%	64.33%
Staff Productivity/Hour per Quarter	$79.74	$82.67	$103.69	$109.39	$93.87

Figure 41-8 Annual productivity statistics.

must be able to grasp basic business concepts and apply them to the eye care industry.

Acknowledgement

The authors of this chapter in the first edition of *Business Aspects of Optometry* were John Rumpakis and Craig Hisaka.

Bibliography

Allergan, Inc: *Pathways in optometry.* Irvine, Calif, 1992, Author.

American Optometric Association: *Career advocate for the new practitioner.* St. Louis, 2001, Author.

Baldwin BL, Christensen B, Melton J: *Rx for success.* Midwest City, Okla, 1983, Vision Publications.

Bennett I: *Management for the eyecare practitioner.* Stoneham, Mass, 1993, Butterworth-Heinemann.

Rumpakis J: Working harder for less? *Optom Management* 33(12):31-5, 1998.

U.S. Small Business Administration: *Business basics for the growing optometric practice.* Washington, DC, 1991, U.S. Small Business Administration, Office of Business Development.

www.sba.gov/library/pubs.html. Web site for the U.S. Small Business Administration, which offers online access to many government publications.

Chapter 42

Estate Planning

John G. Classé and Gary L. Moss

Annual income twenty pounds, annual expenditure nineteen six, result happiness.
Annual income twenty pounds, annual expenditure twenty pounds ought and
six, result misery.

Charles Dickens *David Copperfield*

Although happiness may require more gain than sixpence, misery can quite properly be equated with greater expenditure than income. Indeed, a practitioner's professional life is driven by the necessity of earning more than is spent. Because there also is life after practice, practitioners face the perplexing problem of determining how to use earnings to the maximum advantage for retirement. Like most difficult problems, there are no simple solutions, no easy answers to be followed dogmatically without exception throughout life. Furthermore, the problem is compounded by the lack of experience in financial planning, economics, and money management that is the lot of the average health professions graduate. This lack of experience is probably one of the reasons that young couples argue (and divorce) over money matters more often than any other cause.

There are two ways to try and overcome lack of knowledge: education and experience. Neither way is without cost and neither is–of itself–a sufficient foundation. Both education and experience are necessary to be truly knowledgeable. For the beginning practitioner, education offers an obvious starting point, and there are many sources of information that can be consulted to acquire a working knowledge of financial matters. Because of the complexity of financial planning there is diversity of opinion, even among experts, and it is important to obtain a broad perspective before actually investing money in a plan. Even so, there are certain fundamental concepts that generally are considered the bedrock of any plan. They, in fact, may be used to develop a philosophy of estate planning.

A Philosophy of Estate Planning

For an optometry school graduate entering practice, retirement is a remote goal that is easily relegated to future consideration. In fact, planning for the future may be viewed as being in conflict with more immediate, tangible goals that are related to practice, family life, and financial demands. Such a view is shortsighted, however, and reflects a lack of understanding of the key role that estate planning–preparing for the future–plays in the life of a practitioner. One key aspect of such planning is to ensure that there is financial security, not only for retirement but also for the education of children, in the event of disability, and to protect a spouse left alone by unexpected death. Estate planning provides for both the expected and the unexpected events of life by securing adequate financial resources to manage them if they occur.

Estate planning begins with the following four fundamental steps: adequate income; a home; a cash reserve sufficient to meet emergencies; and affordable, comprehensive insurance coverage. Once these four fundamental requirements have been met, a fifth step may be considered: investment. Each of these steps is briefly described, in the usual order of acquisition.

Income

Although optometry is one of the half-dozen highest paying professions in America, statistics show that individuals in high income brackets overextend themselves with a regularity that is not remarkably dissimilar from that of individuals with more modest incomes.

Therefore, the relative affluence offered by a career in optometry does not insulate a practitioner from the financial tribulations of life. Nor does this affluence, of itself, ensure that a practitioner will be able to attain financial security. It probably does establish great expectations, but these expectations must be tempered by reality.

Studies conducted by the American Optometric Association (AOA) during the past 50 years have created a relatively clear picture of the income levels of optometrists (see Chapter 1). Of course, the great majority of optometrists are in private practice, which represents the most affluent career option in the profession. The net income earned by a private practitioner, however, is related to the number of years that the practitioner has been in practice. Therefore, to obtain an accurate picture of the income that a practitioner should expect to earn, the number of years in practice must be known. The AOA surveys are most useful in this regard.

An optometrist's income is subject to diminution by inflation and taxes no matter the stage of practice, but the income of a beginning practitioner is further diminished by the economics of entry into private practice. The AOA economic surveys have shown that a 5- to 7-year period is required to establish a practice started "cold" and to pay off educational debts. In addition, the usual period that is required to rise from associate to full partner in a practice generally is the same. Payment for the purchase of an existing practice usually involves a period of 5 to 10 years. Surveys also have revealed that, on the average, a private practitioner reaches the national net mean income for optometrists after 10 years. A young practitioner must consider this 5- to 10-year building period when organizing an estate plan and must take care not to formulate unrealistic goals or expectations.

After this initial period is passed, however, net income continues to rise until after 20 years of practice. The relative affluence of this second phase in private practice is challenged by the financial responsibilities of raising a family. After 20 years, net earnings tend to drop slowly until retirement.

These statistics suggest that during the first years of practice a young practitioner should ignore any thoughts of estate planning and instead should concentrate on the demanding task of establishing a financial base. Such a suggestion would, however, be false. In fact, estate planning is vital during the initial period of building a practice, when discipline and a calculated approach toward achieving financial goals are essential. Budgeting of income will be necessary and will have much to do with the practitioner's ability to obtain adequate housing and savings—two prerequisites of estate planning.

A budget is a necessity, both in professional and private life. Effort must be expended to try and stay within the budget's guidelines, which means that income and expenditures must be carefully monitored to ascertain whether that extra "sixpence" is being earned or a deficit is being generated. Good financial recordkeeping will permit adjustments to be made for the cost of living, inflation, and changes in tax laws. It is essential to maintain adequate recordkeeping so that realistic budgeting can be achieved.

There are two simple but important rules of personal budgeting: limit the cost of renting or purchasing a home to no more than 28% of net income and put 10% of net income into a liquid fund that can be used for emergencies. This approach allows 62% of net income to be used for other needs, such as subsistence, servicing of automobiles and appliances, entertainment and vacations, and insurance premiums. Insurance is a particularly important budget item.

Insurance is a necessity that constitutes a fixed charge on income. It is cheapest when acquired at a young age and is an important means of protecting and generating an "estate" if untimely death intercedes. It can cover the loss of a home; personal and property damage involving automobiles; unexpected disability; and accidents or injuries occurring at work, in the home, or elsewhere. Comprehensive coverage should be planned for and acquired, and a reasonable budget should be maintained for insurance premium costs.

Although the statistics compiled by the AOA provide a composite representation of the mean income earned by optometrists, individual circumstances may vary well above or below these averages. No matter what the actual income is, however, it should be adequate to satisfy the following three criteria:

- The income is adequate for the practitioner's budgetary needs, which are based on financial records maintained by the practitioner, and satisfies the practitioner's obligation for a home, cash reserve, and insurance protection
- The income will grow above the eroding effects of inflation and taxation
- The income will be sufficient to allow for investing or participation in a tax-deferred retirement plan.

Budgeting of income for the rental or purchase of a home is one of the first concerns of a young practitioner.

The Home

The choice of where to live usually is based on considerations of personal taste. The selection of a home, because of its potential as an investment, only peripherally enters into the process, despite the assurances of real estate agents that "buying is better than renting." For some individuals, buying is not better than renting because purchasing a home incurs an obligation that extends beyond the cost of a mortgage to include the expenses of furniture, appliances, repairs, remodeling, insurance, taxes, and similar items. There also is the investment of capital into a home–capital that could be used for other purposes, such as the generation of income. Whether the purchase of a home is a good choice depends on the practitioner's circumstances and the economic burden that the payment of home-related expenses represents. If a practitioner makes the choice to purchase a home, however, the decision to do so will exert a significant effect on the practitioner's estate plan.

The purchase of a home provides some unique estate planning benefits, described in the following:

• The home, if well chosen, may appreciate by as much as 8% to 12% annually during the period of ownership; this return on capital is rather substantial, and since a home increases in value with inflation, the eroding effects of inflation are neutralized.
• Interest on a home mortgage is deductible on the owner's personal income tax return.
• The payment of a home mortgage, because it also is a return of principal, actually increases the value of the home to the owner; for each payment made, the debt is reduced, thereby increasing the owner's equity or value in the home.
• Taxes on a home are deductible.

Therefore, a home does provide what may be considered an investment return, thereby providing a benefit to the estate plan. There also are some disadvantages to home ownership, described in the following, that must be considered:

• A home is not a liquid asset and cannot be disposed of quickly; months usually are required before a sale can be transacted.
• The costs required to maintain a home can exceed budgetary expectations and capabilities.
• A home must be held for a number of years before a sizeable financial return can be realized.
• If the selection of a home is not wisely made, it may actually decrease in value.

The cost of a home occupies a central position in the budget of a homeowner. The down payment required to secure a home mortgage generally is 5% to 10% of the home's cost. The size of monthly mortgage payments will be considered by the mortgage company and should be no more than 28% of the homeowner's net income. Payments may be the same from month to month, which is the traditional method of amortized mortgage payment, or they may vary in accordance with the lending rate offered by the mortgage company. Variable rate mortgages have a ceiling, beyond which they cannot increase, and may require "balloon" payments after several years, which could have a large negative impact on budgetary planning.

One other aspect of home ownership that has significance for estate planning is the title. The title to real estate is of particular significance for married couples because the title to real estate can be divided or undivided among the owners. An undivided interest has several advantages because of the right of joint survivorship. A form of title known as *Tenancy by the Entirety* or *Joint Tenancy with Right of Survivorship* considers both spouses to be owners of the entire estate, with the right of joint survivorship. At the death of either spouse, the survivor is considered to be the owner of the home.

Another important consequence of an undivided title involves the rights of creditors. If the title is *Tenancy by the Entirety* or *Joint Tenancy with Right of Survivorship*, creditors cannot satisfy their claims out of the real estate unless both owners are debtors. Therefore, if an optometrist borrows from a bank to finance a practice and is not able to repay the debt, the creditor may proceed against any collateral that the optometrist has used to secure the loan. Unless the optometrist's spouse also has signed the loan agreement, the bank may not collect the amount due from the optometrist by selling the house. The reason is that the spouse has an undivided interest in the realty, and because this interest was not used as collateral for the loan, it cannot be used to collect the debt of the optometrist. For practitioners who are in community-property states, there are special considerations that require consultation with a lawyer whenever property transactions are anticipated.

Besides the acquisition of a home, estate planning also requires the accumulation of a cash reserve for emergencies.

Cash Reserve

A cash reserve provides needed security for a practitioner, particularly in the event of emergencies or other situations that call for the immediate use of cash. The cash reserve can be likened to a piggy bank, which is dutifully filled with an allowance–usually cited as 10% of net income–until 4 to 6 months worth of gross income has been accumulated. After this goal has been attained and insurance needs have been fulfilled, income can be used for investment.

There are several means of accumulating liquid assets that may serve as a cash reserve: savings accounts, interest bearing checking accounts, certificates of deposit, whole life insurance policies, and credit cards.

Savings Accounts. This traditional method of accumulating a cash reserve allows savings to grow, although at a rather modest rate that may not be able to keep up with inflation. Even so, the return of interest is guaranteed, and savings accounts have the advantage of liquidity, which means that money can be withdrawn on demand. In addition, most savings accounts are insured up to a certain maximum, either by the Federal Deposit Insurance Corporation or the Federal Savings and Loan Insurance Corporation.

Interest Bearing Checking Accounts. Beginning in the 1980s, interest bearing checking accounts—known as negotiated order of withdrawal (NOW) accounts—have offered an alternative means of accumulating income in an on-demand cash reserve. The interest paid on NOW accounts is offset by service charges that can be avoided only if a minimum balance is maintained in the account each month. As a result, larger sums have been deposited in checking accounts and lesser amounts into savings accounts.

Certificates of Deposit. Although not truly a cash reserve, certificates of deposit (CDs) are another means of setting aside cash in an interest bearing account so that it is available in times of emergency. The interest paid on CDs is higher than that for savings accounts or interest bearing checking accounts, but to receive the interest payment the CD must be held for a specified period, which may be as short as 6 months or as long as several years. The longer the period, the higher the interest paid. If the CD is cashed in before the period has expired, a penalty must be paid, so CDs do not have the liquidity of savings accounts and NOW accounts.

Whole Life Insurance Policies. These policies acquire cash value in addition to providing insurance protection. Over a number of years the cash value can accumulate to a nice sum. This money can be withdrawn or borrowed, with or without an interest charge, depending on the type of policy and its provisions. The capacity to withdraw or borrow the cash value of a policy should be considered when purchasing whole life insurance as part of an estate plan.

Credit Cards. Although credit cards cannot properly constitute part of a cash reserve, they can provide a source of income—borrowed money—in an emergency. A line of credit is established, based on the income of the cardholder, and the cardholder may draw cash up to the credit ceiling as long as periodic payments are made to reduce the balance. Interest rates, though high, have not been subject to the same fluctuations as the prime interest rate in recent years, and they usually do not compare too unfavorably with the interest rates charged by commercial banks. For a practitioner, credit cards are a necessity, providing identification, immediate credit, and a means of recording professional expenses for tax purposes. They can be abused, however, by individuals who do not have the discipline to restrict their use.

If a practitioner can realize an adequate income, acquire a satisfactory home, and make systematic contributions to a cash reserve, there is one remaining prerequisite—adequate insurance coverage. This last step is a sizeable one, requiring an understanding of the basic types of insurance and their proper use in an estate plan.

Insurance Coverage

Although the fundamental purpose of insurance is to provide financial protection against disaster, insurance also can be used as an estate planning device. Some typical uses of life insurance, for example, include the following:

- For the payment of the costs of death, including debts, taxes and the immediate expenses incurred by the estate
- To create a "nest egg" for the spouse or family of the deceased
- To provide cash for the payment of the mortgage balance on a home through the purchase of a mortgage rider
- To fund a cross-purchase agreement between partners or stockholders of a professional association or corporation
- For the protection of a practice against the death of a "key person"

The primary purpose of life insurance is to provide money in the event of death. In return for payment of premiums the insurance company agrees to pay the face amount of the policy to the beneficiary at the death of the insured. Although some types of life insurance—such as universal life policies—often are referred to as "investments," life insurance primarily provides protection, with some utilization for estate planning.

There are four types of insurance that should be acquired by a practitioner: life, disability, professional liability, and personal (health, automobile, home). Each type of insurance should be thoroughly understood before it is purchased.

Life Insurance

There are two basic types of life insurance, term and whole life. *Term* policies provide only death benefit insurance coverage for a specific period, usually one to five years. The cost of term insurance initially is cheaper than whole life coverage, but the cost increases with age. Term policies usually are not available after age 65. *Whole life* policies provide both insurance and investment return, thereby acquiring a "cash value" that can be borrowed against. The premium is based on the age at which the policy is taken out and does not change. *Ordinary life* policies require payment for the insured's whole life; *limited payment life* policies limit premiums to a certain age, at which time the insurance coverage becomes permanent. *Universal life* is popular with professionals because it combines insurance with reasonable investment return and permits tax-free withdrawals to be made (up to the amount contributed). *Variable life* is a more investment-oriented policy that provides insurance coverage linked to a portfolio of securities. The higher the return on the investments, the greater the death benefit or value of the policy.

Because of its lower cost, term is often the first life insurance that is purchased. An alternative is whole life, with a mortgage payment rider if the insured is a homeowner. This rider actually is a decreasing term policy that pays to the beneficiary the amount owed on the home mortgage at the time of the insured's death. Later in life, term policyholders may convert to a whole life policy or purchase a whole life policy such as universal life.

Payment of the life insurance proceeds is for the face value of the policy, plus any cash value if a whole life policy was purchased. Payment may be in a lump sum, over a fixed period, in fixed installments, or for the life of the beneficiary (as with an annuity).

When attempting to determine the amount of life insurance to purchase there are several factors to be considered, including the earning power of the practitioner, the earning capacity of the spouse, educational obligations to the children or spouse, and the amount of debt that has been acquired. In general, these considerations tend to indicate that life insurance protection should equal 5 to 7 years worth of gross income plus 5 to 7 years worth of debt (such as loans, mortgages).

Disability Insurance

Serious disability is a much more likely eventuality than premature death, yet disability insurance is far less likely to be planned for than life insurance. Policies are expensive, and the benefits vary considerably from policy to policy.

Disability insurance pays the disabled policyholder a guaranteed monthly income, which is expressed as a percentage of earned income before disability. The percentage usually is limited to 50% to 60%; proof of income will be needed to establish policy coverage.

Office overhead insurance is used to cover the expenses of running a practice when a sole practitioner is disabled. The benefits paid are limited to actual overhead expenses (e.g., staff salaries, utilities, office rent) and for a stated period (18 to 24 months). Office overhead insurance does not pay for nonoverhead items such as laboratory bills and the costs of a substitute practitioner.

Professional Liability Insurance

Insurance coverage will be needed to protect practitioners against liability claims and provide for the costs of defense, including attorney's fees and court costs, and for the cost of any judgment or settlement, up to the policy limit. A typical insurance policy will cover claims arising out of negligence, defamation, product liability, premises liability, or vicarious (employee) liability. Extra coverage usually is needed for professional employees (e.g., associate optometrists, opticians), to cover embezzlement, and for injuries to employees (if there is no worker's compensation). The amount of insurance coverage should be at least $1 million per claimant; the purchase of an extra $1 million is worth the usually modest cost.

Personal Insurance

To provide coverage for personal needs, insurance should be purchased to protect health, home, and vehicles.

Health insurance will be needed until age 65, when eligibility for Medicare is attained. Major medical coverage is often a beginning point for young self-employed practitioners, but employed optometrists may be able to secure health insurance as a benefit of employment.

Homeowner's insurance provides coverage for injuries occurring on the property; damage from fire, lightning, and other perils; and loss of personal property. In the event of total loss, the personal effects are valued as a percentage of the coverage on the home (usually 50% to 60%). There is a limit to the value of individual items unless they are "scheduled." Items of special value (such as jewelry, works of art, antiques) should be appraised and listed on a schedule for their fair market value. Of course, an extra premium is paid for these items.

Vehicles should be adequately insured for liability, collision, uninsured motorist, and comprehensive coverage. Coverage should be adequate to protect the policyholder (and family) in the event an accident occurs; generally, the policy limits are increased as the policyholder's economic status improves over the course of years.

Fire and Other Casualty Insurance

Beginning practitioners usually lease office space in a building. To provide protection in the event of fire, coverage of office contents should be obtained. Insurance should be purchased for the replacement value (rather than fair market value) of contents. Receipts, photographs, and other documentation of insured items and their value should be retained. If a practitioner owns a building, adequate coverage must be obtained, both for partial and for full loss. Because buildings appreciate in value, insurance coverage for 80% of the building's fair market value will provide coverage in the event of a 100% loss. Because of appreciation, it also is necessary to adjust insurance limits periodically. Other casualty coverage for burglary, theft, office contents, professional equipment, general liability, and other perils is best purchased as multiperil insurance; comprehensive coverage under such a package often can be cheaper than the purchase of individual policies for these contingencies.

A list of insurance policies should be compiled and used to assess and monitor insurance coverage (Table 42-1).

Once the four basic requirements of estate planning have been satisfied, income may be used for purposes of investment.

Investment

Many variables must be considered when making investment decisions, which are educated projections of the potential economic performance of selected items. Inflation and interest rates must be considered because they will affect how quickly investments will grow, how much buying power the earned income of a portfolio will achieve, and how much buying power the earned income of a portfolio will have at retirement. Safety and risk also are major factors that must be considered when choosing an investment. As a rule, the safer the investment the less the reward (i.e., the lower the earnings), and although with very risky investments it is possible that a large windfall profit could result, it is more likely that all or much of the investment will be lost. (Otherwise, those offering the investment opportunity would not be willing to reward the investor so greatly for assuming the high risk.) Another variable that must be weighed is liquidity, which is the ease with which the investment can be converted into cash. Liquidity affords an investor the opportunity to change investments, typically to a better one, without incurring a significant loss. Investments without liquidity can take months to convert to cash and may result in a loss, such as the sale of real estate in a down market.

There are three general characteristics of an investment that will affect the decision-making process:

Will the investment produce income? Different investments will produce income in different ways; mutual funds, stocks, and bonds will offer dividends; rental property (e.g., an apartment building) will produce cash payments.

Will the investment appreciate? Some investments may not produce an income while they are owned, but instead will increase in value, with profit being realized only when the investment is sold. This type of investment usually is considered speculative in nature and includes gold, gems, or collectible items, which may or may not increase in value as anticipated. Appreciation of these items usually is better during a period of inflation.

Will the investment be convertible? How quickly can an investment be sold and turned into cash without a loss in value? If convertibility is a major concern, investments of a more speculative nature—such as real estate and collectibles—are not a good choice since they will take longer to liquidate in many cases.

There are three basic levels of investment: short term (less than 2 years), intermediate term (2 to 5 years), and long term (greater than 5 years). These different levels of investment must be considered when designing an investment plan. In fact, an

Table 42-1 Summary of Insurance Types and Use

BUSINESS USE		
TYPE	**PURPOSE**	**COST**
Life		
Decreasing term	Security for loan (assigned to creditor)	Moderate
Group term	Benefit for employees	Moderate
Cross or entity purchase	Payment at death of partner	Moderate to high
Disability		
Group or private	Benefit for employees	Moderate to high
Office overhead	Payment for fixed operating expenses	Moderate
Health		
Group or private	Benefit for employees	Moderate to high
Liability		
Professional liability	Liability claims against doctor and employees	Modest
Casualty	Loss of office contents from fire or other peril	Moderate
Worker's compensation	Work-related injuries to employees	Modest
Embezzlement	Theft by employees	Modest
Premises	Injuries to persons in office or on premises	Moderate
PERSONAL USE		
TYPE	**PURPOSE**	**COST**
Life		
Term or whole life	Security for family	Moderate to high
Disability		
Group or private	Payment for loss of capacity to work	Moderate to high
Health		
Group or private	Medical and hospitalization costs	Moderate to high
Home		
Decreasing term rider	Payment of home mortgage at death	Moderate
Premises	Injuries to persons on the premises	Moderate
Homeowners	Loss of home and personal effects from casualty	Moderate
Vehicle		
Liability and collision	Damage to vehicles and injuries to persons	Moderate to high
Uninsured motorist	Personal injury from uninsured driver	Modest
Casualty	Vehicle loss or damage due to fire or theft	Moderate

investment portfolio may be regarded in the same way as a house, with the foundation needing to be strong enough to protect the upper structures. The foundation should be built on the four fundamentals of estate planning, with appropriate protection afforded by basic insurance and ready cash reserves that can be drawn on as necessary. Funding for minor emergency situations should be available from CDs, savings accounts, and cash value in whole life insurance policies. These types of investments have very little risk and can be readily converted into cash if the need arises. Only after this protection is obtained should an investor go on to riskier investments that may yield greater returns. Stocks, bonds, and mutual funds are among the more popular types of investments. These three types of investment differ significantly (Box 42-1).

Another type of low-risk investment that can be used is a tax-deferred retirement plan, such as an individual retirement account (IRA) or a pension plan. These investments grow in value over time and provide income at retirement. The riskiest types of investments should be considered only after a proper foundation has been achieved because they are speculative ventures that may yield little return, such as tax-sheltered limited partnerships in oil, dairy, or equipment leasing companies, or collectibles, such as art, gold, coins, and antiques.

Box 42-1 Types of Investments

Stocks

Stocks are issued by corporations to obtain money to finance the start-up or operation of the corporation. There are two types of stock, common and preferred.

Common stock holders are the owners of the corporation and are entitled to share in the profits—called dividends—of the company. When a corporation first sells its stock, the price is set, but afterwards the value of the stock is based on the prosperity of the company. If the company is well run and profitable, the value of the stock increases; if it is mismanaged and suffers a loss, the value decreases (and there is no dividend). Preferred stock is a more stable investment because dividends are fixed in advance and thus—unlike common stock dividends, which depend on the generation of profits—fluctuations in dividends are minimal. A preferred stockholder is more of a financial backer than an owner, and the stockholder's investment is better protected than with common stock.

The traditional method of earning money from the stock market is to "buy low and sell high." Of course, the successful investor must not only determine that a particular company is solvent and well structured but also that it faces favorable market conditions and industry prospects.

Bonds

Bonds are long-term obligations that pay back a stated amount—the principal—at the end of a term of years (usually 20 or 30 years) and another stated amount—the interest—each year. Bonds are issued to obtain financing for long-term capital investments. The usual sources of bonds are corporations; public utilities; and federal, state, and local governments. The interest paid on a bond is based on interest rates at the time of issue. If interest rates are high at the time of issuance, but they subsequently fall, the bond issuers will want to redeem the bonds because money can be borrowed at lower cost. For this reason, investors may demand "call protection" for high-interest bonds, which prevent the bonds from being redeemed for a period of years.

The bond market constantly adjusts the value of outstanding bonds to compensate for changes in interest rates. If interest rates go up, the value of outstanding bonds goes down, and if interest rates go down, the value of outstanding bonds goes up. No matter how much of a "discount" is placed on the market value of a bond, however, it is redeemable at maturity for the full face value.

Bonds may be held until maturity or they can be bought and sold like stocks, through brokers. Some bonds are tax exempt, such as bonds issued by municipalities; others, such as U.S. Treasury bonds, are exempt from state and local income taxation only.

Whether taxable or tax exempt, the interest on a bond will automatically be paid if the bond is issued in registered form (i.e., the owner's name and address is on the bond), but if the bond is in bearer form (i.e., no name is on the bond) a coupon has to be clipped off and sent in to receive payment.

Mutual Funds

These large investment funds were created to allow small investors to enjoy the advantages of professional money management, reduction of risk, and mobility of investment. Mutual funds are large investment units, composed of the funds of thousands of individuals, which purchase a highly diversified portfolio containing a wide variety of investment vehicles. The size and diversity of these funds protect against large changes in value even when economic indicators shift suddenly. Mutual funds may be classified on the basis of their purpose. Growth funds are used for long-term investments that will appreciate over time; income funds are used to provide more immediate financial return. Funds also can be classified by type of investment, such as specialty funds (which concentrate on certain industries) and balanced funds (which invest in bonds as well as stocks). There also are load and no-load funds. In load funds, a sales charge must be paid at the time the investment is purchased, whereas for no-load funds there is no sales charge.

Mutual funds are used for long-term investment, and the type of fund in which to purchase shares is dependent on the goals of the investor.

An investment portfolio can be built to include all these items, based on the retirement plan of the investor. The ability of these investments to provide for retirement is the guiding force behind the investment strategy.

Retirement Plans

It is essential that retirement planning begin well ahead of retirement, preferably soon after graduation from optometry school. There is a sizeable financial benefit to be derived from beginning retirement planning early, rather than late, in a career (Table 42-2). Retirement planning is an essential part of an estate plan. It is almost certain that any Social Security benefits or employee pension plan payments will be inadequate to satisfy the retiree's needs, especially if the retiree is fortunate enough to be healthy and to live for many years.

There are three key elements involved in planning for retirement: forethought, patience, and specific goal setting. The investor must be able to project expenses and monetary needs 30 to 40 years into the future. Some expenses most likely will decrease, such as housing, food, and taxes. A retiree may wish to spend more time traveling, however, which would be an increased expense. Medical costs also could increase at retirement. In addition, retirement planning will have to take into account the effects of inflation, which will increase retirement costs and necessitate a higher retirement income. The investor must estimate specific retirement needs, set financial goals that will obtain the necessary financial resources, and have the patience to follow the plan over several decades. In constructing a retirement plan, an investor must consider the financial benefits to

be derived from Social Security, work-related pension plans, insurance plans, and personal investments.

Social Security

At present, full eligibility for Social Security begins at age 65, and partial eligibility can be elected at age 62. A retiree receives monthly benefits, which are based on the years of contribution to Social Security by the retiree. An estimate of these benefits can be obtained at any time by directing an inquiry to the Social Security Administration. These payments are modest, however, and inadequate to fund a retirement plan.

Pension Plans

Pension plans are tax-deferred retirement plans in which a certain amount of an employee's income is deducted, placed in an investment account, and allowed to grow without taxation until withdrawal at retirement. These plans usually are available to the employees of corporations (including professional associations, professional corporations, and S corporations)

Table 42-2 Accumulating and Depleting a Retirement Fund

The annual investment needed to accumulate a $100,000 fund for retirement is determined by the amount contributed each year and the percentage return on the investment. The following table illustrates the amount of money, interest rate, and length of time the money would have to be invested to accumulate a $100,000 fund.

INTEREST RATE	5 YR	10 YR	15 YR	20 YR	25 YR	30 YR
5%	$17,236	$7572	$4414	$2880	$1966	$1433
6%	$16,736	$7157	$4053	$2565	$1720	$1193
7%	$16,254	$6764	$3719	$2280	$1478	$989
8%	$15,783	$6392	$3410	$2024	$1267	$817
9%	$15,332	$6039	$3125	$1793	$1083	$673
10%	$14,890	$5704	$2861	$1587	$924	$553

The length of time required to deplete a retirement fund depends on the amount withdrawn each year and the investment return being earned. The following table illustrates the number of years needed to deplete a $100,000 retirement fund, based on a regularly monthly withdrawal.

MONTHLY WITHDRAWAL	INTEREST RATE OF INVESTMENT					
	5%	6%	7%	8%	9%	10%
$600	23	29	*	*	*	*
$700	18	20	25	*	*	*
$800	14	16	18	22	30	*
$900	12	13	14	16	19	26
$1000	10	11	12	13	15	17
$1200	8	9	9	10	10	11
$1400	7	7	7	9	9	9
$1600	6	6	6	7	7	7

*Withdrawals can be made indefinitely at this rate.

and of incorporated multidisciplinary practices (such as heath maintenance organizations). There are two main types of plans: defined contribution and defined benefit.

Defined contribution plans permit a specified amount to be placed in the pension plan each year. These plans can be funded with stock bonuses, profit sharing, and matching contributions from the employer. The most frequently used plan is a 401(k), which permits a limited amount (set by the employer) to be contributed annually to the pension fund. These plans, if begun early in practice, can create a sizable retirement fund for the contributor.

Defined benefit plans are based on actuarial projections and allow contributions to be placed in the pension plan each year, for the purpose of paying a stated benefit during retirement. The amount of the benefit is set by the retiree, and the amount contributed each year is based on this benefit and the anticipated years of retirement that the retiree will have. Because these plans permit large amounts to be contributed, they are most often used by individuals who have a limited number of years before retirement and want to maximize their contributions.

Personal Investments

There are several plans available to self-employed professionals, including IRAs, simplified employee pension IRAs, 401(k)s, and Keogh plans (see Chapter 33).

Individual retirement accounts allow money to be placed in a designated custody or trust account established for this purpose. The two big advantages of a *traditional IRA* are that the yearly contribution can be deducted from income taxes and the contribution earns tax-free interest until it is withdrawn at retirement, disability, or death. With *Roth IRAs*, although income contributed to the account is not tax deductible, all withdrawals are. In addition, there is no age limit for contributions. Contributors to IRA accounts can choose the type of investment (within certain limits) for the IRA funds. The contributor is eligible to start withdrawing income from the IRA at age 59½ and must do so by age 70½. If income is needed before eligibility is attained–other than for disability or death–income tax and a 10% penalty must be paid on the amount withdrawn. Anyone may set up an IRA–employers or employees–and IRA accounts may be established even though the contributor also participates in other types of retirement plans. Although the annual contribution to an IRA account is small compared with that for pension and Keogh plans, if such an account in begun early in a professional's career and is diligently contributed to, a sizeable nest egg may be realized at retirement.

Simplified employee pension individual retirement accounts (SEP-IRAs) are like IRA accounts. A self-employed practitioner or qualified employees may contribute annually to an SEP IRA, and the contributions will be tax deferred until withdrawn at retirement, disability, or death. Like an IRA, the contributions are invested and grow tax free until withdrawn between the ages of 59½ and 70½. However, allowable SEP IRA contributions are much higher than those for traditional and Roth IRAs and thus permit more income to be set aside for retirement.

401(k) plans allow employees to contribute a percentage of income ("salary reduction") to a retirement fund. Employers may voluntarily contribute an additional amount to employees' funds, but both these and the employees' contributions are subject to moderate annual limits. A 401(k) plan can be a profit-sharing plan or a pension plan, or a combination of both. The employee's contributions are excluded from gross income, and all earnings are tax sheltered until withdrawn.

Keogh plans are popular with self-employed practitioners, but eligible employees also must be allowed to participate in the plan, which permits sizable contributions to be excluded from income and contributed to a retirement fund. Like pension plans, there are both defined contribution and defined benefit plans, the latter allowing practitioners who have contributed little to retirement to divert substantial amounts of income, usually late in their careers, to an income-earning plan that is not taxed until proceeds are withdrawn at retirement.

Insurance Plans

When whole life insurance policies are purchased, they provide not only death benefits but also cash value, which can be withdrawn and used as retirement income. The cash value of a policy is dependent on the investment of the premium payment by the insurer and the length of time premiums have been paid. If money is borrowed against the cash value of a policy, an interest charge may have to be paid. At death, the amount borrowed will be deducted from the death benefit paid to the policy beneficiary. The cost of whole life insurance is more than term coverage because of the accumulation of cash value. Whole life policies constitute a type of forced savings plan, which may be preferable for individuals who cannot follow an established budget or investment plan. Whether whole life or term policies are preferable for a given individual depends on that individual's needs, abilities, and retirement plan.

Annuities

Annuities can be used to provide retirement income. At retirement, a whole life insurance policy can be converted into a *single premium immediate annuity*. The annuity is purchased with the cash value of the policy and immediately begins paying an income to the policyholder, either for the policyholder's life or for a set number of years. A *single premium deferred annuity* may be purchased before retirement but also with the cash value of the insurance policy. A loan is taken out, equal to the cash value, and used to pay for the annuity. Like other investment funds, the annuity grows on a tax-deferred basis over time until retirement, when withdrawals may be made. Retirement income is provided for the life of the policyholder or for a period of years, depending on the type of payment option chosen.

Retirement Goals

When considering these various means of funding a retirement plan, the investor should consider the following questions:

- Do I have clear goals in mind as to what I hope to achieve with my retirement fund?
- Will the income from the retirement fund be adequate for my needs?
- Is the retirement plan performing up to my expectations?
- Is the retirement plan set up for maximum tax benefits, both for myself and my heirs?
- Am I sufficiently familiar with the specifics of my plan?
- Have I discussed my retirement plan with my spouse?
- Am I reviewing and monitoring my retirement fund regularly?

Of course, planning is only half of the effort to build an estate; execution of the plan also is necessary. The actual execution of a plan usually requires the advice and assistance of a financial advisor. The wise investor will obtain a knowledgeable professional advisor to assist in the efforts to acquire an adequate retirement fund.

Transfer of Estate

A good estate plan provides for the transfer of the planner's estate at death to the desired heirs with minimum taxation. Federal law imposes a unified transfer tax on lifetime gifts and property that passes at death. A carefully drawn will is essential, not only to minimize taxes but also to ensure that the decedent's estate passes to the appropriate individuals at death.

Wills

A person who leaves a will is said to die testate; if there is no will, the person is intestate. In such a case, state law (referred to as statutes of "descent and distribution") will determine the manner in which the property is to be divided. Relatives of the decedent are specified in these statutes, beginning with spouse and children, and if there are none, to parents and siblings and others of more remote blood relation. Only if there are no heirs that can be found does the property escheat (revert) to the state.

The purpose of a will is to direct how the estate of the decedent is to be distributed. The person given the responsibility to see that the estate is properly divided is called the executor. The will should identify this person and describe the powers to be exercised by the executor in carrying out the provisions of the will. The will must be submitted to probate court, where a judge will ensure that the will is indeed the last testament of the deceased and oversee the administration of the estate by the executor.

Wills should provide for the distribution of the estate if both spouses die in a common disaster. Some states have adopted the Uniform Simultaneous Death Act (all joint property is halved). Wills also need to provide for minor children when both parents die at or about the same time. A trust often is used. The executor transfers the estate proceeds into the trust, which is then administered by the trustee in accordance with the trust instrument's provisions (e.g., for the support and education of the children). A guardian also can be named in the will to serve as the "parent" for the children; however, the probate court is not bound by the will's choice and may select another individual if the judge is convinced it is in the child's best interests to do so.

Complex wills should be drafted by a competent attorney. Holographic (handwritten) wills are enforceable, as long as they have been property executed (signed). The signing of the will must be witnessed; the number of required witnesses varies from state to state but usually is two or three persons. These individuals should be readily identifiable and relatively easy to contact for purposes of attesting to the will's authenticity.

The estate may be subject to both federal and state taxes, which are determined and paid during the pro-

Table 42-3 The Unified Gift and Estate Tax Credit

YEAR	FOR GIFT TAX PURPOSES		FOR ESTATE TAX PURPOSES	
	UNIFIED CREDIT	EXCLUSION AMOUNT	UNIFIED CREDIT	EXCLUSION AMOUNT
2002 and 2003	$345,800	$1,000,000	$345,800	$1,000,000
2004 and 2005	$345,800	$1,000,000	$555,800	$1,500,000
2006, 2007, and 2008	$345,800	$1,000,000	$780,800	$2,000,000
2009	$345,800	$1,000,000	$1,455,800	$3,500,000

Data From: Internal Revenue Service publication 950, Introduction to gift and estate taxes.

bate process. There are some important ways in which the estate can be reduced for purposes of determining the tax, so that heirs can inherit more of the estate and the state and federal government less.

Estate and Gift Taxes

The federal estate tax is imposed on the gross estate of the decedent at death, which consists of the following:
- Property that the decedent owns at death
- Transfers of property that are effective at death (e.g., annuities)
- Transfers occurring within 3 years of death (except certain gifts)
- Life insurance proceeds paid because of death
- Property owned in joint tenancy (e.g., a house)
- Payments from qualified retirement plans (e.g., IRAs)

Generally, the value of the estate is the fair market value of the property that composes the estate at the date of death. The taxable estate is the gross estate, minus the following:
- Administration and funeral expenses
- Claims against the estate
- Casualty and theft losses (if any)
- Charitable deductions (if any)
- Marital deduction

The *marital deduction* is allowed for the value of property in the estate that is passed to a surviving spouse. Therefore, it is limited only to the gifts and bequests made to the spouse; there is no monetary limit. The marital deduction is an important estate planning device since it allows the property transferred to the surviving spouse to be excluded from estate taxes.

Life insurance is subject to special provisions. If the policy was given to a surviving spouse, and the decedent retained no incidents of ownership after the gift, the life insurance proceeds will be excluded from the

taxable estate. If the gift occurred within the 3 years before death, however, it will be included in the taxable estate.

For a home owned as *Tenants by the Entirety* or as *Joint Tenants with Right of Survivorship*, one half of the fair market value of the home will be included in the taxable estate.

The estate tax also is affected by gifts made by the deceased. As of 2002 a gift tax was imposed on gifts that exceeded $11,000 per individual (the "annual exclusion"–this amount is increased annually by cost-of-living adjustments). A gift to a spouse that qualifies for the marital deduction is excluded from taxation. For gifts in excess of the annual exclusion, a return must be filed, Form 709, *United States Short Form Gift Tax Return*, by April 15 of the year after the gifts were made. The gift tax is computed on the return. (The donor pays the tax, not the recipient of the gift.) However, there is a Unified Credit that may be applied to the gift tax. This credit provides a dollar-for-dollar reduction in the gift tax (Table 42-3). Use of the credit enables a donor to avoid paying the gift tax but reduces the credit available to offset estate taxes at death. An example of how this credit may be applied to eliminate the tax on gifts is provided in Box 42-2.

Box 42-2 Use of the Unified Credit To Offset Gift Taxes

Gifts made during year	$570,000
Less annual exclusion	−$11,000
Total taxable gifts	$559,000
Gift tax owed	$178,000
Less Unified Credit	−$178,000
Net gift tax	**$0**

Box 42-3 Use of the Unified Credit to Offset Estate Taxes

Taxable estate	$1,000,000
Federal estate tax owed	$345,800
Less unified credit	−$345,800
Net estate tax	**$0**

Box 42-4 Deduction From Unified Credit of Previous Credit Claimed for Gifts

Allowable Unified Credit (as of 2003)	$345,800
Less previous credit claimed for gifts	−$45,800
Unified Credit remaining for estate taxes	**$300,000**

The Unified Credit also is applied to estate taxes. It may be used to provide a dollar-for-dollar reduction in the estate tax. Because of this credit, estate tax is applied only to estates that have a certain net worth. An example of how the credit may be applied to reduce or eliminate estate taxes is provided in Box 42-3. If part of the Unified Credit has been used for gifts, however, the amount used must be deducted and cannot be used for reduction of estate taxes. An example of how previously used credit for gift tax reduces the credit available for estate taxes is provided in Box 42-4.

Other credits that may be applied to the federal estate tax include the following:
- Credit for state death taxes
- Credit for gift taxes (for gifts included in the taxable estate)
- Credit for foreign death taxes

Expert advice is needed to plan for estate transfers at death. A competent attorney or financial advisor should be consulted.

Conclusion

Estate planning is a complicated but important part of a practitioner's life. It is essential to begin planning early in a professional career; to secure competent technical advisors for guidance; and to develop the estate in a stepwise, orderly fashion. Consistent effort, applied over the course of a professional career, will result in the development of a sizable estate for retirement, protect against the unpredictable likelihood of disability, and ensure that the estate is passed as desired to loved ones at death.

Bibliography

Blackman IL: *Transferring the privately-held business.* Chicago, 1993, Probus Publishing.

Brosterman R, Davis K: *The complete estate planning guide.* New York, 1990, Mentor.

Brown J: *The basics of estate planning.* Colorado Med 2(6): 24-8, 1984.

Commerce Clearing House: *Social Security benefits including Medicare.* Chicago, 2000, Author.

Commerce Clearing House. *Federal estate and gift taxes explained.* Chicago, 2000, Author.

Crumbley DL: *Keys to estate planning and trusts.* New York, 1993, Barron's.

Esperti RA: *The handbook of estate planning.* New York, 1991, McGraw-Hill.

Internal Revenue Service publication 950, *Introduction to gift and estate taxes.*

Kapoor J, Dlabay L, Hughes R: *Personal finance.* Homewood, Ill, 1993, Irwin.

Leimberg S: *The tools and techniques of employee benefit and retirement planning.* Cincinnati, Ohio, 1990, National Underwriter Co.

Lochray P: *Financial planner's guide to estate planning,* ed 3. Englewood Cliffs, NJ, 1991, Prentice-Hall.

www.estateplanninglinks.com. Web site containing many links to information on estate planning.

www.ssa.gov. Web site for the Social Security Administration, which provides information about the Social Security program.